THE WELL-MANAGED HEALTHCARE ORGANIZATION

fourth edition

AUPHA Press/Health Administration Press is a cooperative publishing activity of the Association of University Programs in Health Administration and the Foundation of the American College of Healthcare Executives.

THE WELL-MANAGED HEALTHCARE ORGANIZATION

fourth edition

JOHN R. GRIFFITH

Health Administration Press
Chicago, Illinois
AUPHA Press

03 02 01 00 5 4 3 2

Library of Congress Cataloging-in-Publication Data

Griffith, John R.
The well-managed healthcare organization / John R. Griffith. – 4th ed.
p. cm.
Includes bibliographical references and index.
ISBN 1-56793-102-2 (hard cover : alk. paper)
1. Health services administration. I. Title.
[DNLM: 1. Health Services Administration–United States. W 84 AA1 G816w 1999]
RA971.G77 1999
362.1'068—dc21
DNLM/DLC 98-53990
for Library of Congress CIP

The paper used in this publication meets the minimum requirements of American National Standards for Information Sciences—Permanence of Paper for Printed Library Materials, ANSI Z39.48–1984. ♾™

Health Administration Press
A division of the Foundation
of the American College of
Healthcare Executives
One North Franklin St., Suite 1700
Chicago, IL 60606
(312) 424–2800

Association of University Programs
in Health Administration
1110 Vermont Avenue NW
Suite 220
Washington, DC 20005-3500
(202) 822–8550

CONTENTS

PART II Caring: Building Quality of Clinical Service

LIST OF FIGURES

PREFACE

This book, now in its fourth edition, arises from a deep conviction in the worth of locally managed healthcare and a respect for the organizations that have emerged as central to that care. Originally community hospitals, these organizations have expanded to new roles, embracing more comprehensive services and broader commitments for quality and cost. They have taken new names like "health systems" to reflect their expansion. The new organizations, supported in part by volunteered labor and charitable donations, continue a priceless tradition of neighbors helping one another in time of need. This tradition of Samaritanism is in itself an important contributor to the core concepts of community.

I believe local organizations to manage healthcare are inevitable, improvable, and inherently better than imaginable alternatives. The concepts of local control and Samaritan intent are ones that should be strengthened and expanded. The most important strength of local organizations is their commitment to their communities, and the loyalty that that commitment generates among their users. The most telling evidence of that strength is the rapid response of the community to any perceived threat. The depth of their support is sometimes only clear when there is a danger that the organization will disappear. The central measure of their performance, therefore, is their ability to satisfy local needs, to draw customers, and to bring them back again.

This book offers practical suggestions to strengthen and improve the community healthcare organization. These are based on observation of successful models, searching for the best practices for tasks that clearly must be done if the organization is to succeed. They are organized around a comprehensive and well-supported theory of management, outlined in Chapter 2, and expanded in terms of major systems of activities essential to the organization. I hope they are expressed in terms a beginner can understand, but they are increasingly rigorous and technical. Successful habits and traditions turn gradually to explicit policies, and these become more complex as they are adapted to broader and broader circumstances. What was a handshake for my father is a written, often quantitative procedure for me, and will be a dynamic computerized exchange for my sons and daughters. Simply put, as the world and medicine have become more complex, so has healthcare management.

As the editions mount, it is difficult to keep track of all who have contributed by their examples. My visits to leading institutions, Intermountain Health Care, Legacy Health System, Moses Cone Health System, and Henry Ford Health System, have contributed substantially to my understanding of the best practices, as has my work with Summa Health System and Allegiance Corporation, a physician hospital organization serving my home county in Michigan. I am grateful also for the assistance of my colleagues at Michigan, who read several chapters, and my secretary, Patricia O'Kray, who helped assemble the manuscript.

J.R.G.

CHAPTER

1

EMERGENCE OF THE HEALTHCARE ORGANIZATION

Healthcare Organizations in Transition

Practically everyone in America uses healthcare, or has a close associate who uses healthcare, in any given year. It is personal and sometimes frightening, but it lengthens our lives and makes them more comfortable and more enjoyable. It is also very complicated and very expensive. Healthcare is delivered by about 100 different licensed or certified practitioners, many of whom require substantial amounts of capital equipment. On the average, healthcare consumes nearly $4,000 per person per year, about one-sixth of our income, more than education, defense, welfare, pensions, and justice. Some individuals use several tens of thousands of dollars worth of healthcare in a single year.

Such a large expense must be financed somehow; an unexpected burden of tens of thousands of dollars is beyond almost every family's resources. Healthcare is financed by several insurance-like mechanisms, using employment benefits and both state and federal tax support. The complexity and the financing mechanism diminish the usual market forces that control cost and quality, creating a complex set of social and personal problems.

Forces for Change in Healthcare

In addition to its complexity and cost, healthcare is also rapidly changing. Technology, demography, economics, and politics drive the change, not only as individual factors but interacting to make the rate of change faster. A trip to the doctor's office is noticeably different from a few years ago; a trip to the hospital is even more strikingly changed. Technology develops new drugs, tests, and procedures each year. The population is older and needs more services. These are not new forces. Technological change in healthcare has been important for more than a century, and the population has been aging since public health reforms and immunization campaigns began around 1900. Both change and aging have accelerated in recent decades. Technology is stimulated by the continuing federal support of research through the National Institutes of Health. Partly as a result of successful healthcare, larger numbers of people are living to old age, when they need increasing amounts of care.[1]

Economic and political forces for change arise from the high cost of healthcare and the complex methods of financing it. By the 1990s, the cost of healthcare had been rising rapidly for more than two decades, substantially exceeding the general rate of inflation or the rate of growth of the economy.[2, 3] Federal and state governments found the cost of healthcare eroding their available funds, and employers saw the health insurance benefit reducing their profits. In the 1990s, both acted strongly to curtail the growth of healthcare cost. The issues are value—service received for dollar spent—and access—who can count on, and who is denied, financial assistance.

Political pressures mounted from those dissatisfied with the price and from the growing numbers of uninsured citizens. At the federal level, Congress tied Medicare hospital prices to the federal budget increases[4] and restructured Medicare doctors' fees.[5] Healthcare reform was intensely debated in 1994. The debate reinforced the pressures on Medicare, the largest government program, and stimulated the development of managed care for Medicare, Medicaid,[6] and employer-assisted health insurance.[7] **Managed care** became the term for a broad range of changes in the financing mechanisms for healthcare that transfer the costs back to **providers,** such as doctors and hospitals, and to users, patients, and their families. **Health maintenance organizations (HMOs)** and other new forms of insurance introduced new processes and systems designed to eliminate unnecessary costs and, in many cases, to improve quality and acceptability of service. (Throughout the text, boldfaced words are defined in the Glossary, page 671.)

Healthcare providers found themselves pressed to eliminate expenditures, demonstrate their quality of care, and improve their responsiveness to patient needs. Comparisons to competitors and to **benchmarks**, the best known performance for similar processes, became routine as employers, government agencies, and families began to look for lower cost options. Many community hospitals and their doctors responded with far-reaching reorganizations. **Healthcare organizations**, also called health systems and integrated delivery systems, arose to meet the economic and political pressures. The reason for the existence of healthcare organizations is to address those problems—to ensure that citizens of a community can gain access to healthcare services they need, at high quality and acceptable price.

The leaders in reorganization efforts soon learned that the solution lies in extensive revision of the way healthcare is delivered, with particular attention to how the parts fit together. Traditionally, most physicians worked alone or in small partnerships. They were supported by about 6,000 hospitals, mostly managed by citizens of local communities. Other professions and organizations—podiatrists, psychologists, drug stores, nursing homes, and home health agencies, for example—were even less integrated. Critics called the situation the "non-system" of healthcare and "the last cottage industry."

At the same time, a few healthcare organizations had demonstrated that they can deliver care that is acceptable to large numbers of Americans, at a cost and a rate of cost increase significantly lower than the overall numbers. These organizations have a different style of relationship between the physician, the organization, and the patient, like Henry Ford Health System of Detroit or the Mayo Clinic of Rochester, Minnesota, and Phoenix, Arizona. Reinforcing that relationship, they often have a different health insurance relationship with the patient or the employer, like Group Health Cooperative of Puget Sound or Kaiser Permanente. Organizations like these inevitably emerged as prototypes for the future. But these organizations have been in existence for 50 years or more. They have not been universally popular anywhere, and they have not always succeeded in new locations. It is clear that healthcare organizations will not meet their goals by cloning the prototypes indiscriminately.

The Premise of The Well-Managed Healthcare Organization

Two demands of the marketplace are central to the future development of healthcare organizations. The first is the ability to incorporate into a health insurance package most of the sources of primary care, including office and home care, preventive services, pharmacies, laboratories, and emergency services. The second is the ability to control cost and quality of those services.

Well-managed healthcare organizations will meet these demands. They will start from and improve upon historical models. Many will blend successful hospital organizations with new structures of medical organization and finance. Responding to the marketplace, they will have closer ties to health insurance, sharing in the risk and committing to buyer-determined prices. They will offer the patient a comprehensive array of services, beginning with prevention and routine care at the doctor's office and going through specialized intervention and surgery to rehabilitation and continuing care. They will emphasize their ability to integrate this continuum of care at higher levels of quality and satisfaction with service.

Similar transitions have occurred historically in many other industries. As the business historian Alfred Chandler has noted, the shift is frequently to greater value, not just to lower cost. Greater value usually involves a transfer of responsibilities originally left to the market or the buyer to a more comprehensive organization better equipped to fulfill them. Often the new organization's contributions are in coordinating, integrating, or improving the uniformity of the product or service. It achieves the improvements by designing new technology or new applications.[8] So it will be in healthcare. Instead of individual arrangements with several different doctors and facilities, many Americans will choose healthcare organizations that deliver comprehensive services for competitive package prices.

The transition will go on for decades. New models are sure to be developed. Traditional models may have surprising longevity. But the winners will integrate a broad spectrum of prevention, health maintenance, ambulatory care, acute care, and chronic care, and they will work much more closely with insurance and healthcare financing agencies.

The record of the leaders indicates that success will require the improvement of basic processes by which care is delivered, ensuring the best clinical plan for each patient's condition, flexibility to accommodate varied needs, and responsiveness to the needs of caregivers and workers as well as patients.

This book describes the well-managed healthcare organization in terms of those processes. In the jargon of continuous quality improvement, it is an effort to document "best practice" on the processes critical to organization survival, those that have to work for the organization to succeed. The processes design services, allocate resources, attract patients, ensure quality, and recruit healthcare professionals. They are described in terms of three major system groups: governance and the executive, caregiving itself, and the learning system that supports the continuous improvement necessary for competitive survival.

The emphasis is on integrating these processes and their components into an effective whole. The approach is to identify what each component *must* do to allow the others to work effectively. That is, a caregiving organization must have processes that speed communication about patient needs; select adequately prepared professionals; allow consensus-building discussion of new methods; provide competitive compensation; and deliver the patients, tools, caregivers, and supplies to the right place at the right time. Similarly, governance must decide how big the organization will be, what markets it will serve, what kinds of caregivers it will need, and how it will affiliate with them. The governance and caregiving decisions are based on analyses prepared by planning, marketing, finance, and information processes, and are implemented through human resources and plant services.

The models for the processes are drawn from the experience of leading institutions, those that have built a record of both financial and market success. They are likely to be the best *known* practices; they almost certainly are not the best *possible* practices. They are under continuous improvement at the institutions that developed them, and competitors may make breakthroughs that surpass them. At the same time, the processes as described are consistent with the experience of many thousands of organizations in a variety of fields beyond healthcare. They build on what are now well-established theories of organizations, particularly that the organizations themselves are voluntary associations of people to achieve ends they cannot achieve as well alone, and that organizations function best when they focus deliberately on identifying and meeting the needs of both their customers and their workers. It is a fair statement that no system or process is fully described. Whole books—indeed libraries—of information relevant to each system are omitted by necessity. A modest start on the omissions is provided in the "Suggested Readings" at the end of each chapter.

The Building Blocks: Healthcare Organizations as of the 1990s

Healthcare organizations arise from two ancient and deeply valued social traditions. One is the hospital, the place of shelter for the sick or needy. The other is the physician, or healer, the individual who possesses special talents to promote health. These traditions have occurred in most civilized societies, changing over time and place as needs and opportunities changed. The new healthcare organization can be said to be only the latest implementation of the tradition; it is unique in that it goes further than almost any predecessor in intertwining both concepts. It also is evolving new relationships with the other two parts of modern healthcare, a group of associated industries providing services to patients, and health insurance organizations that are essential to finance such a large portion of personal expenditures.

Hospitals

The idea that a society or community should have a special place for care of the sick and needy is almost as ancient as the "healer" tradition. It is referenced in the earliest writings of major civilizations and is found in some form in every modern society. It found root in the United States before the Revolution, when Ben Franklin founded The Pennsylvania Hospital in 1760[9] and the new federal government constructed hospitals in several other cities. The initial role for these hospitals, and for other hospitals before the late nineteenth century, was to provide a safe place for the ill or impaired to live. Those who had homes did not use hospitals. The visit of the doctor was normally to the home. He often volunteered his time to care for the sick poor, and he came to the hospital only to make those visits.[10]

The rise of hospitals as community resources

Only after the explosion of medical knowledge began did the hospital become an essential partner for the physician. The hospital's ability to provide capital equipment and trained personnel made it important. By the twentieth century, advances in surgery required radiology and laboratory diagnostic facilities, operating theaters, trained nurse assistants, anesthesiologists, and postoperative care. Around the beginning of the century, some doctors attempted to provide these services on their own in proprietary hospitals. It soon became clear that not-for-profit community hospitals had both capital-raising advantages and market advantages because the facilities could be used by many surgeons without the necessity for organizing the surgeons themselves.

As healthcare became more complex, the not-for-profit hospital continued to finance the heavy capital investments, providing facilities and equipment that were paid for by the community and were available to all qualified practitioners. It recruited or trained support staff, pooling demand from many doctors who affiliated with it to provide work for a growing number of healthcare professions and technician groups. After World War II its role was recognized in the Hill-Burton Act, federal legislation that assisted hundreds of communities to build not-for-profit hospitals. Also principally in the postwar era, hospitals began to maintain procedures and systems that ensure quality not just among the healthcare professions they employed, but among doctors who affiliated with them while maintaining private practices.[11] These three elements—capital, human capital, and quality assurance—constitute an organization of healthcare.

By the 1980s, 6,000 community hospitals were society's longest-standing commitment to organizing healthcare. At their peak, about one in ten citizens became inpatients every year, and many others visited emergency rooms or outpatient services. They consumed almost half the total healthcare expenditure. They were found in all but the smallest villages across the nation. In each community, they were the largest resource of facilities and equipment, far outstripping the investment of individual practitioners. They were, and they remain, the leading employers of many of the healthcare professions, including physicians, and they provide systems and procedures that are essential to high-technology medicine. Most important, both the courts and the national organization recognizing good management, the **Joint Commission on Accreditation of Healthcare Organizations (JCAHO)**, have established the hospital as the principal vehicle to control the quality of the healthcare transaction.

Ownership of community hospitals

Hospitals in the United States are owned by a wide variety of groups and are even occasionally owned by individuals. Most hospitals are **community hospitals**, providing general acute care for a wide variety of diseases. There are three major types of ownership.

Government hospitals are owned by federal, state, or local governments. Federal and state institutions tend to have special purposes, such as the care of special groups (military, mentally ill) or education (hospitals attached to state universities). Local government includes not only cities and counties, but also, in several states, hospital authorities that have been created from smaller political units. Local government hospitals in large cities are principally for the care of the poor, but many in smaller cities and towns are indistinguishable from not-for-profit institutions. Both are counted as community hospitals. State mental hospitals and federal hospitals are not classed as community hospitals.

Not-for-profit hospitals are owned by corporations established by private (non-governmental) groups for the common good rather than for individual gain. As a result, they are granted broad federal, state, and local tax exemptions. Although they are frequently operated by organizations that have religious ties, secular, or nonreligious, not-for-profit hospitals constitute the largest single group of community hospitals both in number and in total volume of care, exceeding religious not-for-profit, government, and for-profit hospitals by a wide margin.

For-profit hospitals are owned by private corporations, which are allowed to declare dividends or otherwise distribute profits to individuals. They pay taxes like other private corporations. These hospitals are also called *investor owned*. They are usually community hospitals, although there has been rapid growth in private psychiatric hospitals. Historically, the owners were doctors and other individuals, but large-scale publicly held corporations now own most for-profit hospitals. For-profit hospitals grew rapidly in the 1970s, and again in the 1990s, but never accounted for more than 15 percent of all hospitals. They are much more common in some southern states, and can be a major factor or the sole institution in some communities.

Figure 1.1 shows community hospital statistics compiled by the American Hospital Association (AHA). Because the AHA plays a major role in collecting statistics about hospitals, its classification system is used for most purposes.[12] Several measures of volume are shown in the table, in addition to the number of institutions in each ownership class. Beds, admissions, and expenses can be used to classify hospitals by size. Discharges, which are virtually identical to admissions in the course of a year, and revenue, differing from expenses only by profit or loss, are also used.

Most U.S. community hospitals are small, but as Figure 1.2 shows, larger hospitals provide most of the service. The trend has been for smaller hospitals in urban areas to disappear. They either go out of business or are acquired by larger institutions. In rural areas, there is still a need for a convenient primary care facility, but the role of inpatient care in that facility has diminished. Many hospitals in rural areas have changed to exclusively outpatient services.[13]

Implications of different types of ownership

Both for-profit and not-for-profit ownerships are sometimes referred to as private, to distinguish them from public or government hospitals. However, as a consequence of their commitment not to distribute profits or assets to

FIGURE 1.1 U.S. Community Hospitals by Ownership, 1998

Ownership	Number	Beds 1,000	Admissions 1,000	Expenses ($1,000,000)	Personnel 1,000
Nongovernment					
Not-for-profit	3,045	598	22,542	215.9	2,711
For-profit	759	109	3,684	28.3	359
State and local governments	1,330	155	4,873	49.4	654
TOTAL	5,134	862	31,099	$293.6	3,724

Percentage Distribution (rounded)

Ownership	Number	Beds	Admissions	Expenses	Personnel
Nongovernment					
Not-for-profit	59%	69%	72%	74%	73%
For-profit	15	13	12	10	10
State and local governments	26	18	16	17	18
TOTAL	100%	100%	100%	100%	100%

Reprinted with permission from *Hospital Statistics, 1998–99 Edition* (Chicago: AHA, 1998) Table 2 (pp. 4, 5).

FIGURE 1.2 U.S. Community Hospitals by Size, 1998

Bed Size	Number	Beds 1,000	Admissions 1,000	Expenses ($1,000,000)	Personnel 1,000
6–49	1,168	39	1,041	8.6	145
50–99	1,128	81	2,280	18.4	279
100–199	1,338	189	6,456	53.7	723
200–299	692	169	6,426	56.5	712
300–399	361	124	4,856	46.0	569
400–499	196	87	3,481	35.5	430
500 or more	251	173	6,558	75.0	867
TOTAL	5,134	862	31,098	$293.70	3,725

Percentage Distribution (rounded)

Bed Size	Number	Beds	Admissions	Expenses	Personnel
6–49	23%	5%	3%	3%	4%
50–99	22	9	7	6	7
100–199	26	22	21	18	19
200–299	13	20	21	19	19
300–399	7	14	16	16	15
400–499	4	10	11	12	12
500 or more	5	20	21	26	23
TOTAL	100%	100%	100%	100%	100%

Reprinted with permission from *Hospital Statistics, 1998–99 Edition* (Chicago: AHA, 1998) Table 2 (pp. 4, 5).

any individual, not-for-profit hospitals are legally dedicated to the collective good. Thus, for the vast majority of community hospitals in the United States, the owners, in the sense of beneficiaries, are the communities they serve. The corporation holds the assets, including any accumulated profits, in trust for the citizens of the community.

In part because of the trust relationship, but perhaps in larger part because of the need to be responsive to the same market opportunities, ownership of community hospitals is rarely critical in its overall management. Many hospitals owned by local governments are indistinguishable from not-for-profit hospitals in similar settings. Except for the obvious right to distribute dividends and the obligation to pay taxes, so are those of for-profit owners. In the courts, government hospitals are generally held to slightly higher standards of public accountability and conformity to the Constitution. Because they must honor any citizen's economic rights and religious freedom, they are obliged to provide abortions (if they provide related services),[14] to have open medical staffs, and to respect constitutional guarantees of freedom from participation in religious activities. Private hospitals are obliged simply to use due process and not to discriminate on grounds of age, sex, race, or creed. Other ownership distinctions make similarly minor differences. The only difference in the rights and obligations of religious versus nonreligious not-for-profit owners is that religious owners may favor persons having their own beliefs. (In practice this privilege is rarely exercised.)

Given the narrow range of these distinctions, it is not surprising that studies of the effectiveness of various types of ownership rarely reveal major differences.[15] How well a hospital carries out the process of market assessment and program development depends much more on who manages it and how well than it does on who owns the property. A community hospital can be successful under any ownership if it is effectively managed. The most significant difference is that the results of that success accrue to a **community** in the case of not-for-profit hospitals and to the stockholders in the case of for-profit hospitals. Healthcare systems integrating several hospitals may have an advantage. The range of necessary skills and experience is much broader in a system, and if these virtues can be translated to more effective management, systems will thrive where individual institutions fail. But as in the comparison of for-profit and not-for-profit ownership, evidence of their superiority is not easy to develop.[16]

Healthcare systems

As Figure 1.3 shows, most hospitals, operating 58 percent of beds, are now part of healthcare systems. The nature of the association varies from wholly owned subsidiaries to management contracts and loose affiliations. However, the tendency to aggregation is still continuing. Existing ties are being strengthened and extended, and the number of unaffiliated organizations continues to decline. Affiliation does not change the jobs to be done, nor escape the need to meet the issues of cost control and access. It does increase the influence, capital, and human resources available to smaller institutions. Larger organizations have more clout in political and marketing arenas. They are better able to represent their needs, and their size allows them to command more attention. Economically, they can generate greater borrowing capacity. They can support greater expertise in both clinical and managerial activities. They can develop specialized solutions to problems like information systems, materials management, and plant and equipment maintenance.

Healthcare systems can be described in terms of two categories. Geographically scattered systems have a small market share in each of many

FIGURE 1.3
U.S. Healthcare Systems

Ownership	Number of Systems	%	Beds* (1,000)	%
Church-Related	57	21%	128	26%
Other Not-for-Profit	171	64%	218	44%
For-Profit	39	15%	153	31%
TOTAL	267	100%	499	100%

*Includes beds owned, leased, managed by contract, and sponsored.
SOURCE: American Hospital Association *Guide to the Health Care Field, 1998–99 Edition* (Chicago: AHA, 1998) Tables 1 and 3 (p. B63).

different healthcare regions. Many of the Catholic healthcare systems follow this model. The original for-profit corporations also followed this model, building small hospitals in a large number of cities stretching across the Sun Belt. Geographically focused systems attempt to capture substantial market share in one or a small number of geographic areas. They are often formed by merger or acquisition of previously independent institutions. Many of the larger systems following this model are also closely affiliated with HMOs. Their large market share in a specific place makes it possible for them to sell and service large risk-sharing contracts, whereas the systems operating in geographically scattered sites have had difficulty meeting specific customer needs. Kaiser Permanente, by far the largest healthcare system in the nation, has replicated the geographically focused model in many different sites. Several other large systems are geographically focused in one or a few sites, such as Intermountain, serving most of Utah and parts of adjacent states; Mayo, with operations in Minnesota, Arizona, and Florida; Uni-Health in southern California, Henry Ford in southeast Michigan, and Geisinger in Pennsylvania. Focused systems have generally thrived in recent years, and many of their processes are models for this text.

Along with the trend to healthcare systems, hospitals have recently moved to alliances to increase their political and economic influence and help them improve their cost and quality performance. Unlike systems, which generally involve merger of assets and permanent transfer of some governance decisions to a central organization, alliances are contractual arrangements that can be terminated on relatively short notice. Despite sound theory which suggests that they are inherently transient vehicles,[17] 12 systems reported serving 2,400 hospitals and systems.[18] The Premier Health Alliance was by far the largest, serving 1,400 members.[19]

Physicians

The notion of the healer with special powers can be traced to the witch doctor or shaman of prehistoric civilizations. Early healers provided herbal remedies, surgical intervention, and psychological support for patients and families. Their knowledge and skills were extensive, and some treatments remain in use today. Traditional medical knowledge occurs in the early writings of both eastern and western civilizations. Hippocrates began the codification of disease and treatment for western civilization in 260 BCE. A long line of clinical investigators added slowly to Hippocratic knowledge.[20]

The rise of specialization

In the mid-nineteenth century, the discovery of anesthesia and the germ theory of disease greatly extended surgical opportunities. An explosion of surgical capability continued through the twentieth century. Beginning in the 1930s, vastly more effective pharmaceuticals were discovered for anemia, diabetes, and a wide variety of infectious diseases. In the later decades, immunizations for many serious epidemic diseases were developed, and oral contraceptives became available. Radiologic, chemical, and electronic diagnosis were perfected. Endoscopic diagnosis and treatment as well as direct visualization and manipulation of internal organs through small surgical incisions became commonplace near the end of the twentieth century.

The rapid increase in knowledge was paralleled by a restructuring of medical education and the development of medical specialties. Although American physicians are licensed by state governments to practice any form of medicine or surgery, the vast majority now practice in only one or two of more than 30 different specialties. Certification for these specialties is provided by a system of specialty boards that supervise training programs, maintain life-long periodic examinations, encourage research and publication in their area, and stimulate continuing education for their members.[21] Specialty certification is rapidly becoming a condition for practice, especially in organized medical settings.

The specialties can be grouped several ways, but the most useful for the purposes of healthcare organizations may be that which emphasizes four main divisions: primary care, medicine, surgery, and diagnosis. **Primary care** doctors hold themselves out as the first point of contact for the patient, doctors who can identify diagnoses, provide treatment directly for most problems, and select appropriate specialists for the balance. The latter three groups receive many or all of their patients on referral from other physicians. They are called the **referral specialties**. Figure 1.4 shows a list of specialty boards in the United States and their 1990 membership in active practice. It also shows the number of multiple specialties reported by individual doctors and the number of doctors not certified by any board. Two important generalizations are supported by Figure 1.4. First, most physicians are now certified. A small and declining fraction is in what used to be called "General Practice."[22] Second, fewer are certified in primary care than in the referral specialties. It is generally believed that there are significant shortages in primary care and surpluses in many referral specialties.[23]

The actual practice of these specialties is different on almost every dimension. Some doctors (e.g., rheumatologists) practice principally by evaluating and understanding the course of disease; some (orthopedists) make dramatic interventions with elaborate technology. Some (pathologists) rarely communicate with patients as individuals; others (anesthesiologists) relate to them almost incidentally in the course of treatment; still others (psychiatrists) must establish an intimate ongoing relationship. Some (intensivists) cannot practice outside the hospital; others (family practice) rarely use the hospital themselves. There is also a substantial difference in earnings. Until the 1990s, primary care doctors earned less than half the income of those who rely on the most expensive technology. Not surprisingly, there are also substantial differences in temperament, lifestyle, and values between specialties as well as between individuals.

FIGURE 1.4
Distribution of Physicians in Active Practice by Specialty Certification, United States, 1996

Specialty	Number of Physicians (1,000)	Specialty	Number of Physicians (1,000)
Primary Care	**217.2**	**Surgery**	**99.8**
Family practice	51.5	Anesthesiology	21.3
Emergency medicine	12.5	General surgery	23.5
General internal medicine	71.4	Neurosurgery	3.1
General pediatrics	33.7	Ophthalmology	14.2
Obstetrics/gynecology	26.0	Orthopedics	16.4
Psychiatry	22.1	Otolaryngology	7.1
Medicine	**64.3**	Plastic surgery	4.6
Cardiology	17.0	Thoracic surgery	2
Dermatology	7.2	Urology	7.6
Endocrinology	2.8	**Diagnosis**	**21.5**
Gastroenterology	8.8	Pathology	14.0
Geriatrics	1.4	Radiology	7.5
Pediatric sub-specialties	3.5		
Neurology	7.8	Deduction for multiple certification	−31.5
Radiation oncology	2.8		
Physiatry	3.8	Practicing without certification	221.3
Pulmonary medicine and intensive care	6.2	Total active physicians	655.6
Rheumatology	3.0		

SOURCE: American Medical Association, *Physician Characteristics and Distribution in the US.* 1996 ed. (Chicago: AMA, 1996), Tables B-8 and B-12; American Osteopathic Association, 1996 *Yearbook and Directory of Osteopathic Physicians*, 87th. Ed. (Chicago: AOA, 1996) Statistical Tables on the Osteopathic Profession, Numbers of Current (Active) Osteopathic Certificationbs.

Figure 1.5 shows the distribution of U.S. physicians by type of practice as of 1996. The majority of those in office-based practice were in small, single-specialty groups or independent practice, and most of the financial arrangement was in individual fees. While it would be wrong to say these forms are not organized, they are small organizations with limited capability. The larger, more organized models of medical practice included:

- multispecialty group practices open to fee-for-service and HMO financing, such as the Mayo Clinic and Henry Ford Medical Group;
- group practices limited to HMO financing such as Kaiser Permanente;
- **independent physicians associations (IPAs)** organized to allow doctors practicing independently for fee-for-service financing to collaborate to serve managed care contracts;
- **physician hospital organizations (PHOs)** including hospitals or health systems and **physician organizations**, and generally accepting both fee-for-service and managed care financing;

- government programs such as the Army and the Veterans' Administration; and
- university medical school faculties.

Other Healthcare Providers

Hospitals and doctors provide about two-thirds of all healthcare. The balance is provided by a wide variety of other practitioners and organizations.

Healthcare professions

About 50 professions other than physicians provide health services to patients. The list of professions reported by the U.S. Department of Labor is shown in Figure 1.6. Most are licensed or certified by state agencies and have professional associations providing evidence of appropriate training. They work as employees in hospitals, clinics, and nursing homes, but many also practice independently under fee-for-service compensation. As insurance becomes more comprehensive, the trend is for these professions to move toward employment in healthcare corporations. The greater the interaction between the profession and other forms of care, the faster this movement is likely to be. For the patient, integration offers increased assurance of quality, greater convenience, and reduced danger of confusion or conflict between caregivers. For the insurer or healthcare organization, integration improves cost, quality, and utilization control.

Other provider organizations

Also paralleling the growth of medical technology, many other sources of care emerged in the twentieth century. They include public clinics, nursing homes, pharmacies, specialty hospitals, visiting nurse and home care programs, home meal programs, hospices, and durable medical equipment suppliers. Many of these are affiliated with general hospitals and clinics, but many operate as independent entities. Most are small businesses operating in a single community. Some, such as the for-profit nursing home chains, are multi-state corporations. The public clinics are generally operated by local government. In addition to these identifiable businesses, there are voluntary organizations and

FIGURE 1.5 Practice Arrangements of Active U.S. Physicians, 1996

Practice Arrangement	Number (1,000)	Percentage
Office-based practice	446	69%
Hospital-based practice	57	9
Residents and fellows	96	15
Teaching, administration, and research	42	6
Other	3	neg.
Total active physicians	644	100%

SOURCES: American Medical Association, *Physician Characteristics and Distribution in the United States: A Survey of Practice Characteristics* (Chicago: AMA, 1997, p. 19).

FIGURE 1.6
Healthcare Professions Other Than Physicians

	Number (1,000)	Percentage
Providing general care:		
Licensed practical nurses	699	16%
Nurse practitioners	30	1
Physician assistants	64	1
Registered nurses	1,971	44
Total	2,764	62%
Providing care limited to specific organs or diseases:		
Chiropractors	44	1%
Dentists	162	4
Optometrists	41	1
Podiatrists	11	0
Psychologists	143	3
Social workers	59	1
Total	460	10%
Providing care limited to specific modalities:		
Dieticians	58	1%
Electroencephalograph technologists	6	0
Electrocardiograph technologists	32	1
Emergency medical technicians	150	3
Laboratory technologists	285	6
Occupational therapists	57	1
Pharmacists	172	4
Physical therapists	115	3
Radiologic technologists	174	4
Recreational therapists	38	1
Respiratory therapists	82	2
Speech therapists and audiobiologists	87	2
Total	1,256	28%
GRAND TOTAL	**4,480**	**100%**

SOURCE: U.S. Dept. of Labor, Occupational Outlook Handbook, Bulletin 2500, 1998.

support groups that provide substantial healthcare. Alcoholics Anonymous is the oldest and one of the most successful.

Many of these care organizations became important industries in themselves, while remaining relatively small parts of the total expenditure for healthcare. The prescription drug industry is a useful example. The amount spent per person per year mounted from $15 in 1960 to $25 in 1970 to $226 in 1997.[24] The increase paid for all the antibiotics; oral contraceptives; anticoagulants; hypertensive agents; vaccines for polio, measles, and whooping cough; and cancer drugs. Drugs are produced principally by a few large multinational companies and distributed principally by hospitals and 50,000 licensed pharmacies. Although many pharmacies were independent small businesses, retail drug chains began rapid growth in the 1970s and by the 1980s provided 65 percent of the non-hospital market. Drugs provided in the hospital were insured in early private health insurance plans. Traditional Medicare and private health insurance programs did not cover outpatient drugs, but managed care plans generally do.

The nursing home, home care, and hospice industries have important parallels to pharmacies. They generate commercial opportunities for small local businesses and national supply corporations. The local businesses are often acquired by larger, publicly listed stock companies who form geographically scattered systems. These seek economies of scale by mastering the details of care delivery and supporting local operations with training, supplies, and capital. Some healthcare organizations offer these services as well, but independent, geographically scattered organizations tended to dominate.[25]

Health Insurance Organizations

It is clear that modern healthcare can be financed only in the context of health insurance or related risk-sharing mechanisms. Most Americans have a mechanism to finance their healthcare. Most working families receive health insurance as an employment benefit. The aged participate in Medicare, a universal government health insurance, and most of them have supplementary private insurance. Some, but not all, poor receive Medicaid, a state and federal insurance. A few people purchase health insurance individually, or through groups other than employment. Coming from so many different sources, it is not surprising that the insurance varies widely in the details of the protection it provides, or that some people fall through the cracks. About 15 percent of the population have none of these mechanisms, and additional millions had insurance that was inadequate for their needs.

The coverage itself is administered by about 2,000 different companies. A much smaller number are economically important in geographically specific marketplaces. These are mostly large voluntary HMOs, **Blue Cross and Blue Shield Plans**, and commercial insurance companies who administer many different kinds of programs for employers and government. Technically, many of these programs are not insurance because the employer or the government accepts the financial risk for the group in question, and the health insurance organization acts as **intermediary**, seeing that care is provided according to the contracts and pays the providers. Medicare is the largest single example. The federal government holds the insurance risk, through the Medicare Trust Fund. Intermediary insurance companies administer the plan in each state. There are often two intermediaries, one for Part A, covering mostly hospital expenses, and one for Part B, covering medical and other practitioner expenses. Similar complexities describe the private market. Large employers often self-insure their groups. They frequently turn to intermediaries to administer the healthcare benefit.

Health insurance companies initially identified their function as bearing risk, marketing, subscriber billing and service, and claims payment. They often avoided any selection of providers and accepted the providers' judgment on both appropriate treatment and fair price. The Medicare Act Preamble, which called for "reasonable costs" to pay hospitals and "usual, customary and reasonable" fees for physicians,[26] was widely accepted as a model. Traditional health insurance still fulfills these functions. Under pressure to improve cost performance, managed care plans added negotiation of fees and various mechanisms to ensure quality and minimize cost. The large intermediaries offered these and even pioneered in their development, so that they now offer a range of products and services from traditional health insurance to HMOs, with several risk-sharing alternatives.

However necessary it might be, insurance itself contributes to the increase in costs. Insurance divorces the payment mechanism from the point of service and removes the economic consequence of decisions by both the caregivers and the patients. When the premium is paid by employers and is subject to tax preferences, the consequence is doubly or triply removed.[27] The issue is how to design insurance that simultaneously provides the necessary financial protection and minimizes the inflationary consequences of the divorce.

Devices to achieve cost control have become increasingly sophisticated in the past 20 years, since the passage of the HMO Act in 1973. They fall into three major categories: limits on payment, limits on provider selection, and provider risk sharing.

1. Limits on Payment
   - *To patients.* **Deductibles** delay insurance participation until a specific amount has been spent by the patient and **copayments** put the patient at some financial risk at each step of care. The deductible is a standard feature of catastrophic or major medical insurance contracts, where it serves to rule out routine medical expenses. Copayments are often a feature of **indemnity insurance** which pays cash benefits for specific services received, up to a limited amount for each healthcare event. They are also used in HMOs to reduce premiums or discourage unnecessary or inappropriate use.
   - *To providers.* Fee-for-service payment to providers discounted below what is perceived to be the market rate. This approach has been routine in Medicaid and is used in managed care financing. Medicare payments to hospitals and physicians were restricted by Congress in the 1990s.
2. Limits on Provider Selection
   - Most advanced healthcare financing plans limit the patient to a panel of providers approved in advance. **Preferred provider organization (PPO)** and HMO contracts are designed around this feature. **Point-of-service (POS)** plans offer unlimited choice of provider with substantial financial incentives for the patient to use panel providers.

3. Provider Risk-Sharing
   - Risk-sharing plans use financial devices to encourage providers to eliminate unnecessary services. They include bundled prices such as **diagnosis-related groups (DRGs)**, where payment is based on the patient's condition rather than what was done for each patient. They also include a variety of payment mechanisms, such as withholding a fraction of the payment to distribute if utilization targets are met or providing other incentives for meeting targets.
   - In its most advanced form, risk-sharing pays providers **capitation**, a fixed dollar amount for each month the patient remains under contract. This requires an explicit selection of provider by the patient, even though the patient may not seek care at all. The provider, usually a hospital–physician group combination, accepts full risk for managing the patients' care.

The most sophisticated insurance products use several of these devices simultaneously. HMOs frequently combine copayments, provider selection, bundled payment, and provider capitation. POS plans offer the patient a choice of provider for a price but use copayments deliberately to channel care to selected providers with whom they have risk-sharing contracts. Even traditional contracts have increasingly elaborate devices to influence both patient and provider behavior. Because the individual customer or group of customers can select the product they want, each successful product must attract a reasonable share of the market. No product will be perfect; there are real choices in front of the customer. The most important choices center around the provider panel and price considerations. Obviously the more attractive the panel is, the larger market share it will attract at a given price, and the more effective at cost control the panel is, the lower price it can offer. Panels that are both attractive and cost-effective will attract large numbers of patients and achieve further economies through their size.

The health insurance market has undergone significant changes in the 1980s and further rapid change is likely through the 1990s. All forms of cost-controlling products are growing in market share. The more flexible POS products are growing most rapidly. In some cities they have achieved substantial market shares, and where this has occurred, healthcare has been revolutionized and healthcare organizations have flourished. When providers must meet cost and quality standards to be selected, and when they share in the risk that costs will exceed premiums paid, strong incentives are established to change patterns of practice and seek new economies. The providers' energies are turned to devising lower-cost ways to achieve equivalent or better quality of care. They reorganize the array of existing hospitals, physician practices, other professionals, and other provider organizations to meet that challenge.

The Vision of the Well-Managed Healthcare Organization

The well-managed healthcare organization described in this book is an evolving organization, building upon its predecessors and continuously striving for an ideal. One can summarize the ideal on four dimensions: access, technical quality, satisfaction, and cost. Simply stated, the ideal healthcare organization will provide convenient access to sound, comprehensive, and appropriate quality of care, please all its patients, and be affordable to its community. There are inevitable tradeoffs between these four dimensions. The well-managed organization must make the tradeoffs in a manner that its customers will call satisfactory.

The customer voice for change has intensified and clarified in the past decade. The four dimensions have become more clearly articulated. The feasible levels of performance have become more visible, and standards that the well-managed organization must meet have become clearer and more challenging.

Access

Customer demands for access have several important dimensions to the well-managed healthcare organization. First, the process of care will be **vertically integrated**. The ideal healthcare organization will strive for seamless service to the patient from the initial contact for preventive services and health promotion, through routine care to crisis episodes and the management of chronic illness. It will encourage healthy lifestyles through education and advertising. It will offer convenient access through organized primary care. It will organize referral specialists, clinical support services, and inpatient care to make the most expensive episodes of care cost-effective. It will improve efficiency and quality of other professions and provider organizations, integrating pharmacies, nursing homes, home care, hospices, and the professionals who work in them.

Primary care assumes a special prominence because of its frequent contact with patients and its control of the referral process. The success of a specific insurance plan frequently rests on the panel of primary care providers available to the customer. People want providers who are sensitive, are responsive to questions, and have convenient hours and parking. If the plan is to grow, some providers must be open to new patients. Many of the contacts must be for prevention of disease and promotion of health. Primary care practitioners must be able and willing to assist customers on smoking, contraception, immunization, child safety, diet, and emotional health. Effective cost control begins with programs to reduce illness and the need for healthcare.

Frequently used referral specialists and clinical support services like cardiology evaluations and imaging must also be convenient. Although people are willing to go further for hospital and less common referral care, they clearly prefer to stay in the community where they shop or work. Excessive delays, long drives, and multiple trips discourage customers and reduce reenrollment. They also reduce word-of-mouth endorsement.

Second, the ideal healthcare organization will serve all patients and will strive to capture as large a share of each form of health insurance as it can. Because healthcare organizations and even individual physician providers have high fixed costs, high volumes lead to lower costs. Because much healthcare is highly specialized, large numbers of primary care patients are necessary to support each specialty. Both economies of operation and marketing advantages accrue to the organization that actively recruits all possible patients, even though some of them may be financed at less than full cost. Various experimental programs suggest that most healthcare organizations will have specific programs for access by low income groups. They will include convenient clinics for primary care, emergency and walk-in care, and outreach activities emphasizing early treatment and prevention.

Third, the ideal healthcare organization will be **horizontally integrated**. Several important healthcare services, like obstetrics, coronary care, emergency care, and expensive diagnostic services, and services supporting the care process, like education, marketing, information systems, and finance, are less costly when spread over larger bases. Each organization will strive to be as large as it can within its geographic community. The more cost-effective organizations will tend to acquire or dominate less efficient ones. The trend to healthcare systems will continue.

Quality of Care

The ideal healthcare organization will provide and document uniformly high quality of care, as measured by conformity to standards for care processes and desirable outcomes. Considerable evidence exists that the quality of the present healthcare is highly variable. Customer pressure for uniform high quality is mounting, matched by increasing sophistication in measurement.[28] Employers and insurers purchasing care and assembling panels of providers will insist on technical quality. Well-designed organizations can make major gains in quality, and they will do so to capture larger market shares.

The principles of quality management are now well-documented and understood. They emphasize meeting customer demands, relying on measurement of outcomes, and empowering caregivers to agree on **protocols** or **guidelines**, specific processes that will ensure those outcomes. The very notion of agreement between individual practitioners and different professions is radical to some concepts of individual professional integrity. Advanced organization and human relations skills are essential to achieve consensuses and implement protocols. Reward systems, including both monetary and nonmonetary rewards, are essential to encourage compliance. A substantial portion of the administrative structure of the ideal healthcare system will be devoted to quality infrastructure—information systems, incentive systems, and continuous improvement processes.

Customer Satisfaction

The ideal healthcare system will emphasize customer satisfaction as the best way to build and retain market share. Direct measurement of satisfaction will be detailed, comprehensive, and commonplace. There will be high expectations for the simpler elements of customer satisfaction, like sensitivity to patients and waiting times. Failure to satisfy patients on these elements will be as serious as departures from technical quality. Many caregivers will find that they have two customers, the patient and the referring primary provider. Both will have substantial authority to dictate the terms of service.

Beyond the initial determinants of good service, customer satisfaction is likely to take on a deeper meaning. Much of medical care involves choices between alternatives, sometimes with enormous consequences. Through most of the twentieth century, responsibility for these choices was vested solely with physicians. The trend toward informing the patient about his or her disease and its management alternatives began with informed consent for surgery in the 1960s,[29] and has grown steadily since.

Where traditional medicine was likely to recommend or prescribe a certain course of action, managed care will present it as an option more or less strongly urged as the clinical situation suggests. Defensive medicine, the policy of protecting against rare but high-cost eventualities, will be replaced with watchful waiting approaches that reserve the more expensive and invasive actions for cases in which clear threats develop, unless the patient expresses a clear and coherent desire for more action. Patient choice is likely to become a major part of managing care of aging and chronically ill patients, resulting in the expanded use of hospice care and deaths outside the acute hospital.[30]

Affordable Cost

The ideal healthcare organization will deliver care at costs determined by the customer. For 25 years following the passage of Medicare and Medicaid, costs passed to the customer or payor were determined mostly by the providers. The Medicare guidelines, reasonable cost and usual customary and reasonable fees, turned out to be highly inflationary as interpreted by the providers. Healthcare costs mounted at double-digit rates throughout the period. It is clear that these guidelines and rates are no longer acceptable.

Effective demands for cost control began in 1983, when Medicare established fixed prices for individual inpatient DRGs. The demand for non-Medicare cost control was expressed mainly by shifts to HMO and PPO insurance. It spread rapidly in some cities but hardly at all in others throughout the next decade.

Prevention

Many illnesses and problems can be prevented. Tobacco usage adds about $100 billion a year to national expenses, in both healthcare and lost wages. Alcohol abuse, domestic violence, traffic safety, unplanned pregnancy, workplace safety, other substance abuse, obesity, lack of exercise, and unprotected sex also contribute substantially to the cost of care.[31] Managed care insurance and risk-sharing by providers create strong incentives to address these issues. Most healthcare organizations have improved their prevention activities. The leading ones are developing systematic programs of collaboration with other community agencies to reduce these hazards. These programs work with other community agencies to identify and prioritize risks, and develop collaborative programs to reach the highest-risk individuals. Because many of these risks are associated with low income, the programs are targeted to disadvantaged populations.[32]

The ideal healthcare organization will be very good at all these jobs. Its primary care physicians will be easily accessed and responsive to patient demands. Its hospitals will be efficient units just big enough to meet the needs of its insured population. It will encourage truly cost-effective medicine by selecting and rewarding physicians and other practitioners who practice it. It will move patients easily across several sites for care, from primary care sites to specialty treatment centers, hospitals, home care, rehabilitation, and long-term care. It will stress health promotion and illness prevention for all, and will have special programs for populations at higher risk. Doing all five jobs will require close cooperation between the various caregivers, and between the organization and other agencies. It will require faster and more complete communication, improved information to evaluate care, shared financial and professional incentives, and new levels of communication among caregivers and between caregivers and the organization itself. That is the vision of the healthcare organization.

Using This Book

This book is a basic text on building and managing organizations that directly provide healthcare. It is deliberately designed to identify the major functions that any caregiving organization must perform and to describe the way the most successful organizations accomplish those functions, emphasizing the common elements of leading practice. Where possible, it adds a commentary on known shortcomings of existing methods and discusses experimental solutions. It should thus serve as a guide and a starting point for those operating healthcare organizations. The approaches described here will work, and they will provide the basis for continuous improvement tailored to local needs.

Structure of the Book

The essential functions are organized into three major groups of activities: governing, caring, and learning. Within these groups, each system and process is described not as the insider performing the task would see it, but rather as the other systems require it. That is, each system is described in terms of what it must do to make the whole effective.

Governing: making healthcare organizations responsive to their environment

Any successful organization must have a boundary spanning function that relates it effectively to its environment.[33] The function is called "governance," and in all but the smallest healthcare organizations it is carried out by a governing board. Part I examines what it means to relate to the environment, how successful governing boards establish policies that improve the organization's response, and how executive offices implement the policies.

Modern organizations execute policy decisions through an elaborate structure deliberately designed to encourage two-way communications and to identify, evaluate, and resolve conflicting opportunities and opinions. The leadership of the executive system performs a critical function in designing the way decisions are made, expanding participation in each decision.

Caring: building quality of clinical service

The defining characteristic of healthcare organizations is the actual provision of healthcare; it is an individualized, deeply personal activity unlike any other in modern life. It is, and must remain, the responsibility of autonomous practitioners, but it must respond dynamically to customer needs. The mechanisms that reconcile autonomy and responsiveness are built upon a century of effort. Part II describes how they work, beginning with the tested and proven approaches and distinguishing the structures for physicians, nurses, and other clinical support professions, continuing care, and outreach and prevention.

Learning: meeting planning, marketing, finance, and information needs

The modern organization is dynamic, constantly changing in response to new demands from its environment. Peter Senge has called it the "learning organization."[34] Elaborate fact-finding, performance measurement, and analytic activities support the learning organization. Information is used as a resource, like money. Part III describes the structure that supports learning, including the learning necessary to make specific decisions. It describes functions of planning, marketing, and finance and the information services necessary to support decision making and clinical care. Learning requires human resources activities that recruit, select, train, compensate, and motivate its workers. Learning also requires an effectively controlled environment, provided through plant services.

How to Use the Book

The book is designed to be both a text and a reference. Beginners should read through it as it is written. Even if they choose to start with some part other than governance, there is value to seeing how the processes of managing a complex organization unfold. Starting at the beginning means starting with an understanding of the kinds of forces operating on the organization and the role of governance in identifying and responding to those forces. Even the most detailed study of another major system will be incomplete without that understanding.

Experienced executives should already understand the governance process, at least at an intuitive level. They might skip to whatever system is of interest, to see what desirable practices are on a question of interest. The parts of the book are designed to be self-contained for the sophisticated reader. There is an index and a glossary to track important terms across the parts. Clinical practitioners who want to understand how the organization affects their lives directly can begin with Part II on caring. But again, the issues of governance are essential to a well-grounded understanding.

Notes

1. L. A. May, "The Physiologic and Psychological Bases of Health Disease and Care Seeking." Ch. 2 in *Introduction to Health Services*, S. J. Williams and P. R. Torrens, eds. 5th ed. Albany, NY: Delmar Publishers (1999)
2. National Health Expenditures by Type of Service and Source of Funds: Calendar Years 1960–96. Health Care Financing Authority website: www.hcfa.gov (October 1998)
3. K. R. Levit, H. C. Lazenby, and B. R. Braden, "National Health Spending Trends in 1996: National Health Accounts Team." *Health Affairs* 17(1):35–51 (Jan–Feb, 1998)
4. *Tax Equity and Fiscal Responsibility Act of 1982.* (P.L. 97-248)
5. *Omnibus Budget Reconciliation Act of 1989.* (P.L. 101-239)
6. R. Blankenau, "Forging Ahead with No National Reform, States Look to Tackle Medicaid Issues." *Hospital & Health Networks* 68(22):40, p. 43 (November 20, 1994)
7. R. H. Miller and H. S. Luft, "Managed Care Plans: Characteristics, Growth, and Premium Performance." *Annual Review of Public Health* 15, pp. 437–59 (1994)
8. A. D. Chandler, *The Visible Hand: The Managerial Revolution in American Business.* Cambridge, MA: Belknap Press (1977)
9. B. Franklin, *Some Account of the Pennsylvania Hospital*, I. B. Coker, ed. Baltimore: The Johns Hopkins Press (1954)
10. C. E. Rosenberg, *The Care of Strangers: The Rise of America's Hospital System.* New York: Basic Books (1989)
11. R. Stevens, *In Sickness and In Wealth: American Hospitals in the Twentieth Century.* New York: Basic Books (1989)
12. *Hospital Statistics.* Chicago: American Hospital Association (published annually)
13. W. D. Helms, D. M. Campion, and I. Muscovice, *Delivering Essential Health Care Services in Rural Areas: An Analysis of Alternative Models.* Washington, DC: Alpha Center Health Policy and Planning, Inc (1991)
14. A. F. Southwick, *The Law of Hospital and Health Care Administration.* Chicago: Health Administration Press, pp. 455–56 (1988)

15. B. H. Gray, ed., *For-Profit Enterprise in Health Care*. Washington, DC: National Academy Press (1986)
16. S. M. Shortell, "The Evolution of Hospital Systems: Unfulfilled Promises and Self-Fulfilling Prophecies." *Medical Care Review* 45(2), pp. 177–214 (1988)
17. H. S. Zuckerman and T. A. D'Aunno, "Hospital Alliances: Cooperative Strategy in a Competitive Environment." *Health Care Management Review* 15(2), pp. 21–30 (Spring, 1990)
18. American Hospital Association, *The AHA Guide, 1998–1999*. Chicago: American Hospital Association, pp. B163–91(1998)
19. Premier Health Alliance website: www.premierinc.com (November 13, 1998)
20. H. E. Sigerist, *The Great Doctors; A Biographical History Of Medicine*, translated by E. and C. Paul. Garden City, NY: Doubleday (1958)
21. D. G. Langsley, M.D., ed., *Legal Aspects of Certification and Accreditation*. Evanston, IL: American Board of Medical Specialties, pp. ix–x (1983)
22. American Medical Association, *Physician Characteristics and Distribution in the U.S.,* 1992 ed. Chicago: American Medical Assocation, Table A-29, Update (1992)
23. J. A. Schroeder, "Training an Appropriate Mix of Physicians to Meet the Nation's Needs." *Academic Medicine* 68(2), pp. 118–22 (1993)
24. National Health Expenditures by Type of Service and Source of Funds: Calendar Years 1960–96. Health Care Financing Authority website: www.hcfa.gov (October, 1998)
25. American Hospital Association, *Hospital Statistics,* 1993–94 ed. Chicago: American Hospital Association (1993); M. A. Davis, "Nursing Home Ownership Revisited." *Medical Care* 29(11), pp.1062–68 (November, 1993); A. J. Kania, "Hospital-Based Home Care: Integral to Seamless Service." *Health Care Strategic Management* 11(8), p. 21 (August, 1993)
26. *Social Security Amendments of 1965*, Preamble. (P.L 89-97)
27. P. J. Feldstein, *Health Care Economics*, 4th ed. Albany, NY: Delmar Publishers, Inc., p. 546 (1993)
28. *Health Plan Employer Data and Information Set (HEDIS)*. Washington DC: National Commission on Quality Assurance (1994)
29. A. F. Southwick, *Law of Hospital and Health Care Administration*, 2nd ed. Chicago: Health Administration Press, p. 361 (1988)
30. J. Arras, "Ethical Issues in Emergency Care." *Clinics in Geriatric Medicine* 9(3), pp. 655–64 (August, 1993)
31. K. A. Phillips and D. R. Holtgrave, "Using Cost-Effectiveness/Cost-Benefit Analysis to Allocate Health Resources: A Level Playing Field for Prevention?" *American Journal of Preventive Medicine* 13(1):18–25 (Jan–Feb, 1997)
32. J. R. Griffith, *Designing 21st Century Healthcare: Leadership in Hospitals and Healthcare Systems.* Chicago: Health Administration Press (1998)
33. H. Mintzberg, *The Structuring of Organizations, A Synthesis of the Research.* Englewood Cliffs, NJ: Prentice-Hall (1979)
34. P. Senge, *The Fifth Discipline: The Art and Practice of the Learning Organization.* New York: Doubleday/Currency (1990)

PART

I

Governing: Making Healthcare Organizations Responsive to Their Environment

The need for an organization to deliver modern healthcare is obvious. Hardly any disease or condition, beyond the very simplest, can be treated by a single individual; almost everything requires a team, and often special facilities. A systematic, collective effort of many different people is clearly needed to provide all these services. But a collective effort must serve collective goals. How do we as citizens make sure the effort goes in directions we want? The answer, in healthcare as in other enterprises, is that we delegate the question in two ways—first to individuals to make their own choice, usually between competing organizations, and second to a group of people called the governing board. The board, sensitive to the reality that they must be the choice of a substantial number of individuals to succeed, establishes the direction of the collective enterprise. They hire an executive to implement their decisions, and the executive negotiates a series of agreements with the caregivers and others. Those agreements are made through a largely formal structure that we call "the organization." Increasingly, the agreements and even the underlying direction are quantitative; goals and performance are measured; numbers drive much of the discussion that goes into identifying goals, building consensus, and agreeing on expectations. Overall, the process that shapes the collective effort toward the needs of the individual patients is called governance.

Part I of the text discusses the governance process from the origins of the collective effort itself, through the contributions of the governing board and the executive, the design of the organizational structure, and the measurement of performance. Hidden within the complexities of these processes is a pattern of behavior that gets repeated over and over again, from the highest levels of strategy to the care of an individual patient. The pattern describes how an organization sets goals, selecting some objectives over others. As shown in Figure I.1, the pattern is one of search for possibilities or opportunities, discussion to build consensus among the participants, and agreement about a course of action and an expected result. The pattern begins again when the result is evaluated and the new possibilities are identified.

Leading institutions are good at implementing this pattern at all levels. They bring large numbers of people, open minds, and innovative ideas to the search step. They conduct broad and free-ranging discussion, airing potential disputes rather than concealing them, so that a large number of people

FIGURE I.1
Pattern of Goal Selection in Organizations

Setting goals and objectives, eliminating obstacles, defining processes, specifying realistic outcomes

Reviewing hopes and dreams, seeking ideas, analyzing problems, understanding interrelationships, comparing to similar situations

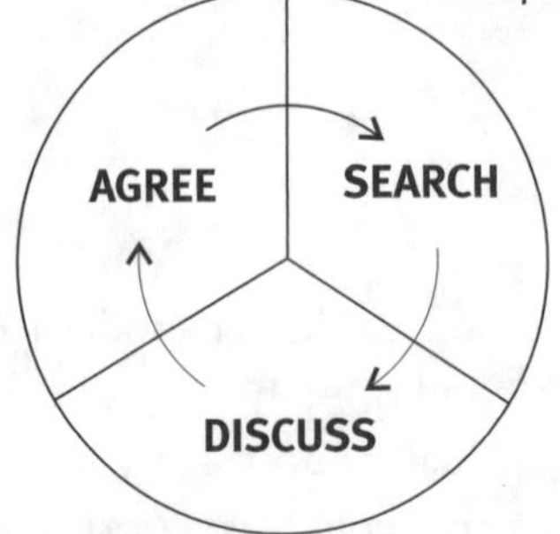

Considering viewpoints, searching for commonalities, weighing priorities, identifying and resolving differences

understand not only what the goal is, but what its limits are and why it was selected. Finally, they agree on actions that are realistic within the range of agreement, and generally achieve them.

CHAPTER

2

HOW HEALTHCARE ORGANIZATIONS RELATE TO THEIR ENVIRONMENT

Organizations are creations of and by human beings to accomplish goals they might otherwise be unable to reach. They emerged contemporaneous with civilization itself,[1] are often unsuccessful, and in the last century have become noticeably more complicated.[2] Healthcare organizations are no exceptions to these statements. This chapter outlines the vocabulary, taxonomy, and premises describing the relationship of the organization to its environment. The chapter

1. develops a four-part theory of management selected to represent the actual activities of successful healthcare organizations, but consistent with general studies of organizations;
2. applies the theory to the modern healthcare organization, identifying the many individuals and groups it serves and illustrating its activities;
3. identifies the motivations of customers of healthcare organizations, and shows how these motivations affect activities; and
4. identifies the core motivations of people who use and work in healthcare organizations.

Understanding the Forces Shaping Organizations

A large number of theories are useful to understand organizations and their activities.[3] The distinction between well-managed organizations and those not so successful appears to begin with the underlying theory guiding the actions of their leaders.[4] This chapter develops a theory based on four concepts that are widely accepted among the most successful healthcare organizations and that have been found useful in the study of organizations generally.[5] The first is the concept of **open systems**, which suggests that organizations depend on their ability to attract resources, such as financial support of customers and the effort of employees. They thrive only because they are successful at attracting these resources, and fail when they are unable to attract one or more resources. The second concept is that of **community-focused strategic management**, the notion that the organization itself repeatedly asks the questions what is our community's goal, why, and how does the organization serve it? "We" is the community being served by the organization. The third concept, **continuous improvement**, suggests that equilibrium will never be fully achieved, that the organization is, in fact, always striving toward a moving goal. The fourth, **scale,** implies that comprehensive organizations meeting a broad spectrum of health needs for large markets have the best chances for long-term success.

Open Systems

Open systems theory implies that any organization can be described in terms of processes that meet demand and earn income by transforming certain resources, basically labor, supplies, and equipment, into new products and services with added value. Any successful organization is dependent on all elements of the set, that is, demand, income, labor, supplies, and equipment, and is limited by the element in shortest supply.

The transactions between the elements, such as hiring, buying, and selling, are exchanges. An **exchange** is a transfer of goods, services, or purchasing power that occurs legitimately when both parties believe themselves to benefit from it. Exchanges occur constantly in society, and in a certain sense they ultimately can occur only between individuals. As a practical matter, however, a great many exchanges occur through formal groups of people, such as governments and organizations that represent and have the commitment of their members. **Exchange partners** are individuals or groups who have an existing commitment to an organization, including at least customers, workers, and suppliers. Partners can be classified according to the nature of their exchange. One very useful classification of partners is between **customers** and providers. Customers are all those partners who use the services of the organization and generally compensate the organization for those services. Providers are all those who provide services and generally are compensated by the organization for their efforts. (Compensation in either case may be something other than money.)

A simple organization, say a hamburger stand, exists because it has resources—cooks, meat, buns, a grill, and skill at cooking burgers—and demand—customers who perceive that there is value added (that is, they are willing to pay at least slightly more than the cost) for the output—hamburgers. Open systems theory says that all of these elements must be present, and that the size of the hamburger stand will depend exactly on the level of the scarcest one. That is, the stand will sell as many hamburgers as customers want, or as many as it can make from the available meat or buns, or as many as the cooks can grill, whichever is smallest.

The concept of open systems is closely related to the theory of the firm in economics. Like the theory of the firm, open systems theory forces the operator to consider prices, quality, and value for the customer; and a similar list for the suppliers, including employees, the organization, and its owners. The two lists inevitably conflict, but they must be integrated as a totality, seeking a solution that is acceptable to all. The solution is always compared to realistic alternatives, that is, competition. If it is not as good as other alternatives, the organization will shrink and fail; if it is better it will grow and thrive.

Open systems theory is particularly useful in a market economy and a free society because it reveals the importance of satisfying people who voluntarily contribute to the exchange. That is, it teaches hamburger stand operators that they are always dependent on the customers, the cooks, the butcher, the baker, and any other exchange partners, like the government agencies that permit the stand to sell hamburgers. None of the exchange partners are forced to make their contribution; the operator must convince each of them to cooperate. Because convincing them will inevitably involve some compromise, they have **influence,** that is, the ability to change or shift the organization. Influence is gained by controlling a resource. The more complete the control and the more critical the resource, the greater the influence. Those people who can affect the success of the organization are called **influentials.** (Particularly important influentials are called **stakeholders**.) Open systems management, then, is the constant search for the solution that is optimally attractive to the influentials.

Influence is relative among the partners and variable across time and place, although national, regional, and community trends and events dictate considerable similarity at any particular time. Change is driven by changes in the desires of the influentials and changes in the relative importance, or **power**, of the influentials.

Community-Focused Strategic Management

Strategy is the systematic response to the changing conditions surrounding the enterprise. The concept of strategic management implies that the organization is deliberately guided toward an explicit purpose, and that one of the functions is to ask persistently three questions: (1) What is our purpose, or why are we here? (2) Why did we select that purpose and is it the best choice? (3) How do we best achieve our purpose?[6] The pursuit of these questions serves a dual purpose; it forces the organization to a continuing survey of its environment and its relation to it, and it provides a mechanism to promote consensus among the people supporting the organization. The "we" underlying these questions is the stakeholders, but under open systems theory it becomes clear that they must answer in a broader context if their organization is to thrive. In for profit companies (and the hamburger stand) the broader context is "customers." Not-for-profit healthcare organizations are owned by, and serve, communities, so that becomes the context for their decisions. A community focus including all potential exchange partners and is essential to provide a broad base of continuing support.

Because environments are constantly changing, the search for answers to the three questions is an ongoing one. **Boundary-spanning** activities, those through which the organization selects its exchanges, look outward to define what the organization must do to thrive. Strategic management includes a deliberate effort to identify people, both providers and customers, whose needs are not met and bring them into the consensus. The organization searches for ways to expand, partly because expansion increases the rewards to the exchange partners and partly because it is protection against shrinking.

The hamburger stand is set up where customers want to buy hamburgers and the cooks are comfortable cooking them. It learns the price, quality, and service combinations that please the most customers, and trains and supports its workers to meet them. If the combinations change, the organization will deliberately evaluate the change and adapt its operations in the direction that seems most fruitful. This means that if the customers express a desire for chicken nuggets, or if the owners decide the customers can be convinced to buy them at a profitable price, the organization will deliberately weigh a change that takes it outside its original hamburger mission and technology.

The organization must translate the desires of the external world, learned by boundary-spanning activities, into effective responses. It does this by identifying specific expectations for its processes and activities. Even in a very simple hamburger stand, there are a great many expectations—for example, the size of the burgers, the availability of condiments, the wrappers or utensils, the cooking methods, the number of burgers one cook can cook in one hour, the level of customer satisfaction anticipated, the sale price, the appearance of the finished order, and its bacterial content. The **operating system** specifies them and makes them clear to the workers. (And recognizing the workers' status as influentials and stakeholders, it tries to gain worker acceptance, or consensus about them.) It also measures what actually happens and compares that to the expectations. It strives to bring the two into agreement by manipulating various parts of the organization. Its success must be fed back to the organization as one consideration in the boundary-spanning activities and selection of future exchanges. That is, if the stand is having trouble meeting some expectations, then either the expectations or the process must be changed.

Both boundary-spanning activities and operating systems use systems of control and communications to seek equilibrium. The outward-looking, broader-reaching, more ambiguous boundary spanning identifies potential directions. These are translated into the more immediate, narrow, and precise expectations used by operating systems. The results of operations are fed back into boundary spanning for the next round of revisions.

Continuous Improvement

If influentials and exchange partners were unchanging in their needs, strategic management would lead to a stable, more or less permanent relationship, a condition called **homeostasis**. Homeostasis happens occasionally for organizations, usually in smaller communities for limited periods of time. For most of the world it is unrealistic. The desires of the exchange partners change, the relative influence of various stakeholders change, and the goals of the organization must change in response. So pervasive is change in modern society that most successful organizations expect to change constantly. Homeostasis becomes a goal that is never reached. The organization is designed around a concept of continuous improvement, that the organization will set expectations that it can and will achieve, but that will be set at a better level each year. Continuous improvement concepts were developed in Japan[7] and became widely accepted in the United States during the 1980s and 1990s.[8] They add several important dimensions to the theory.

Customer initiative

First, continuous improvement places the customer—that is, the one who starts with the money—in the position of defining the good or service the organization supplies. Without in any way ignoring the needs of the worker, it notes that success depends on convincing customers to use the service (and part with their money). If the customers want soy burgers instead of beef burgers, that is what the stand will make. This concept has three advantages. It provides a focus for boundary spanning and expectation setting. It gives a rule for settling disputes. Most important, the focus and the rule are consistent with free market and democratic principles. All of us are both customers and servers.

Worker empowerment

Second, continuous improvement relies heavily on the workers. It **empowers** workers, encouraging them to take control of the operating system and revise it as necessary to meet or improve upon the expectations. Empowering workers requires effectively translating the results of boundary spanning to specific expectations. It also requires a reward system and a unique style of management. The forces supporting the workers' empowerment—adequate training, effective logistics (supplies, tools, equipment), and response to questions—must be supplied by management. Management's responsibilities are derived from worker needs, rather than the other way around. In the hamburger stand, the workers are free to act as they please, so long as the needs of the other influentials, including other workers, are met. In practice, this means management must explain the goals and coach about how to meet them, rather than give orders without explanation. It also means that management is responsible for the stand, the meat and bun supply, advertising, and answering any question the worker has.

Process focus

Third, as a result of the authority accorded to customers and workers, the focus of improvement itself is on revision of **process**, that is, the series of actions or steps that transform inputs to outputs. If there is a gap between what the customer is willing to buy and what the operation can produce, the production process is the focus for revision.[9] If the customer is willing to pay 49 cents for a burger but it costs 50 cents to make one, the process must be changed. The ingredients must be obtained more cheaply or prepared more cheaply. Considerable experimentation could go into finding a way to eliminate that one penny difference. New formulations of the burger, new ways of cooking it, wrapping it, or handling the condiments might all be considered. The possibilities to increase volume, such as faster service at peak hours, longer hours, advertising, and relocation, have to be evaluated. Other requirements like taste, appearance, and the food sanitation rules cannot be ignored. The workers would be expected to come up with the solution if possible, but management must answer all their questions and provide appropriate logistics.

Process revision typically follows the **Shewhart cycle** called **"Plan Do Check Act" (PDCA)**, shown conceptually in Figure 2.1.[10] PDCA suggests that process revision is approached by careful study of the problem with a deliberate effort to uncover the most fundamental possible corrections (Plan); an idea, or proposal for revision that is developed to attack the problem (Do); a trial, where the idea is systematically field tested (Check); and implementation (Act). The cycle is a robust methodology for a team or an individual searching for a way to improve a process.

Factual basis

Fourth, workers are guided in their search for improved processes by facts and factual analysis. Facts (i.e., measurements from the real world) define the specific goals of improvement, and factual analysis identifies the shape it might take. Facts are the arbiters for the inevitable disagreements between and among the customers and workers. The search for facts is far ranging. Science, the study of the factual world, is central. The organization will do what is factually sound and scientifically proven. Most applied activities, even including hamburgers, integrate several different sciences in the creation and marketing of their product or service. The hamburger stand will fail without at least intuitive understanding of the relevant issues in nutrition, bacteriology, accounting, economics, and psychology. If the stand succeeds and grows larger, chemistry and statistics will be added to the list, and the depth of understanding must increase for all.

FIGURE 2.1
Shewhart Cycle for Process Improvement

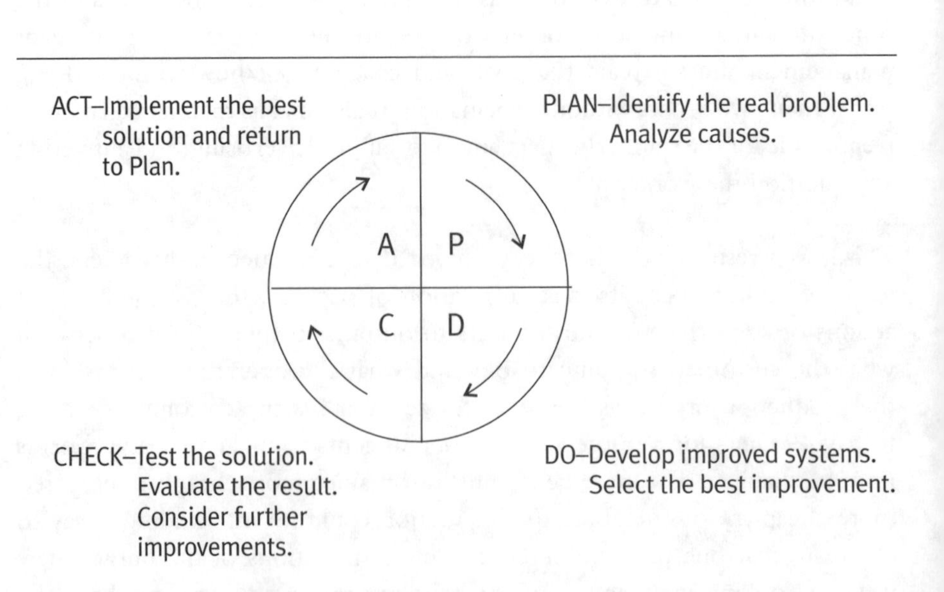

A team of empowered workers will do better if it gains skill at using facts to analyze and understand actual performance and to make choices between alternative goals and processes. Analyzing performance calls for measurement, data collection and recording, data manipulation, and display. For example, as shown in Figure 2.2, the hamburger stand striving for the essential one-cent margin might study what size hamburger is satisfactory to its customers (Part I of the figure). Then, recognizing that smaller burgers can drive away customers and bigger ones erode profits, it might measure actual burgers to identify how many burgers are different than the minimum, and design a patty-making process that ensures uniformly satisfactory size (Part II of the figure).

Statistics will figure heavily in this analysis. Samples of customers will be drawn to identify the satisfactory size. Samples of burgers will measure the process. Because both the average size of the burger and the variation in size are important, both the mean and the standard deviation of the process sample must be analyzed. Further, because most of us are not statisticians, graphic devices will be necessary to show everyone what performance is.

Using facts to make choices between alternative goals and processes is a philosophical commitment, as important as—and quite different from—the ability to analyze the facts themselves. There are competing philosophies, such as religion or ethics (which may forbid certain businesses entirely, or under certain circumstances), authority (whatever the boss says), power (a test of wills between management and union), and simply tradition (we've always done it this way). The theory of this book suggests that the more reliance is on facts, the greater the organization's chance of success. Most people are unwilling to make a complete commitment to follow facts blindly, and therefore make certain religious or ethical constraints. The successful organization integrates these effectively into its mission and uses facts to identify the best solutions within a domain defined by religion, ethics, and law.

The hamburger stand might have several proposals for improving profits, such as buying a higher quality of beef, expanding its advertising, or improving its worker training. Each of these will add to costs. Profits will increase only if new sales or reduced costs exceed the cost of the proposal itself. If the stand is a continuous improvement organization, it will use facts and the Shewhart cycle to assess the proposals. It will survey customers and make trials of new advertising, revised beef specifications, and training programs. Finally, it will select the opportunities that increase profit. It will not decide the question on the owner's opinion or the threat of a strike, and it will not allow inertia to stifle all three opportunities.

The organization that follows continuous improvement theory quickly comes to know more about its business than anyone else. It is likely to be the first to discover or invent new opportunities that go beyond the customers' range of knowledge, but that will fill customer needs. Sony's Walkman is the example most often cited, but Henry Ford's Model T is the most striking. Nobody was asking for a Walkman or a Model T before they were built.

FIGURE 2.2
Use of Facts f
Management
Decisions: Ho
Big Should a
Hamburger B

Part I. Customer Wishes—Data from Customer Surveys

A. Known elements affecting overall satisfaction with product
  Burger: price, size, condiments, roll, cooking time
  Wrapper: convenience
  Service: server attitude, hours, location, parking, amenities
  Other: other meal items, side orders, drinks

B. Customer survey

McDougal's Burgers

Overall, how would you rate this trip to McDougal's?

	Great	Good	OK	Poor	Awful
Now tell us about the details:					
Wrapper	Great	Good	OK	Poor	Awful
Roll	Great	Good	OK	Poor	Awful
Burger size	Great	Good	OK	Poor	Awful
Burger cooking	Great	Good	OK	Poor	Awful
Condiments	Great	Good	OK	Poor	Awful
Fries	Great	Good	OK	Poor	Awful
Desserts	Great	Good	OK	Poor	Awful
Drinks	Great	Good	OK	Poor	Awful
Service	Great	Good	OK	Poor	Awful
Parking	Great	Good	OK	Poor	Awful
Location	Great	Good	OK	Poor	Awful
Hours	Great	Good	OK	Poor	Awful

C. Multi-variate analysis

$$\text{Customer Satisfaction} = \beta_1 \text{(Wrapper)} + \beta_2 \text{(Roll)} + \beta_3 \text{(Size)} + \beta_4 \text{(Cook)} + \beta_5 \text{(Cond)} + \beta_6 \text{(Fries)} + \beta_7 \text{(Desserts)} + \beta_8 \text{(Drinks)} + \beta_9 \text{(Service)} + \beta_{10} \text{(Parking)} + \beta_{11} \text{(Location)} + \beta_{12} \text{(Hours)} + \varepsilon$$

Part II. Burger Size Control

A. Actual burger sizes

Daily Burger Weight Sample

Burger #	Size (Lbs.)
3	.275
14	.243
27	.258
35	.260
49	.243
•	
•	
•	
Average	.250
Std. Dev.	.065

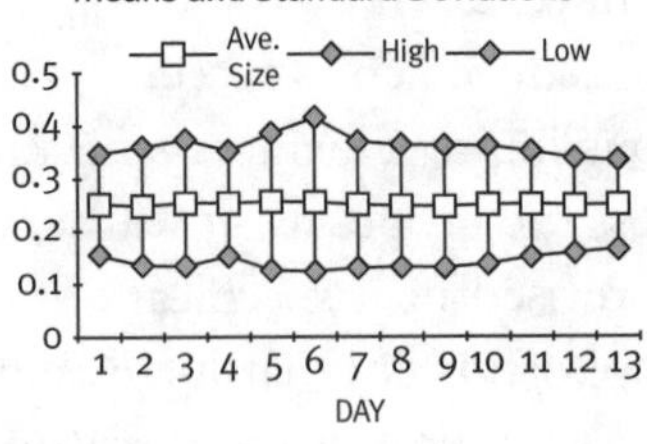

B. Desired burger size: 240 pounds, +/– .065 pounds

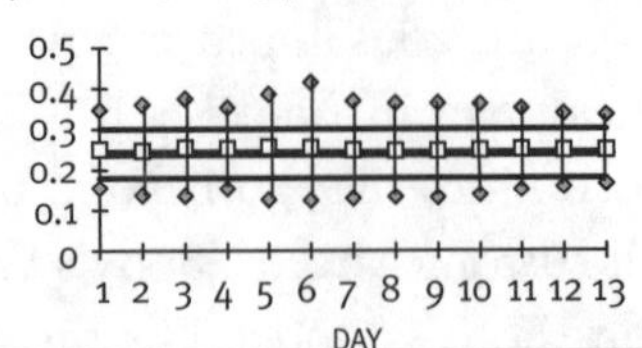

After people saw them, tried them, and became convinced that they worked, the market for them exploded. Organizations deeply knowledgeable in their products and the markets involved are positioned to make these kinds of advances.

Scale

The three principles of resource dependence, community-focused strategic management, and continuous improvement taken in combination imply substantial size and scope of operations. Large, even very large, organizations are the rule in many fields, including hamburger stands. The modern organization has grown precisely because size has proven to be an asset in following the principles. How did McDonald's emerge from something so simple? The answer is that there is a large market for inexpensive hamburgers, and a not-so-simple technology that made them profitable. The technology is based rigorously in a broad range of science. The contribution of McDonald's—"over 100 billion sold"—is scale. Ray Kroc, the founder, ran a hamburger stand. McDonald's uses television to advertise to mass markets, sophisticated franchising and stock structures to gain capital, standardized equipment and supplies to control cost and quality, concentrated purchasing power to gain price advantage, and central education to teach its franchisees and workers. These kinds of activities are not accessible to the small organization.

When Kroc converted from a hamburger stand to McDonald's, he discovered how to put the advantages of scale to work. He copied the history of several other industries (transportation, petrochemical, communications, steel)[11] in inventing a new, larger scale approach to hamburgers. McDonald's as an idea did not exist before he created it, and it is obviously something much different from simply a collection of hamburger stands. Independent hamburger stands still exist, of course. They sell hamburgers that are several times more expensive, and they count their sales in thousands, not billions. They have become what is called a niche market.

Applying the Theory to Healthcare Organizations

This four-part theory of open systems, community-focused strategic management, continuous improvement, and large scale is one that successful healthcare organizations follow aggressively. They recognize their dependence on customers and workers, seek areas where the community can benefit, measure their performance against expectations, and strive for continuous improvement. They have built up consistent ways of implementing the theory through years of experimentation. Those solutions are the content of the book. The four concepts appear and reappear in methods these organizations use to solve the day-to-day issues that arise.

Open Systems

Exchanges and exchange partners

Healthcare organizations have a particularly complex set of exchange partners. The importance and cost of the service lead to both the customer and the provider exchanges that are far more complicated than for hamburgers. Figure 2.3 summarizes the exchange partners.

Customer partners: patients and families

Patients are the most important exchange partners. They anticipate appropriate, high-quality medical care, and they hold the healthcare organization responsible for supplying it. Friends and family aid most patients in their hospitalization. In some cases, healthcare organizations must establish close and direct relations with friends and family (for example, with the fathers of newborn, the next-of-kin of the dying, and the family of chronically impaired patients). The healthcare organization is responsible for amenities, safety, parking, and on-site mobility for both patients and families.

Customer partners: payment partners

In modern industrial societies, patients rely on a variety of insurance mechanisms to pay for care. Insurance intermediaries are essential exchange partners. As noted in Chapter 1, there are several different forms, including a variety of managed care options and traditional insurance. In most communities a few large intermediaries each offer a full range of these forms.

Two large governmental insurance programs are at least indirect exchange partners with most healthcare organizations. **Medicare** deals with healthcare organizations through its intermediary, usually the local Blue Cross/Blue Shield Plan. **Medicaid**, a state-federal program financing care for the poor, is run by the state **Medicaid agency**, but the agencies are increasingly turning to intermediaries.

Customer partners: buyers

Much insurance is provided through employment. Because healthcare insurance is an increasingly expensive employment benefit, employing corporations have become important exchange partners. Historically, unions played a major role in establishing health insurance as an employee benefit. Federal, state, and local governments purchase insurance for special groups of citizens and also buy as employers. In the past decade, buyers have been concerned about the cost of health and hospital care and have taken action to restrict the growth of costs, with only partial success.

Customer partners: regulatory agencies

Healthcare is judged by society to require collective supervision via government regulation. As a result, governmental regulatory agencies are exchange partners at least nominally acting on behalf of the patient and buyer. Licensing agencies are common, not only for hospitals and healthcare professionals, but sometimes for other facilities such as ambulatory care centers. Many states have certificate of need laws requiring permission for hospital construction

FIGURE 2.3 Major Exchange Partners of Healthcare Organizations

Customer Partners
- Patients and families
- Payment partners
  - Insurance carriers and intermediaries
    - HMOs
    - IPAs
    - PPOs
    - TPAs
    - Medicare
    - Medicaid
  - Buyers
    - Employing corporations
    - Unions
    - Federal, state, and local governments
  - Regulatory partners
    - Government regulatory agencies
    - Peer review organizations
    - JCAHO
  - Community partners
    - Police
    - Social service agencies
    - Local government
    - Charitable, religious, educational, and culture organizations
    - Citizens at large
    - Media

Provider Partners
- Members
  - Employees
  - Medical staff members
  - Trustees
  - Volunteers
- Member groups
  - Unions
  - Professional associations
- Suppliers
- Other providers
  - Community clinics
  - Mental health and substance abuse clinics
  - Mental hospitals
  - Home care agencies
  - Drug stores
  - Long-term care facilities
- Government agencies representing members
  - Occupational safety
  - Professional licensure
  - Environmental protection
  - Equal employment opportunity

or expansion. **Peer review organizations (PROs)** are external agencies that audit the quality of care and use of insurance benefits by individual physicians and patients for Medicare and other insurers.

Most insurers mandate two outside audits of hospital performance, one by the JCAHO or its osteopathic counterpart, the American Osteopathic Association, and the other by a public accounting firm of the healthcare organization's choice. HMOs themselves are accredited by the **National Commission on Quality Assurance (NCQA)**. Healthcare organizations have exchange relationships with these agencies.

Customer partners: community groups

The healthcare organization makes certain exchanges with governments, community agencies, and informal groups. These are numerous, varied, and far reaching. They provide babies for adoption; receive the victims of accidents, violent crimes, rape, and family abuse; and attract the homeless, the mentally incompetent, and the chronically alcoholic. These activities draw them into exchange relations with police and social service agencies.

Healthcare organizations take United Fund charity. They facilitate baptisms, ritual circumcisions, group religious observances, and rites for the dying. They provide educational facilities and services to the community, such as health education and disease prevention programs and assistance to support groups. These activities often make them partners of charitable, religious, educational, and cultural organizations. Prevention and outreach activities draw healthcare organizations into alliances with governmental organizations such as public health departments and school boards.

Healthcare organizations require land and zoning permits; they use water, sewer, traffic, electronic communications, fire protection, and police services. They are subject to environmental regulations. In these areas, healthcare organizations often present special problems that must be negotiated with local government. Healthcare organizations are frequently one of the largest employers in town, and not-for-profit healthcare organizations often occupy land that, if taxed, would add noticeably to local tax revenues. As a result, the electorate and the local government hold the healthcare organization to certain standards; they, too, can be viewed as exchange partners. Communication with the electorate often involves the media—press, radio, and television coverage, as well as purchased advertising.

Provider partners: members

The second most fundamental exchange, next to patients, is between the healthcare organization and its **members**, those people who give their time and energy to the organization. Healthcare organization members are employees, medical staff members, trustees, and other volunteers. Employees are compensated by salary and wages. Medical staff members (for example, physicians, dentists, psychologists, podiatrists, etc.) may receive monetary compensation either through the healthcare organization or directly from patients or insurance intermediaries. Trustees and a great many others volunteer their time to the healthcare organization, their only compensation being the satisfaction they achieve from their work. The compensation must be economically competitive. Also, whether participation is compensated or volunteer, the individual must receive some satisfaction beyond earnings. Otherwise, volunteers will stop volunteering, and doctors and employees will leave for other organizations that can better fulfill their needs.

Provider partners: member organizations

Members are often organized into groups, and their groups manage their exchanges to some extent. Unions and professional associations represent members. Physicians often form associations and practice groups, and healthcare organizations make formal contracts with them. Any subunit of the healthcare organization—the doctors specializing in neurology, for example—can become a group representing its members to the healthcare organization. Group membership is itself an exchange; it is fruitful for individuals because they can meet some needs that would otherwise go unmet. The success of the groups depends on the set of exchanges that commits the individuals to their groups.

Provider partners: suppliers

Healthcare organizations use significant quantities of goods and services, from artificial implants to banking. The suppliers of these are exchange partners. Suppliers of certain critical goods and services—such as electrical power, communications, and human blood—are particularly important exchange partners.

Provider partners: other providers

In the course of meeting patient needs, healthcare organizations have considerable contact with other providers, including competing healthcare organizations and agencies whose service lines may be either competitive or complementary, such as mental health and substance abuse clinics, mental hospitals, home care agencies, drug stores, and long-term care facilities. The vertical integration of healthcare providers, the tendency to cover the broadest possible spectrum of healthcare rather than a single service such as hospitalization, has led to increasingly formal relationships with these organizations, ranging from referral agreements through joint ventures to acquisition and operation of services. It is not uncommon for two healthcare organizations to collaborate for certain activities, such as medical education or care of the poor, and compete on others. Even competitors with almost exactly the same service lines negotiate contracts with each other. Negotiation between competitors is regulated by federal and state antitrust laws, but the prohibitions are specific and other communication is permitted.

Provider partners: government agencies representing members

Government agencies of various kinds monitor the rights of member groups. Occupational safety, licensure, and equal employment opportunity agencies are among those entitled to access to the healthcare organization and its records. The healthcare organization is obligated to collect Social Security and federal income taxes. Records and taxes are examples of exchanges between healthcare organizations and government agencies.

Networking

Each of the exchange partners of the healthcare organization has relationships with exchange partners of its own. These interactions lead to **networks** of exchange relationships. The healthcare organization is always located in a web of such networks. Understanding and respect for these networks is one of the keys to success. Exchange partners can participate more readily, and on more generous terms, in activities that do not require them to revise other important relationships. Conversely, proposals that threaten established relationships tend to move slowly, and at high cost. Figure 2.4 shows a greatly oversimplified network relationship of healthcare organization exchange partners. A healthy organization will make a great many network ties, and will act in such a way as to keep them intact whenever possible.

From an individual perspective, patients create exchanges with their families, with health education and promotion services, doctors, drug stores, hospitals, other care providers, and support groups. Primary care practitioners—doctors in family practice, general internal medicine, pediatrics, obstetrics, and psychiatry; nurse practitioners and midwives—are the most common formal contacts for healthcare. Emergency services of hospitals and clinics fill a similar role for the poor. Referral specialists tend to see patients referred by primary care doctors and to care for them on a more limited and transient basis. They are more likely to manage episodes of inpatient hospital care. Several diagnostic and treatment services, also called **clinical support**

FIGURE 2.4
Network of Exchange Partners in a Community

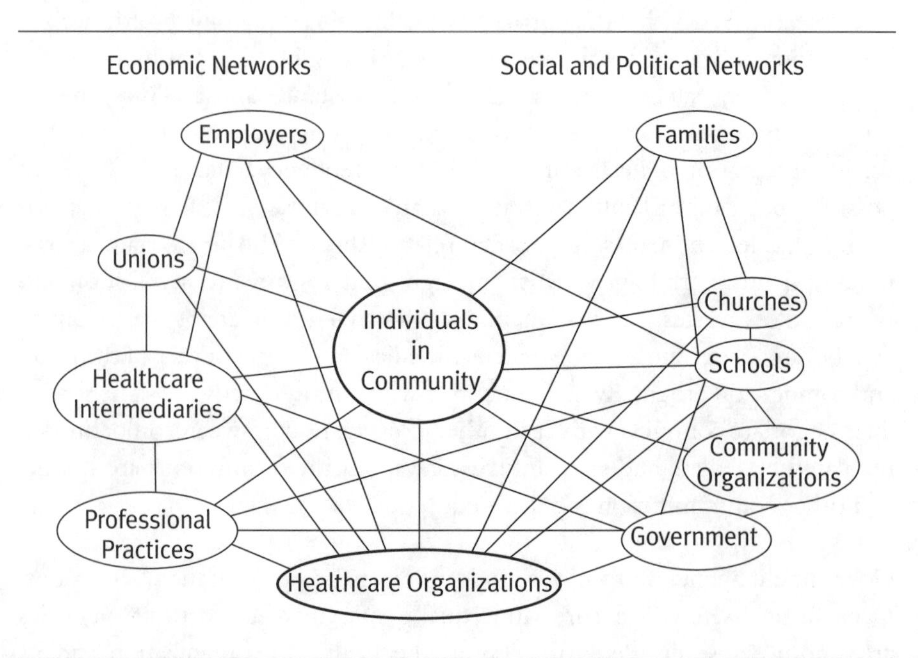

services, are used by both primary and referral doctors. They are available to patients at the most appropriate site: hospital, home, or office.

Most people expect all of these services to be available when needed, and particularly older people have several established relationships. As a result, all of these caregivers are drawn together around patient needs. The healthcare organization is the result of formal contracts between a reasonably comprehensive set of these needs.

The network financing care is also important. Most people relate to employers who in turn select intermediaries. Viewed from the perspective of the employment network, healthcare is important, but it is obviously only a small part of the total relationship. Changes in the general economy, chiefly in the diminished ability of the United States to compete in world trade led first to stagnation of wages and profits. In the 1980s, as part of a widespread response to this problem, the buyers stimulated profound shifts in the exchanges between intermediaries and employees. New forms of insurance and financing were developed; the risks associated with the cost of care were redistributed, bringing the providers into the search for improvement. The redesign process continued to the present day.

A third important network is the one relating to government. Governments have multiple exchanges with healthcare organizations, as well as exchanges among themselves (for example, state and federal governments) and between units such as Medicaid and the regulatory agencies. There are obvious relations among governments and employers, unions, and the citizenry. When people are dissatisfied with their exchange relationship with healthcare organizations, they can choose either governmental or non-governmental routes to relief. Government difficulty paying for Medicaid and Medicare costs has already led to a series of new rules aimed at finding more cost-effective solutions. As of 1998, consumers were pressing for redress against perceived problems of HMOs through government regulation. The problems had their origins in the redesign process stimulated by the buyers.

Influence

For the typical healthcare organization, thousands of individuals affiliate with hundreds of organizations that form a handful of important networks. The organizations can be classified by their influence. Member partners with critical skills, such as doctors, have considerable influence, as do partners with whom there are frequent exchanges, such as payment partners. Buyers have developed influence through their role as trustees, through intermediaries, and through buyer groups. Some partners have very specific or temporary influence, but it may still be powerful. Public health licensure officials, for example, can close a healthcare organization for an emergency situation. A group or even an individual who relates to the institution only infrequently can sometimes acquire startling influence for a short period of time. Pickets or the media are examples.

Community-Focused Strategic Management

In healthcare, strategy involves the deliberate tracking of changing needs and power among the networks of influentials. The origins of the modern healthcare organization can generally be described as one of steadily increasing numbers of influentials and a gradual shift away from the dramatic curative episode. The "doctors' workshop" of the first decades of the twentieth century accurately captures the influence existing then—influence limited almost exclusively to physicians, particularly surgeons. The spread of technology beyond surgery, the growth of employment-based health insurance, and government finance led to demonstrable increases in the lists of influentials. But professional judgment and medical technology continued to capture widespread respect. The money and the influence went to high-tech medical services largely in acute general hospitals through 1990.

Over time, dissenters to the high-tech consensus slowly gained more influence.[12,13] One of the obvious weaknesses of high-tech medicine was its cost. A large number of states investigated regulatory agencies approaches to control costs in the 1970s, and some states implemented them. They had only mixed effectiveness, so the pressure for cost control continued to grow.[14] In 1983, the federal government changed the hospital payment for Medicare from a "reasonable cost" concept to a fixed amount per discharge, with annual increases based on the federal budget. Because Medicare revenue constituted 35 to 40 percent of most hospitals' income, the government's influence was unquestionable.

Driven by some of the same underlying causes, some employers became more aggressive in addressing the cost of health insurance premiums. Many firms avoided providing insurance, creating a pool of uninsured persons. Others reduced the scope of coverage or demanded partial payment by the employee. Lack of health insurance, or the fear of it, became a political force in itself. Employee premium sharing generated opportunities for managed care insurance that could offer better financial protection for less cost. The net result of these actions was a significant rise in the influence of payment partners. At the same time, certain kinds of government regulatory agencies, particularly the health systems agencies, lost influence because they were not effective.

This change in the influence structure established the grounds for extensive revision of healthcare delivery. The leading hospitals and medical group practices responded to it as it emerged, making substantial changes to improve the efficiency of inpatient services. HMOs capitalized on these improvements and demanded their spread to outpatient care. Because the cost of care involves the clinical decisions about what services to use, reorganizations soon began to focus heavily on the medical staff. Attention to outpatient care and integration of the medical staff are the elements that distinguish the healthcare organization from its predecessors.

Well-managed hospitals entered the period of extreme change with three assets: First, they had the resources that accrued to successful institutions prior to the change; second, they had a background of goodwill and effective communications with their medical staffs and other exchange partners; and third, they had better sensing, forecasting, and consensus building mechanisms that allowed them to perceive trends and respond to them faster. The perception and response capability is the essence of strategy.

The contribution of community focus

It is often argued that America's healthcare system does not handle its strategic decisions well. Not only are costs not controlled, but the system spends a large amount of money on an infrastructure that only facilitates equilibrium between the demands of the participants and does not itself deliver care.[15] Much of this equilibrium building cost is related to the local nature of healthcare organizations. Yet given the diversity of the country, and the difficulty of gaining consensus on issues such as healthcare, a local approach may be the most feasible. Accountability is transferred to the local level; if cost is high or quality low in a given community, those most at risk are the ones who must change the system. The decision makers are accessible. Political, social, and economic avenues are open to those who wish to make changes.

The terms "community focus" and "customer initiative" imply a point of view about the strategic management, that priority belongs to the patient and the community as a whole, rather than a select group of owners or workers. That perspective is adopted deliberately by many healthcare organizations. They are legally incorporated for the benefit of the community they serve, usually granted tax advantages in return for the service, and their strategies are deliberately responsive to that community.

The mission of community focused healthcare organizations is usually stated as improving the health of the community, rather than simply providing healthcare to it. Broader mission statements incorporate perspectives of prevention and health promotion that until recently were rarely emphasized by hospitals or medical group practices. These perspectives hold great promise for cost reduction, particularly among poor and disadvantaged populations. Counseling on child-rearing, safety, smoking, alcohol and other substance abuse, safe sex, and nutrition can reduce the cost of care itself and improve health and productivity. Among the elderly, management of disease is intermingled with social needs—housing, nutrition, and assistance with daily living.

These perspectives have led to a new concept of an **integrated health system**, an organization that strives deliberately to meet all the health needs of its community at minimum cost. (The terms "integrated health network" and "integrated delivery system" are also used.) As Figure 2.5 shows, services of the organization begin with those aimed at keeping the community well and continue through several levels of disease or condition management. At each stage, the objective is to return the patient to the well population at the lowest possible cost. Thus, the bulk of disease is treated on an ambulatory basis. The services of the healthcare organization extend through continuing nursing home care, where the goal is to maintain as much independence as possible, to the end of life, where the patient is encouraged to determine the outcome as much as possible.

For-profit healthcare organizations cannot ignore community focus. They must satisfy the same customer requirements, including cost control. The preventive and health promotion activities have the same return for them. Their strategies are tempered by the need to return profits to their shareholders, but the difference tends to be one of degree.

The contribution of ethical values

The best-managed healthcare organizations begin with ethical concepts that minimize conflicts between customers and providers. They seek members who share certain ethical values:

- A love of human life and dignity, which is expressed as a willingness to give service and to respect each patient's rights and desires. Love and respect extend to members of the organization as well. Members are accepted as individuals and are respected for their contributions.
- Quality of service to the patient or customer is taken as primary and inviolate. The well-run healthcare organization satisfies all reasonable expectations of quality and requires adequate quality as the immutable foundation of any activity it undertakes.
- Quality of service is multidimensional and must include access, satisfaction, continuity, comprehensiveness, prevention, and compliance,

FIGURE 2.5 How the Healthcare Organization Sustains Its Community at Minimum Cost

Condition or Disease State	Kind of Healthcare	Management Objective	Example
Well Population	Health promotion/ Disease prevention	Promotion of healthy lifestyles	Immunization, environmental safety, nutrition, exercise
↓			
Disease or Condition Risk	Detection and secondary prevention	Encourage effective use of care	Smoking cessation, prenatal, well-baby care
↓			
Ambulatory Management (Acute or Chronic Condition)	Health maintenance	Maximum functioning	Infectious disease, AIDS, asthma, trauma, arthritis
↓			
Acute Management	Episodic care	Cure, repair, limit disability	Surgery, radiation, ICU, obs. delivery
↓	Restoration	Prompt, full return return to	Exercise, retraining, prostheses
Rehabilitation Management			
↓	Support	Maximum independence	Nursing home, home care
Continuing Care			
↓			
Death	Assistance	Most satisfactory end of life	Hospice, self determination

as well as the narrow technical issues of accurate diagnosis and treatment.[16] Because all of the dimensions of quality of service are important to the patient, the well-managed healthcare organization attempts to consider them all in its mission, plans, and expectations.
- Members of the organization are expected to search for improvements that serve both customers and members, and to derive satisfaction from identifying and achieving these improvements.

Well-managed healthcare organizations strive to attract and encourage people who share these values. They announce their ethical commitment through their mission and their public statements, and reinforce it through their actions. They praise acts of kindness and foster a caring environment. They avoid and discourage those who disagree, particularly those who are unable to express love and respect for individual dignity. A broad spectrum of incentives, including recognition, encouragement, praise, promotion and monetary compensation, rewards dedication to these values. Sanctions are used rarely, in cases in which the individual's behavior threatens the quality of care or the continued effectiveness of the work group.[17]

The role of the organization

The organization, the superstructure beyond the intimate healthcare transaction itself, has a role that is harder to understand than the doctor's or the patient's. It must carry out a series of functions that identify and maintain the equilibrium. These are functions clearly different from caregiving.

- The organization conducts an ongoing search and evaluation process that identifies mutually acceptable exchanges between customers and providers.[18] The best exchanges are those that society wants most, as measured by its willingness to commit resources, and those that the healthcare organization can deliver better than any other source. All objectives, goals, or purposes, even the mission of the healthcare organization are set as a result of this search.
- The organization acquires the necessary resources. That is, it markets services, recruits people, purchases supplies, and collects revenue. (These are often called logistic functions.)
- The organization facilitates solutions. That is, it supports communications, clarifies responsibilities, assists in building consensus, encourages performance, and resolves conflicts.
- The organization controls its customers and its providers so that it usually meets the customers' expectations. Control of customers is achieved through the selection and location of services. Control of providers is achieved via agreement with empowered workers, about designed processes and detailed expectations. Control is achieved by building consensus with customers and providers, not by enforcing compliance.

These functions remain secondary to the exchanges of medical care itself. Success for the organization is the reward for fulfilling the exchanges society sees as most useful, and society gets little benefit from the organizational activities per se. On the other hand, the organization is essential, because it provides services direct caregivers cannot do by themselves.

Organizational failure can occur in four ways:

1. The organization can misread society's desires and select the wrong exchanges.
2. The translation of exchanges into expectations can contain errors.
3. The delivery units can fail to meet their expectations.
4. The demands of society can move away from those the organization can fulfill.

Continuous Improvement

The concepts of continuous improvement are the most recent additions to the theory of healthcare organizations. The individual components of customer initiative, worker empowerment, process focus, and factual basis have long histories and were both scientifically and practically supported before what is called "the quality movement" began. The movement reinvigorated the elements and tied them together effectively.[19]

Patients, the primary customers of healthcare, were historically viewed as passive recipients of treatment they did not understand and could not evaluate.[20] They have emerged as the final arbiters of both cost and quality. Leading healthcare institutions survey their patients constantly, seeking evidence of satisfaction with the care process, the amenities surrounding it, and the results.[21] Documented outcomes of treatment and efforts at prevention and health promotion are now required by employers.[22] The financial realities of healthcare delivery enhance the power of relatively small groups of customers. High fixed costs, particularly the training of specialists and the capital equipment they require, must be supported by large patient volumes. Each specialist and specialty service, therefore, must optimize income by attracting the largest possible group of patients. Few can afford the luxury of denying their service to any group.

The quality movement stresses the importance of empowered workers who can modify their jobs to meet customer needs. Healthcare may have the largest number of different professional skills of any industry. Specialization has provided great benefits, but it has created a world in which many professions compete for power. Effective integration of several dozen specialists (several may be involved even in a single case) has not been easy. The creation of multispecialty teams focused around specific diseases has been important. It coordinates specialties around scientifically defensible objectives. It replaces both authoritarian bureaucracies and the dominant voice of the physician.

The emphasis on process revision has led to analyzing patterns of care and devising general guidelines or protocols. It allows workers to review factual and scientific evidence, debate alternatives, and reach agreement about processes of care. As they do, they learn and implement new approaches. The use of protocols is widespread in inpatient care and growing rapidly in outpatient applications. The contribution of the protocols is measured by an increasing number of quality indicators, including those developed by HEDIS. The measures make benchmarking—the comparison with the best known practice—possible. The combination of prospective process evaluation and benchmarking opens the possibility of major gains in quality in the next few years.

The attention to factual data and scientific evidence has transformed information into a strategic resource for the organization.[23] Its importance is recognized among leading healthcare organizations, as evidenced both by survey of management[24] and capital expenditure plans.[25] Measured performance is rapidly becoming the focus of accreditation. The capture, archiving, analysis, and communication of information has become a major element in the contribution of the healthcare organization.

Scale

Healthcare organizations have traditionally been small, as Chapter 1 illustrates, but in the future, well-managed healthcare organizations are likely to be large in size (number of patients or annual dollar volume) and scope (variety of services). Large organizations supported by large markets generate returns to scale, the ability to finance technology of all kinds that smaller firms cannot afford. The emerging healthcare organization requires technological resources for clinical and business operations. The list of different skills to produce patient care is much longer than for hamburgers, requiring large, diverse worker groups and physical facilities. The technology to process facts also provides returns to scale.

Scale generally requires mass markets; healthcare organizations tend to serve as large a fraction of the community as possible. At the same time, healthcare remains a uniquely personal service delivered by one human being to another. The technological imperative is to invent the larger scale approach that retains the personal touch. There will be a role for niche providers, small independent hospitals, and medical practices. They will trade the returns to scale for specific advantages in specific markets. Although some analysts feel they hold great promise,[26] comprehensive healthcare organizations have advantages in their ability to meet multiple needs of patients and families and their ability to steer patients to specialties.

Important Customer Motivations

If the open systems concept is correct, healthcare organizations have grown in importance because customers perceived that they fulfilled certain needs more effectively than did the available alternatives. Organizations as widespread as these must respond to needs that are nearly universal, and it ought to be possible to identify what they are. Benjamin Franklin, conducting the fund drive for the first community hospital in North America (The Pennsylvania Hospital, founded in 1760), eloquently built his case on five arguments.

1. We need a refuge for the unfortunate, and Christianity will reward you for your generosity to this cause. (Although Franklin did not say so, Judaism, Islam, and Buddhism also praise charitable behavior.)
2. You might need it yourself this very night.
3. Among other things, we can keep contagious people off the streets.
4. We can certainly handle this better as a community than as individuals.
5. Grants from the Crown and the Commonwealth will lower the out-of-pocket costs. (He might have added that the grants were "new money" that would eventually end up in Philadelphians' purses.)[27]

Little has changed in 200 years except the language. Four of these arguments appear in most twentieth century fundraising literature. The fifth, control of contagious disease, is a contribution of healthcare organizations to public health. It was reduced in importance when antibiotics came into widespread use, but it has received increased attention recently.

In fact, the history of hospitals and the emergence of healthcare organizations clearly reveal multiple and powerful motivations in the communities that built them.[28,29] Although other taxonomies could be created, it is useful to think of these motivations in Franklin's five groups.

1. *Samaritanism and support of the poor.* A desire to aid the sick and needy because the aid itself has value or intrinsic merit. In advanced industrial nations, Samaritanism has two forms: tax-supported government programs and voluntary charity.
2. *Personal health.* A desire to improve the health of oneself and one's loved ones, and to deal more effectively with disease, disability, and death.
3. *Public health.* A desire for health as a collective or social benefit; to reduce contagion; ensure a healthy work force and military force; and reduce the tax burdens associated with disease, disability, and death.
4. *Economic gain for the community.* A desire to use the healthcare organization as a source of income and employment to make the community as a whole economically successful.
5. *Control of costs and quality of healthcare.* A desire to ensure certain levels of quality and costs for healthcare, now expressed through the insurance premium as well as out-of-pocket payments.

These five motivations are the permanent support for community healthcare organizations. The debates that occur in every generation are about the relative importance of each rather than the introduction of new ones.

Samaritanism and Support of the Poor

Whether Samaritanism deserves first place in a list of motivations for healthcare organizations is debatable, but a claim for prominence can be based on the long history and diversity of examples. It does not apply to for-profit healthcare organizations, but these are a minority. The urge to help one's fellow man is widespread, although it appears to wax and wane at various times and places. It is one of the characteristics that distinguishes man from animals. "It is more blessed to give than to receive" is an important principle in most major religions and ethical systems. A world without charity would be palpably less civilized.

The word "hospital" has the same root as the words "host" and "hospitality" and "hotel," reflecting the ancient role of places called hospitals as refuges. Samaritanism still occurs in twentieth-century citadels of high technology. Healthcare organizations in most communities cannot ignore uninsured or underinsured patients. Emergency services must accept and at least stabilize any patient they receive. As a practical matter, it is difficult to turn acutely ill patients away, although they are often concentrated in a few facilities in large cities. They accept them with little distinction from paying patients. Not-for-profit healthcare organizations are granted tax advantages to assist with this burden.

Samaritanism includes personal contributions of both service and funds. Charity to the sick and injured is particularly appealing to many citizens of the community. The opportunity to give or serve is part of the exchange; people gain rewards from charitable activities. The sick have an obvious need, and concerns with the worth of the recipients can be set aside more easily than they can, for example, in the case of criminals or unwed mothers.[30]

The contributions of time and effort are not easily measured, but they probably exceed monetary gifts by several times when the efforts of providers are included. **Volunteers** provide amenities and assistance in most community healthcare organizations. The service of trustees is almost entirely volunteered; tax law for not-for-profit corporations requires that they receive no direct profit from their efforts. Many hours of medical staff activity are unpaid as well. Although one can argue that doctors are compensated by the privilege of using the organization in caring for patients of other economic advantage, it is clear that many doctors contribute their time just because they want to. Often overlooked is the charitable impulse of employees at all levels in healthcare organizations. Aiding the sick is in itself a reward of their job, a compensation that sometimes offsets low wages. Whenever a healthcare organization employee or doctor spends time at activities that would be better compensated elsewhere, a charitable donation has occurred.

Donated funds amount to less than 2 percent of all income, but they are important in research, education, and buildings. Added to an earned surplus, they allow levels of flexibility and amenities that might otherwise be impossible. They are important sources of unrestricted capital.

Not all charitable motives are altruistic. Donations to healthcare organizations are a way to relieve feelings of guilt about wealth, advertise the better characteristics of the donor, and, since 1913, reduce income taxes. Donors seek to meet needs that could be more those of the giver than of the recipient. For example, children's hospitals are more appealing to donors than an objective observer might expect. Donor satisfaction is as important to the exchange as the use to which the gift is put; if donors are not satisfied, gifts will not continue.

Local, state, and federal governments grant healthcare organizations tax exemption. The exemption is at least partly in support of the charitable endeavors.[31] The exemption is periodically challenged, and uncompensated care is a major argument for retaining it. The value of this exemption varies but is on the order of 3 to 5 percent of annual expenses, an amount larger than contributions and often equal to net profits. The burden of care for the poor has been increasingly assumed by government programs. State and federal funds are combined in the Medicaid program, now the largest source of funds for care of the poor. Medicaid can be viewed as Samaritanism; in fact, it is often justified politically in that way. They also have more mundane motives. Government funds distributed through a community's healthcare organization create jobs, simultaneously fulfilling the economic gain motivation.

Personal Health

Most Americans would say that the purpose of healthcare organizations is to provide personal healthcare, but until a century ago, hospitals and doctors had almost no contribution to make toward restoring health, and the actual lifesaving abilities of a healthcare organization are probably still less than most people think. Personal health comes from several sources; education and lifestyle are important along with self-care, family care, and care from organizations. The healthcare organization can be viewed as supplying what other sources cannot provide or fail to provide.

High-tech healthcare

Highly technical interventions are the economic mainstay of healthcare organizations. The hospital operating room was the first such service to emerge. By 1870, new technology was providing safe and pain-free surgery, greatly improving the patient's chance of surviving what are today's routine procedures. Cesarean section ceased to be immediately fatal to the mother. Hernia repairs, trauma repairs, and removal of diseased organs in the abdominal cavity became dramatically safer. The cost, difficulty, and need for trained personnel put this technology out of reach of most individual doctors. The new opportunities for truly valuable care via the hospital led to the first great growth period for American hospitals.[32]

After a new service leaves the research stage, it often becomes an activity that occurs solely in the hospital on an inpatient basis. As the technology is improved and its limitations understood, the service gradually moves to the outpatient clinic before finally migrating to the doctor's office, at least for the less complicated cases. Many of the surgical procedures responsible for the rise in the hospital's importance a century ago are now done without overnight hospitalization. Some are done in doctors' offices, and some have been replaced by nonsurgical treatment.

High-tech services consume at least half of national health expenditures, even though they are received by less than 5 percent of the population. A community's investment in healthcare organizations is dramatically affected by attitudes toward the desirability of new technology. Within surprisingly broad ranges, the level of technology chosen is not reflected in measurable differences in health. One reason is that healthcare benefits are difficult to measure. Another is that patients can usually go to another community that has the necessary technology, if it is not provided in the local community. It may be less convenient to drive Grandmother to the state university hospital for care; it does not measurably affect her health, and it clearly does not affect her longevity.

The high-touch alternative

The popular image of healthcare organizations is high-tech. Stopped hearts are restarted, airways are reopened, arteries are sewn, babies are rescued, rampant infection is overcome. The day-to-day reality is relief of distress that is not life threatening. Not only are few patients at death's door when they seek care, few are cured when they leave. The patient with cardiovascular disease is much more often in the hospital for continuing support of an impaired heart than immediate treatment of a heart attack. Chronic lung disease is more common than the occasional dramatic stoppage of breathing. Alcoholism, a principal cause of accidents, remains after the bone is set and the artery is sewn. Prenatal care and prevention of unwanted pregnancy are both cheaper and more effective than dramatic interventions at birth. Increasingly, healthcare organizations are emphasizing a "high touch" program of prevention, health maintenance, and management of chronic illness.

The steady transition of technology to less complex applications and the move to "high touch" care have led to a proliferation of new delivery mechanisms—multispecialty facilities for outpatient diagnosis and treatment; increased use of psychologists, nurse practitioners, social workers, and other nonphysicians; group educational activities for prevention and case management; services and equipment delivered to the home; hospices; and long-term care facilities.

Public Health

The distinction between public and personal health is conceptually clear but sometimes hard to trace in real situations. Personal healthcare is that given directly to the individual, while public health emphasizes activity for groups, such as maintaining a pure water supply. A public benefit also occurs, however, when care is given to individuals, and maintenance of a healthy work force and a healthy army are important public health goals.

The historical example of hospitals' public health role was care of contagious disease. Quarantine of persons with a contagious disease was one of the important exchange contributions of hospitals until the twentieth century. Hospitals were relied on for care of persons with a long list of contagious diseases, beginning with tuberculosis and leprosy and including scarlet fever, polio, and infant diarrheal diseases. These diseases have now been nearly eliminated by vaccines or reduced greatly in severity by antibiotics.

Today, AIDS (acquired immune deficiency syndrome) is one of the few numerically important infectious diseases, and, once again, the healthcare organization is expected to provide public health support. Tuberculosis (TB) is recurring as an antibiotic-resistant disease. Management of contagion is part of the job of the healthcare organization. Both AIDS and TB as public health problems relate to people's risk habits and treatment habits. The new issues of public health are related to behavioral issues. Laws, regulations, education, taxation, and subsidies remain important vehicles for containing or eliminating these diseases, as they were for TB, pneumonia, and syphilis a century ago. Modifications of personal healthcare are also important and they are the domain of healthcare organizations.

Healthcare organizations contribute to public health by providing personal health services for these diseases. They also have an important role in prevention, because they normally reach people when they are especially receptive to learning better health habits and care for their continuing disease or disability. Many healthcare organizations also provide preventive education for parents: safe pregnancy, avoidance of drugs injurious to the infant, nutrition and breast feeding, psychological aspects of child rearing, the importance of immunization, and family planning are topics frequently covered. They also assist the aged and chronic sick with programs for blood pressure control, substance abuse, nutritional habits, exercise and rehabilitation. Each preventive success eliminates a potential financial burden on the individual or the community. Collaboration with public health agencies to meet the prevention needs of the poor has become more common; the trend will continue so long as healthcare organizations accept risk for the cost of care through Medicaid HMOs and similar financing.[32]

Economic Gain for the Community

Funds spent on healthcare organizations generate non–health-related economic gains for their communities, both directly and indirectly. Directly, healthcare organizations create jobs, particularly for unskilled workers, who are an employment problem in many communities. Healthcare organizations also generate income for some local **suppliers**. If the money that pays for these expenditures comes from outside the community, the community as a whole benefits. Indirectly, the recipients of these funds spend them within the community on more goods and services. It is estimated that each dollar of hospital expenditure generates two dollars of total community wealth.

A healthcare organization can attract outside dollars in four basic ways:

1. by selling services to patients from other communities;
2. by attracting federal and state funds and donations from foundations outside the community;
3. by providing service to local people whose insurance is paid by sources outside the community; and
4. by attracting new industry.

Healthcare can be sold as interstate or even foreign exchange. Rochester, Minnesota, and Boston, Massachusetts, are extreme examples of communities that attract dollars through healthcare. Sales to local customers bring in new money when the funding comes from a larger pool. For example, if a community provides more treatment to Medicare patients than other communities do, it earns more than it pays in Social Security tax. A similar example exists where a plant or division of a large corporation shares a common health insurance cost with other units in other communities.

The fourth case is more complicated. Many U.S. communities have aggressive programs to recruit new industry. New industry brings new people and new wealth to town, but the new people want satisfactory healthcare organizations and doctors. Concerned industrialists are now seeking economy, quality, and access in healthcare. When employers locate new plants or expand old ones, they examine the resources that each competing site offers. A respected healthcare organization and its doctors are one of the assets of an attractive community.

Healthcare organizations also provide training opportunities. Although few are associated with medical schools, many assist in the training of other clinical specialists. As such, they open vocational opportunities within the community for young people who would otherwise move away.

The Healthcare Organization as a Control Organization

One function of organizations is to ensure uniformity of performance, that is, to control. Government regulation, intermediary contracts, and the courts have assigned healthcare organizations responsibility for maintaining quality, cost, and access to their services. The best results are achieved by organizations following continuous improvement principles of empowerment, process improvement, and factual assessment.

Quality of service

Facility licensure to ensure the safety of hospitals has a long history, but many states acted only when they were forced to by the Medicare law. The states wrote different standards and adopted different approaches to enforcement. Licensure focuses heavily on fire safety and sanitation. While these are important in hospitals, as they are in other dormitory settings, the most serious risks lie in the practice of medicine and nursing. These were not often addressed by licensure programs.

A voluntary certification program undertook the evaluation of clinical practice, introducing the notion of peer review—that a group of caregivers can assist themselves in improving quality. The American College of Surgeons (ACS), an association of surgeons seeking to improve their profession, began in 1917 to certify hospitals that could demonstrate that they kept adequate records and routinely reviewed at least the more serious results of care.[33] Not incidentally, certification also required that surgical practice be limited to qualified surgeons. Membership in the ACS was not the sole measure of qualification, but it certainly was an acceptable one. Much is made of the self-serving character of the ACS concepts, but the ACS program was successful. Hospitals became steadily safer places, and under ACS leadership much surgery by unqualified surgeons was eliminated.

By 1951 the certification program had grown beyond the ACS's capabilities. At ACS's invitation, a joint commission made up of the ACS, the American Medical Association, the American Hospital Association, and the American College of Physicians was formed to accredit hospitals. A process of extending and improving the criteria for accreditation was begun. The importance of achieving accreditation increased dramatically when Blue Cross included accreditation as a condition for payment of insurance benefits. By the late 1950s, Blue Cross had become the dominant private insurance carrier, and its endorsement of accreditation meant that few hospitals could do without it. Amendments to the Medicare Act in 1972 recognized the voluntary system of accreditation as one of two ways in which a hospital could be certified to receive Medicare funds. It is almost impossible for a community hospital to survive without Medicare certification, and more than 95 percent of U.S. hospitals are accredited.

The accrediting organization broadened its scope to other kinds of delivery organizations and changed its name in 1987 to the Joint Commission on Accreditation of Healthcare Organizations (JCAHO). It now accredits hospitals, integrated delivery networks, ambulatory facilities, nursing homes, home care organizations, behavioral health organizations, and clinical laboratories. JCAHO has the influence to enforce minimum standards on every community hospital and, through that, healthcare systems.[34]

Throughout the 1990s, JCAHO emphasized the development of measures of healthcare performance. In 1995, it established the National Library of Healthcare Indicators (NLHI) and requested submissions. By 1998, the NLHI had accumulated 225 measures, with definitions, applications, and other descriptive material.[35] JCAHO identified 42 measures for its IMSystem, "a comparative performance measurement system that meets the national mandate for meaningful measures of patient outcomes."[36,39] By 1997, the system was in active use, with 800,000 records in its comparative database.

JCAHO also began evaluating and listing systems of performance data collection and reporting. In 1997, JCAHO initiated a requirement for hospitals, networks, and home care programs to document outcomes measurements covering at least 20 percent of patients. The percentage of patients covered is scheduled to rise at regular intervals.

Arguments that JCAHO was biased toward providers led to the appointment of consumer representatives in the early 1970s, but it remains a provider-dominated organization. In the late 1980s, employers became interested in quality assurance and began to seek broader measures of quality. Their efforts led to the National Commission on Quality Assurance (NCQA), which accredits managed care organizations. NCQA is a consumer-dominated organization. It developed, and puts heavy emphasis on, a series of measures of population health and overall effectiveness of healthcare called Health Plan Employer Data and Information Set (HEDIS).[37]

In 1998, JCAHO, HEDIS, and an accreditation program for individual physicians run by the American Medical Association announced the formation of a Performance Measurement Council to coordinate their measurement activities. As a result of a decade of effort by JCAHO and HEDIS, the use of outcomes measures of performance was mandated for healthcare organizations. Any healthcare organization that wants to survive must document its performance and stand comparison against competitors and the nation.

Third, the malpractice lawsuit became an important pressure to maintain quality. A strong public interest has been expressed in protection of individuals who might have received injury through the healthcare system. Relief is provided through the courts, where suit can be brought against both the healthcare organization and the doctor for malpractice. Charitable immunity and governmental immunity protected hospitals from malpractice liability through World War II. Beginning about 1950, the courts began holding hospitals financially responsible for the consequences of their negligent acts. The number of suits won by former patients increased, but the number instituted rose even more spectacularly.

By 1980, community hospitals were clearly responsible not only for any negligence of their employees, but also for any negligence of their physicians. These changes in the legal exchange relationships had profound implications for the organization of hospitals. They forced the development of means for controlling physician behavior and encouraged consensus on standards of practice for diagnosis and treatment. Most hospitals chose to respond by using peer review, reinforcing the JCAHO quality assurance structures. Peer review as originally conceived was a retrospective review of cases that had seriously departed from the expected. Under continuous improvement, it has moved to a prospective evaluation of the best way to approach similar medical problems, embodied in protocols. Ironically, a landmark survey, the Harvard Medical Practice Study in 1990, found malpractice claims themselves to be a clumsy weapon. Although adverse clinical events occur in about 4 percent of all inpatient hospitalizations,[38] there is little relation between them and court decisions. Less than 3 percent of adverse events could be documented as malpractice claims, and "most of the events for which claims were made in the sample did not meet our definition of adverse events due to negligence." These facts led the study group to conclude that "medical-malpractice litigation infrequently compensates patients injured by medical negligence and rarely identifies, and holds providers accountable for, substandard care."[39]

Cost control

The amount of money to be devoted to healthcare is a function of income and the desire for healthcare relative to the desire for other services, such as food, defense, and education. The decision should be a function of a marketplace or political forum that balances those needs against the needs of providers. In the United States, both buyers and taxpayers delegated this process to providers for many years, but began to restore the marketplace as the controlling vehicle around 1990. This means that the price of healthcare in a community is set by a market, and not by individual healthcare organizations. Similarly, many characteristics of the healthcare system—its rules for charity, fascination with technology, and response to malpractice liability, for example—are statements from the marketplace rather than issues to be debated in healthcare organizations.

Buyers and governments tend to demand economy; customers and providers tend to seek service. Advocates of economy have two serious problems: the economy they seek involves the loss of somebody's job, and it may seriously impair service. Advocates of service must attract the funds from competing opportunities. Economy advocates have pursued two approaches, regulation and competition.

Regulatory approaches

Public Law 89-749, the Community Health Planning Act of 1966, established a set of locally oriented review boards for hospital capital expansion. Public Law 93-641 and Public Law 93-602, eight years later, reinforced local review board decisions by requiring state **certificates of need (CON)** for construction and federal approval for Medicare and Medicaid payments. Thus, in most states, hospitals could not construct additional facilities or open new services without approval. Public Law 93-602, also in 1974, took an additional step: it established professional standards review organizations (PSROs), local physician-controlled groups responsible for utilization review monitoring both the quality and the appropriateness of hospital care under the Medicare program. In 1983, the PSROs were reorganized into **professional review organizations (PROs)**.

Unfortunately, neither planning nor utilization review worked particularly well. Repeated studies had trouble demonstrating that gains exceeded program costs.[40] Thus, while the drive for economy was blunted temporarily, the motivation became stronger as costs continued to mount.

After 1975, the states developed a strong interest in hospital economy, not only because of the views of their citizens, but more directly because of difficulties in funding their share of the Medicaid program. More than half the states had rate regulation programs by 1980. They differed markedly. Only about four states (New York, Massachusetts, New Jersey, and Maryland) were rigorous in their approach. Only the New York program actually documented real dollar savings. Rate regulation in most other states was a less pressing issue. As a result, legislation gathered less widespread support, and the programs were weaker in design and less effective in controlling costs.

The competitive movement

Around 1980, the forces for economy turned to marketplace mechanisms, with a rapid growth of interest in organizations directly controlling the cost of care and guaranteeing a certain insurance premium. A limited total cost per person per year, or capitation, is central to the concept. The recession of 1981–1983, combined with the implications of international manufacturing competition, stimulated buyers to adopt the capitation concept. In addition, difficulties in funding the Social Security Trust Fund for Medicare led the federal government to limit payment to hospitals through the **prospective payment system (PPS)** (Public Law 98-21, Social Security Amendments of 1983). The federal program was a payment program, not rate regulation. It differed from the capitation approach by focusing on each hospitalization, setting a price based on categories of illness called diagnosis-related groups (DRGs). A similar program limiting physician fees, the resource-based relative value scale (RBRVS) was implemented in 1992.[41]

Under the competitive movement, the prices paid for healthcare moved to market control, where they remain. The concept was effective. Many companies saw their health insurance premiums stabilized for the first time in decades. The growth of national health expenditures, in double digits for several years in the 1980s, fell to 3 percent, only slightly more than inflation, by 1996.

After 30 years of experimentation, devices were found that hold healthcare organizations accountable for quality (through NCQA, HEDIS, and the interconnection of poor quality and low efficiency) and cost (through the market). The implication is that the organizations themselves must control their operations, matching or exceeding competitive alternatives. This is nothing new in most industries, but it is one of the major forces creating healthcare organizations. The preceding forms of organization were not able to handle the task.

Important Member Motivations

No one is forced to work for a specific institution.[42] Healthcare organization members, whether volunteers, physicians, or employees, voluntarily exchange their services to fulfill their personal needs. This is true in two senses. Any member can legally (though perhaps not conveniently) leave but, more important, members' enthusiasm and commitment determine the amount of effort they contribute to the organization's goals. The well-managed institution attracts and keeps the best members because it understands what members seek from their work and provides those rewards copiously enough to gain enthusiastic participation.

Member rewards are both psychological and monetary. Although most members require a competitive monetary compensation, the extra enthusiasm and commitment that make the difference between excellence and mediocrity tend to come from psychological rewards. These may also be more difficult to provide, and only a well-run institution can offer extensive psychological rewards. As a result, they should come first in any analysis of member motivation. While the list can be arranged in different ways,[43] the following is a convenient summary of the psychological and monetary rewards many members seek. (There is further discussion of incentives and programs for building an effective work force in Chapter 15.)

1. *Samaritan satisfactions in treating the sick.* Both the caring role and the curing role are intrinsically enjoyable, and they are also recognized and respected in human societies. Religious recognition is particularly strong. A surprising number of healthcare organization workers feel that God will reward them for their efforts, but many others simply believe that their work is part of a good life and, therefore, wish to do their jobs well. This satisfaction is not limited to professional caregivers; unskilled workers also enjoy knowing that they are contributing to the Samaritan motive.
2. *Acceptance by the work group.* Work is an important social event for most people, and the comradeship of the work group is an important reward. To use this reward for the benefit of the organization as a whole requires careful control of the corporate culture, but it is not impossible. Healthcare organizations have advantages over many kinds of commerce in that their professional groups already share a common socialization and they can attract people who share belief in a Samaritan motive.
3. *Professional or craftsmanship rewards.* Similar to the Samaritan motive is the intrinsic reward offered by the power and technology of modern medicine. At a very fundamental level, it is rewarding to do a surgical procedure or see a patient get well. Craftsmanship applies as well even to menial jobs, which can be a source of pride if well done. Proper training, tools, work plans, and supervisory attitudes are supplied by management, and they allow workers to take pride in their work.
4. *Personal and public recognition.* Recognition of satisfactory performance is an essential psychological reward in organizations. The member's immediate superior must recognize the member's effort and show a discriminating appreciation for it. The approval of peers is also important

and stems from the socialization of the work group. Beyond this personal recognition, public acknowledgment can be achieved in a variety of ways, as appropriate to the service, such as recognition of the achievements by professional organizations.

5. *Compensation, incentive compensation, and promotions.* These constitute the tangible rewards of healthcare work. The possibilities of using compensation as a reward for extra effort are limited because each member's base compensation must be at a competitive level. Theoretically, additional rewards can be given to individuals who help units achieve their expectations. Relatively small bonuses or annual increases based on merit, rather than time in grade, are common ways to do this. However, elaborate incentive compensation systems are difficult to use and have not been proven effective.

The healthcare organization rewards the member and completes the exchange agreement by fulfilling these needs. Well-managed operation can be understood as fulfilling the largest possible set of exchanges, simultaneously meeting the members' needs and customer partners' needs described above. The well-managed healthcare organization must fulfill more member needs than its competitors. Reviewing the list shows several opportunities, but simultaneously reveals the complexity of the task.

Healthcare organizations that have difficulty motivating their personnel often have problems with the second, third, and fourth incentive groups. They lack the kind of complex systems necessary to provide comfortable environments, pride of profession and craft, and explicit recognition of good performance. Lack of clear expectations and consensus on goals are probably the most common causes of disincentive. A feeling that the real rewards will be handed out on a basis other than achievement of the publicly stated goals may be the most destructive counter incentive. Boards and executive officers whose actions are unpredictable or inconsistent are in danger of generating this result. Cynical statements such as "It's not what you do, but who you know," or "The doctors (or the surgeons, or the unions, or any other special-interest group) really run this place; they get what they want, and the rest of us get leftovers," reflect the alienation that causes failure. To correct these problems, one must look to the organization structure and management technology as well as to the incentives.

Suggested Readings

On Organization Theory

Laumann, E., and F. Pappi. 1976. *Networks of Collective Action: A Perspective on Community Influence Systems.* New York: Academic Press.

Pfeffer, J. 1994. *Competitive Advantage Through People: Unleashing the Power of the Work Force.* Boston, MA: Harvard Business School Press.

Pfeffer, J., and G. R. Salancik. 1978. *The External Control of Organizations: A Resource Dependence Perspective*. New York: Harper & Row.

Scott, W. R. 1992. *Organizations: Rational, Natural, and Open Systems*. Englewood Cliffs, NJ: Prentice Hall.

Thompson, J. D. 1967. *Organizations in Action*. New York: McGraw-Hill.

On the History of Hospitals and Healthcare

Ginzberg, E. 1996. *Tomorrow's Hospital: A Look to the Twenty-First Century*. New Haven: Yale Univerity Press.

Griffith, J. R. 1998. *Designing 21st Century Healthcare: Leadership in Hospitals and Healthcare Systems*. Chicago: Health Administration Press.

Rosenberg, C. E. 1987. *The Care of Strangers: The Rise of America's Hospital System*. New York: Basic Books.

Starr, P. 1982. *The Social Transformation of American Medicine*. New York: Basic Books.

Stevens, R. 1989. *In Sickness and In Wealth: American Hospitals in the Twentieth Century*. New York: Basic Books.

Vladeck, B. C. 1992. "Healthcare Leadership and the Public Interest." *Frontiers of Health Services Management* 8 (3): 3–26.

Notes

1. W. H. McNeill, *The Rise of the West: A History of the Human Community*. Chicago: The University of Chicago Press, pp. 53–58 (1963)
2. A. D. Chandler, *The Visible Hand: The Managerial Revolution in American Business*. Cambridge, MA: Belknap Press (1977)
3. W. R. Scott, "The Organization of Medical Care Services: Toward an Integrated Theoretical Model." *Medical Care Review* 50(3), pp. 271–303 (Fall, 1993)
4. M. Arndt and B. Bigelow, "Vertical Integration in Hospitals: A Framework for Analysis." *Medical Care Review* 49(1), pp. 93–115 (Spring, 1992)
5. J. Pfeffer, *Competitive Advantage Through People: Unleashing the Power of the Work Force*. Boston, MA: Harvard Business School Press (1994)
6. W. R. Scott, "The Organization of Medical Care Services: Toward an Integrated Theoretical Model." *Medical Care Review* 50(3), p. 293 (Fall, 1993)
7. M. Imai, *Kaizen: The Key to Japan's Competitive Success*. New York: Random House (1986)
8. W. E. Deming, *Out of the Crisis*. Cambridge, MA: Massachusetts Institute of Technology, Center for Advanced Engineering Study (1986); J. M. Juran, *On Leadership for Quality: An Executive Handbook*. New York: Free Press (1989)
9. V. K. Sahney and G. L. Warden, "The Quest for Quality and Productivity in Health Services." *Frontiers of Health Services Management* 7(4), pp. 2–40 (Summer, 1991)
10. W. E. Deming, *Out of the Crisis*. Cambridge, MA: Massachusetts Institute of Technology, Center for Advanced Engineering Study (1986)
11. A. D. Chandler, *The Visible Hand: The Managerial Revolution in American Business*. Cambridge, MA: Belknap Press (1977)

12. I. Illich, *Medical Nemesis: The Expropriation of Health*. New York: Pantheon Books (1976)
13. P. Starr, *The Social Transformation of American Medicine*. New York: Basic Books, pp. 379–88 (1982)
14. C. C. Havighurst, *Deregulating the Health Care Industry: Planning for Competition*. Cambridge, MA (1982)
15. S. Woolhandler and D. U. Himmelstein, "The Deteriorating Administrative Efficiency of the U.S. Health Care System." *New England Journal of Medicine* 324(18), pp. 1253–58 (1991); D. U. Himmelstein and S. Woolhandler, "Cost Without Benefit: Administrative Waste in U.S. Health Care." *New England Journal of Medicine* 314(7), pp. 441–45 (1986)
16. A. Donabedian, "Explorations in Quality Assessment and Monitoring," Vol. 1, *The Definition of Quality and Approaches to Its Assessment*. Chicago: Health Administration Press (1980)
17. C. C. Haddock, "Transformational Leadership and the Employee Discipline Process." *Hospital & Health Services Administration* 34, pp. 185–94. (Summer, 1989)
18. G. O. Ginn, "Strategic Change in Hospitals: An Examination of the Response of the Acute Care Hospital to the Turbulent Environment of the 1980s." *Health Services Research* 25(4), pp. 565–91 (October, 1990)
19. J. R. Griffith, V. K. Sahney, and R. A. Mohr, *Reengineering Health Care: Building On Continuous Quality Improvement*. Chicago: Health Administration Press (1994)
20. R. L. Coser, "Alienation and Social Structure," in *The Hospital in Modern Society*, E. Freidson, ed. Glencoe, IL: The Free Press, pp. 231–65 (1963)
21. R. A. Carr-Hill, "The Measurement of Patient Satisfaction." *Journal of Public Health Medicine* 14(3), pp. 236–49 (September, 1992)
22. ———, "Health Plan Employer Data and Information Set (HEDIS) 2.0: To Provide Standard Performance Data for Health Plans." *QRC Advisor* 9(9), pp. 6–7 (July, 1993)
23. J. R. Griffith, "Reengineering Health Care: Management Systems for Survivors." *Hospital & Health Services Administration*, 39:451–70 (Winter, 1994)
24. R. R. Gillies, S. M. Shortell, D. A. Anderson, J. B. Mitchell, and K. L. Morgan, "Conceptualizing and Measuring Integration: Findings from the Health Systems Integration Study." *Hospital & Health Services Administration* 38(4), pp. 467–89 (Winter, 1993)
25. J. R. Griffith, V. H. Sahney, and R. A. Mohr, *Reengineering Health Care: Building on Continuous Quality Improvement*. Chicago: Health Administration Press (1994)
26. R. Herzlinger, *Market-Driven Health Care: Who Wins, Who Loses in the Transformation of America's Largest Service Industry*. Reading, MA: Addison-Wesley Pub. (1997)
27. B. Franklin, *Some Account of the Pennsylvania Hospital*, I.B. Coker, ed. Baltimore, MD: The Johns Hopkins Press (1954)
28. C. E. Rosenberg, *The Care of Strangers: The Rise of America's Health Care System*. New York: Basic Books (1989)

29. R. Stevens, *In Sickness and In Wealth: American Hospitals in the Twentieth Century*. New York: Basic Books (1989)
30. C. E. Rosenberg, *The Care of Strangers: The Rise of America's Health Care System*. New York: Basic Books, pp. 337–52 (1989)
31. J. D. Colombo and M. A. Hall, *The Charitable Tax Exemption*. Boulder, CO: Westview Press (1995)
32. *Ibid*, pp. 142–65
32. T. G. Rundall, "The Integration of Public Health and Medicine." *Frontiers of Health Services Management* 10(4), pp. 3–24 (Summer, 1994)
33. P. A. Lembcke, "The Evolution of the Medical Audit." *Journal of the American Medical Association* 199 pp. 543–50 (1967)
34. Joint Commission on Accreditation of Healthcare Organization's activities are extensively described at its website: www.jcaho.org
35. ———, *National Library of Healthcare Indicators*. Oakbrook Terrace, IL: The Joint Commission on Accreditation of Healthcare Organizations (1998). Also available on the JCAHO website: www.jcaho.org
36. *National Library of Healtcare Indicators*, Introduction
37. NCQA and HEDIS programs and a list of accredited plans are available at the NCQA website: www.ncqa.org
38. T. A. Brennan, L. L. Leape, N. M. Laird, L. Hebert, et al, "Incidence of Adverse Events and Negligence in Hospitalized Patients: Results of the Harvard Medical Practice Study I." *New England Journal of Medicine* 324(6): 370–6 (Feb 7, 1991)
39. A. R. Localio, A. G. Lawthers, T. A. Brennan, N. M. Laird, et al, "Relation Between Malpractice Claims and Adverse Events Due to Negligence: Results of the Harvard Medical Practice Study III." *New England Journal of Medicine* 325(4): 245–51 (Jul 25, 1991)
40. R. Lohr and R. H. Brook, *Quality Assurance in Medicine: Experience in the Public Sector*. Santa Monica, CA: Rand (1984)
41. ———, "Medicare Program: Fee Schedule for Physicians' Services—HCFA. Final Rule." *Federal Register* 56(227): 59502–811 (Nov 25, 1991)
42. C. I. Barnard, *The Functions of the Executive*. Cambridge, MA: Harvard University Press (1938)
43. R. M. Steers and L. W. Porter, *Motivation and Work Behavior*, 3rd ed. New York: McGraw-Hill (1983)

CHAPTER

3

THE GOVERNING BOARD

Because their responsibilities are so important and because most people have only infrequent contact with them, governing boards tend to be surrounded with mystery. In fact, however, they are units of bureaucratic organization and are more similar to than different from the other units. They are committees by design—individual board members have no authority per se—and they are subject to all the usual problems of committees. Like the simplest manufacturing unit, the governing board can be described in terms of its purposes, functions, membership, and internal organization and the measures by which its performance is judged. In addition, the chapter discusses some of the strategies pursued to maintain excellence at the board level.

Society has established, through law and tradition, two basic criteria for the actions of governing boards. The first is that the yardstick of action is prudence and reasonableness rather than the looser one of well intentioned or the stronger one of successful. Board members should be careful, thoughtful, and judicious in decision making. They need not always be right. The second is that the board members hold a position of trust for the owners. They must not take unfair advantage of their membership and must, to the best of their ability, direct their actions to the benefit of the whole ownership. Board members must avoid situations that give special advantage to some owners, particularly the board members themselves. In not-for-profit corporations, the board members must attempt to reflect the needs of all individuals in the community who depend on the institution for care.

The topics addressed by board members are complex, ambiguous, multidimensional issues that demand both knowledge and judgment. Boards rarely act alone; the fact-finding and analysis required usually comes from the executive management and the organization at large. The executives themselves spend a great deal of time assisting boards to understand the content of the issues before them. Executive staffs in finance, planning, marketing, and information also support the board as well as other organization members. This chapter tries to illuminate the decisions the board must make. Chapter 4, "The Executive Office," and Part III, on the learning organization, detail the kind of support that is required.

Purpose

The basic purpose of the governing board is to be accountable to the owners and to identify and carry out their wishes as effectively as possible. Two long and relatively clear traditions, one for-profit and the other not-for-profit, amplify this deceptively simple statement. It is fair to say that the differences between the two forms of organization are clearer at the governing board level than anywhere else.

In the for-profit tradition, the focus is on maximizing profit. Board members, usually called directors, are compensated for their efforts and are usually given strong financial incentives for success. Subject to legal restrictions designed to protect the owners, directors may choose to maximize profit in either the long run or the short run. They should select among opportunities for expansion on the basis of the expected profit. They may sell all or part of the assets whenever that is the most profitable course of action. They may discontinue all parts of the business and are obligated to liquidate the assets when profit can be enhanced by investment in some other area or activity.

In the not-for-profit tradition, the owners are the members of the community served. The concept arises from legislation and the courts and is less precise than the marketplace concepts defining for-profit boards. The assets must be used for the healthcare needs of the community. They must usually be protected, and in recent decades healthcare boards have accepted the need for at least a small profit to ensure continued capability.[1] The governing board members are often called **trustees**, rather than directors, reflecting their acceptance of the assets in trust for the community. They are rarely compensated except for out-of-pocket expenses. It is illegal and unethical for them to benefit financially as individuals. They should expand the organization in directions that best fulfill community healthcare needs. They may sell assets or discontinue services only when these are no longer necessary, and there are important legal barriers to their liquidating or transferring the entire assets of the healthcare organization.

The governance functions (i.e., the responsibilities that the governing board normally assumes) must always be met, but the growth of multi-unit healthcare systems has opened a variety of structural solutions. Some have centralized the governance functions, while others have divided the governance functions in various ways between subsidiary boards and a central corporation. The structural forms are still evolving, but there appear to be two keys to their success: completeness and total clarity in the division of responsibility. No governance function may be omitted or left ambiguously to more than one group.[2]

Functions

In both legal and organization theory, responsibility can never be completely delegated. Thus one statement of the governing board's responsibilities is that the board is responsible for everything that goes on in the healthcare organization, as well as things that did not go on but might reasonably have. Under this theory, the board is responsible for all decisions and their consequences. Whether the organization thrives or fails, the board is responsible. In fundamental and inescapable ways, these statements are true. No one active in healthcare organizations should ever forget the ultimate, all-inclusive responsibility of the governing board.

On the other hand, the all-inclusive viewpoint seems to contradict the foundation of bureaucratic organization, which is to subdivide tasks to allow for many participants and to gain the benefits of specialization. While the board may be responsible for delivering babies safely, the plain fact is that most board members know nothing about delivering babies. This dilemma can be resolved by looking at responsibility as a multidimensional concept and finding those elements that can be done best by each participant. Then the list of functions of the governing board is the list of things it can do best. With the governing board and many other units, the list of functions begins with those activities *only* it can do.

Many writers have tried to list unique or appropriate board functions. Their lists reflect the diversity of opinion across the nation, the developments of thinking over time, and the subtlety of the question. At least three perspectives on the functions of boards exist. Managerial perspectives trace activities or decisions necessary by the board to support the organization as a whole. Political perspectives view the organization as a source of largesse and establish rules for the distribution of resources. A third resource perspective establishes the board's function as the contributor of critical resources.

Most real organizations probably balance all three perspectives. This chapter examines all three. Managerial perspectives are emphasized, under the theory that without successful discharge of these functions, the organization will collapse and the other functions become moot. Like the four-part theory adopted in Chapter 2, this approach parallels that of the most successful healthcare organizations. The dynamic appears to be that winning organizations tend to attract the resources they need and generate sufficient resources for all, so that contribution and distribution perspectives become less significant.

There is now little or no disagreement about the following list of essential managerial functions shown in Figure 3.1.[3] These five functions describe the governance needs of almost any sized healthcare organization, from a small home care company to a large integrated system. Smaller organizations may not have boards; however, their leaders must still accomplish these functions. As community hospitals transition to integrated delivery systems, the list does not change. The answers may be more difficult, the risk of failure grows, and the need for effective performance is greater.[4]

Appoint the Chief Executive

Typical board members have full-time occupations, volunteer their services, and have only limited time for the organization. They will serve only a few years and will be replaced by others. Board decisions are made by committee, whereas implementation requires an individual. All of these factors—the

FIGURE 3.1 Managerial Functions of the Governing Board

1. *Appoint the chief executive.* Select an executive, establish an effective relationship, evaluate performance, and reward success.
2. *Establish the mission and vision.* Agree on common goals and core values of the organization and articulate them as a guiding concept.
3. *Approve the long-range plans and the annual budget.* Decide major lines of investment consistent with the mission and vision, balance them against financial realities, and develop plans for implementation.
4. *Ensure quality of medical care.* Identify quality goals as part of the long-range plans and annual budgets, and support a medical staff structure that will attract and retain the most competent physicians.
5. *Monitor performance against plans and budgets.* Review progress measured against goals and events in the community to identify improvement opportunities.

competing obligations of board members, the lack of continuity, and the need for an individual to implement the will of the majority—demand an executive. Except in very small organizations, the **chief executive officer (CEO)** is a full-time paid position. In larger healthcare organizations, an executive office supports the CEO with up to several dozen deputies and staff.

The functions of the CEO are developed in detail in Chapter 4. They are far-reaching and critical, making the selection of the CEO an extraordinarily demanding board decision. In summary, the CEO selects and supervises all other employees of the organization; coordinates the design and operation of the governance system, the caring system, and the learning system; and represents the board internally and externally. CEOs act for the board in all emergencies and countless small, unforeseen events, where they must divine and do what the board would have wanted. The CEO generates almost all the internal facts the board sees and influences what external facts are brought to the board's attention. Finally, the members of the executive staff are often the only people in the community professionally trained in healthcare delivery. That training covers technical questions of need, demand, finance, quality, efficiency, law, and government regulation that are not included in the training of doctors, lawyers, or business persons. As such, the executive staff is the sole routine source of information in this complex and rapidly changing area.

Appointing the chief executive is actually a two-part function: it involves the selection of the CEO and the development and maintenance of a sound working relationship later.

Selecting the CEO

Many persons would say selecting the CEO is the most important decision a board will make, principally because of the impact the CEO has on other board decisions. The decision is also exceptionally difficult. It involves judging the future skills of individuals, always a hazardous undertaking. It is made without the assistance of a CEO, whereas other decisions have the benefit of the CEO's counsel. It is made infrequently, and the people who make it may never have selected a CEO before.

How does a board make such a difficult decision? The best way is to follow with extra thoroughness and care the rules that improve all high-level personnel decisions. There should be a description of duties and responsibilities, even though for this job they are ambiguous. The job description should be translated into selection criteria identifying the desired skills and attributes of the individual. The priority or importance of these criteria and the ways in which these skills will be measured in specific applicants should be specified.

The job description should include typical CEO functions (see Chapter 4), but it should also be tailored to the mission, vision, and long-range plan, because these identify directions the board believes are important. Selection criteria are derived from the available personnel pool (also discussed in Chapter 4) and the needs developed in the long-range plan. Sometimes the board is seeking a CEO because it is dissatisfied with the long-range plan, so a key part of the new CEO's job would be to develop a plan. The criteria in such a case would emphasize planning skill.

A wide-ranging search for applicants should be undertaken. Large healthcare organizations usually search nationally, or over large regions. "The best possible training and experience" is now preferred as a criterion over "knowledge of local customs." For most U.S. organizations, the law requires not only equal opportunity on the basis of race, age, sex, and handicap, but affirmative action in seeking candidates disadvantaged on those grounds. An unbiased procedure relying on the judgment of several people should be used to select among the applicants. Formal reporting of independent opinions is often sought, both to encourage conformation to the selection criteria and to avoid bias. The interviews and activities used to acquaint the board with the candidates must also be used to acquaint the candidates with the job opportunity and convince them to accept it if offered.

Given the rigor and complexity of these procedures, it is not surprising that many boards fail to follow them completely. To the extent that they fail, they rely on good luck to find the executive they need. Increasing numbers of boards have found that using consultants trained in executive recruitment is effective. Consultants have substantial experience with the process, knowledge of how to complete the procedures efficiently, objectivity regarding local history, and familiarity with candidates and their demands. They lack knowledge of local needs. Like any other group of people, they differ in skill and motivation, but their record can be assessed by talking to previous clients. Evaluating consultants is easier by far than evaluating executives.

CEO evaluation and retention

One way to minimize the difficulties and risk of CEO selection is to keep a sound relationship with the current CEO. While this is obviously a complex matter, there are four guidelines for improving the effectiveness and prolonging the tenure of CEOs. Not surprisingly, these are similar to the guidelines for all participants in bureaucratic organizations.

1. The board and the CEO should have a mutual understanding of the employment contract. There is always a contract between the board and the chief executive. The formality of that contract depends on the situation, but more formal, written contracts have become popular in recent years.[5] The contract should specify any departures from the usual duties of the CEO, mechanisms for review of performance, and compensation and ways in which it can be changed. It also should state the procedures for terminating the relationship, including appropriate protection for both the organization and the CEO. Properly performed, the CEO's job is now and always has been a high-risk one.[6] Thus, even handshake agreements should include appropriate protection if the CEO must leave the institution.
2. The board and the chief executive should agree on short-term (usually one-year) goals and expectations and should review progress toward them at the end of the period. The expectations for the CEO are related to the goals of the institution as a whole. They emerge from other activities of the governing board, particularly establishing the long-range plan and approving the annual budget. The CEO's performance should be formally reviewed annually, based on the short term goals and expectations. The expectations for the CEO are more ambiguous than those for others in the organization, and they are also more subject to unexpected outside influences. They must occasionally be revised radically in midcourse. Even in extreme cases, however, it is far easier to evaluate the accomplishments of the CEO when the desired directions have been established in advance.
3. Compensation should be based on market conditions. As a general rule, the only fair and reasonable guideline for designing a compensation package is the marketplace, that is, what the institution would have to pay a similarly prepared person and what the person could earn in similar employment elsewhere. This statement is true for all employees, but particularly for CEOs. The high visibility of CEOs in the community and their relatively high income tempt unsophisticated board members to use other criteria, but these are likely to encounter difficulty. The marketplace used to determine pay should be the same one used in the selection procedure. For almost all large healthcare organizations, and for increasing numbers of small ones, this is the national market for people trained and experienced in healthcare management.

   Compensation includes payments in addition to salary that frequently are unique to the CEO. A compensation package can consist of a salary, the employment benefits offered to all employees, special benefits offered the chief executive, the terms under which bonuses and merit increases will be paid, an agreement on the disposition of any incidental income the CEO might earn as a result of related professional activity, and an agreement on both voluntary and involuntary termination compensation. Special benefits usually exploit both the mutual interests of the organization and of the CEO and the income tax laws. Many different items can be included, such as payment of housing, transportation, education, association, and club membership costs and deferred income provisions.

4. Incentive compensation is increasingly common for CEOs of larger healthcare organizations. The incentive should be based on the overall achievement of the organization, and can be based either on a previously agreed formula or an annual evaluation against previously agreed criteria. A small standing board committee, the compensation committee, usually reviews executive performance and establishes both any monetary reward for performance and the compensation for the coming year. The payment can be quite large, on the order of 50 percent of total compensation. It may be better to minimize base salary and use performance-based compensation both to motivate the executive and to provide convincing explanation of the total compensation. Incentive-based compensation may be more palatable to the general public than high salary.

Establish the Mission and Vision

Modern corporations work by a process of goal setting, assessment, adjustment, and achievement. They repeat this process many times and in many ways, striving for three ideal conditions derived from open systems theory, strategic management, and continuous improvement:

1. The goals of the organization as a whole are those that the larger society of customers and providers will appreciate and reward.
2. A clear corporate strategy is consistently translated to a readily visible goal for each unit of the organization.
3. The goals and achievements of the organization are assessed and amended at frequent intervals.

No organization ever achieves the ideal. Good organizations spend more thought and effort determining what society will appreciate, and more time communicating and coordinating goals among units. They assess and adjust more thoroughly at all levels.

The goal-setting process for a large corporation begins with the establishment of the mission and vision, continues through the amplification of the mission into a strategic plan, tests the reality of the plan with a carefully developed financial plan, and uses the plans to guide annual budgeting exercises, which establish the expectations for individual work units.

The first step toward these ideals is the identification of an explicit mission for the healthcare organization, and a vision of how it will be carried out. The mission and vision are core beliefs about the organization that serve as moral and practical guides to many decisions. Properly developed and written, the mission and vision express the common beliefs that bind the members together. They are symbolic statements designed to extract an emotional commitment. They advertise beliefs to potential customers and suppliers, serve as guides for evaluating practical alternatives, and are frequently referenced to test ideas about future directions. They are widely disseminated public statements that are only infrequently changed.

The **mission statement** is a statement of the basic purposes and activities of the organization. Most people tend to think of the **vision statement** as broader, more emotionally and morally based, and more difficult to achieve than the mission.[7] Both perspectives are essential, but terminology differs. Some combine mission and vision into a single document, and others make slightly different assignments between the terms. Some add a section on values to expand moral commitments. Taken together, they express not only what the organization is committed to do (here called the mission), but what it hopes to do (here called the vision). Examples of missions and visions are shown in Figures 3.2 and 3.3, from two very large and successful healthcare organizations.

The organizational mission

The mission statement of a healthcare organization should specify three things:

1. *Community.* What geographic, demographic, religious, or financial group is to be served? Under free choice of physician and healthcare

FIGURE 3.2
Mission and Vision Statement of Henry Ford Health System

MISSION

Henry Ford Health System is dedicated to developing and providing the highest quality, compassionate health care to serve the needs of the Southeast Michigan community. The System's services will be the most comprehensive, efficient, and clinically effective in the region, supported by nationally recognized Henry Ford education and research programs.

VISION

Henry Ford Health System will

- Evolve into the highest quality, most comprehensive and integrated health system in the region.
- Develop a Center for Health Sciences that will be engaged in leading-edge tertiary care, research, and teaching.
- Provide virtually all of the health care needs of the population served, from primary care to highly specialized tertiary care.
- Offer a range of health insurance and managed care programs that meet the diverse needs of the population and payors.
- Think of itself as an entity to which the users of its services belong. Administrative systems will emphasize the ease and convenience of use by the members.
- Be a responsible member of the community and assume leadership in developing sound health care policies at the local, state, and national level.

FIGURE 3.3 Mission Statement of Intermountain Health Care

Our Mission
Excellence in the provision of health care services to communities in the Intermountain region.

Our Commitments

- *Excellent service* to our patients, customers, and physicians is our most important consideration.
- We will provide our services with *integrity*. Our actions will enhance our reputation and reflect the trust placed in us by those we serve.
- *Our employees are our most important resource.* We will attract exceptional individuals at all levels of the organization and provide fair compensation and opportunities for personal and professional growth. We recognize and reward employees who achieve excellence in their work.
- We are committed to *serving diverse needs* of the young and old, the rich and poor, and those living in urban and rural communities.
- We will reflect the *caring and noble* nature of our mission in all that we do. Our services must be high quality, cost-effective, and accessible, achieving a balance between community needs and available resources.
- It is our intent to be a *model health care system*. We will strive to be a national leader in nonprofit health care delivery.
- We will maintain the *financial strength* necessary to fulfill our mission.

The mission of Intermountain Health Care's nonprofit hospitals is to provide quality care to those with a medical need, regardless of their ability to pay. For more information about qualifying for financial assistance, call the business office of any Intermountain Health Care Hospital.

organization, the organization often indicates an offer or an intent to serve a community. The measure of how well it actually serves that community is represented by its market share. A broad statement would be, "All the citizens of XYZ County and those who seek our care from elsewhere." A narrow statement would be, "All children (or some other limited population) who live in XYZ County."

2. *Service*. The full scope of potential services of healthcare organizations is shown in Figure 3.4. A strong base in traditional acute care, almost always including acute inpatient care and at least some outpatient care, is the usual starting point. Larger healthcare organizations are expanding outpatient activity, mental health and substance abuse programs, chronic care, and prevention and health education. Some are also extending their services beyond health-related issues to include residential care and social services, particularly for the aged. Some healthcare organizations identify specialized missions or services such as teaching and research. Some include health insurance and healthcare financing activities. Multi-institutional systems operating over broad markets, like Henry Ford and Intermountain Health Care, generally have the most comprehensive mission statements.

FIGURE 3.4 Scope of Services of an Integrated Delivery Network

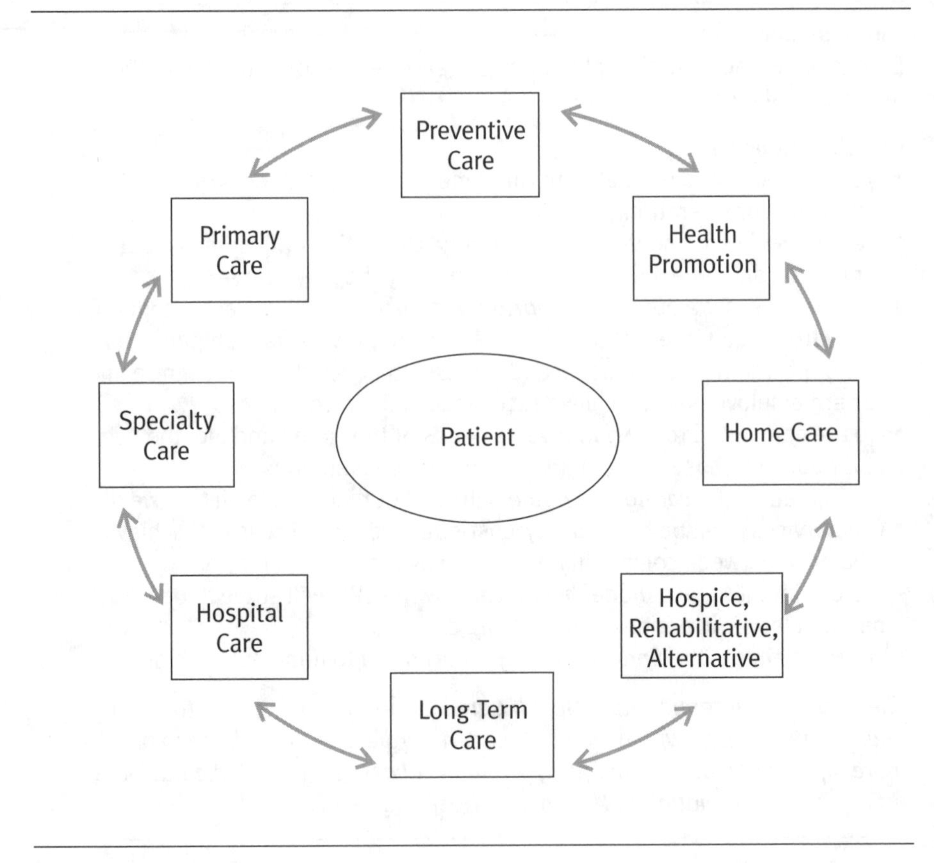

Smaller organizations are usually constrained by resources or market size from undertaking a broad mission. They focus on a niche among the potential services, usually acute ambulatory or inpatient care. A narrow statement, typical of the only hospital in a small community, might be

- "acute inpatient care for diseases routinely encountered and for procedures routinely undertaken by primary care physicians and general and orthopedic surgeons;
- referral arrangements for diseases requiring more specialized resources;
- ambulatory surgical and emergency services; and
- assistance to private primary care physicians."

Even this statement is broader than the traditional inpatient hospital, although it covers only the left three activities of Figure 3.4. (Note the explicit references to primary care and referral arrangements.) Small healthcare organizations also focus on other parts of the figure, providing long-term care in nursing homes, home care and hospices, and expanding their missions toward nonhealth services for the aged. Some emphasize primary and preventive care. A few focus on specific specialty care, as cancer treatment centers, or more comprehensive missions for limited populations, such as women's health centers.

3. *Financing*. Financial constraints should be explicitly stated. The amount of unfunded or underfunded work the institution is willing or able to undertake often limits certain activities. It is often wise to set the exact amount annually, but recognize the existence of a constraint. Thus, a broad mission would be: "Provide services to the paying public at the lowest price consistent with long-term financial needs and provide charity care to the identified community to the extent resources permit. The board of trustees will establish eligibility criteria for financial need and charitable care annually." A narrow mission might be: "Services will be priced competitively but must earn the return on equity required by market conditions. Service will be offered to all those who can demonstrate sufficient resources."

Too broad a mission makes planning decisions difficult and potentially inconsistent. A more serious problem is that it can dilute limited resources to the point where no job is done well. Too narrow a mission can cause the organization to overlook important community needs and opportunities. These usually are met by the competition, which may then supplant the original institution in other areas as well.

Extending the mission to a vision

The vision should make clear what the organization hopes to achieve, what constraints it recognizes, and how it does business. It typically includes:

- *How the organization should be viewed by members and outsiders.* Concepts such as "caring," "charitable," "customer-oriented," "friendly," and "reliable" are often used to convey a patient-centered focus. Many not-for-profit organizations emphasize their effort to embrace all members of the community. Religious organizations frequently state their spiritual commitments explicitly.
- *The organizational philosophy that guides operations.* Most organizations state their commitment to high-quality care. They emphasize equal rights for all employees and the dignity of work. They may recognize the importance of diversity, freedom of speech or opinion, or a spirit of tolerance. Some "strive to be best," but care must be taken to identify what "best" means. "Striving to be the best healthcare organization" may not be as meaningful as "Striving to have the best quality of care and patient satisfaction."
- *The organization's concept of its strengths and weaknesses.*[8] Many recognize a need to be cost-effective, prompt, and convenient. Some state a certain business strategy, such as a medical group practice, or a commitment to research and the most advanced technology.

Vision statements deal with hopes as much as with realities, but they must stay close enough to the possible to be perceived as sincere. A vision that is seen as pious or hypocritical can trigger a cynical response opposite from the one desired. The vision imposes an obligation upon the board members and corporate leadership. Their actions speak louder than words; if they often act contrary to the spirit of the vision, the other stakeholders see the statement as phony.

Developing the mission and vision

Writing the vision is difficult because of the need to be credible. The process of setting the mission and vision is complex and political. There are obvious conflicts, for example between the scope of service and the need for financial constraint. A good mission-setting procedure is based on an accurate and comprehensive view of the desires of the exchange environment and the interests of stakeholders. The unique responsibility of directors or trustees is to pick, from all the possible things the organization might do, those that society will appreciate and reward most. The perspective they bring to the task is more that of an outsider than an insider. They rely on the CEO and the planning staff to provide alternate formulations of mission and vision and to amplify the selected phrases into exchange needs and resources. In the end, the trustees must balance what is wanted with what is practical.

Although final responsibility for the mission and vision rests almost exclusively with the governing board, the purpose of mission and vision development process is twofold:

1. To establish a mission and vision that is consistent with the community needs and desires, so that customers and providers will prefer the organization over other alternatives.
2. To educate as many members of the organization as possible about the mission and vision, encourage them to consider the choices they represent, and come to a full understanding and acceptance of them.

Corporations like Henry Ford and Intermountain use their missions and visions as a central educational device. They are prominently displayed and periodically reviewed by large numbers of managers to promote consensus and commitment. They are referenced in debate about future alternatives and become the starting point for the development of long-range plans.

Approve the Long-Range Plans and the Annual Budget

The mission and vision are translated into plans that express the commitments of the organization in increasingly specific terms as time horizons grow shorter. They are often translated first into broad general directions or strategies that sketch important initiatives in terms of technology, markets, products, or affiliates—for example, to be the largest provider in an area, to offer nursing home care, to expand into healthcare finance, to achieve technological excellence in certain services, to collaborate with other organizations. The strategies in turn are accomplished through plans—to merge with competitors, purchase land, build buildings, acquire equipment, recruit personnel—that take several years to implement. The plans finally are translated to budgets that specify expectations for individual work groups for the next year or two.

These are **resource allocation decisions,** distinguished from the mission and vision by the commitment to expend resources in certain directions. Resources are finite; no organization can do everything. Selecting the opportunities to pursue means foreclosing others. The board shapes the evolution of the corporation through the series of planning activities from strategic plans to specific plans to annual budgets to the design of specific processes and activities. As the decisions get more specific, the involvement of the board becomes more general; the board is usually directly and deeply involved in strategic decisions but provides only general oversight of the annual budget. Specific processes and activities are left to internal teams that must reach solutions consistent with the more general commitments. That is, a team working on a process must stay within the budget, be consistent with previously adopted plans and strategies, and conform to the mission and vision.

Strategic planning

A dynamic, successful enterprise will develop dozens, even hundreds of new business opportunities and ways of meeting old goals. The board concentrates on maintaining consistency, responding to short-term changes in the environment without losing sight of the mission and vision. Governing boards retain final authority over major decisions that disburse or obligate the organization's assets, such as long-term borrowing, disposal or construction of buildings, and changes in the mission.

Strategic decisions are best approached by developing several scenarios. Scenarios often begin with sketches of various outcomes for the community: Several of the common topics for these scenarios are shown in Figure 3.5. The scenarios can be quite abstract and ambiguous, but they evaluate alternative **strategic opportunities**. These generally involve quantum shifts in service capabilities or market share, usually by mergers, acquisitions, and joint ventures or by very large scale capital investments. Strategic opportunities require careful evaluation. Because they often are triggered by events external to the organization, and because they often require rapid decisions, the governing board of the well-run healthcare organization quietly but thoroughly evaluates the more probable strategic scenarios in advance and is therefore prepared for prompt action when required.

Strategy is successful when it meets market needs. Thus there is no blueprint for strategies, other than the brief checklist of recurring possibilities shown in Figure 3.5. The initiative for identifying strategic opportunities comes from **environmental assessment,** the formal and informal review of the trends occurring in the local area, from community health needs to competitor activities. The more thorough the assessment is, and the more people consider its implications, the more scenarios will be suggested. The most realistic of these should be developed and evaluated.

Long-range plans

Once strategies and priorities are set, the planning effort largely leaves the board level. This delegation is important to empower the personnel who operate the organization, and it is made possible by the clarity of the mission and vision. Virtually the entire management group contributes. The chief executive, the chief financial officer, clinical leaders, and a staff of the governance system dedicated to planning and marketing make especially important contributions. The processes by which these contributions are made are described in detail in Part III, Chapters 12 through 17. The board reenters the decision process when a final set of proposals has been developed and documented. It ratifies the list or selects among the final proposals. The board's initial role, establishing the strategic direction and outlining the specific goals to be met, is far more important than their final ratification.

Most of these decisions depend on a certain level of consensus within the organization to succeed. They require a great many people to consider the

FIGURE 3.5 Illustrative Scenario Questions for Healthcare Organizations

ISSUE	SCENARIOS	CRITICAL QUESTIONS
Local Affiliations	Specific Affiliation Opportunities	Size and strength of competitors Impact on cost and quality Ability to support high-tech specialties Existing physician affiliations Antitrust considerations Regional affiliation opportunities
Regional Affiliations	Specific Affiliation Opportunities	Impact on local market share Total cost to patients and insurers Scope of services and medical specialization Total local expenditures Likely size of local healthcare organizations Local political issues
Relation to Insurers	Contract Joint Venture Own	Market response Retention cash flow Variety of plans available to local buyers
Physician Organizations	Contract with: Physician Organization Medical Service Organization Physician-Hospital Organization Foundation	Extent of HMO coverage Primary care physician preferences Specialist preferences Existing group practices

implications. Their implementation requires several years, and their impact lasts for decades. (Bonds, for example, are usually issued for 30 years or more.) At the same time, decisions must be timely. Real opportunities arise and disappear; once lost they may never return again. The management of these decisions must accommodate their complexity. This is done through a **planning** process that specifies how the board and others will make strategic decisions and implement them through **long-range plans**. The process establishes orderly review of opportunities, details the kinds of information that will be collected, and specifies who will be involved. Because the issues are so specific and so different, well-managed organizations have general guidelines on these questions that they adapt to the needs of each issue. The plans are documents that record decisions made, usually in the form of actions or events that are expected to occur at specific future times.

Long-range financial plans

The test of the strategic and long-range planning activities comes when the financial impact is assessed. This involves realistic assumptions about future market share, prices, and costs that are used to build a **long-range financial plan** showing earnings, debt, and capitalization for at least the next seven years. The plan is actually a sophisticated financial model that can quickly calculate the implications of major decisions.

The plan tests the reality of the planning process. It accepts estimates of the cost and demand for various strategic opportunities and shows the impact on profit and debt structure under the market and price assumptions. The alternatives that generate the most favorable combination of market share and capital structure can be identified. The interactions are complex because all the elements are interrelated. A new service affects cost, prices, market share, and profits, and the planner can structure it various ways to change the effects. Figure 3.6 shows the relationships built into the financial plan.

Approve the annual budget

The budget is the final step through which the mission, vision, and plan are translated into reality. Like the long-range plan, the budget is a detailed, complicated construction that requires substantial staff work and several months to complete. The budget includes both operating and capital expenditures. In well-managed organizations it is being broadened to incorporate an expanded array of measures reflecting the multiple dimensions of corporate success (discussed below in "Measures of Board Effectiveness"), including quality, demand, efficiency, revenue, and profit, as well as costs. (The details of preparing the annual budget are described in Chapter 14, because in most organizations they are coordinated by the finance group.)

Quality and scope of service and cost are determined by the annual budget. For example, hours of operation affect access to care; number and type of staff affect waiting time; expenditures on supplies and maintenance affect amenities offered; and investments in education, capital equipment, and information systems affect the technical quality of many aspects of care. Well-run organizations use the budget exercise as a way to improve quality, market

FIGURE 3.6 Relationships Shaping Strategic Plans

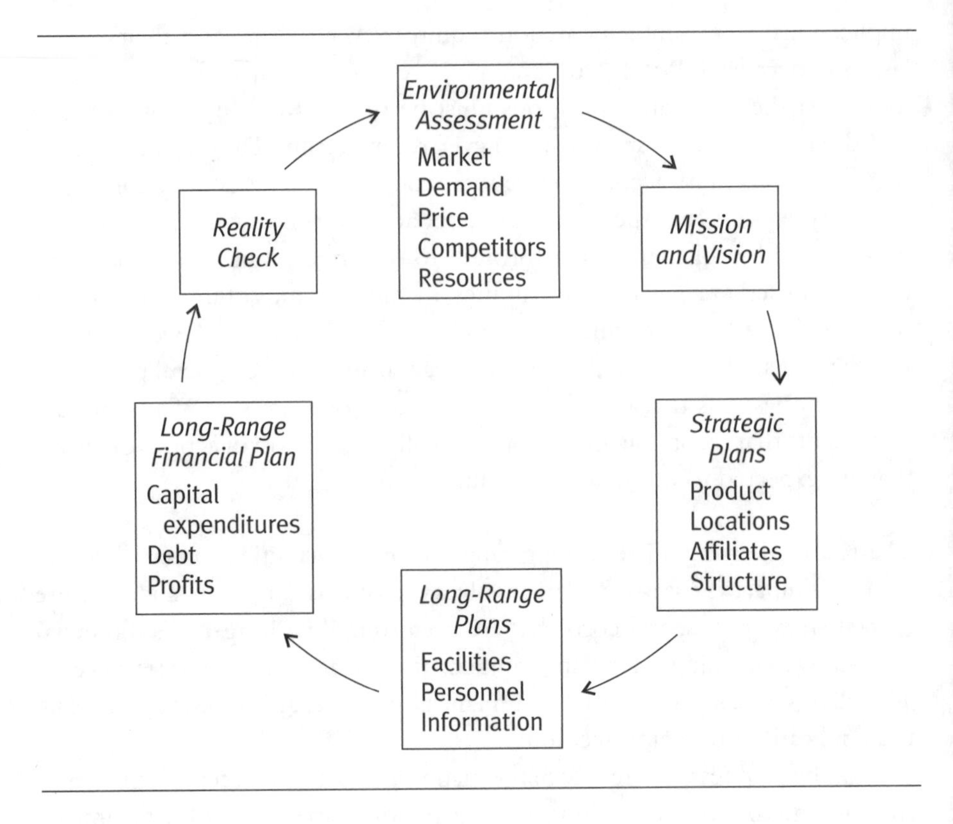

share, and productivity. The board's insistence on quality forces management to seek innovations that often improve both quality and productivity. Its insistence on productivity forces innovations that decrease price and increase market share.

The board is involved at two critical points in the budget development. At the outset, board committees are deeply involved in establishing guidelines. At the conclusion, the board makes the final choices among competing opportunities and approves the finished budget. Final approval should be anticlimactic; a well-managed budget process conforms to the guidelines and settles most questions before the board's approval.

Budget guidelines

The budget requires effort by almost every member of the well-run healthcare organization. The board's role is often implemented through its planning and finance committees. There will be important decisions among strongly defended alternatives that the board must resolve as the community's or stockholders' agent. To coordinate such widespread activity, the board sets desirable levels of key indicators, called **budget guidelines:**

1. The total expenditures, including total employment and compensation of employees.
2. The pricing structure, and with it both the total revenue and the amount to be paid out-of-pocket by local citizens.

3. The expenditures on new programs, plant, and capital equipment, and with these much of the cost increases that will occur in future years.
4. Goals for measures of quality, patient satisfaction, and physician and employee satisfaction, including programs to improve specific deficiencies. (These are a recent addition to the budget process. As well-managed organizations rely more on objective measures, the desired values are being translated to guidelines.)

The profit or surplus to be earned is determined by items one and two, and the amount of indebtedness to be incurred is determined by items one, two, and three. The alternatives must be selected by weighing the impact of a specific decision—say higher costs—on the other measures, including prices, quality, profits, debt capacity, and market share. All of these elements are interrelated, as shown in Figure 3.7. The guidelines provide initial direction to the management, which will develop a budget within them.

The operating budget prepared by management is a book-sized document that starts with global summaries and establishes expectations for every unit of the organization. A companion capital budget lists all major capital expenditures (Chapter 14). They normally meet the guidelines, but the board finance committee may wish to understand where the greatest difficulties were encountered and what the tradeoffs were. Capital projects are normally ranked in the priority recommended by management; the board may wish to debate the priorities as well as revisit its capital expenditure guideline. In general, however, the final review is a fine-tuning exercise within the guideline intentions.

Ensure Quality of Medical Care

The fourth essential duty of the governing board is unique to healthcare organizations. The governing board is legally responsible for ensuring the

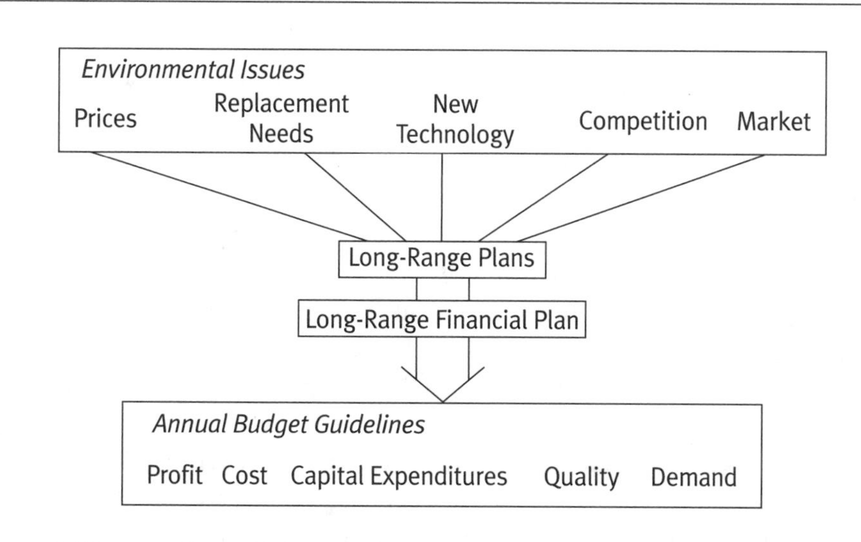

FIGURE 3.7 Relationships Shaping Annual Budget Guidelines

quality of medical care.[9] In carrying out this function, the board implements the community's specific desires and capabilities for quality of care and makes an important positive statement about the "corporate culture."[10] The board is responsible for failing to exercise due care on behalf of the patients and the community and on behalf of physicians desiring to participate, and the organization as a whole is liable for damages should they fail. In addition to these legal requirements, JCAHO has specified many of the structures by which the board and the hospital medical staff discharge this duty. Those traditions often form the basis for more comprehensive healthcare organizations.

At the same time, the board's duty is increasingly discharged through the budget process and documented through specific clinical performance measures. The JCAHO is moving away from its former emphasis on structure and strongly encouraging the use of outcomes measures of care. Also, with the growth of independent physician organizations, many of the duties are now delegated to those organizations, particularly for outpatient care. The delegation does not excuse the board from responsibility to ensure high-quality care in its community, but it changes the approaches that are taken.

For inpatient care and care delivered through employed physicians, the board has the following five obligations:

1. Approval of the **medical staff bylaws**, a formal statement of the governance procedures for physicians providing inpatient care and all employed physicians.
2. Appointment of medical executives at all levels.
3. Approval of the plan for medical staff recruitment and development, a part of the long-range plans.
4. Approval of appointments of individual physicians, after review according to the bylaws.
5. Approval of contracts with physician organizations.

The board's role in these functions is limited. The core concept is one of **peer review**, that the care of all patients is subject to review by a group of similarly trained physicians. The initial development of all five steps is carried on by groups of peer physicians, whose work is integrated by the medical staff organization and the executive. The board assures itself that the result is consistent with the mission, vision, and plans. A well-run board will review the documentation and ask enough questions to protect its interests and the public's. The board also serves as a final arbiter in case of disputes, but these should be rare. The board depends heavily on the CEO in discharging its oversight function; it is his or her obligation to make sure all the components of medical staff management are effectively implemented. As continuous improvement principles are applied, the board's role in monitoring quality will change. Stronger consensus among caregivers and better measures of performance should mean higher quality, but also less need for board intervention.[11]

Some basic facts heighten the importance of the board's medical staff activities. First, the healthcare organization is an expensive capital resource made available to the doctors by the owners in return for either profit or community healthcare. The board has an obligation to see that the owners receive fair value for the use of the resource. The courts have interpreted that obligation to include limiting privileges to the competence of each doctor.[12] Second, doctors are a uniquely expensive and critical resource for the community. A shortage of doctors in a community can be as serious as giving privileges beyond a safe level of competence. A surplus may encourage marginally necessary treatment that is both costly and dangerous. If community demand is low relative to the supply, costs will mount drastically, and lack of practice may impair quality. Third, most doctors would find their income severely reduced without participation in a healthcare organization. Doctors deserve fair treatment and equitable opportunities to participate. The process of peer review can be subverted for the personal gain of some members[13]; the board's responsibility is to see that this does not occur. In short, the issues involve a sensitive balance of community and professional needs on both quality and economic dimensions.

Approval of medical staff bylaws

The procedures of medical staff governance are formally governed by bylaws that cover the structure of the medical staff, the charges for its standing committees, other mechanisms for medical staff representation, rules for selection of committee members and medical staff leaders, and rules for granting **privileges**—the right to practice as a physician in the organization. The privileging process, also called **credentialing**, is designed to ensure the qualifications of practicing physicians. Because it involves basic issues of quality for the community and important sources of income for the physician, privileging is highly sensitive and extensive formal procedures have been adopted. (These procedures are discussed in Chapter 8.) Most lawyers believe that sound, well-implemented bylaws are the best protection against litigation, either for malpractice or for unjustifiable denial of privileges.[14] The bylaws are drafted by legal counsel, with the active participation of medical staff representatives, and approved by the board on advice of counsel and the CEO.

Appointment of medical staff leadership

Medical staff members are organized according to the various specialties. Each specialty (or group of similar specialties comprising an adequate number) has a leader and reports upward through a formal hierarchy. Medical staff leaders play an increasingly direct role in assessment and control of quality. As care has been more directly managed, sophisticated information systems are providing measures of the quality and cost of care. One role of staff leaders, for which they may be held accountable, is the setting and achieving of expectations on these measures.

At the same time, the **medical staff organization** can be viewed as a collective bargaining organization for doctors. From that perspective, the best leader may be the person who best represents the doctors' viewpoint. Thus, members of the medical staff and the board may disagree not only on the specific people who should lead, but also on the criteria for leadership. In practice, successful organizations resolve this disagreement in two ways. They seek people who meet both criteria, and they identify other opportunities for representation of and communication with the medical staff. Boards of successful organizations have steadily increased their influence in selecting medical staff leadership within this framework.

Approval of medical staff recruitment plan

To ensure that the community has the correct number of various kinds of physicians, the board often approves a **medical staff recruitment plan** as an element of its long-range plans. The appropriate numbers and specialties of doctors are based on careful forecasts of community demand. The medical staff must be integrated with the services the organization provides. Each medical specialty requires certain kinds and quantities of clinical support services, and, conversely, most hospital services require certain specialties on the medical staff. Each service must attract sufficient volume to support its fixed costs at a price the community can afford. Individual doctors must have enough work to maintain their skills, and the group must generate enough demand on support personnel that they too remain proficient.

The plan is normally developed by the planning staff, with extensive consultation from the medical staff. (A medical staff of physicians in independent, competing practice should not approve the plan, because that action might constitute a potential antitrust violation: the doctors can be voting collectively to restrain entry of other doctors into the local community.)

Trustees must weigh four questions in adopting the plan:

1. whether sufficient volume will exist to maintain skill levels of doctors and support personnel;
2. whether the proposed services are compatible with each other;
3. whether the estimated cost of the proposed scope of service is consistent with community desires; and
4. whether the community's funds can better be spent by a different scope of service.

The first two questions are of quality. Infrequently used skills and services with small demand tend to have poorer results than high-volume activities.[15] The array of services must be carefully balanced. For example, cardiovascular surgery requires strong cardiology, a nonsurgical specialty, and increased capabilities in clinical and cardiopulmonary laboratories, anesthesia, and imaging. The second pair of questions relates to optimal use of resources. With modern transportation, any specialized service is available to any patient.

It is not a question of access, but one of convenience. The price paid for convenience must come from something else. It is the board's job to weigh whether having an expensive service in town is worth the convenience, and to select the profile of services that best meets the community's desires and resources.

The plan adopted guides the recruitment efforts of the medical staff and the executive. The best organizations always recruit, recognizing that the first step to effective medical staff relations and to quality of medical care is to attract good doctors who are sympathetic with the mission and vision. Being competitive in recruitment usually requires significant financial investments. Doctors are financially assisted in a variety of ways at various times in their careers. Funds for this support become part of the financial plan and are approved by the board as part of the recruitment plan.

Annual appointment of physicians

Good practice now limits the appointment of each physician to a 12-month term. Appointment includes privileges to treat patients that are limited to the physician's demonstrated areas of competence. Annual reappointment follows a review of all areas of contribution to the organization's goals, but the emphasis is on the quality of care given individual patients. (Hospitals owned by governments must appoint any licensed physician but may restrict privileges based on competence.[16] Certain states have similar requirements on HMO participation, called "willing provider" laws.[17])

The board role is the final review, after several levels of professional review. The board should assure itself that review has been appropriately thorough on grounds of quality, but also that it has followed due process. Due process means adherence to the organization's own bylaws, assurance of adequate supporting facilities and trained personnel, avoidance of discrimination based on race, age, sex, or (in most cases) religion, and avoidance of restraint of trade.

Approval of contracts with physician organizations

Traditionally, the relationship of physicians to hospitals was an individual one, even when the physicians belonged to groups or partnerships. With the evolution of managed care, physicians began to form formal organizations for the purpose of acquiring and managing patient care contracts. A variety of structures have emerged. They are subject to varying state law and are still evolving, but in general they attempt to ensure both the quality and cost of care, a purpose consistent with the goals of healthcare organizations. These organizations require the collaboration of the healthcare organization and are often stimulated by it as a way to achieve comprehensive, easily accessible care.

A formal contract should exist between the two organizations, and it should have governing board approval. The board's role in approving the contract is to encourage high-quality, cost-effective care. It therefore seeks contracts that build on the first four obligations, providing formal procedures, selecting strong leaders and holding them accountable, encouraging representation, planning the physician supply in a systematic, cost-effective manner, and fairly and carefully credentialling individuals.

Monitor Performance Against Plans and Budgets

The well-managed healthcare organization is future oriented. It stresses discussion and agreement about future events, expressed in scenarios, plans, guidelines, and expectations, and works on the assumption that carefully developed agreements about expectations will generally come to pass. Monitoring becomes principally an activity to find insights for the next round of future agreements. The board's monitor role in that context is built into the annual environmental assessment, identifying the gaps between actual and desired that should be priorities for action. Only rarely is it necessary for the board to correct or discipline.

Two traditional monitoring functions remain important. The first is routine surveillance of performance data to detect important departures from plan. The second is acceptance of reports from outside agencies.

The measures used in routine surveillance are discussed below in "Measures of Board Effectiveness." The norm is that the expectations will be met. When variations occur, it is important to give management the time and freedom to correct them. Board intervention should not occur unless the variation is drastic, or it has gone on for several periods. Even then the first question is: What does the executive plan to do about the variation? Anything else draws the board into details of management it is not equipped to handle. Worse, it draws the board away from the future-oriented tasks it can do better than any other part of the organization.

Several outside agencies monitor performance from a public perspective and report directly to the board. The most important are the **external auditor** and JCAHO. The financial auditor attests that the accounting practices followed by the organization are sound and that the financial reports fairly represent the state of the business. A **management letter** is directed to a board-level officer. It points out real or potential problems that might impair either of these two statements in the future. The management letter is the board's best protection against misrepresentation, fraud, or misappropriation of funds. The JCAHO reviews the medical staff process and other elements of the hospital promoting quality of care. Its recent emphasis has been on identifying specific measures of quality and productivity useful in improving performance in the various areas of hospitals. As of 1998, JCAHO accredits the components of integrated healthcare organizations—hospitals, behavioral care organizations, ambulatory facilities, home care, clinical laboratories, long-term care, and rehabilitation units. It has recently begun accrediting "healthcare networks," essentially the same concept as "healthcare organization" used in this book.[18] NCQA accredits HMOs, including both their insurance and provider activities. It does not accredit provider organizations without insurance activities.[19] The board should also receive the reports of any accrediting or certifying examinations for its physician organization partners.

These are activities designed as much to prevent misdoing as to detect it. Many boards establish an audit committee to receive and review such reports. Well-managed organizations expect "clean" reports; exceptions must be treated in proportion to their seriousness.

Resource Distribution Functions of the Board

The list of board functions can be lengthened by adding duties otherwise assigned to the executive, but more fruitfully by examining different perspectives on the board's role. Alexander has argued that the five functions above represent a managerial perspective on board function. An alternative perspective sees the board not as a strategically-oriented body, but as a "political arena wherein competing interest groups vie for control of resources." Under such a model, "the satisfaction of critical constituencies such as the medical staff management and the community in terms of their involvement in the resource allocation process, becomes a more appropriate effectiveness outcome."[20]

Board members as interest group spokespersons

If board members are viewed as resource distributors, questions of equity of expenditures are highlighted vis-à-vis questions of patient service. Most of the organization's expenditures are income to various members of the community, and they represent an important economic resource to those members. The healthcare organization will be among the largest employers, and a large share of its income will come from outside the community (see Chapter 2). The ability of the board to represent the socioeconomic character of the community becomes important. Physician, supplier, and employee representation must be considered in addition to representation of the owners as users of healthcare.

There is much about this model that is realistic and important. Distributional equity is a matter of constant concern, and politics is chiefly devoted to it. In healthcare it clearly takes two forms—who gets the care itself, and who gets the income generated by it.[21] Relocating a hospital to the suburbs makes care more accessible to the rich and less to the poor. For the large number of low-income workers, it also means more travel time and costs, more work for less pay. Similarly, an emphasis on high-tech specialties moves both income and service away from the pressing needs of the disadvantaged, toward the more marginal ones of the wealthy. (The income of some specialist physicians is more than 20 times minimum wage).

From a resource distribution perspective, healthcare organizations are clearly suspect. Most board memberships are heavily weighted toward higher social strata. Physician members automatically represent the highest income group in healthcare, and nonphysicians tend to be drawn from corporate executives.[22] They are chosen for their exceptional skill at the managerial functions, and skillful people in U.S. society almost always earn comfortable incomes. If they exploit their position, they will pull resources toward the "haves" away from the "have-nots."

Accommodating the political model

Well-managed healthcare organizations use three strategies to accommodate the realities of the political model:

1. *Reliance on open systems and community-based strategic management theory.* One problem with the resource distribution model is its emphasis on distribution. It is clear that equity in dividing the pie is not the only factor determining how big a piece each group gets. The size of the pie is also important. Open systems and strategic management suggest that the better managed the institution is, the greater the rewards in total. Many people are willing to tolerate some inequities if they feel their needs have been met. What supports the continued appointment of corporate executives and physicians to governing boards is their ability to make the organization successful.
2. *Deliberate identification and correction of dissatisfaction.* Well-managed organizations deliberately monitor satisfaction of all social groups. Patient and family satisfaction measures can easily be stratified by proxies for social class. Employee satisfaction can be monitored by skill and income level. Spokespersons from disadvantaged groups can be added to the board itself. Focus groups can explore attitudes of specific groups in depth. Specific problems can be identified and corrected. Strategies can be developed that deliberately redress important inequities. Affirmative action programs in employment and community clinics for care of the poor are examples. These targeted programs can have striking results and can win considerable support.[23]
3. *A commitment to Samaritanism.* The underlying motive of Samaritanism is important here. It implies, as Franklin did (Chapter 2), a universal, rather than a class, concern. These programs can easily deteriorate to tokenism or be ignored if that motive is allowed to die out. It is often the task of individual leaders, particularly including the chair and the CEO, to make sure Samaritanism and equity get appropriate attention.[24]

Resource Contribution Functions of the Governing Board

Yet a third perspective views board members as contributors of resources to the organization. This is in contrast to Alexander's perspective, which views the organization as a source of resources. The resource-contributor model emphasizes the funds or services the board members may donate, or the influence they can bring to bear on critical external relations. Naming the richest family in town to the board, or the mayor's spouse, are examples of resource-contributor approaches. So is the appointment of a leading lawyer in the hope of reduced legal fees. There is evidence that organizations that can gain support from various parts of their communities do better than those that cannot.[25]

Board members as resource contributors

If board members are viewed as resource contributors, three functions must be added to the initial list. Although each of the additional functions has merit and many board members perform them well, they have to be ranked as less important than the five decision-making functions. Among the three, board members as influentials is probably the most important.

1. *Board members as influentials.* Open systems theory holds that the board represents access to resources the organization must acquire to succeed. Thus, board members must know people who can give large sums of money, have entry to political offices where the organization can be helped or hurt, and be able to speak for the organization at other centers of community power, such as the boards of major employers. In short, board members are influential people who use their influence to help the organization achieve its mission.
2. *Board members as figureheads and donors.* Board members are expected to exhibit loyalty to their organization and to speak well of it whenever possible. In that sense, all board members participate in public relations. Some individuals are so well known that the use of their names is in itself an endorsement; thus, their first service to the organization is simply the lending of their names. Similarly, some board members can afford to make major gifts to the institution.
3. *Board members as specialists.* A slightly different theory of resource contribution holds that board members are selected for their particular skills—in law, finance, medicine, and so on. Such people are expected to contribute their professional perspectives to board deliberations rather than or in addition to a general understanding of community needs and values and broad experience making complex decisions.

Accommodating resource contribution perspectives

The resource-oriented perspectives obviously have both theoretical merit and practical application. Many board members are in fact selected because they can contribute and others are chosen to represent differing perspectives in the community. The theoretical case against the resource perspectives is simple: the five managerial functions are more important. Influence and resources should come from success of the organization, not be borrowed from board members. If the organization is managed well, it won't need to solicit help; if it is not, no amount of help will matter.

The theory seems to be correct in general, but not necessarily in the specifics. Organizations that are diligent at environmental assessment and strategic planning tend to identify specific resources that they can gain by selective board representation. Thus, some members are selected because they have the ability to deliver a critical resource. Resource contribution becomes a secondary criterion of membership.

Membership

The capability of the board of directors or trustees may be the central factor in a healthcare organization's success or failure. Well-qualified boards tend to make more effective decisions, and they encounter less difficulty when they present their case to others in the community. They attract well-qualified executives and doctors, as well as other well-qualified board members. Thus, success feeds on itself.

The issue of board membership is a continuing search for qualified, interested members, followed by ongoing programs to help those members make the biggest possible contribution. This section discusses board selection criteria, selection processes, compensation, education, and support. It also addresses two special issues of membership: conflicts of interest for board members, and roles for doctors and CEOs on boards.

Membership Criteria

Skill and character criteria

The first criterion for board membership should be ability to carry out the five managerial functions. If the board is well chosen by this criterion, the community will have a healthcare organization closely tailored to its needs and wants. Without question, such excellent organizations exist. Their doctors and managers are capable, and their board members bring to each meeting good judgment based on an acute sense of the directions the community as a whole would feel were appropriate. What characteristics predict these critical skills?

- *Familiarity with the community.* The raison d'être of community boards is their ability to relate healthcare decisions to local conditions. This means insight into how much money the community should pay for care, how to recruit professionals to the community, how to attract volunteers and donations, how to make community members feel comfortable in their organization, and how to influence local opinion and leadership. Most communities are composed of many different groups whose views on these questions differ. A board can accommodate differing viewpoints both by having representatives of different groups as members and by having members whose grasp includes the diversity of the community. Desirable board members are those whose understandings transcend their own sex, race, and social group. (See the discussion of the representation criterion, below.)
- *Familiarity with business decisions.* Most board decisions are multimillion-dollar commitments. They are measured and described in business terms. Healthcare organizations are part of the commerce of the

community and therefore must communicate in the languages of accounting, business law, finance, and marketing. These languages incorporate sophisticated forecasting and statistical analyses. The healthcare organization board room, like other board rooms, is a place where technical language is frequently used to communicate complex concepts. Thus, board members need to be familiar with the languages and styles used to make these decisions.

There is also an emotional component to multimillion-dollar decisions. Although concepts from household management are important, and householders can make excellent board members, moving from hundred-dollar decisions to million-dollar decisions takes some practice. Both for familiarity with the languages and for psychological preparation, previous experience at decision making is important.

- *A record of success.* Candid managers will confess that selecting people for any job is difficult, and selecting them for jobs like board membership is exceptionally risky. The best predictor, more important than general experience or formal education, is how well the person has done on similar assignments. This indicator is important after the individual has joined the board, as well. Effective members should be promoted to higher board offices. Reliance on achievement is a way of overcoming biases in selecting board officers. Objective criteria open opportunities for capable women and members of minority groups.
- *Reputation.* The general reputation or character of an individual is important in two senses. First, like the record of success, it is an indication of what the individual will do in the future. Second, it serves to enhance the credibility of the individual. Persons with reputations for probity frequently gain influence because of that reputation. What they say is received more positively. Boards have a legal obligation for prudence. The appointment of people whose reputation is suspect could be construed as imprudent.

Representation criteria

Representation criteria stem from the resource distribution functions of the board. As noted above, these functions are important. By law and tradition, the healthcare organization is an institution for persons of all races, creeds, and incomes. Many people support the political argument that only a member of a certain constituency can understand truly how the organization treats that group. And constituencies are usually pleased by recognition at the board level. They believe a good board should have representation from women, the poor, important ethnic groups, labor, and so forth. The concept of representation can be extended to include employees, doctors, religious bodies involved in ownership, and other groups.

Several caveats must be attached to the representation criterion. Most important is that representatives who lack the necessary skills and character are unlikely to help either their constituency or the community at large. Second, the board acts *by* consensus *for* the community as a whole. The concept of resource distribution tends to foster adversarial positions and compromise instead of consensus—and the compromise process may be inferior to consensus. Third is the problem of tokenism. A seat on a board, particularly a single seat, does not necessarily mean influence in the decisions. Finally, the appointment itself changes the individual. The lessons of the board room are not available to their constituents, and over a period of time, the board members are coopted from the view for which they were selected. Tokenism and cooptation can be deliberate adversarial strategies to diminish a group's influence.

Affirmative action to ensure that competent individuals are not excluded from board membership is encouraged under the law and seems likely to make organizations more successful. A balance can best be struck if two points are kept in mind:

1. Board members are appointed as individuals, not as representatives. They should be competent to serve in their own right, regardless of their position in the community.
2. Board members act on behalf of the community as a whole. This does not rule out special considerations of groups with unusual needs, but it places those considerations in a context—they are appropriate to the extent that they improve the community as a whole.

Selection Processes

Selecting board members involves issues of eligibility, terms, offices, committees, and the size of the board as well as the actual choice of individuals. Officers and committee chairs have more power than individual members, so their selection is equally important.

Appointment to membership and office

Most healthcare organizations have **self-perpetuating boards**. That is, the board itself selects new members and successors. Other methods include election by stockholders, the prescribed procedure in stock corporations, and election by members of the corporation who sometimes are simply interested members of the community. Boards of government institutions are frequently appointed by supporting jurisdictions or, rarely, through popular votes. Boards of subsidiaries in multicorporate systems are usually appointed by the parent corporation, with local nomination or advice. Boards generally elect their own officers. In addition to the officers, a number of committee members and chairs must be appointed, a job usually left to the chair, but sometimes subject to discussion or approval.

Role of the nominating committee

Nominees are usually asked beforehand if they will serve, and the best candidates frequently must be convinced. Keeping the job within limits that make it attractive is an important consideration. On most boards and similar social structures, truly contested elections and overt campaigning are rare. Many organizations nominate only one slate for boards and board offices. The existence of formal provisions for write-in candidates and nominations from the floor is an important safeguard in the corporate structure. They are rarely utilized. In the normal course of events, selection occurs in the **nominating committee**. The committee often proposes not only board members, but also corporate and board officers and occasionally chairs of standing committees.

The nominating committee is usually a standing committee with membership at least partially determined by the bylaws. It is common to put former officers on the nominating committee. Such a strategy emphasizes continuation of the status quo in the organization, so organizations wishing fresh ideas broaden nominating committee membership and charge the committee with searching more widely for nominees. It is typically in the confidential discussions of the nominating committee that individuals are suggested or overlooked, compared against criteria, and accepted or rejected. This makes the nominating committee one of the most powerful groups in an organization. Sophisticated leaders generally seek membership in it, or at least a voice in it. A key test of power in an organization is who nominates the nominating committee? While the formal answer may be found in the corporate bylaws, the real answer reveals the most influential people in a well-run organization.

Size, eligibility, and length of terms

The number of nominations to be made each year is a function of the number of board members and the length of their terms. There is little consensus on these issues. Board sizes range from a handful to a hundred, although between 10 and 20 members are most common.[26] The size of not-for-profit hospital boards has dropped,[27] although perhaps not as much as the demands for downsizing to make the board more efficient would suggest.[28] A theory that boards should be small and business-focused competes with one that says they should be broadly representative and structured to meet the needs of component stakeholder groups.[29] The Henry Ford Health System has a structure with 14 subsidiary boards involving 150 members, reporting up to a system board of 44 members[30] (see Figure 3.11).

Terms are generally three or four years, and there are usually limits on the number of terms that can be served successively. Lengthy terms or unlimited renewal of terms can lead to stagnation; it is difficult for the nominating committee to pass over a faithful member who wants to serve another term unless the rules forbid it. Too-short terms reduce the experience of officers as well as members. (It is possible to allow officers to extend their service beyond the normal limits.) Inexperienced officers rely more heavily on the CEOs, thereby increasing their power, but the entire board is more prone to error because of its inexperience.

The size, terms, and limits are related. If there are 15 members, three-year terms, and a two-term limit, there will be five nominations each year, but only two or three new people will be added in most years. The median experience of board members will be about three years. (Some members will not serve two terms, of course.) Similarly, 16 members, four-year terms, and a two-term limit will add two new people a year, and the median experience will be near four years.

In addition to a length-of-service eligibility limit, many organizations have eligibility clauses related to the owning corporation. For-profit boards can require stock ownership. Church-sponsored organizations, even when they are operated as secular community institutions, can require that board members be from the religious group. Some government and voluntary not-for-profit institutions require residence in the political jurisdiction for board membership. Other eligibility clauses include phrases like "good moral character," although so much judgment is implied that they are more selection than eligibility criteria.

Compensation

Board compensation is rare among leading healthcare organizations. About 20 percent of all nongovernment hospitals compensate members. For-profit and not-for-profit hospitals do not differ; about one-third of government hospitals provide compensation. The dominant form of compensation is a per-meeting fee, apparently to cover costs of attending. Although there has been discussion of the importance of compensation to attract members and to allow lower income participants,[31] the concept has not spread. Rates of compensation declined between 1985 and 1989.[32]

The rewards for serving on healthcare organization boards are complex. They include the satisfaction of a Samaritan need, pride in professional achievement, public recognition, association with community leaders, and some commercial opportunities that relate indirectly to recognition and association. They do not include significant direct financial reward. People serve on healthcare organization boards because they want to, because they enjoy the work.

Education and Support for Board Members

Successful organizations have both formal and informal programs for the education of board members. New members need education in several unique aspects of healthcare management. There are also issues unique to the particular institution. While new members should bring fresh perspectives, they should not operate in ignorance of history. Evidence from California voluntary hospital boards shows that educated boards achieve greater financial success.[33]

Formal programs are limited principally by the time available to incoming members. They include tours, introductions to key personnel, conveyance of written documents and texts, and planned conversations and presentations. A typical list of subjects is shown in Figure 3.8.

To be effective, formal programs for board members should follow certain rules. Brevity is essential. Small segments should be scheduled for each specific topic. Most important, the member should be a participant. Questions

FIGURE 3.8 Outline for Orientation of Trustees

Mission, Role, and History of Healthcare Organizations
- Difference between for-profit, not-for-profit, and government ownership
- What healthcare organizations give to the community

How Healthcare Organizations Are Financed
- Operating funds
  - Private insurance
  - Government insurance
  - Uninsured patients
- Capital funds
  - Donations
  - Use of earned surplus
  - Sources of long-term debt

Healthcare Organizations–Physician Relations
- Nature of contract between doctors and healthcare organizations
- Concept of peer review
- Trustee responsibilities for the medical staff
  - Approving bylaws
  - Annual appointments
  - Maintaining communication with the medical staff
    - Need for communication
    - Why communication should go through channels

Duties of Trustees
- Appoint the CEO
- Approve the long-range plan
- Approve the annual budget
- Appoint the medical staff
- Monitor performance

Legal Issues in Trusteeship
- Trustee liability
- Trustee compensation
- Conflict of interest

should be encouraged, the style should be conversational, and the discussion should be extended over several sessions.

Most board member learning is on the job. Well-organized boards make committee appointments carefully, allowing new members to become acquainted with the organization in less demanding assignments. They fill chairs with experienced members. They use chairs and organization executives to help members learn as they serve. The three critical committees, executive, finance, and long-range planning, should be composed of the more seasoned board members, and their chairs should be members nearing the end of service. The nominating committee is frequently the last service of a board member.

Board members are supported by the executive, who has responsibility for developing facts and arguments about issues, making recommendations, answering questions, and achieving expectations. In a larger organization, a substantial staff is committed to this work. The board member of a well-managed organization can expect accurate, thorough documentation and a reliable discussion of the alternatives as background for most important issues.

Board members can be sued as individuals, although such suits are rare. They are technically liable for failing to take due care, for deliberate self-serving, and for unnecessarily risky behavior. By definition, these events cannot occur in well-managed institutions. The corporation should maintain directors' and officers' liability insurance that provides legal and financial assistance against suits that might be placed.

Special Issues of Board Membership

Three issues of board membership have been prominent in many communities. They are issues on which there is room for substantial difference of opinion, but in each case a national consensus seems to have emerged. The latter two, doctor and CEO membership on boards, are philosophically related to the first, conflict of interest.

Conflict of interest

The law and society assume that members of governing boards are serving on behalf of owners and that they should not serve when their personal interests conflict with the owners'. Conceptually, this is clear enough. In practice, difficulties crop up quickly. The local banker meets all other criteria for board membership—should the community deny the bank the profits of the organization account, or deny itself the benefit of the banker's volunteered service? The mayor's wife is knowledgeable, popular, and successful. It happens that she and her husband own a tract of land critical to the organization's future expansion. Should she be invited to serve on the board? Unfortunately, the criteria for board membership make it likely that situations analogous to these will arise frequently. It is hard to find people who meet the skill, character, and influence criteria but have not also become involved in activities that eventually will conflict. Conflict of interest is inherent in any democratic structure and it cannot be permanently resolved. Law and good practice allow persons with conflicts to serve, but require that potential conflicts of interest be recognized, and that the individual not participate in the specific decision where a conflict may exist. Well-run boards solicit a list of each member's major activities and holdings annually and make the list available for inspection. Individuals are expected to disqualify themselves, but they may be encouraged to do so by the chair or another member. Most organizations find practical solutions to the selection problem on a case-by-case basis, judging whether the benefits to the community outweigh the possible cost of self-interest. Individuals with such extensive conflicts that their service to the organization would be impaired are not appointed.

CEO membership

The CEO is always an active participant in board deliberations. Because their principal livelihood is from employment at the organization, most CEOs have fundamental conflicts of interest in serving on the board. The conflict is particularly apparent when possibilities for merger or closure of the institution are considered. It also occurs when other employees or doctors present grievances against the CEO. Although less obvious, CEOs can influence the board by controlling the information it receives (including the minutes) and by their role in suggesting the agenda.

Most hospital boards make the CEO an *ex officio* member, and there has been a steady trend toward giving them the right to vote.[34] In some cases, they hold prominent offices, such as chair of the executive committee or president of the corporation. The justification lies in the same rule governing other conflicts, that the community's potential benefit exceeds its potential loss. It appears to be correct; there is evidence that organizations that deeply involve the CEO in strategic decisions have better financial performance.[35]

Physician membership

Physicians practicing at the healthcare organization also have clear conflicts of interest. The national consensus, however, is even clearer for physicians than for CEO board membership; in fact, the JCAHO recommends physician representation. There is empirical evidence that hospitals that have physicians in board roles have better mortality and morbidity performance, that is, their scores on important measures of quality of care are superior[36] and their financial performance improves.[37] Physician representation improves overall success: the board needs to hear the viewpoint of doctors, and doctors need to know their views are being expressed. Many organizations set seats aside for doctors and solicit nominations from the medical staff. It is not uncommon for the medical staff to elect its representatives to the board. Physician representation is usually limited to a few seats.[38]

The resolution leaves behind some new problems. One or two doctors cannot reasonably represent the view of all doctors on important issues. Their technical, economic, and political views are influenced by their specialties. Family practitioners generally earn more of their income outside the hospital than surgeons, are paid less overall, collect less from health insurance and more from patients directly, and are paid more on the basis of day-to-day services than on episodes of illness. It is unlikely that a surgeon would effectively represent a family practitioner on important board issues, or that any family practitioner would feel reassured being represented by a surgeon. Other mechanisms must still be found to ensure communication across the broad spectrum of medical skills and interests.

Recent developments in medical staff relations (Chapter 12) have raised the possibility of much higher physician representation fractions, approaching 50 percent. Not-for-profit corporations actively including physicians are subject to three different and often conflicting legal concepts. **Inurement rules** protect against the distribution of assets of a community corporation to individuals or small groups within the community. Regulations for these formerly called for no more than 20 percent physician membership, but these have been relaxed by the IRS to eliminate a numerical test and rely on explicit rules to avoid inurement.[39] Antitrust considerations forbid doctors (or other vendors) from collusion in restraint of trade. Independent practitioners (those who are not employed by the organization) cannot use the organization board to further their economic advantage. Medical practice acts in some states forbid "corporate practice of medicine," which can be construed to mean that a majority of the board of any organization employing physicians for direct medical care must be physicians. Healthcare organizations seem to be using hierarchies of subsidiary and affiliated corporations to resolve these issues.[40] They also use a variety of other mechanisms for physician participation, emphasizing the decisions most immediate to each doctor's practice. These include participation in the decisions regarding care procedures (Chapter 12) and in operating and capital budget decisions (Chapter 14).

Organization of the Board

Board organization involves two major questions—how the governing board of the corporation as a whole organizes to ensure effective completion of its functions, and how governance structures are arranged for subsidiaries.

Structure for an Effective Corporate Board

An effective board must be thorough in its environmental assessment, imaginative in its search for solutions, and deliberate in its eventual actions. It must also be timely, responding to issues promptly, and efficient, not wasting the time of its own members and other participants in the decision process. Well-managed organizations meet these criteria better than their competition. They do so by a strategy of priorities, preparation, focus, and delegation. The strategy generates the structure of the board.

Priorities A board fails to the extent that it mishandles the managerial functions. The boundary-spanning and leadership roles the board alone can fulfill include understanding what stakeholders require to sustain their commitment. Ineffective boards fail to set clear missions or to back them with practical, attractive plans, or allow other members to implement those plans. They allow political dissatisfaction to fester and grow, rather than deal with it. The first step in a successful board organization, therefore, is one that assigns priority to these functions.

The managerial functions are generally handled by a permanent calendar. As suggested in Figure 3.9, a systematic annual progression through them will occupy much of the board's available time.

The schedule should not be inflexible. Reports of political dissatisfaction or strategic opportunities will frequently draw the board off schedule, but a well-managed board returns to it rigorously. On the other hand, the calendar encourages the aggregation of similar and interrelated topics. One

FIGURE 3.9 Calendar for Managerial Functions of Governing Boards

QUARTER*	ACTIVITY	INVOLVEMENT
1	Final review of performance	Finance, whole
	Executive review and compensation	Compensation
	Medical staff leadership appointments	Medical staff, executive staff
	Special projects assigned to ad hoc committees	Planning, ad hoc
	Matters arising	As indicated
2	Audit committee report	Audit, whole
	Monitor performance to date	Finance
	Environmental assessment	Planning, executive staff
	Review of strategic plans	Planning, executive staff
	Reports from special projects	Ad hoc, planning
	Initial update of long-range financial plan	Finance
	Matters arising	As indicated
3	Annual review of mission, vision, strategic plans, long-range plans	Whole plus guests
	Monitor performance to date	Finance
	Revise long-range financial plan	Finance, whole
	Establish budget guidelines	Finance, whole
	Matters arising	As indicated
4	Monitor performance to date	Finance
	Nominations for coming year	Nominations, whole
	Approve final budget	Finance, whole
	Matters arising	As indicated

* Quarters start with fiscal year.

response to any proposed agenda item is: "Would that fit well into our forthcoming discussion on ______? Is there anything we should do to prepare for a discussion then?"

The actual agenda management falls heavily to board chair and CEO. Both topics and allotted time are developed in advance. The purpose of board discussion and the kind of results desired are made clear to the board at the start of the discussion. Results can include information, discussion and clarification, delegation to committee, and action. A major issue may come before the board for each of these results as the issue evolves, is understood, and is finally resolved.

Preparation

CEOs and their staffs are responsible for preparing appropriate backup for every agenda item. They have heavy responsibility for the environmental assessment and ongoing surveillance of the environment, for identifying issues, for analysis and development of proposals, and for understanding the needs of the community. Staff are also used extensively in disputes, both to gather and disseminate facts and to negotiate or eliminate conflicts. The CEO may be criticized for failing to identify an issue in time for appropriate action, for failing to develop the background properly, and for failing to identify potential conflict.

The other aspect to preparation is general rather than specific to the issues at hand. Most issues take meaning from context; the better the environment and the usual processes are understood, the better the specific decision is likely to be. Thus, board selection and education are important preparation. Well-managed boards pursue these matters diligently. In addition, they are careful to balance the importance of the issue to the team managing it. They frequently pair inexperienced and experienced members to facilitate on-the-job learning.

Focus

Successful boards tend to focus on major issues one at a time, attempting to comprehend all aspects of the single issue and reach a consensus understanding of it. Meetings and retreats feature a few or even a single issue in depth, rather than a superficial review of several topics. Focus promotes understanding and is a prelude to an effective decision; even if a minority is opposed to the final outcome, the members understand the logic that determined it and are convinced that the process was appropriate.

Retreats are effective as devices to focus board attention. They can be held in comfortable off-site settings, emphasizing the departure from usual practice. Longer sessions allow fuller presentation of issues and background. Additional representatives of medical staff and management can be invited, facilitating understanding, acceptance, and implementation of the final decision. Consultants and guests from the community can be used to expand knowledge of factual and political issues.

Delegation

Successful institutions are delegating more and better, to gain the benefits of broader intelligence, participation, and consensus. Board committees serve several functions. They set priorities by weighing the importance of various issues, identifying interrelationships and combining or separating issues, and dispensing with issues that do not require full board attention. They prepare by fact-finding and educating board members and others with special interests. They focus by developing an expertise in a given area, such as finance. They often expand representation, routinely including staff not invited to the board itself. They solicit and evaluate differing political perspectives, a job employed staff may find difficult. Finally, they can take on especially sensitive issues, such as compensation, nomination, auditing, and medical staff membership, in a more discreet setting.

Well-managed boards delegate routinely to **standing committees**. These are permanent units of the board, established in the bylaws of the corporation. As shown in Figure 3.10, finance, compensation, audit, and nominations committees are almost universal. Planning committees are also common. A committee on medical staff relations is probably the next most frequent. It is possible to have too many standing committees. Each standing committee should have a clear, recurring agenda that cannot be handled as well by other structures. The use of an executive committee appears to be diminishing among the smaller boards, where routine use of an executive committee is unnecessary. The overall tendency is toward a small, active board, with a few important standing committees. The counter trend of organizations like Henry Ford Health System is to a large network of boards and subsidiary boards, but with an executive committee and a few other standing committees.

Beyond the few standing committees, well-managed boards of all sizes use **ad hoc committees**, formed as appropriate to the issue at hand, for a specified time period. An organization often has several ad hoc committees working simultaneously and reporting to the board, its standing committees, or operating units. Large numbers of people can be involved. Effective use of ad hoc committees results in an accountable delegation, deliberately passing authority down to the lowest relevant level, using broad representation and clear goals or acceptable solution parameters. "Accountable" protects the right to have one's view heard if necessary. Stakeholders understand that they have a reliable mechanism to a fair hearing on any question, at their discretion. "Delegation" assigns decisions to the people most important to their implementation. Within accountability limits, delegation is complete.

FIGURE 3.10 Typical Standing Committees of the Governing Board

COMMITTEE	FUNCTION	MEMBERSHIP
Finance	Long-range financial plan, debt structure, initial budget guidelines, monitor budget performance	Treasurer, chief financial officer, potential future chairs
Planning	Environmental assessment strategic plans, long-range plans	Chief planning officer, potential future chairs, medical staff representatives
Compensation	Review executive performance, award increases and bonuses	Officers, former officers
Audit	Review financial audit, JCAHO audit	Officers, former officers, medical staff representatives
Nominations	Nominate new board members and board officers	Senior board officers

The boundaries of an acceptable decision are established in advance, and decisions within the boundaries are accepted without debate. The decisions are not "micromanaged" by meddling or ritualistic reviews. The committee receiving the delegation knows it must produce a solution within the parameters if possible, and report back for further instructions if it cannot.[41] An effort is made to limit the number of committee levels; ad hoc committees should not report to each other.

Subsidiary Boards and Their Roles

The original concept of a governing board was of the ultimate authority for an independent corporate unit. The managerial and resource functions identified above derive from that concept. They must be referred to the most central level to be properly coordinated. The nature of hierarchical organizations is such that one can affiliate several corporate units, and establish governance functions for the affiliates, setting up boards that report to boards. For example, a healthcare organization that operated two hospitals, a medical group practice, and a health insurance company as subsidiaries would need at least one board, as shown in Figure 3.11A, over the whole organization, but it might have five, four, or three, as shown in Figures 3.11B through 3.11D. (Technically, any separately incorporated unit must have a board, but the requirement can be met by a small group of officers from the subsidiary and the parent. The discussion here is of boards that include other stakeholder representation.)

Subsidiary boards make four contributions that have made them popular in larger healthcare organizations:

1. They expand geographic representation, allowing local preferences to be reflected in operating decisions and local leaders to retain a sense of influence over their institution.
2. They expand the time and resources important to manage complex ventures like HMOs more effectively, permitting the appointment of outside specialists, and also recognition of inside operating executives who would normally have board access if their corporation were freestanding .
3. They permit joint ventures with other corporations and partnerships with the medical staff.
4. They allow identification of taxable endeavors and protect the exemption of activities qualifying under the Internal Revenue Code.

Subsidiary boards operate under the concepts of "reserved powers" and "accountable delegation." **Reserved powers** are held permanently by the corporate board. They include enough specific power to make sure the subsidiary continues to follow the central mission and vision, and to resolve conflicts between subsidiaries. These powers usually include the rights to buy

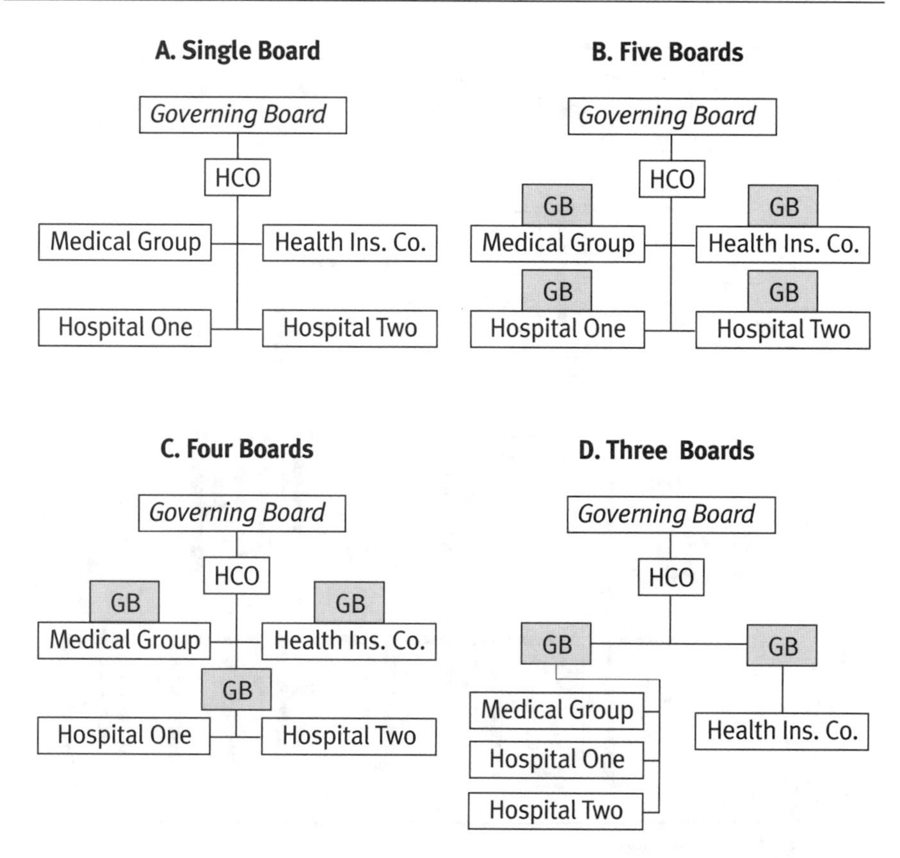

FIGURE 3.11 Board Possibilities for a Multi-Unit Healthcare Organization

or sell other corporations and real estate; issue stock or debt; approve long-range plans, financial plans, and budgets; appoint or approve board members and the chief executive; and approve bylaws. Within the limits imposed by reserved powers and accountable delegation, subsidiary boards tend to work as corporate boards do. They carry out the managerial and resource-related functions for their organization, making recommendations to the parent board on the reserved matters.

Figure 3.12 shows the board structure of Henry Ford Health System. The several boards allow almost 200 people to participate in the activity of the corporation, which serves about 20 percent of the metropolitan Detroit market of 4.5 million people. It is sufficiently flexible to allow the system to operate a successful insurance company, participate in a variety of partnership activities with several other large healthcare providers and insurers in the area, as well as to operate healthcare organizations oriented to specific local communities and reflecting their histories and preferences.

Alliances and Affiliations

The search for sufficient scale of operations and the ability to address specific problems has led to a variety of organization forms short of parent-subsidiary

FIGURE 3.12
Henry Ford Health System Governance Structure

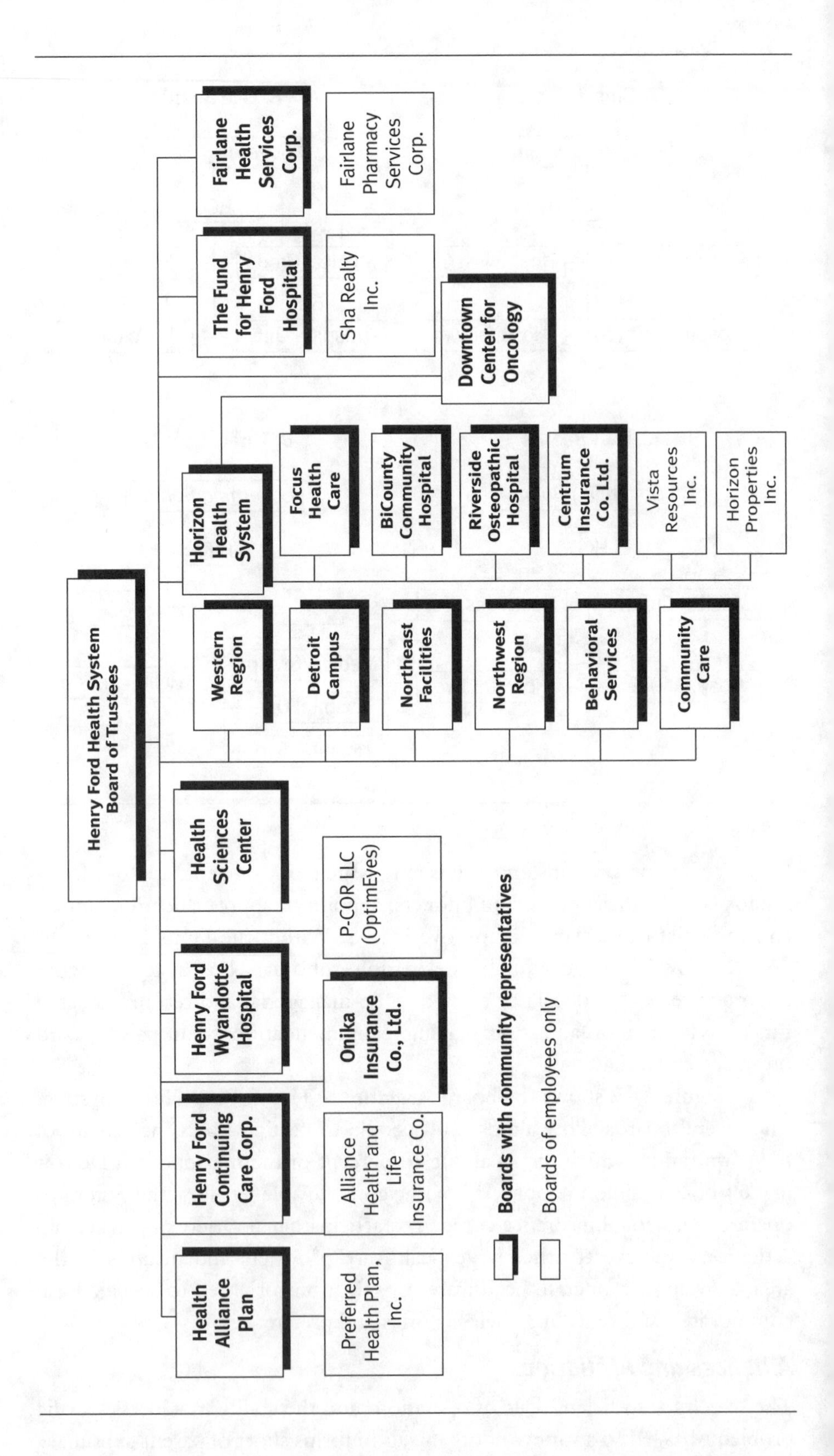

relationships. These are called alliances and are implemented in general by contracts, rather than corporate charters or bylaws. The distinction is less a matter of corporate form than of the strength of the reserved powers. Alliances can be reversed; mergers in general cannot. Alliances must continually balance individual with group needs, and they expend some energies in that process that more centralized forms can avoid.[42] Despite their limitations, they are popular devices to achieve lower prices on purchased supplies, provide certain services that are not easily supplied to remote geographical areas, represent similar organizations in state and national lobbying, and negotiate contracts with national and regional health insurance providers. About 1,300 institutions are affiliated with the two largest alliances, Voluntary Hospitals of America and Premier Alliance. More than 2,900 hospitals belong to alliances in total.[43]

Regional affiliations are also popular. They provide opportunities to market health insurance to companies with regional distribution of workers and to arrange comprehensive coverage of services under managed care insurance. Large teaching hospitals in central urban areas affiliate with suburban and more remote institutions. The affiliation formalizes referral relationships, providing convenient specialty services to the hinterland and higher volumes to the central institution. Affiliations between regional systems and insurance carriers are becoming more common. These amount to contracts specifying cost, quality, and volumes healthcare organizations are expected to provide. The carriers handle subscriber services and marketing.

It is important to understand competition, even in hotly contested local markets, as a form of cooperation. For healthcare, competition is regulated by federal and state law, which generally encourages rivalry to win customers under specified conditions such as licensure, fair advertising, and avoidance of collusion or discrimination. The law permits a variety of kinds of collaboration. Healthcare organizations are learning to exploit both aspects of regulated markets. Thus, they can and do compete and collaborate with each other simultaneously. In Detroit, for example, Henry Ford Health System and Mercy Health Services have developed several effective collaborations, and their collaborative effort is expanding. In Portland, Oregon, Oregon Health Systems in Collaboration brings the three providers and public health agencies together to work on problems such as prevention and medical education.[44] Arrangements like these are formed because they offer routes to market advantages that are more practical than other available alternatives.

Measures of Board Effectiveness

The board is to a large extent self-governing. Other than financial audits and inspection by licensing and accrediting agencies, there is no routine surveillance. It is therefore incumbent upon the board to have a rigorous program of self-assessment. The essential question in assessing the board's performance is whether owners' wants have been satisfied as well as realistic alternatives would permit. The board's performance is the corporation's performance. When the corporation is for-profit, performance is the long-term potential profit. When the owner is the community at large, as is the case for not-for-profit corporations, performance is measured in terms of the effectiveness of the interaction between the organization and its exchange partners. Conceptually, the healthcare organization must find the balance equitably satisfying to all. Realistically, such a balance is as hard to measure as it is to achieve. The first step is to understand the kinds of measurement necessary. As Kaplan and Norton have noted, these go well beyond simply accounting and financial reports, even for for-profit firms.[45]

Scope of Corporate Performance

Following the multidimensional concepts introduced by Kaplan and Norton restated in healthcare terms, one might begin with four major categories of performance measures. Figure 3.13 shows several different measures, reflecting differences in the meaning of good performance to different stakeholders. The goal of board reporting is to cover all influential perspectives, so that no important perspective goes unreported. The omission of a perspective is potentially destructive, but the list of numbers should be as short as comprehensive coverage permits. The categories and labels are not likely to be critical so long as everything is reported and understood. It is frequently useful to present the values graphically to allow quick detection of changes, successes, and potential problems.

Profit, market share, cost, and staffing, the first-listed measures in each category of Figure 3.13, are direct reflections of the acceptability of the organization to important stakeholders. While these constitute an acid test of the exchange relationships, they also may be slow and insensitive to important changes occurring in the environment. Additional measures are used to provide more diagnostic information on stakeholder demands and to improve the speed of response. Put another way, by the time profit, market share, cost, or staffing shows a clear deterioration, it may be too late.

Healthcare organizations are beginning to measure many of the Figure 3.13 concepts.[46] Figure 3.14 shows the measures in use by the corporate board of Henry Ford Health System, and Figure 3.15 shows their summary reporting system.

These reports are designed to give the governing board a current assessment of overall performance. The Ford "spider" or **radar chart** measures are expressed relative to established expectations, from the budget process, allowing a uniform reporting for very diverse measures. The specific measures can be carried down the organization. There are "spiders" for each subsidiary and most operating units, with some changes in detail. Ford management reports that the spiders are a powerful device to unify the large organization around common goals. They also note that the measures require substantial

FIGURE 3.13 Dimensions of Satisfactory Corporate Performance

DIMENSION	MAJOR CONCEPTS
Financial Performance	Adequate profit to sustain long-term growth or viability Satisfactory credit rating and financial structure
Patient and Family Satisfaction	Market share Positive responses to unbiased surveys Acceptable levels of positive outcomes Appropriate coverage of specialized and chronic needs Satisfactory access for disadvantaged groups Approval of appropriate regulatory agencies
Buyer Satisfaction	Competitive costs of care Satisfactory claims and membership services
Provider Satisfaction	Acceptable staffing levels and recruitment success Positive responses to worker and physician surveys

maintenance. So much depends on them that definitions and data collection must be carefully monitored as well. As the Ford managers put it, there must be "a source of truth" for each measure.[47] At Legacy Health System, which uses a similar approach to measurement, a single senior management team member has responsibility for all performance measurement except finance.

Guidelines for Evaluating Performance

In addition to current reports of values for the measures, the board needs referents or standards by which to evaluate them. There are four conceptual referents, listed here in increasing rigor or difficulty.

1. *Trends.* Last year's value or a time series of several years provides an initial baseline and allows judgment on the direction of the measure.
2. *Competitor and industry comparisons.* What other similar organizations are achieving provides crude guidelines, even if the available information is not strictly from competitors.
3. *Expectations.* A formally developed, agreed-upon expectation of an achievable goal allows integration of trends and comparisons with an analysis and improvement of process. Expectations for many of the measures should arise from the budget process discussed in Chapter 8.
4. *Benchmarks.* "Best practice," the best value reported by any organization using the measure. The benchmark value may be from an organization entirely different from the governing board's, as for example, the standards for financial ratios that are driven by the total bond market, not simply healthcare bonds, or the healthcare cost levels of a country with a different system.

Most boards use all four, but well-managed organizations are moving toward expectations and benchmarks.

FIGURE 3.14
Henry Ford Health System Balanced Scorecard Performance Measures

1. External Customer Satisfaction
- A. Percentage of patients dissatisfied or very dissatisfied
- B. Percentage of voluntary disenrollment
- C. Access indicators
- D. Physician satisfaction survey
- E. Business attitude evaluation

2. Clinical Process—Outcomes
- A. Accreditation and regulatory approvals
- B. Health status (SF-36)
- C. Number of claims and litigations
- D. Patient falls
- E. Nosocomial infection rates
- F. HCFA-derived disease-specific mortality rates

3. Financial Performance
- A. Net operating income
- B. Cost/enrollee or cost/case (case mix adjusted)
- C. Patient days/1,000 members
- D. DRG margin
- E. Bond rating

4. Philanthropy
- A. Total donations received (including commitments)
- B. Net philanthropic collections (net of expenses)
- C. Philanthropic expense ratio

5. Community Dividend
- A. Uncompensated care
- B. Contribution in voluntary efforts including such activities as community education (man hours, $ value)

6. Growth
- A. Equivalent population served
- B. Market share

7. Business Strategic Advantage
- A. Cost leadership
- B. Distribution system
- C. Product offerings
- D. Process improvement teams—accomplishments

8. Innovation
- A. Percentage revenue from new products
- B. Percentage revenue from new markets

9. Internal Customer Satisfaction
- A. Employee satisfaction surveys
- B. Labor turnover
- C. Diversity goals

10. Academic (education and research)
- A. NIH grants received
- B. Total external funding
- C. Resident match results
- D. Student satisfaction with educational programs

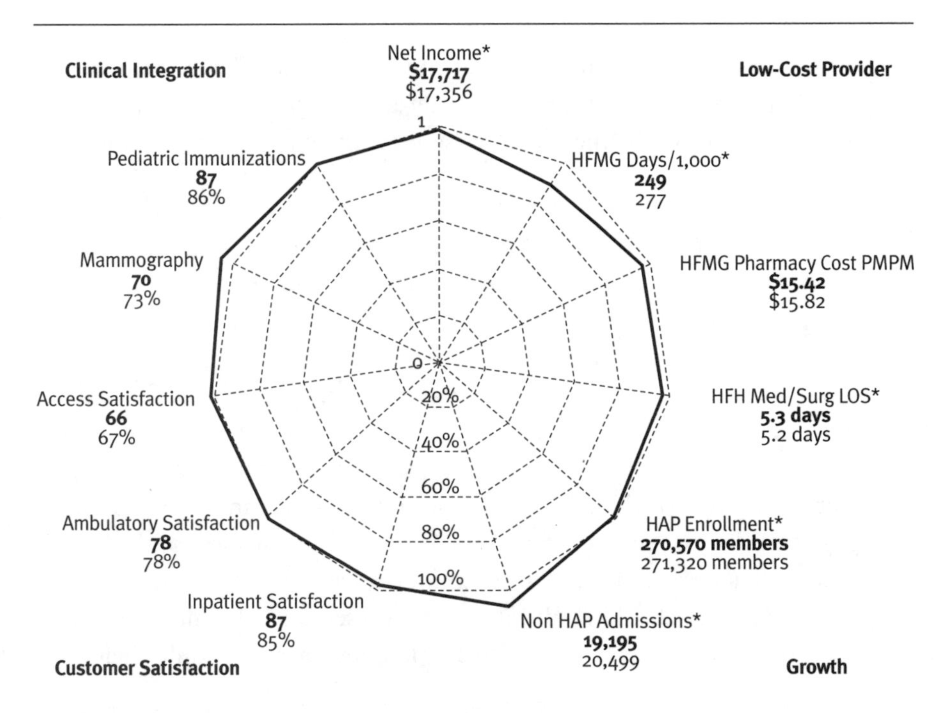

FIGURE 3.15 Henry Ford Health System "Spider" Performance Report

Targets are in bold face. Actuals in light face.
Each measure is expressed as a ratio of target and actual, expressed to show shortfalls as less than 100 percent.
*Asterisked items for current month, year-to-date. All others lagged two months.
HFMG: Henry Ford Medical Group; PMPM: Per member per month for HAP members; HAP: Health Alliance Plan.

Annual Performance Review

The process of setting expectations in advance and comparing performance to them appears to be superior to the simpler retrospective survey at all levels of the organization, including the governing board. Leading boards are learning to emphasize expectation setting as the stimulus to progress. An annual report on the measures, including historic trends, competition, and benchmarks, provides a basis for setting expectations. Well-managed organizations undertake such exercises at the start of the organization's annual budget cycle. The executive will supplement the measures themselves with a narrative of achievements, departures from plans, and opportunities for the future. Introspective review of this information and other information from environmental surveillance identifies necessary revisions to the mission and long-range plan and identifies the general goals guiding the organization's budget activity.

Failures of Governance and Their Prevention

Well-managed organizations encourage board performance by pursuing the time schedule and procedural matters identified in the preceding section and by foreseeing and forestalling difficulties. Despite their best efforts, they occasionally encounter problems; less well-run organizations tend to encounter the same kinds of problems more frequently and in more serious forms. There are no easy solutions, but these failures suggest the corrections required.

Membership failures

- *Representation.* The views of the board drift toward some groups in the community, such as the current medical staff and board members, or families under age 65 or families with health insurance. The solution lies in board education, more effective environmental assessment, and nomination of new members.
- *Judgment.* Board members lack the knowledge and experience for their roles. The causes can include excessive turnover, poor selection, or poor member development. The corrections usually require finding a few leaders and role models and revising the agenda and committee structure.
- *Motivation.* Board members fail to recognize the seriousness of the decisions. They are absent, or absentminded, when critical decisions are made. Improved selection, education, and presentation by management are solutions. Logistics such as regular and convenient schedules help.

Structural failures

- *Overcentralization.* Power becomes concentrated in a small group within the larger body. The solution is more use, and more effective use, of standing and ad hoc committees.
- *Overdelegation.* Too many committees debating each question involve so many people that decisions are no longer made expeditiously and peripheral views get excessive attention. The solution is better management of committee agendas, including training for committee chairs.
- *Individualism.* Board members forget that their authority derives only from consensus and that they serve all owners rather than a special-interest group. (When board members act as individuals, they automatically become executives; conflict with the appointed executive is an immediate danger.) The solution is education, and re-education in specific instances. The chair of the board plays a key role.
- *Insufficient reserved powers.* Too much power in the subsidiaries is reflected in conflicts, delays on critical corporate-wide decisions, and general loss of market share, provider satisfaction, or profitability. The solution is performance measurement, which helps identify and publicize the problem, expectation setting, and increased reserve powers.
- *Excessive reserved powers.* Too little power in the subsidiaries is often reflected in declining satisfaction among stakeholders with interests in specific subsidiaries. The solution is usually expanded expectation-setting processes, drawing subsidiary interests in at an earlier stage of the process.

Process failures

- *Identification of issues.* Critical trends are not identified quickly enough to deal with them satisfactorily. It is the chief executive's obligation to identify critical issues, but a badly managed board can ignore the executive's warning. Board members are also able to identify issues, and the well-managed organization encourages them to do so.
- *Inadequate staff preparation.* The CEO and executive staff fail to present concise, complete descriptions of problems and analysis of facts. The solution can be expansion or replacement of executive staffs and the CEO.
- *Poor control of agenda.* Ineffective management of agendas omits key viewpoints, fails to specify the opinions solicited, or allows committees to delay projects by inaction or by spending excessive time on less critical functions. The solution usually requires collaboration between the chair and the CEO.
- *Repetition.* The board unnecessarily recapitulates debates and decisions of subcommittees and subsidiaries. The solution is improved agenda control and requires training a capable chair.

Well-managed organizations devote considerable attention to preventing these kinds of problems and to containing them when they occur. Trouble-free performance is an ideal, achieved only by rigorous attention from the chief executive and the board leadership. The various difficulties and their corrections are interrelated. If motivation is weak, an extra effort to clarify the question and present the background concisely may help. If a standing committee has exercised questionable judgment, an ad hoc supplement may be in order. If recapitulation of debate has no other benefit than to ease the pain of defeat for a major constituency, it may be the right action.

Suggested Readings

Alexander, J. A., and L. L. Morlock. 1997. "Power and Politics in Health Services Organizations." In *Essentials of Health Care Management*, edited by S. M. Shortell and A. D. Kaluzny, 256–85. New York: Delmar.

Annison, M. H., and D. S. Wilford. 1998. *Trust Matters: New Directions in Health Care Leadership.* San Francisco: Jossey-Bass.

Goodspeed, S. W. 1998. *Community Stewardship: Applying the Five Principles of Contemporary Governance.* Chicago: AHA Press.

Griffith, J. R. 1998. *Designing 21st Century Healthcare: Leadership in Hospitals and Healthcare Organizations.* Chicago: Health Administration Press.

Holland, T. P., R. A. Ritvo, and A. R. Kovner. 1997. *Improving Board Effectiveness.* San Francisco: Jossey-Bass.

Seay, J. D., and B. C. Vladeck. 1988. *In Sickness and In Health: The Mission of Voluntary Healthcare Institutions.* New York: Mc Graw-Hill.

Shortell, S. M., R. R. Gillies, and K. J. Devers. 1995. "Reinventing the American Hospital." *Milbank Quarterly* 73 (2): 131–60.

Notes

1. J. D. Seay and B. C. Vladeck, "Mission Matters," in *In Sickness and In Health: The Mission of Voluntary Health Care Institutions,* J. D. Seay and B. C. Vladeck, eds. New York: McGraw-Hill pp.1–34. (1988)
2. Sisters of Mercy Health Corporation, *Integrated Governance and Management Process Conceptual Design*. Farmington Hills, MI: Sisters of Mercy Health Corporation (1980)
3. A. R. Kovner, "Improving the Effectiveness of Hospital Governing Boards." *Frontiers of Health Services Management* 2, pp. 4–33 (August, 1985). See also commentaries by R. F. Allison, R. M. Cunningham, Jr., and D. S. Peters.
4. J. A. Alexander, H. S. Zuckerman, and D. D. Pointer, "The Challenges of Governing Integrated Health Care Systems." *Health Care Management Review* 22(3), pp. 53–63 (Summer, 1997); S. M. Shortell, R. R. Gillies, and K. J. Devers, "Reinventing the American Hospital." *Milbank Quarterly* 73(2), pp. 131–60 (1995)
5. Witt Associates, Inc., *Contracts for Health Care Executives.* Oak Brook, IL: Witt (1984)
6. D. M. Kinzer, "Turnover of Hospital Chief Executive Officers: A Hospital Association Perspective." *Hospital & Health Services Administration* 27, pp.11–33 (May–June, 1982)
7. R. L. Ackoff, "Mission Statements." *Planning Review* 15(4), pp. 30–31 (1987)
8. C. K. Gibson, D. J. Newton, and D. S. Cochrane, "An Empirical Investigation of the Nature of Hospital Mission Statements." *Health Care Management Review* 15(3), pp. 35–45 (1987)
9. A. F. Southwick and D. A. Slee, *The Law of Hospital and Health Care Administration*, 2nd ed. Chicago: Health Administration Press, p. 597 (1988)
10. M. R. Greenlick, "Profit and Nonprofit Organizations in Health Care: A Sociological Perspective." In *In Sickness and In Health: The Mission of Voluntary Health Care Institutions*, J. D. Seay and B. C. Vladeck, eds. New York: McGraw-Hill, pp. 155–176 (1988)
11. B. J. Weiner and J. A. Alexander, "Hospital Governance and Quality of Care: A Critical Review of Transitional Roles." *Medical Care Review* 50(4), pp. 375–410 (Winter, 1993)
12. A. F. Southwick and D. A. Slee, *The Law of Hospital and Health Care Administration*, 2nd ed. Chicago: Health Administration Press, p. 585–89 (1988)
13. P. V. Burgess et al., No. 86–1145, Supreme Court of the United States
14. A. F. Southwick and D. A. Slee, *The Law of Hospital and Health Care Administration*, 2nd ed. Chicago: Health Administration Press, Chapter 14 (1988)
15. D. Bayta and M. Bos, "The Relation Between Quantity and Quality with Coronary Artery Bypass Graft (CABG) Surgery." *Health Policy* 18(1), pp. 1–10 (June, 1991)
16. A. F. Southwick and D. A. Slee, *The Law of Hospital and Health Care Administration*, 2nd ed. Chicago: Health Administration Press, pp. 589–98 (1988)

17. J. Anderson, "Perspectives: Any Willing Provider Battles Heat Up in States." *Faulkner Gray's Medicine and Health* 48(18): supplement 4 (May, 1994)
18. Joint Commission on Accreditation of Healthcare Organizations: www.jcaho.org. (November 2, 1998)
19. National Commission on Quality Assurance: www.ncqa.org (November 2, 1998)
20. J. A. Alexander, "Governance for Whom? The Dilemmas of Change and Effectiveness in Hospital Boards." *Frontiers of Health Services Management* 6(3), p. 39 (Spring, 1990)
21. B. Ehrenreich and J. Ehrenreich, *The American Health Empire: Power, Profits, and Politics.* New York: Random House (1970)
22. J. A. Alexander, *The Changing Character of Hospital Governance.* Chicago: The Hospital Resource and Educational Trust, pp. 5–6 (1990)
23. ———, "Partners in the Community." *Quarterly Newsletter*, Henry Ford Health System Department of Community Development, Detroit, MI (Summer, 1994)
24. J. R. Griffith, *Designing 21st Century Healthcare: Leadership in Hospitals and Healthcare Organizations.* Chicago: Health Administration Press, Ch. 2, pp. 57–66 (1998)
25. I. Belknap and J. Steinle, *The Community and Its Hospitals.* Syracuse, NY: Syracuse University Press (1963)
26. J. A. Alexander, "Current Issues in Governance." *The Hospital Research and Educational Trust, Hospital Survey Series.* Chicago: American Hospital Association (1986)
27. *Ibid*, 220
28. R. C. Coile, Jr., *The New Governance: Strategies for an Era of Health Reform.* Chicago: Health Administration Press, pp. 27–44 (1994)
29. G. T. Savage, R. L. Taylor, and T. M. Rotarius, "Governance of Integrated Delivery Systems/Networks: A Stakeholder Approach." *Health Care Management Review* 22(1), pp. 7–20 (Winter, 1997)
30. J. R. Griffith, *Designing 21st Century Healthcare: Leadership in Hospitals and Healthcare Organizations.* Chicago: Health Administration Press, Ch. 4., pp. 155–158 (1998)
31. R. Umbdenstock and W. Hageman, *Hospital Corporate Leadership: The Board and Chief Executive Officer Relationship.* Chicago: American Hospital Publishing Company (1984)
32. J. A. Alexander, "Current Issues in Governance." *The Hospital Research and Educational Trust, Hospital Survey Series.* Chicago: American Hospital Association, p. 25 (1986)
33. C. Molinari, L. Morlock, J. A. Alexander, and C. A. Lyles, "Hospital Board Effectiveness: Relationships Between Board Training and Hospital Financial Viability." *Health Care Management Review* 17(3), pp. 43–49 (Summer, 1993)
34. J. A. Alexander, "Current Issues in Governance." *The Hospital Research and Educational Trust, Hospital Survey Series.* Chicago: American Hospital Association, pp. 12–13 (1986)
35. C. Molinari, L. Morlock, J. Alexander, and C. A. Lyles, "Hospital Board Effectiveness: Relationships Between Governing Board Composition and Hospital Financial Viability." *Health Services Research* 28(3), pp. 358–77 (August, 1993)

36. S. M. Shortell and J. P. LoGerfo, "Hospital Medical Staff Organization and the Quality of Care." *Medical Care* 19(10), pp. 1041–52 (1981)
37. J. B. Goes and C. Zhan, "The Effects of Hospital-Physician Integration Strategies on Hospital Financial Performance." *Health Services Research* 30(4), pp. 507–30 (October, 1995); C. Molinari, M. Hendryx, and J. Goodstein, "The Effects of CEO-Board Relations on Hospital Performance." *Health Care Management Review* 22(3), pp. 7–15 (Summer, 1997)
38. J. A. Alexander, "Current Issues in Governance." *The Hospital Research and Educational Trust, Hospital Survey Series.* Chicago: American Hospital Association, pp. 15–18 (1986)
39. R. Whitehead, Jr. and B. Humphrey, "S Eases Rules for Physician Representation on Governing Boards." *Healthcare Financial Management* 51(3): 36, 38–39 (March 1997)
40. L. R. Burns and D. P. Thorpe, "Trends and Models in Physician-Hospital Organization." *Health Care Management Review* 18(4), pp. 7–20 (Fall, 1993)
41. J. R. Griffith, "Reengineering Health Care: Management Systems for Survivors." *Hospital & Health Services Administration* 39(4): 451–70, (Winter, 1994)
42. H. S. Zuckerman and T. A. D'Aunno, "Hospital Alliances: Cooperative Strategy in a Competitive Environment." *Health Care Management Review* 15(2), pp. 21–30 (Spring, 1990)
43. American Hospital Association, *Guide to the Health Care Field 93.* Chicago: American Hospital Association (1993)
44. J. R. Griffith, *Designing 21st Century Healthcare: Leadership in Hospitals and Healthcare Organizations.* Chicago: Health Administration Press, Ch. 3 and 4 (1998)
45. R. S. Kaplan and D. P. Norton, "The Balanced Scorecard—Measures That Drive Performance." *Harvard Business Review* 72(1), pp. 71–79 (January–February, 1992)
46. C. W. Chow, D. Ganulin, O. Teknika, K. Haddad, and J. Williamson, "The Balanced Scorecare: A Potent Tool for Energizing and Focusing Healthcare Organization Management." *Journal of Healthcare Management* 43 (3): 263–80 (1998)
47. J. R. Griffith, *Designing 21st Century Healthcare: Leadership in Hospitals and Healthcare Organizations.* Chicago: Health Administration Press, Ch. 4, pp. 176–82 (1998)

CHAPTER

4

THE EXECUTIVE OFFICE

The executive office supports the governance system both in facilitating the decisions of the governing board and in seeing that the board decisions and plans are effectively implemented. As a result, it relates to every part of the enterprise and is an inescapable part of any bureaucratic organization. It is a major component of the processes described in Part I, Governing, and it works intimately with the staff functions described in Part III, Learning. This chapter describes the purpose, functions, personnel, design, and evaluation of the executive office. The following chapter covers organizing the enterprise as a whole.

The executive office is led by the chief executive officer who is supported by an operations team. Although the team does not make a large number of decisions itself, it acquires considerable influence through its focal position in so many important communications. In larger healthcare organizations the team includes key line executives who manage the clinical activities, leaders of the major staff functions described in Part III, and corporate support such as the general counsel and development officer. Smaller organizations may contract executive functions in whole or in part to outside firms. In very small healthcare organizations, the job of CEO can be part time, either with other organizations or with other jobs such as chief nursing officer or CFO.

Purpose

The purpose of the executive office is implementation. (The word "executive" itself comes from a Latin root meaning to carry out.) Implementation rests on three kinds of two-way exchange shown in Figure 4.1. The executive maintains effective commerce to and from the external world, the governing board, and the systems that support the care process. Effective commerce in this context must include whatever steps are necessary to achieve successful exchange relationships. Communication must occur in both directions; environmental assessment must report changing needs; and agreements must bring necessary resources. The executive office is responsible for almost all information formally supplied to the board, for all implementation of board decisions, and for all relationships with the medical staff and the employees. It is also responsible for a number of outreach and boundary-spanning functions, such as public relations, government relations, and fundraising.

Two conflicting stereotypes may confuse persons trying to understand what executives do. One is that the executive is a communicator, bringing

FIGURE 4.1
Channels of Executive Implementation

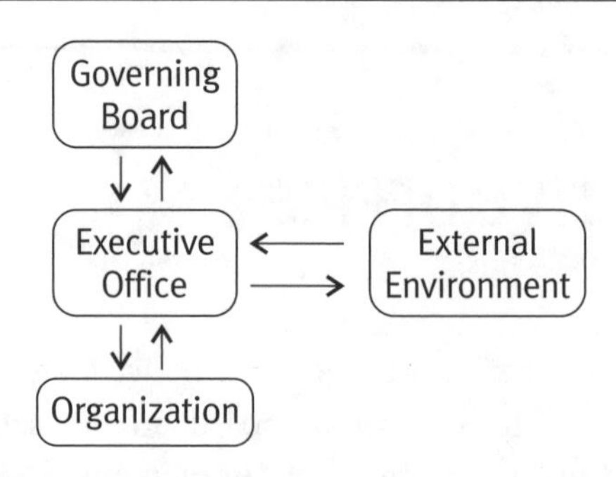

people together to discuss their problems. While this stereotype is an excellent beginning in defining the executive function, it is incomplete. Discussion is not enough to create "effective commerce." Action must result, and it must be constructive in terms of the exchange relationships. Executive responsibilities do not end until constructive action occurs. The other stereotype is that the executive is the chief decision maker. In reality, decisions of great importance are made at every level of the organization; the most far-reaching are influenced by large numbers of stakeholders. The executive is not a stakeholder; he or she is the agent for the stakeholder consensus established by the governing board. The character of executive decisions is different as well. Rather than dealing directly with actions, they tend to deal with the structures and processes that support good action decisions. Executives do not decide questions so much as design methods by which questions are decided.

The success of the executive function lies in decisions understood, accepted, and implemented in the organization. It lies in helping many people outside the executive office to participate in making the decisions. It lies in changes foreseen far enough in advance to allow a smooth transition—crises avoided rather than crises resolved. The best executive offices (though not necessarily the people in them) become almost invisible. So smoothly does the organization respond to the pressures of the outside world that the hand of the executive office is noticed by only the most observant. For most members of well-managed organizations, the front office is not a source of authority; it is a resource and a guide.

Functions

The executive function in bureaucratic organizations has proven quite difficult to describe, although many texts have striven to clarify it (see, for example, the introductory chapters to Shortell and Kaluzny[1] and their bibliography, in the Suggested Readings). The unlimited scope of executive responsibilities is a major source of the difficulty: the executive can be held responsible by the board for almost anything the board chooses. A second source of difficulty is the collaborative nature of executive behavior. The commerce between many groups indicated in Figure 4.1 requires prodigious flexibility. On the other hand, that same effective commerce requires that the general functions of the executive office be clear to other members of the organization and to the outside world. The functions discussed in this chapter delineate what an outsider, a doctor, an employee, or a board member should expect from the executive office. They can be summarized under the headings "lead," "support," "represent," and "organize," as shown in Figure 4.2.

Leadership

Leadership can be understood as cognitive, moral, and inspirational. All three are important.

Cognitive leadership

Like lawyers, engineers, and managers in other fields, healthcare executives exercise leadership by virtue of an intellectual area of study. The executive team, and particularly the chief executive officer, have training in a combination of healthcare finance, economics, marketing, and measurement that allows

FIGURE 4.2 Executive Office Functions

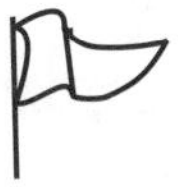	**Lead**	Identify trends and implications. Provide the initiative for action. Emphasize the importance of an issue. Provide or reward examples of ethical behavior. Encourage, reassure, motivate.
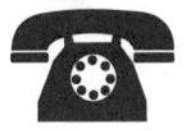	**Support**	Provide training, supplies, and facilities. Provide information. Provide special counsel or outside funding or both.
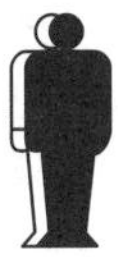	**Represent**	Form alliances with like-minded organizations. Affiliate with organizations providing supplementary services. Form joint ventures with potential competitors. Contract with financing intermediaries.
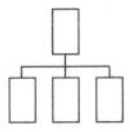	**Organize**	Assign accountability for operations. Form ad hoc committees, task forces, and work groups. Reconcile conflicts.

them to understand the needs of various stakeholders and the implications of alternatives. They are important as observers and commentators on the external environment, and as sources of ideas, perspectives, suggestions, and solutions. The importance of this contribution cannot be overlooked; there is rarely any local source for a substitute.

Cognitive leadership activities include identifying trends, articulating visions, designing responses, clarifying alternatives, developing criteria and measures, and answering questions. These often are introduced as seeds for collaborative development of an activity. By the time agreement is reached on the final product, the original idea is often unrecognized and sometimes unrecognizable. The initial ideas are critical to effective commerce because they provide starting points for agreement. Cognitive leadership also includes developing and presenting educational programs. Examples include developing education programs for board members and other managers, providing examples from other institutions, bringing outside consultants and guests, and explaining the implications of legislation, regulation, and market developments.

As an illustration of cognitive leadership, the concepts of the "balanced scorecard" measures (Chapter 3, Figures 3.14 and 3.15) do not spring to the minds of doctors or board members. Formal education is necessary to establish a consensus as to their value. The questions raised about the concept and the specifics to implement it must be resolved to the stakeholders' satisfaction. The concepts are not useful until specific measures have been found, tested, and installed. The measures do not collect themselves; elaborate systems are necessary for most of them. When faced with the cost of measurement, governing boards ask why the cost is justified, and the executive office is the only point in the organization equipped to give a comprehensive answer. The skills involved in the balanced scorecard include heavy doses of statistics, measurement, economics, accounting, finance, and marketing, all in the context of healthcare.

Moral leadership

The chief executive and the executive office are highly visible. Their behavior is widely copied and admired. Their character eventually colors the organization as a whole. The **organization culture**, the style of its daily interactions at levels ranging from honesty and mutual respect to dress and etiquette, is strongly influenced by the executive office.[2]

Serious problems in areas such as ethnic, religious, and gender discrimination, theft and conversion of assets, fraud and misrepresentation, and even unnecessary death and disfigurement of patients is known to be related to moral leadership failures.[3] Conversely, many healthcare organizations have maintained admirable records. Intermountain Health Care, founded by the Mormon Church and now operated as a secular institution, is an example. Values that run counter to the Mormon tradition of communal support and mutual respect simply do not flourish in the Intermountain culture. An etiquette of respect and politeness pervades the organization, but at the same time its leaders emphasize the need for rigorous response to economic reality.[4]

The executive office establishes moral leadership by profession, in written and oral statements of all kinds, and by actions. Among the actions, the selection of other leaders who clearly agree with the professed moral positions is one of the most telling. The personal behavior of the team is always important. The often-subtle signals to discourage unwanted moral behavior are also influential. For example, candor and gender equality are reflected frequently in many small actions. Moral leaders try to be candid and non-sexist in all their own actions, but they also deliberately encourage those traits in others and discourage their opposites. Many people test the sincerity of the organization's public ethical professions. Their initial tests are tentative and limited, and they are sensitive to appropriately limited responses. From the consistent small responses of the executive office, a culture is built where most people simply conform without thinking about it. The dramatic, serious challenge does not often arise.

Inspirational leadership

Leaders also inspire by charisma and personal example.[5] Separate from the cognitive and moral aspects of organizational life, there is an emotional component, whether the work is satisfying or stultifying, important or trivial, invigorating or daunting; and whether the work place is enjoyable or unpleasant, comforting or threatening, collaborative or contentious. Leaders not only understand that open systems, strategic management, and continuous improvement models call for constant change in the organization, they also understand that many people find the change itself frightening. Leaders not only trace the cognitive aspects of response, they spend time helping people overcome their fears. They present change, like the work itself, as a rewarding challenge. Rhetoric and attitude are as important as the cognitive content in many ventures that test the mettle of organizations and their members.

Support

In a sense, the three forms of leadership support the organization, but there are other essential activities. The executive office provides support to all the other systems of the organization, and it is responsible for several activities undertaken for the good of the whole.

Functions supporting stakeholder needs

The executive office is accountable to each of the other systems of the organization for their workplace, tools, and supplies. It is accountable for the information necessary to do the job, including some of the specific training. If any of these elements fail, workers cannot do their best. Figure 4.3 shows the major support services reporting to the executive office and the important needs of various stakeholder groups. The provision of these services is so complex that they constitute Part III, "The Learning Organization," in this text. All of these activities are accountable to, and coordinated by, the executive.

FIGURE 4.3
Major Support Functions Reporting to the Executive Office

Function	Needs of Special Importance by Stakeholder Group		
	Patients and Customers	Governing Board	Medical Staff and Clinical Services
Strategic:			
Planning		Environmental assessment, development of investment proposals	Preparation of new equipment and facility proposals, development of staffing plans
Marketing	Promotion of services	Maintenance of affiliations and alliances	Assistance with individual service marketing
Financial:			
Accounting	Billing, credit, and collection	Cost of specific actions	Cost of specific actions
Finance		Cost and revenue performance	Individual cost and revenue performance
Information:			
Clinical	Knowledge of quality, amenities	Knowledge of quality, amenities	Knowledge of quality, amenities
Management	Knowledge of prices	Benchmarks, competitor information	Benchmarks, competitor information
Human Resources	Reliable, responsive personnel	Staffing, recruitment, and training	Staffing, recruitment, and training
Plant	Safety, convenience	Safety, convenience effectiveness	Safety, convenience effectiveness

Patients and families need knowledge of the services offered, comprehensible bills, access to and protection of confidentiality of medical records, and assurance of quality. At a much different level, the governing board needs an environmental assessment, detailed analysis of all major proposals, and quality, accounting, and financial reports in sufficient depth to make realistic financial plans and to monitor progress. The medical staff and clinical services need information similar to what is supplied the board, but often in greater detail. All stakeholders need effective work teams and safe, comfortable physical facilities. The executive is responsible for making all these things happen.

Functions supporting the organization as a whole

Legal counsel

Legal advice has become increasingly important in preventing law suits and reducing settlements for damages. Most large healthcare organizations have an office of the general counsel available to assist in difficult issues of patient care, employment, medical staff relations, affiliations, and supplier contracts. Smaller ones usually have a retainer arrangement with a private law firm. When necessary, specialist firms are employed on a fee basis.

Public relations and fundraising

The CEO and members of the executive staff are normally the public spokespersons for the healthcare organization. They routinely present its mission, vision, achievements, and needs to the community through speeches, meetings, and interviews. They also identify and establish communications with key individuals in the community—political leaders, business leaders, major donors, and important figures in religious, charitable, and cultural activities. Often the most successful individual relationships are established with potential leaders in each of these activities. Although much important public relations is based on individual contact, it is also necessary to manage the presentation of the organization in the media. This is done through formal releases, designated spokespersons, and planned advertising.

Funds for expanding healthcare organization activities come from loans and gifts as well as past operations. The newer forms of corporate structure involve equity capital (stock and partnership agreements) as well. The CEO is generally expected to present the case for major new capital from any of these sources. Success frequently depends on earlier general communication and individual relationships.

Larger healthcare organizations appoint professional staff for public relations and fundraising. This staff is part of the executive office. Although it handles routine communications and relations with the news media and provides essential support for fundraising, it does not eliminate the need for direct participation of the CEO and other ranking officers.

Legislative and regulatory representation

Local, state, and national governments all directly affect healthcare delivery.[6] Their activities include laws restricting and encouraging different forms of activity, licensure of facilities and personnel, taxes and subsidies of various kinds. These are laws and administrative regulations:

- *governing caregivers and facilities*, such as federal education programs, state licenses, and local building permits;
- *shaping health insurance*, such as federal ERISA (Employee Retirement Income Security Act) legislation and state enabling acts for HMOs and PPOs;
- *defining patient rights*, such as federal civil rights laws, drug and medical device regulation, and state laws governing liability and patient self-determination;
- *protecting employee rights*, such as federal social security, unionization and equal opportunity laws, state employment security, and worker's compensation requirements;

- *offering subsidies for certain activities and taxing others*, such as federal and state subsidies for certain services, long-term finance, and certain construction sites, and federal income, state sales, and local property tax exemptions; and
- *paying directly for patient care*, such as the federal Medicare, and federal employee programs, state Medicaid, and local support.

Healthcare organizations are important parts of political constituencies, entitled and obligated to represent their views in the legislative environment and to seek the most favorable possible decisions in regulatory activities. (The obligation is twofold. First, legislators and regulators depend on the healthcare organizations to protect their interests; they cannot be expert in all the implications of their actions. Second, the organization owes it to its owners to take full advantage of all opportunities.) Larger organizations often support lobbyists who monitor government activities. Smaller ones rely on trade associations and alliances. In either case, understanding the implications of actions and supplying information useful in presenting positions is an executive responsibility.

Accreditation

Although accreditation by the JCAHO (or the **American Osteopathic Association**) is technically voluntary, it is closely related to certification for Medicare payment and thus essential to most institutions. The JCAHO survey every three years is the most rigorous inspection the institution undergoes at the hands of an outside agency. Preparing the documentation and coordinating a team visit, which usually spans several days, is the responsibility of the executive. Other voluntary accreditation is often equally important. It is the executive responsibility to make the requirements clear and arrange for review.

Disaster Planning

Providing care during civil disaster is an important and respected function of community healthcare organizations. Warning, medical needs, and severity of injuries differ greatly depending on the disaster. The most common disasters are storms and large-scale accidents, such as fires and mass transport crashes. Fortunately, in many cases the larger the number of injured, the lower the percentage of very serious or fatal injuries. When disaster strikes, people turn instinctively to the hospital. Victims are brought by rescue vehicles, in private cars, or by other means. Even a large emergency service can face 20 times its normal peak load with very little warning. Disaster management is not limited to the clinical team. Word of disaster spreads quickly, particularly under the stimulus of television and radio. The hospital may be inundated with visitors, families, and well-meaning volunteers in addition to the sick and injured. Communication with other community agencies is essential, and normal channels are often overwhelmed or inoperable.

Response to disaster requires a detailed plan that must be rehearsed periodically to comply with JCAHO regulations.[7] The design of the plan is a major project requiring the coordinated efforts of all management except members of the finance system.[8] The elements of the response include:

- rapid assembly of clinical and other personnel;
- reassignment of tasks, space, and equipment;
- establishment of supplementary telephone and radio communication;
- triage of arriving injured; and
- provision of information to press, television, volunteers, and families.

Representation

The executive office is responsible for negotiating, monitoring, and maintaining relationships with other organizations that complement, supplement, or compete with the mission. With the vertical integration of healthcare services, the representation function of the executive has greatly expanded. For larger organizations, each relationship begins with a **make or buy decision**: the organization can employ individuals or acquire subsidiaries skilled in the activity, "making" it a part of the core capability, or it can negotiate contract arrangements of various sorts relying on the collaboration of an independent corporation, effectively if not actually "buying" the service in question. The profile of makes and buys is a set of key strategic decisions. No known organization can make everything, and one that buys too much ends up with no core capability. Neither extreme is feasible. The executive office manages a panoply of relationships with outside corporations. (It is possible to view the relationship with the medical staff as a form of representation, but this text will treat it as part of the core capabilities, discussed in depth in Chapter 8.)

Alliances with similar non-competing organizations

As noted in Chapter 2, many well-run healthcare organizations now have relations with similar corporations through contractual membership in alliances. These relations are designed to accomplish important goals the participants could not do as well on their own. They are with similar organizations in other geographic markets, so the members do not compete directly. The services tend to expand the capability of the executive office itself, rather than increase the scope of services or directly affect market share. Important activities include:

- *joint purchasing agreements,* using the leverage of many buyers to obtain favorable prices;
- *educational and consulting programs,* where several organizations can collectively support highly trained and specialized skills;
- *benchmarking and comparative data,* where organizations agree on common definitions and a method of reporting values, and sometimes the sharing of best practices;

- *medical research*, where a consortium of organizations can provide statistically reliable samples of patients specific diseases or conditions;
- *general public relations*, as is common with trade associations; and
- *legislative and regulatory representation*, where the participants must all be in the same governmental unit.

Alliances of this type are reasonably stable and provide useful services. The form of affiliation is usually an annual contract. The contract is normally undertaken with a longer term expectation and involves substantial financial commitments, both to pay significant fees and to commit participation volume. General trade associations such as the American Hospital Association also perform some of these activities for members, but generally for lower fees and less commitment. The more recent growth of alliances such as Premier or Voluntary Hospitals of America has shown the increased power of grouping organizations with comparable missions and less danger of direct competition.

Affiliations with competing healthcare organizations

It is more difficult to maintain collaborative relationships with organizations that are directly competing in the same geographic market, but important opportunities exist. They include:

- *postgraduate medical education*, where several institutions can support specialty training;
- *highly specialized clinical services*, where neither of the partners can support the volumes necessary, such as programs for the disadvantaged or, in smaller communities, shared expensive diagnostic facilities; and
- *collaboration to capture markets*, where two competing healthcare organizations agree to combine provider lists to attract employer groups.

The form of collaboration is usually contract for medical education and joint venture for other activities. The relationships may be prelude to merger or acquisition.

Affiliations with complementary healthcare organizations

Vertical integration calls for service across all healthcare needs. Hospitals and doctors, the largest two groups of providers, historically avoided several services important to patients, including nursing homes, assisted living facilities, home care agencies, mental health and substance abuse services, preventive and public health services, social services for groups with special needs, medical equipment suppliers, and hospices. These services complete the comprehensive character of the integrated delivery network shown in Chapter 3, Figure 3.4. Separate, usually small organizations sprang up in many communities to fill these needs. As insurance and financing mechanisms improve, ownership of these facilities will become more attractive to larger healthcare organizations. Not surprisingly, the better financed services—chiefly home care and medical equipment—have attracted ownership by acute care organizations. In the meantime, there are important advantages to affiliations by contracts.

The largest healthcare organizations now have at least token ownership in all of these services, but smaller organizations often choose affiliation. The goal of the contract is to ensure customers' seamless access to all necessary services and to maintain control of cost and quality. The affiliation contract needs to include explicit programs to monitor all three dimensions of access, cost, and quality, and it must be placed with agencies capable of meeting market goals. Otherwise, it becomes preferable for the healthcare organization to provide the service itself.

Alliances with healthcare insurers

The majority of all patient care is financed through insurance carriers and intermediaries. The ability of the provider organization to increase or maintain market volumes depends directly on the success of intermediary relationships. Under managed care, the intermediaries are increasingly selective in their contracts. Some intermediaries deliberately separate hospital from physician contracting, but many prefer to contract with a **common provider entity** or **medical service organization (MSO)** making comprehensive services available. The federal government is apparently moving the Medicare program, the largest purchaser for most hospitals and many doctors, toward common provider contracts.[9]

Because there are large potential savings under managed care by reducing inpatient hospital, medical specialist, and clinical support services, contracts are increasingly restrictive on these items. To win the contracts, most provider organizations must restructure at lower prices and volumes and reduce resources for these services. Negotiation of the contracts requires an ability to commit the organization to effective restructuring.

Organization

The relationship of the parts of the organization to each other, and the rules and incentives that bind them to a common goal, are an area of decision making requiring knowledge, skills, and experience rarely possessed by clinicians or trustees. The design of the organization is one of the very few areas where the executive office normally takes an authoritative position. Because of the complexity and technicality of the issues involved, it is the subject of the following chapter.

Selecting Executive Personnel

Large healthcare organizations now have several levels of healthcare executives, clinical executives, and specialists in the support services. Chief executives lead a team, hiring or promoting individuals as they mature. Clearly the quality of the team is a major determinant of the organization's success. Because it also determines the experience of future CEOs, it may be critical to the success of its members as individual professionals as well. Issues in the selection and development of that team are the subject of this section. While the experience and skill required are discussed from the perspective of a younger executive planning a career, the same perspective should be useful to a superior seeking a subordinate executive.

Career Opportunities

The management of large healthcare organizations presents substantial opportunities. There are about 29,000 members of the leading professional association, the **American College of Healthcare Executives (ACHE)**,[10] and an unknown but not insignificant number of others. Masters programs now produce about 2,000 graduates per year, suggesting a total pool of about 60,000. While many professional executives work in government, health insurance companies, and other activities not directly involved with patient care, about three times as many are in caregiving organizations.

A career in healthcare management, like other management careers, should present an opportunity for continuous growth and for a lifetime of personal and psychological rewards. Financial rewards should reflect the increasing skill and contribution of the individual, with major increases in compensation reserved for those few who wish to be and are capable of being successful CEOs. Healthcare management supplies both of these needs.[11] There are opportunities for limited responsibility, specialization, and demanding senior executive roles reachable only after 25 years of learning. The financial rewards are commensurate, reaching annual compensation 10 to 12 times entry level professional salaries.[12]

The evolution of the industry from rapid growth to controlled growth and from small provider organizations to large integrated ones can be expected to produce major changes in both the number and roles of executives. Executive positions for clinicians will unquestionably increase, and there will be a shortage of qualified physician and nurse executives for some time to come. The steadily increasing sophistication of the field has led to a continuing demand for accountants, lawyers, information specialists, and planning personnel. As corporations grow larger, opportunities for highly skilled and well-compensated general executives will increase. On the other hand, restructuring in the early 1990s emphasized elimination of management layers, reducing lower level opportunities for both clinical and general managers.

Careers in healthcare management are generally an end in themselves; people come into healthcare management at various ages from various prior roles much more often than they leave the field for some other activity. Entry from senior clinical levels is much more common, for example, than return to clinical practice. Lawyers and accountants who come to specialize in healthcare applications tend to stay with the specialty, either improving their specialty skills or moving into general healthcare management as they are promoted.

Career Education

Graduate education

Graduate education is increasingly the norm for all but the lowest levels of executive activity. Although exceptional individuals occasionally arrive through other routes, successful completion of graduate education is evidence of general intellectual ability, energy, and perseverance. High class standing or a degree from a particularly competitive school is usually a predictor of future success. Entry to healthcare management is from one of three sources. Many young people enter by way of a masters program in the field, gaining experience before and after their degree in junior management positions. Others enter from established careers in caregiving professions, chiefly medicine and nursing. The third, and probably smallest group, enter from general business, law, accounting, or other specialties. All develop their skills by continuing education and experience.

The kind of graduate education influences the knowledge and skills acquired. Clinical and legal education emphasize skills other than management, and the knowledge these educational specialties impart is only partly relevant to healthcare. Finance, marketing, organizational design, and human relations are topics dealt with only in management-oriented graduate programs. A factual and analytic review of the healthcare system is generally available only in healthcare administration programs. The odds for young persons seeking a career in healthcare management favor those with graduate education in the field at the most selective school they can get into. For those who possess other graduate education, an alternate strategy would be to acquire missing skills through experience and missing knowledge through continuing education.

Additional formal education is particularly important for caregivers transferring to management roles. It is useful for people whose prior work has been outside healthcare. General healthcare managers often seek additional learning from the fields of business and law. A few master clinical professions after beginning a general career.

Continuing education

Regular participation in formal continuing education programs is a requirement for membership in the ACHE, as it is for many professional associations. Continuing education has three roles in an executive career: remedial, complementary, and supplementary. Remedial education addresses oversights in previous formal education. Evening courses, weekend programs, extended summer conferences, and study on one's own can do much to expand skills and knowledge. The diligent student can acquire or expand important concepts and skills in medicine, law, finance, management engineering, statistics, marketing, and other important skills through programs available at local colleges and books in nearby libraries.

Complementary education often consists of factual knowledge of new developments. The most common examples are factual presentations on various new laws, regulations, and business opportunities. New analytic techniques can also be learned. Forecasting, using discounted cash flows, or installing patient-scheduling systems are examples. Most complementary education is in the form of one- or two-day conferences, but home study and participation via electronic media are becoming more common. The ACHE has developed an extensive series of conferences, home study programs, and publications.

Supplementary education is the least formal of the three forms, but not necessarily the least important. It broadens perspectives beyond the normal professional limits. Study of the healthcare systems of other nations is relatively popular. Some universities offer summer courses in comparative healthcare. Religious and liberal arts studies are important supplementary education. Some executives read literature, history, biography, and philosophy. The broader perspectives gained from these pursuits are useful in evaluating the changes in the environment and the opportunities they suggest. They are also useful in coping with the frustrations inherent in management. Among executives fully qualified in professional knowledge and skill, a broad perspective distinguishes the exceptional from the adequate.

Career Experience

Those seeking an executive want both formal education and the skills that are the distillate of successful experience, but the skills are harder to appraise. Decision support experiences include roles in information systems, planning, marketing, and supporting the board and medical staff. Decision-implementation experience includes organization design and direction of successful units or corporations. Different jobs have different balances of requirements, and advancing executives seek a cumulative profile that matches their interests and the needs of the positions to which they aspire.[13]

Decision support experience

Decision-oriented experience relates to the processes that help the organization set its expectations. The skills involved are largely analytic and often require quantitative techniques. Beginners often do fact-finding and preliminary work on budgets and long-range plans. These exercises are particularly fruitful because they show the range of possibilities and restrictions of the organization so well. They also are not sensitive; the inevitable beginners' mistakes will almost certainly be caught in subsequent reviews.

More seasoned executives move to activities closer to final decisions: negotiating expectations with middle management and primary monitors, ranking new program activities, developing plans to implement broad goals, specifying information requirements, and designing systems to produce them. Mature executives, often CEOs, address the most sensitive and difficult decisions: weighing the importance and permanence of environmental changes, recommending budget guidelines, and resolving serious disputes. As executives progress, the cost of error mounts, but so do their skills, wisdom, and emotional maturity.

Implementation-oriented experience

Implementation experience focuses more clearly on the ability to convince others and to gain their cooperation. The skills involved in implementation transcend human relations, although they require effective interpersonal abilities. In the healthcare world, where little gets done without a team, implementation experience is learning how to make teams effective, getting people to accomplish goals because they see it as in their own best interest. One famous textbook put it:

> The essential task of management is to arrange organization conditions and methods of operation so that people can achieve their own goals best by directing their own efforts toward organizational objectives.[14]

Implementation skill is almost impossible to teach in formal settings. (Efforts like this book can lead people away from the wrong ideas, but they cannot build skills at the right ones.) What does seem reliable is that implementation skills are apparent early in most leaders and that they are improved by practice. Experience for healthcare executives can appropriately begin before the professional career, with college activities, for example, and can include experience outside healthcare, if time permits. Smaller voluntary organizations, local government, and charitable fund drives are common examples. So are state and national professional organizations.

Implementation skills are developed by leading work groups, including cross-functional teams and task forces. The traditional role of the "supervisor" of a work group is replaced by a "team leader" concept in continuous improvement. The group leader's role is to help the group achieve their goals, whether that be the improvement of a process design, or the actual work itself. For CEO-level skills, the composition of the group led is probably more important than its size. Opportunities to lead groups containing doctors and other extensively educated individuals or groups of leaders, such as trustees, are valuable. It is important to understand that several jobs traditionally labeled staff—especially consulting, planning, and board and medical staff support—can develop these skills as well as the line tradition of supervision. Certainly good staff work requires analytic skills, decision-making skills, and the ability to bring a group to timely and enthusiastic consensus. The ultimate skill, the ability to project values and describe goals so that they are attractive to large numbers, is the characteristic that distinguishes the highest ranks of executives. The opportunities to practice it in advance are rare; the chance comes as the individual reaches the ranks just below the top.

Mentoring

An important aspect of experiential education is guidance and feedback. Ideally, senior executives coach junior ones, giving them guidance on how to approach problems, evaluations of performance, insights into hidden complexities, reassurance, and encouragement. It is generally wise for beginning executives to seek not one but several mentors, shifting among them as their situations change.[15]

Assessment of Professional Skills

Honest assessment of one's skills is a powerful tool. Maturing executives should develop profiles of their personal skills and knowledge, along with their professional goals. The profile, together with an effort to identify and analyze the requirements of jobs desired in the future, helps set learning goals and priorities. The ACHE offers an instrument to assist in self-evaluation, but it is a better beginning than final guide.[16] A realistic test of the profile is to compare it with actual job descriptions of open positions.

In the final analysis, skillful executives are those whose groups do a good job. In addition to personal profiles, executives should have an ongoing sense of how well they are doing their job. The annual round of expectation setting and review of performance usually included a review by superiors and provides an opportunity for self-assessment. Leading institutions are moving to "**360-degree reviews**" that add evaluations by subordinates and customers as well. Good executives monitor their own performance continuously. If the information conveyed at an annual review is a surprise, that in itself is a symptom that needs to be explored. Good mentors can offer tips about potential growth and improvement, as part of the annual review and when indicated throughout the year.

Recruiting Effective Executives

Executive level personnel are mostly recruited through search firms, consulting companies that specialize in locating and evaluating executive talent. A good firm helps articulate job descriptions and selection criteria, advises on compensation and relevant experience, pursues affirmative action policies, develops the richest possible list of candidates, and conducts initial selection using interviews, references, and biographical information. The healthcare organization usually makes the final selection from a small panel of persons found qualified by the search firm. Probably more important than the final selection are the organization's actions to describe the job and the selection criteria. It is impossible for the search firm to know the details of the local needs, and easier to find a good candidate for the wrong job than vice versa.

Most chief executives are now offered written contracts specifying the terms of employment.[17] These include a general description of the work obligations (it is almost impossible to describe an executive job specifically), salary compensation, incentive compensation, employment benefits, rights to products developed on the job, and extension and termination arrangements. Executives below the CEO are often covered under the organization's general supervisory-level employment agreements, with letters confirming verbal contracts unique to the position. Although service of executives is at the pleasure of the CEO, or the board for the CEO position, it is increasingly common to have clauses protecting the executive against unexpected termination.

Executive compensation is determined by competitive markets. The usual domain of comparison is the national market place of organizations of similar size and type. Compensation in general parallels the earning opportunities of the lower-paid medical specialties. The opportunity to acquire equity, commonplace as an element of compensation among for-profit firms, is not available in healthcare organizations with a nonprofit structure. Thus, although salaries tend to parallel comparable responsibility in other industries, total compensation is lower.

Because of the specialization of executive office personnel, healthcare organizations are often forced to recruit from outside. The largest healthcare organizations often follow a policy of promoting to the executive office from within. This reduces the risk associated with hiring outsiders and provides opportunities and incentives for lower managers in the organization. It also builds an executive office with detailed familiarity with the organization. The disadvantages are the dangers of inbreeding and complacency. An organization composed solely of people who have worked there all their lives can easily lose touch with innovations occurring elsewhere. It also can become willing to accept local compromises that others would reject and, in the worst cases, can build a culture of deference to its more persuasive or powerful members that obscures the important resource dependencies and market trends. The disadvantage can be overcome by an explicit policy of seeking outside education, consultation, comparison, and advice.

Organization of the Executive Office

The executive office is small relative to other units of the healthcare organizations. In small organizations it may be only one or two people; even in large ones the office accounts for only a small percentage of total payroll costs. Despite its size, it presents several important design problems, principally because of its role in integrating the other systems and the complexities of being the focal point of commerce as indicated in Figure 4.1. This section discusses representative examples of executive office organization and the responsibilities of key executives, with special attention to the accountability of the CEO and the chief operating officer (COO).

Design of the Executive Office

Organization charts for executive units depict reality poorly, largely because they show only permanent formal accountability, while many activities take place in committees and informal relationships. Figure 4.4 shows the elements that must relate through the executive office of a large healthcare organization operating a broad scope of services and in several geographic locations. The nine support activities represent common groupings of the executive office functions described above. Marketing includes customer-related activities, alliances with competing and complementary organizations, and relations with buyers and intermediaries. It might mean operating a health insurance plan, but it also includes partnerships with other providers and insurance

FIGURE 4.4
Relationship Problem of a Large Healthcare Organization

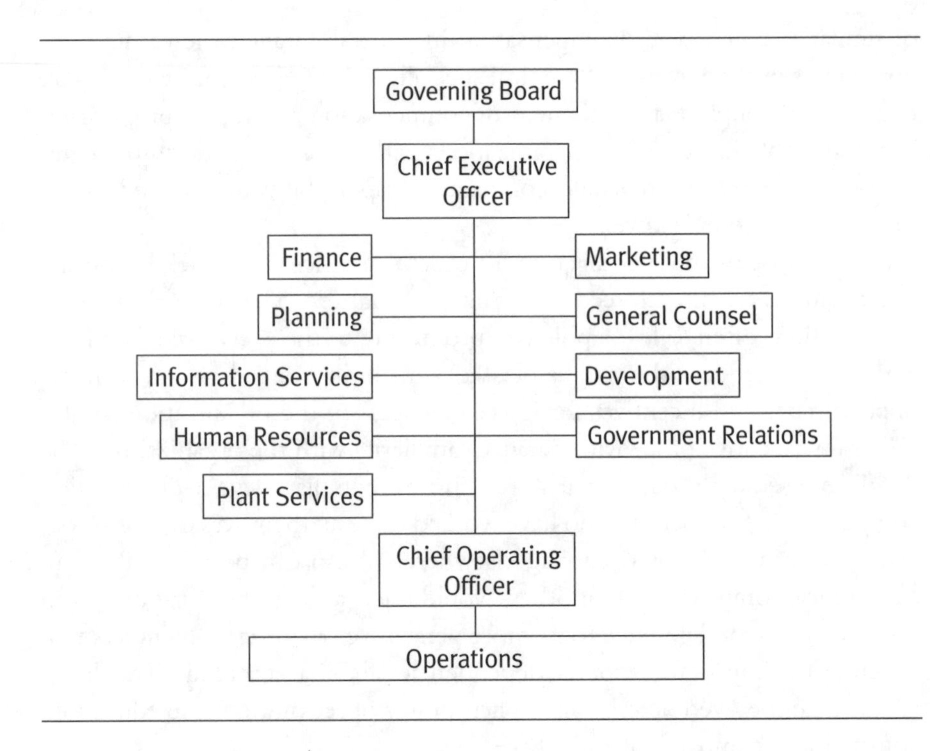

intermediaries such as Blue Cross. It is the newest entry on the list, and its activities are expanded in Chapter 7.

Figure 4.4 as it stands almost certainly would not be effective. Assuming a vice president for each box, CEOs would have 11 or 12 people reporting to them directly, an unmanageable load given the complexity and importance of the issues. What is worse, the figure shows no direct, face-to-face communication between the administrative support units themselves or with the operations. It implies information flows to the governing board only through the chief executive and to operations only through the operating officer. The limits of what these two individuals can realistically process fall far short of what a modern organization requires. This problem, how to bring a very large number of activities together into decision-making groups that are effective both in size and in representation, is a critical one for larger healthcare organizations.

Real organizations are learning to solve the problems of Figure 4.4. The test is the organization's ability to respond to the changes in the marketplace. The winners succeed because they can effectively deliver the administrative services to their caregivers, enabling them to be more desirable in the market place than the earlier forms. It is clear from market trends that some organizations are winning, but the solutions they use are not simple or easy to describe.

The leading institutions create fluid organizations that pass authority easily from one function to another, depending on the issue. The solution emerging, shown in Figure 4.5, establishes groupings around common problems and team assignments. The nine support functions work in three operational groups and form permanent or ad hoc teams to address specific issues. Operations units and cross-functional participation in specific teams is expected.

Information flows between the individuals as well as through the formal lines. The result is a different perspective on leadership and new roles for the members of the executive office. The traditional concept of the executive implied great power stemming from the office itself. The classical thinking reflected the rigid formality of Figure 4.4; the chief executive was assumed to dispense decisions to which there often was no appeal, and the subordinates held similar authority in their respective domains. The new solution suggests that few questions are answered by one person, that authority comes from reaching a consensus on a viable solution.

The strength of the teams is their ability to develop consensus between powerful groups, mutual commitments that will ease the implementation once the decision has been reached. Power, rather than being viewed as intrinsic to the office, is viewed as intrinsic to the resources.[18] Solutions become tradeoffs between potentially competing sources of power for mutual gain. This perspective puts considerable emphasis on negotiating skills. The teams must accept accountability; it is understood that effective solutions will be reached on timely schedules. The support function leaders and members must understand the commitment. Their job is no longer simply to provide their particular skill or service; it is to participate in building an effective solution.

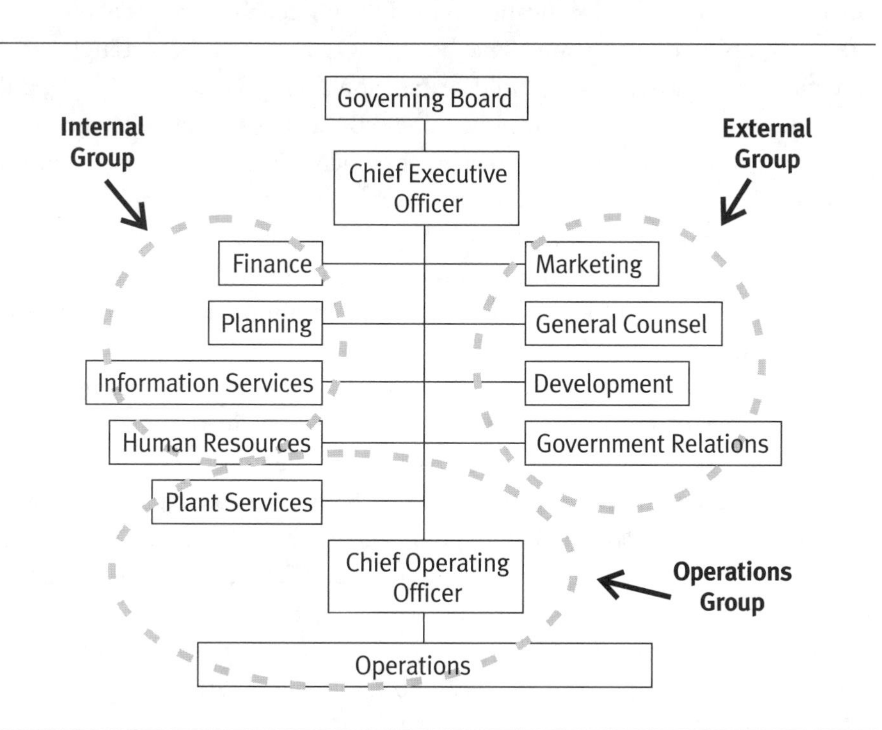

FIGURE 4.5 Hierarchical Groupings of Executive Office Functions

Those who lead teams to the biggest gains get promotion opportunities. They may not be the individuals with the greatest technical understanding or the most powerful entry position.

Responsibilities of Executive Officers

The members of the executive office (often called the **senior management team**) are responsible as a group for the same global corporate success elements as the governing board (Chapter 3). The emphasis expands from identification of issues and solutions to include implementation. Several of the executive office members have specific duties, including support for various governing board activities, as shown in Figure 4.6. Dual titles such as President and CEO or Executive Vice President and COO are increasingly common. The office of the general counsel can serve as secretary of the corporation, managing bylaws, charters, corporate reports, minutes, and other formal documentation. Chief financial officers (CFOs) commonly report to both the CEO and the finance committee of the board. They may hold the office of treasurer, although it is sometimes assigned to a volunteer board member in not-for-profit organizations. The chief medical officer usually has a board seat as well.

Unique responsibilities of the chief executive officer

The CEO is uniquely responsible for leadership of the executive office, for representing the organization to the outside world, for relations with the governing board, and for leadership of the organization as a whole. Leadership of the executive office is exercised through intellectual superiority, gained through experience and education and through coaching and encouraging other members of the team. The best CEOs are often surprisingly non-directive. They frame issues, build teams, applaud successful proposals, and raise questions about less promising ones. By acting in this way, they promote true delegation. A non-directive approach allows alternative opinions, dialogue, and innovation, when more assertive stances would have the subordinates simply agreeing to the CEO's view. Their directive statements are at the most strategic level, such as proposals for initial budget targets, strategies for crucial negotiations, major restructuring, and stimulation of task forces to study new ideas.

CEOs are usually the principal spokespersons for the organization, representing it to the other organizations and forces in the community, in regional and state associations, and to its own members. The direct CEO contact is often critical to a certain level of exchange relationships. Accessibility to community business, charitable, political, and financial leaders determines how comfortable those leaders are in sharing their views about important issues. When community leaders lose comfort, the stage has been set for actions not in the organization's interest. Such actions might include aiding competing institutions, denying access to funds or real estate resources, and taking restrictive political steps.

FIGURE 4.6
Duties of Executive Staff Members

Officer	Governing Board Committee Assignment	Major Duties
Chief Executive Officer	Executive, ex officio on all	External relations, governing board, leadership, ceremonial functions
Chief Operating Officer	Executive, Planning	Operations, selection, and support of other line officers, coordination of staff support
Chief Financial Officer	Finance, Executive, Planning	Finance, accounting, protection of assets
Chief Medical Officer	Executive, Medical Staff Relations, Planning	Medical staff relations, medical education, medical staff recruitment, physician-hospital organization
Chief Nursing Officer	Planning	Nursing staff planning and recruitment, inpatient care, outpatient facilities management
Chief Information Officer	Planning	Information services, information planning, medical records
Vice President for Planning and Marketing	Planning, Finance	Planning support, marketing to intermediaries and buyers
General Counsel	Executive, Finance	Bylaws, major contracts, risk management, board minutes, and documentation
Vice President for Human Resources	Compensation, Planning	Work force planning, recruitment, benefits management, training programs, compensation programs
Vice President for Plant Services	Planning	Facilities planning, space allocation, plant operations, plant services

External relations now include a variety of agreements and contracts with other agencies. The CEO often initiates and finalizes these contracts, even though the detailed negotiation is left to others. The CEO remains active in most joint venture, merger, and acquisition discussions. The negotiation of contracts specifying privileges and responsibilities between subsidiaries and parent or between partner organizations must involve the chief executive.

Successful chief executives also always play an active role in the affairs of the governing board. CEOs usually have voting membership on the board, but these activities are much more influential than a single vote. They monitor the agenda, making sure it is complete and efficient. They provide full factual support for all agenda items, almost always including a recommendation. They brief the chairs of the major committees on likely debate and its management. They maintain profiles of current and potential board members, suggest new board members, and provide criteria for selection. They guide orientation and training programs. They identify promising members and develop them through committee assignments. They make themselves available for informal discussion at the instigation of members, and they facilitate direct communication with their own subordinates and leaders of the other systems. Many of these duties cannot be delegated, but the most effective CEOs find ways to use board members and lower executives in these activities, both to save themselves time and to increase training opportunities.

The CEO is also spokesperson to, and leader of, the organization at large. The meaning, implications, and importance of major directions should be explained to the organization at large by the CEO, but the process of expanding the ideas into specific expectations is left to the rest of the executive office. The continuous improvement concept is one example. Enthusiastic support from the CEO is generally felt to be essential. The CEO is also sometimes the final point of appeal for dissatisfied members, but this role increasingly falls to other members of the executive office.

The best CEOs seem to lead their organizations in an ongoing, three-part process. First, they establish themselves and then their subordinates as respected sources of problem solving. That is, they make the management structure responsive to its employees, doctors, trustees, and patients. Beginning in the front office, but spreading as rapidly as possible to all management, they emphasize the concept of service. This improves performance, but, equally important, it raises the confidence of members and exchange partners. Second, CEOs work to open and expand conversations about the organization so all ideas can be discussed; they put a premium on useful innovations. This climate results from candor and objectivity, virtues that are themselves achieved by effective staff support and information systems. It also results from CEOs who share credit for progress with others. Third, the CEO uses the momentum of growing confidence and achievement to explore external threats to and opportunities for the organization—issues too frightening to debate openly in poorly run organizations—in ways that allow innovative and rewarding responses. The CEO's sound relationships and personal grasp of external issues are essential to completing this process.

Unique responsibilities of the chief operating officer

The role of the COO is less specific than that of the other officers, and some organizations operate without a designated COO. Clinical leaders such as the Chief Medical Officer or Chief Nursing Officer can serve as COO. When there is a COO, these positions must work in close collaboration with it. The traditional COO role is an inside, implementation focus complementing the CEO's external one. In this model, the chief operating officers are accountable to deliver on the short-term expectations for cost, demand, quality of care, and quality of work life. They are accountable for any failure of structure or process in medical staff organization, clinical care, recruitment, collective bargaining, non-financial records, and plant safety. In addition to these obligations, traditional COOs perform a "linking" function; they participate actively in strategic processes and are the main source of information about future performance and potential operating problems. They must maintain close relationships with information services, finance, and intermediary contracting, because these services directly affect operations.

Traditional COOs will participate directly in the recruitment of executive personnel other than the CEO. They will coordinate all issues of formal organizational design and work to overcome the inevitable design weaknesses. Finally, COOs will want to play the central role in both the design and the administration of compensation and reward systems. Management of the reward system is a logical extension of the COO's role in providing direction and control, and it also provides an opportunity to increase the loyalty of subordinates.

Properly understood, the traditional COO role is a focal point in the executive office almost as significant as the CEO, differing more in internal versus external focus than scope. It is hard to see how such a crucial role could ever disappear, but some institutions have had success with an operations team. The team would form anyway around the implementation issues and would comprise the major contributors to operational success, as shown in Figure 4.7. To succeed, the team must be able to work as effectively without a COO as it could with one.

Three elements are likely to be important in the success of the operations team, with or without a COO. First, the team members must be compatible, and must work at prompt identification and resolution of potential conflicts. Second, the support staff in information, accounting, and intermediary contracting must be effective, so that team energies can be devoted to creating solutions rather than fact-finding and analysis. Third, the overall scale must be such that the CEO can participate actively and can handle the linking functions to external questions. In short, the "no COO" operating team is more likely to succeed in smaller organizations that are richly staffed. The best examples may be hospitals and clinics that are subsidiaries of larger integrated systems.

Measures of Executive Performance

Measures of performance of the executive office as a whole are identical to those used by the governing board. In addition, there should be explicit expectations, reviews, and rewards for all individual executives, from the CEO to the beginning assistant. The measures should be appropriate subsets or components of the general measures, and should be as quantitative as possible.

FIGURE 4.7
Members and Agenda of the Operations Team

Members	Chief operating officer, if named Chief medical officer Chief nursing officer Director of ambulatory services Director of human resources Director of plant services
Agenda	Communicate budget guidelines to individual units. Establish improvement priorities. Commission improvement teams. Establish cross-functional clinical teams. Supervise preparation of capital budget. Work with planning team on facilities and human resources plans. Work with information services on new information systems. Recruit new management personnel. Coach managers. Review compensation scales. Coordinate renovations, expansions, and major new equipment. • • • Etc.

The higher the rank of the executive, the greater importance should be placed on response to and management of external issues. At the CEO level, and for the vice president of marketing, external issues could be considered more important than current operating performance. Evaluation of external issues can be based on objective measures, but subjective assessment of what is feasible is inescapable.

Outcomes Performance Measures

Figure 4.8 shows the quality compass measures developed in Chapter 3 as they might be assigned to specific executives and expanded to more detail. Most of these items are now measured routinely by well-managed institutions. They are outcomes, or external measures that can be individually compared to benchmarks and quantitative expectations agreed upon at the start of each budget year. Taken as a whole, they constitute an overall measure of the executive office. When each measure is related to an expectation, the set can be presented as a radar chart as shown in Figure 3.14.

Well-managed institutions use an annual process like the following:

1. They use the measures suggested by Figure 4.8, and expectations and goals for each.
2. They compare performance to expectations and develop a radar chart such as Figure 3.14.

FIGURE 4.8
Measures of Executive Performance

DIMENSION*	CONCEPTS	EMPHASIS**
Financial performance	Profit	CEO, CFO
	Credit rating	CEO, CFO
	Financial structure	CFO
Patient and family satisfaction	Market share	CEO, Mktg., Plng.
	Survey scores	COO, CMO, CNO, Plant
	Clinical outcomes	CMO
	Scope of services	CEO, Plng.
	Access for disadvantaged	CEO, Plng.
	Regulatory approvals	COO
Buyer satisfaction	Costs	COO
	Intermediary and member service	Mktg., CIO
Provider satisfaction	Staffing and recruitment	HR, COO
	Employee and physician surveys	COO, CMO, CNO

* See Chapter 3 for concepts of dimensions.
** Executive office members having increased direct responsibility.
CEO: Chief executive officer; CFO: Financial; CIO: Information; CMO: Medical; CNO: Nursing; COO: Operating; HR: Human resources; Mktg: Marketing; Plng: Planning; Plant: Plant services

3. They use board committees (usually finance and compensation) to evaluate the overall results, pronouncing them excellent or acceptable or worse.
4. They use the judgment and the specifics as input for next year's expectation setting.
5. They use the overall judgment and the comparisons to evaluate performance of individuals in the executive office. (This step ties the performance of the individual to that of the entire executive group, a critical linkage.)
6. The executive office members repeat the process for their subordinates. It spreads through the organization, using progressively more detailed measures, but retaining the emphasis on the overall achievement.

The central concepts here are the use of objective measures, the central role of the judgment for the organization as a whole, and the application of the results both for feedback to the next round of expectations and the evaluation of individuals. Objective measures permit detail, precision, and reliability that cannot be approached by subjective assessments. The governing board role is central to the board's power to carry out its functions. It is by interpreting performance that the board illustrates the mission and vision and puts reality into the planning process. Often the board makes explicit statements about what will or will not be acceptable. Rules conditioning the assessment on the most global measures, such as outcomes quality, patient satisfaction, or profit, help organization members understand the real priorities of the board. Finally, using the assessment both as feedback and for individual performance evaluation closes the loop. It shows priorities for next year's improvement, and it makes clear that individuals must first contribute to the success of the whole. Without this message, it is easy for individuals and units to optimize their own needs at the expense of the whole. This is an important way to encourage the opposite behavior. (It is sometimes stated very strongly: No department or individual bonuses unless the corporation as a whole does well.)

Other Performance Measures

Process measures

Particularly at levels below the CEO, there are numerous measures of individual processes that contribute to global outcomes measures. These are useful in several ways. They permit diagnosis of trouble spots, assist in designing improvements, and allow assessment of individuals and activities that are only components of the whole. They can be used to supplement outcomes measures in evaluating the executive office and its members. They do not replace outcomes measures. The association between good process and good outcomes is usually imperfectly understood, and to omit direct measures of critical success elements is imprudent.

Statements describing professional quality of work can be found in textbooks for many areas of executive activity, such as planning, community relations, advertising, information systems, and law. Where these standards exist, a series of questions or criteria can be developed to indicate acceptable practice, and actual practice compared against it. However, there are few published commentaries on the CEO's obligations to represent the organization, to maintain contact with influential persons in the community, and to assist in board selection and development.[19]

The Process of Evaluating Executives

The reality is that executive worlds are ambiguous and executive behavior is complex. The central question in evaluating performance of the office and its members is how to use the measures most effectively. A single score could be constructed from the radar chart by weighting each element. (A simple average assigns a weight of one to each element.) Assigning weights is almost impossible, and the weights may change radically over time. A profile including subjective evaluations may be more useful. It leads to an analysis and specific plans for improvement that provide more insights than a batting average. It discourages competitive ranking against peers, a practice that is destructive in the executive office, where constant collaboration is essential.

Often the board compensation committee and one or two top executives guide the evaluation of the CEO, a few of the top officers, and the plan for evaluating other management personnel. The executives evaluate their subordinates according to the plan. Self-evaluation is essential; an employee should have the opportunity to prepare a self-evaluation before a conference with superiors. It is increasingly common for the evaluation of the top tiers of managers to be used for merit pay increases and bonuses. A retrospective evaluation with subjective components is probably preferable to more mechanistic reward systems that pick a few of the many measures in advance and automatically reward achievement on those measures. The richness of subjective evaluation, profiling, and retrospective review add information and perspective missing in prospective schemes.

Encouraging Effective Executive Office Performance

The issues an organization deals with come and go rather quickly. The organization makes appropriate responses and thrives, or inappropriate ones and declines. However important the issues of today, they will be replaced by others tomorrow. It is the structure for dealing with this stream of transient issues that is the constant and the key to success. Although the executives of well-run organizations are always deeply involved in the issues of the day, it is their ability to relate those issues to the underlying structure and improve it that makes them exceptional. Using the specific issues as opportunities, they work tirelessly to achieve certain characteristics of structure. These criteria for excellence are like the organization's vision statement. They are never fully met; the continuous effort brings the organization closer to the ideal. Three important elements of this "Executive Vision" are the appropriate use of power, effective timing, and the development of a supporting culture or style.

Using Power

Alexander and Morlock have pointed out that many healthcare executives have serious and possibly disabling ambivalences about power. They recognize its existence and importance, but they fear that it will subvert official goals.[20] Alexander and Morlock agree with Pfeffer, who argues for the deliberate use of politics and power to advance the goals of organizations of all kinds.[21] This perspective calls for an intimate familiarity with the needs and viewpoints of all the stakeholders. Positions are made explicit, needs and rights are recognized, conflicts are identified and resolved as feasible. In some cases, power of individual stakeholders is accepted, and the vision of others is trimmed to the political reality. The organization accepts openly what it would accept tacitly in a more traditional structure.

Well-managed organizations do as these authors suggest. Their assessments identify individual and group goals, and their strategic plans recognize realities stemming from technical, economic, and regulatory advantages. They build coalitions, make deals, and compromise collective goals to achieve as much as possible within feasible limits. They are, in short, political in the deepest sense of the word, politics as a method of resolving conflict within a group.

One implication of this perspective is that external events drive improvement, rather than the governing board or the executives. On some of the most critical issues of the day, such as the extent of managed care, the treatment available to the disadvantaged, or the centralization of management, the prevailing view of the community is accepted. The power that drives change is the power of the marketplace. The legitimacy of any issue and the criteria for its solution are defined by the customer. The topics that are selected for change are those where the largest forces can be assembled or, in some cases, where the weakest defenses lie. The executives of well-managed organizations say, "The customer is demanding these changes." They do not say, "The board wants this done," or worse yet, "The boss wants this."

The weakness of this approach is that some important items may escape notice by the customer. One of the tasks of the executive group is to identify overlooked topics that might offer major threats or opportunities in the future, and prepare for their emergence.

Timing the Response

A consequence of the pragmatic use of power is that the ultimate control of the agenda passes to the customer. But this approach naively pursued could lead to a chaotic expediency, rather than effective response to customer needs. The American marketplace is a babel of conflicting demands. It would literally be impossible to respond to them all. So well-managed organizations not only listen to the marketplace, they weigh and filter what they hear, responding to the set that they believe will be optimally satisfactory in the long run. Finding the optimum is a difficult, time-consuming challenge. Well-managed organizations identify the issues far enough in advance to allow full exploration.

Ideally, an organization should perceive each new external or exchange demand before it becomes a serious concern, to respond as it is articulated rather than when it becomes critical. The well-managed organization is rarely surprised or unprepared; change without crisis is the mark of successful management. An organization that has drifted toward crisis management must make hasty decisions and impose them on its members. The farsighted organization can afford the time to educate, debate, and innovate in formulating its response. The special skills and knowledge of the CEO and the executive office are vital to the farsightedness of the organization.

Management Style

Executive attitudes in the best healthcare organizations are more positive, more helpful, more open, and more encouraging in their relations with others. A participative, rather than an authoritarian, style of management is permanently embedded. The best executives coach; they don't order. They praise before they criticize. In the end, there is more to praise and less to criticize because the executives have established a system that helps people do well.

Six elements of style that are repeatedly cited as important in organizational literature are predictability, candor, responsiveness, persuasiveness, conflict resolution, and participation.

1. *Predictability.* Much of an organization's success depends on teamwork, and teamwork depends on knowing the role of others. Thus, an organization that handles similar decisions in similar ways and follows predictable cycles of behavior reduces stress and enhances the contribution of its members. An organization that is unpredictable is harder to deal with than one that is predictably dysfunctional.
2. *Candor.* An ever-present temptation in organizations is to tell people what they want to hear rather than the truth. Unfortunately, they all want to hear something different, and the practical result of lack of candor is chaos. The withholding of information is as self-defeating as overt distortion; yet many poor managers do it, whether accidentally or deliberately. Ignorance leads first to guesswork and surprises and shortly thereafter to suspicions and paranoia. In well-managed organizations, one can easily find out what one wants to know and rely on what one hears. Good executives encourage this characteristic by personal action, repeated reference to its importance, and reward for its practice.
3. *Responsiveness.* One obligation of management is to respond to subordinates' questions and concerns. It is clear that the more effectively the superior responds, the greater the productivity and performance of the subordinate will be.
4. *Persuasiveness.* An ability to articulate objectives, describe potential rewards, explain how difficulties can be overcome, and inspire confidence is a valuable tool in building consensus and motivation. The impact is enhanced by predictability, candor, and responsiveness. Persuasiveness is often based less on rhetoric than on a thorough understanding of both people and concepts, backed by a record of success.
5. *Conflict resolution.* Closely related to responsiveness is the ability to resolve conflicts in ways that are predictable and reasonable, but also as constructive as possible. Predictability applies both to the method of conflict resolution and the result. Understanding the likely outcome tends to minimize the conflicts. "Reasonable" is a better criterion than "fair," because many conflicts must be resolved in the organization's favor rather than in that of an individual. Polzer and Neale offer a typology of conflicts applicable to healthcare organizations, and a discussion of how to resolve many kinds of conflicts.[22]
6. *Participation.* Generally speaking, an organization that solicits the opinion of its members, both formally and informally, as a matter of course will do better than one that discourages member participation. This is especially

true in hospitals, where the constant variation in patient needs places a great many decisions at the bedside or at lower levels of the organization.

Suggested Readings

Pfeffer, J. 1992. *Managing with Power: Politics and Influence in Organizations.* Boston, MA: Harvard Business School Press.

Pointer, D. D., and J. P. Sanchez. 1997. "Leadership: A Framework for Thinking and Acting." In *Essentials of Healthcare Management, edited by* S. M. Shortell and A. D. Kaluzny, 99–132. Albany, NY: Delmar Publications.

Kovner, A. R., and D. Neuhauser (eds.). 1998. *Health Services Management: Readings and Commentary*, Fifth Edition. Chicago: Health Administration Press.

Shortell, S. M., and A. D. Kaluzny. 1997. "Creating and Managing the Future." In *Essentials of Healthcare Management,* edited by S. M. Shortell and A. D. Kaluzny, 478–500. Albany, NY: Delmar Publications.

Steers, R. M., and L. W. Porter. 1987. *Motivation and Work Behavior.* New York: McGraw Hill.

Tyler, J. L. 1998. *Tyler's Guide: The Healthcare Executive's Job Search,* 2d ed. Chicago: Health Administration Press.

Notes

1. H. S. Zuckerman and W. L. Dowling, "The Managerial Role"; and S. M. Shortell and A. D. Kaluzny, "Organization Theory and Health Services Management," *Health Care Management Organization Design and Behavior*, S.M. Shortell and A.D. Kaluzny. Albany: Delmar Publishers, 3–53 (1994)
2. M. Alveson, *Cultural Perspectives on Organizations.* New York: Cambridge University Press (1993)
3. J. R. Griffith, *The Moral Challenges of Health Care Management.* Chicago: Health Administration Press, 95–148 (1993)
4. J. R. Griffith, V. K. Sahney, and R. A. Mohr, *Reengineering Health Care: Building on Continuous Quality Improvement.* Chicago: Health Administration Press, Chapter 6 (1995)
5. D. D. Pointer and J. P. Sanchez, *Leadership: A Framework for Thinking and Acting*, in Shortell and Kaluzny, 85–112
6. G. Anderson, R. Heyssel, and R. Dickler, "Competition versus Regulation: Its Effect on Hospitals." *Health Affairs* 12(1): 70–80 (Spring, 1993)
7. Joint Commission on Accreditation of Healthcare Organizations, *Accreditation Manual for Hospitals.* Chicago: Joint Commission on Accreditation of Healthcare Organizations, published annually.
8. Joint Commission on Accreditation of Healthcare Organizations, *Emergency Preparedness: When the Disaster Strikes.* Oakbrook Terrace, IL: Joint Commission on Accreditation of Healthcare Organizations, 1990
9. G. C. Faja, "Package Pricing Project Improves Hospital-Physician Relations." Interview by Donald E.L. Johnson. *Health Care Strategic Management* 10(10):14–19 (Oct, 1992)

10. American College of Healthcare Executives: www.ache.org (revised August 1998; Oct. 18, 1998)
11. D. F. Fahey, R. F. Myrtle, J. L. Schlosser, "Critical Success Factors in the Development of Healthcare Management Careers." *Journal of Healthcare Management* 43:(4) 307–20
12. L. Scott, "Facilities Spread the Cash Around." *Modern Healthcare* 23(24): 39 (June 14, 1993)
13. B. B. Longest, "Managerial Competence at Senior Levels of Integrated Delivery Systems." *Journal of Healthcare Management* 43:(2) 115–134.
14. D. A. McGregor, *The Human Side of Enterprise.* New York: McGraw Hill (1960)
15. T. C. Dolan, Mentoring in the 1990s. *Healthcare Executive* 8(6):3 (Nov–Dec 1993)
16. M. B. Silber, "CEO-ship: Avoiding the Rocks of Self-Malpractice." *Healthcare Executive* 7(6):26–27 (November/December, 1992)
17. American College of Hospital Administration, *Report on the Committee on Contracts for Hospital Chief Executive Officers.* Chicago: American College of Hospital Administrators (1982).
18. J. A. Alexander and L. L. Morlock, "Power and Politics in Health Services Organizations," in Shortell and Kaluzny, 212–338.
19. The Foundation of the American College of Healthcare Executives, *Evaluating the Performance of the Hospital in a Total Quality Management Environment.* Chicago: American College of Healthcare Executives (1993).
20. J. A. Alexander and L. L. Morlock, "Power and Politics in Health Services Organizations," in Shortell and Kaluzny, 215.
21. J. Pfeffer, *Managing with Power: Politics and Influence in Organizations.* Boston: Harvard Business School Press (1992).
22. J. T. Polzer and M. A. Neale, "Conflict Management and Negotiation," in Shortell and Kaluzny, 113–33.

CHAPTER

5

DESIGNING THE HEALTHCARE ORGANIZATION

Organize: . . . provide with the structure and interdependence of parts which subserves vital processes. . . . Oxford English Dictionary[1]

A healthcare delivery organization creates a whole from several hundred or thousand well-intentioned individuals. It provides a structure called a **bureaucratic organization**, which recognizes and capitalizes on those individuals' interdependence, using specialization to enhance the individual contributions, so that the whole is substantially more valuable than anything they could achieve on their own.[2] Most of the economic activity of modern society is carried out by bureaucratic organizations (as is most religious, artistic, and social activity; the Catholic Church, the New York Philharmonic Orchestra, and the Boy Scouts of America are bureaucratic organizations). Although the term "bureaucratic" is often used pejoratively, this application is purely descriptive, coined by researchers to describe a form of human endeavor in which individuals and groups bring different skills to bear on an objective in accordance with a formal structure of authority and responsibility.

The purpose of bureaucratic structure is to facilitate responsiveness to the environment. The structure allows the enterprise to gain the benefits of specialized labor and capital, understand its resource dependencies, establish strategies to deal with them, and undertake continuous improvement. Building the bureaucratic structure—organizing the healthcare delivery enterprise—is one of the four functions that must be performed by the executive office.

Structure is provided in several ways. First, in social behaviors common to any human group, people learn to respect the power if not the rights of others, to share information and gratification, to make partnerships and friendships, and finally to divide and specialize the work. Any long-standing group develops an **informal organization** as a result of these processes. Second, in what is called the **formal** or **hierarchical organization**, people are granted authority over certain activities, held accountable for certain results, and given incentives for achieving them. Third, to operate in a dynamic environment the hierarchical organization must specify rules for collaboration to solve arising problems and reach certain decisions. These rules create a collateral organization of group activities, committees, task forces, and work groups with assignments and methods of operating different from the formal organization. All three of these are ongoing, evolving parts of even a small healthcare operation.

Beyond these interactions of people, it is possible to organize organizations. If a number of people are organized effectively to be a medical group, and a second set is organized to be a hospital, the two can affiliate with each other and then with a second, similar pair, and so forth. **Multi-unit organizations** interrelate several organizations of similar or complementary services. A variety of multi-unit healthcare structures have emerged, differing not only in size, services, and the geography of their components, but also in their formality and the way they distribute power and authority among their members.

This chapter reviews how well-managed healthcare providers build and use their organizations. It starts with the informal organization and proceeds to the hierarchical organization and the collateral organization of a single provider unit such as a hospital or clinic. Following history, the chapter then reviews the organization of several such provider units into healthcare systems, alliances, and other multi-unit structures.

The goal of the chapter is modest: to provide a framework that describes what successful healthcare organizations are doing. The framework should provide healthcare managers with a useful beginning and allow healthcare providers and others who work within organizations an understanding of what lies behind the structures of daily work life. The subject of organization is easily a lifetime's study. Despite a century packed with major milestones of understanding, it is clear that there is much still to be learned. The Suggested Readings at the end of the chapter are themselves condensations of dozens of other works.

The Informal Organization

All groups of people working together develop informal organizations. They consist of the communication networks and agreements the members establish for their own reasons. In smaller organizations informal structures are often more important than the formal ones. As size, distance, and complexity grow, informal organizations lose some of their power, but they never disappear and should never be ignored. Healthcare organizations of all sizes have extensive informal organizations. They are exceptionally important, because healthcare requires that small groups of caregivers have great latitude to deal with patients' varying needs. Much of the interaction of caregivers is the result of informal organization. The three-shift operation of hospitals is another factor encouraging informal organization. The night crew is almost certain to encounter situations in which it must devise its own answers. Informal structures also arise among large numbers of people with common interests or similar rank, such as doctors.

Although it is usually impossible to describe the informal structure in detail, the best formal organizations not only recognize their informal shadows, but also exploit their strengths and overcome their weaknesses.[3]

In other words, the formal organization strengthens the informal one and does what the informal one cannot. Simultaneously, it relies on the informal organization to do what it cannot. Informal organizations are powerful, if not always reliable, communications links. They spread facts, falsehoods, and opinions quickly. They encourage and discourage selected behaviors, setting both high and low limits on work output in certain situations, rigidly defining job roles in others. Informal structures can exert powerful forces where formal ones would be intolerable.[4] They can cause consensus around important ideas, such as how patients are approached, what can be said to a person of higher formal rank, who the leaders are, and who can be trusted.

The informal organization is used in several ways by well-managed healthcare enterprises. Direct participation in the communication provides a view of what is important to organization members. Potentially troublesome information can be "leaked" so that reactions can be judged without attribution or confrontation. Informal leaders can be identified.[5] Recognized leaders can be kept abreast of issues as a way of keeping the "rumor mill" accurate. They can be brought into critical decisions, so that the outcome adequately reflects member needs, and so that they can convey marketplace realities to their colleagues. A number of important issues of management style get designed and transmitted through the informal organization. Peters and Waterman have documented its power in several case studies.[6]

The Accountability Hierarchy, or Formal Organization

The Accountable Work Group

Responsibility centers

The smallest aggregate of formal organizational activity modeled is usually the first level at which a formal, monitored **accountability** appears. That unit has several labels, **responsibility center (RC)** probably being the clearest. **Work group** is also used. Healthcare work groups can be formed around similar skills, such as a nursing station staff, or around patient needs, such as a primary care practice.

Several examples of work groups are shown in Figure 5.1. Hospitals and large clinics will typically have a work group for each care unit, such as a nursing floor or clinic. They divide large departments in single geographic locations into work groups on the basis of technical function (for example, the laboratory is divided into chemistry, hematology, bacteriology, and histology work groups). They may organize a 24-hour service, such as security, into shifts. They divide a dispersed activity, such as housekeeping, into geographic areas. Laundries and operating rooms are organized around equipment—wash wheels and irons, heart pumps and lasers. Work groups are generally fewer than 15 people. Very large healthcare organizations will have hundreds of work groups.

FIGURE 5.1 Examples of Healthcare Responsibility Centers

Inpatient Nursing Unit Head nurse (BSN) Clinical specialist (BSN) Staff nurses (RN) Licensed practical nurses Nurse aids Clerks	*Intensive Care Unit* Physician manager (MD) Head nurse (BSN) Clinical specialists (BSN) Staff nurses (RN) Licensed practical nurses (LPN)
Primary Care Office Primary care physician (MD) Nurse practitioner (MSN) Office nurse (RN or LPN) Clerks	*Housekeeping* Supervisor Housekeeping personnel
Clinical Laboratory Chief pathologist (MD) Laboratory manager (MS or PhD) Certified technicians (BS) Assistant technicians Clerks	*Home Care Team* Team manager (BSN, RN) Home care nurse (RN, LPN) Physical therapists (BS, RPT) Home health aid Clerks

The accountability commitment

The work group makes certain commitments to the central organization and receives certain assurances in return. These commitments are called **expectations** throughout this text. The assurances and expectations constitute an informal contract that describes the relationship. Many of the expectations covering measures traced directly from the balanced scorecard concepts (Chapter 3) are formalized. A quantitative expectation is negotiated to reflect a mutual understanding of what must be done to fill the strategic management goals (Chapter 2). The group is empowered in the sense that it has authority to change its work conditions to fulfill the expectations.

In traditional management, an accountable leader for the group was always designated, called generically the **work group leader, responsibility center manager,** or **first-line supervisor**. Often the group leader has a title, such as head nurse or foreman, related to the type of work the group does. Under continuous improvement, it is not always necessary for the group to have a formally designated leader. A trend has grown to use team or group accountability, sharing negotiation of the expectations, design of the work, and rewards of achievement. Large groups working in dynamic environments such as patient care usually need some designated spokesperson. The practical result is that the leader remains, but the group becomes more participative and democratic. The leader's role now emphasizes coordination, coaching, and external communications.

The newer approach has proven successful for a number of leading healthcare organizations.[7,8,9] It is important to understand how it differs from traditional thought about accountability. Figure 5.2 emphasizes the key distinctions. The agreement is negotiated, not imposed. The leader coaches, not commands. The measures of performance reflect the full range of strategic needs, not simply output and cost. The team is encouraged, not threatened. It is expected to understand both the origin and validity of the goals and the ways to manipulate the work environment to improve goal achievement. In short, it is dramatically different from the traditional view of organizations as top-down, authoritatively driven structures.[10,11,12]This view is not only prevalent among leading healthcare organizations, it is highly consistent with what has been learned about organizations and the motivation of people in them during the twentieth century.[13]

Criteria for work group design

Design of work groups is one of the organizing tasks. It is usually carried out under the supervision of the executive office, with each level designing its subordinate groups. The design criteria for each responsibility center are:

FIGURE 5.2 New and Traditional Accountability Approaches

NEW	TRADITIONAL
Shared Vision Management and workers understand their mutual dependence on customers and share a common vision of how they will succeed.	*Adversarial Competition* Management and workers view themselves as dividing a fixed set of resources and competing for shares.
Negotiated Agreement Workgroup participates in analyzing open systems needs and work processes, commits itself to a realistic level of achievement.	*Imposed Decision* Superiors in organization use authority to tell RC workers what production goals must be.
Coaching Management provides information, answers questions, makes suggestions to workers who design new processes.	*Commanding* "The boss tells you what to do."
Full Performance Measures Quality, patient/customer satisfaction, worker satisfaction, output, cost, and contribution to overall profit all considered in designing process, assessing performance.	*Partial Performance Measures* Usually just cost and output. RC team could "game" by cutting quality and satisfaction.
Encouragement Workers trained to solve problems, encouraged to try, praised for success, and often given monetary incentives for meeting goals.	*Threats* Workers punished for failures, sometimes even when they weren't at fault.

1. *To assign every necessary task to a single work group.* If tasks are assigned to more than one work group or to no work group, there is no way of ensuring accountability.
2. *To assign related tasks to the same work group.* If related tasks are assigned to different work groups, problems of continuity and coordination may arise.
3. *To assign tasks requiring similar skills to the same work group.* A work group and a manager with a common background can communicate with each other more easily.
4. *To limit each work group to a reasonable overall set of tasks.* The work group must be able to maintain control of the activity by direct communication of group members, imposing time, geographic, technical, and size limits on work groups.

These criteria are more difficult in reality than they sound on paper. The design of work groups is related to the identification of tasks. A thorough effort to define and assign tasks will complete the first criterion. The second and third are harder. Tasks are related in many different ways, but only one assignment is possible. At a conceptual level, all care of each patient is interrelated, suggesting that the unit of organization should be the patient. At the same time, it is impossible for one person, or even one team, to master all the skills necessary to care for seriously ill patients, suggesting that the unit of organization should be skill or function. Figure 5.3, a partial list of routine needs of a recovering surgical patient, illustrates the problem. In the real world of healthcare, criterion 2, relating tasks, and criterion 3, relating skills, are intrinsically in conflict. One calls for an organization around patients with similar needs (as exist in ICUs, nurseries, primary care clinics, etc.). The other calls for organization around similar skills (as also exist in therapy departments, pharmacies, diagnostic services). The trend in healthcare for many years was toward the right side of Figure 5.3—specialists proliferated to master specific tools and skills. The recent trend has been in the opposite direction, cross-training workers in a single site so that they can meet all patient needs for a specific group of patients, usually defined by diagnosis.

Similar conflicts exist with geography and function. There are frequently two geographic units with similar functions, or two functions in the same geographic area, or two skills required for the same function. Is it better to put all the therapists in one place, or one in each ambulatory care site? Should the hospital pharmacists be located on the floors, as part of the patient floor work group, or the pharmacy work group? If the pharmacists are assigned to pharmacy (the most common solution), how big is the organization when it becomes desirable to split the pharmacists into two work groups?

As a result, there is no such thing as a perfect set of work groups. The conflicts arise again and again and must be met with supplementary arrangements to ensure an acceptable overall quality and cost. And, because

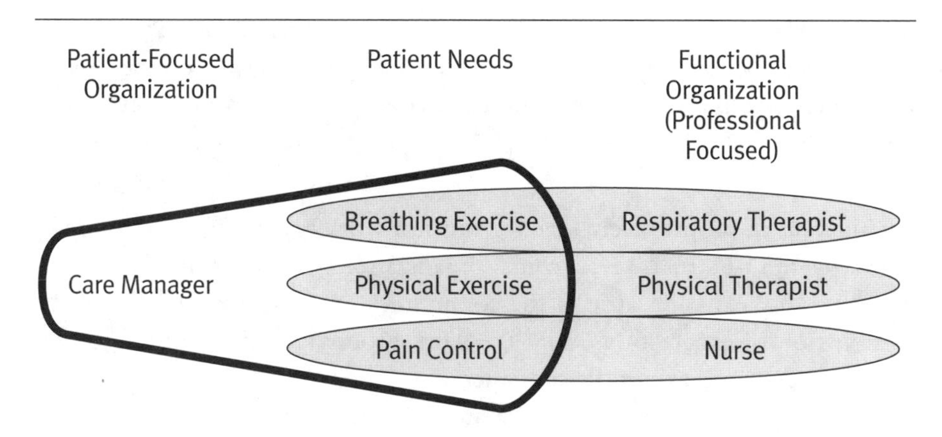

FIGURE 5.3 Patient Need and Professional Skill Conflicts

conditions change, there is no permanent solution. Thus, organization design is an ongoing process (see Figure 5.4).

Implementing the criteria

In every case where these conflicts arise, tradeoffs must be made to resolve them. Well-run hospitals consider the next two steps of organization design—setting the reporting hierarchy of middle management and building collateral communications—as ways of overcoming the weaknesses of a specific set of work groups. When the work group design process is properly done, it generates three results:

1. It specifies the work groups and the group leaders.
2. It identifies the tradeoffs, or departures from criteria, that were made to resolve particular conflicts.
3. It suggests hierarchical and collateral relationships that will optimize these tradeoffs.

In other words, there are always three avenues to organizational improvement: changing the work groups, revising the middle management structure, and strengthening collateral relationships.

Grouping Work Groups

Once work groups are formed, they can themselves be grouped, creating the traditional hierarchical accountability structure fanning outward from the

ANY REAL RESPONSIBILITY CENTER CONTAINS INHERENT CONFLICTS FROM THE DESIGN CRITERIA.

FIGURE 5.4 The Inherent Conflict in Responsibility Center Design

governing board. There are many ways to accomplish this, and local conditions are always an important factor in the final result. The two most common issues are structuring the organization as a whole and structuring the operations components.

Structuring the organization as a whole

The linking of progressively larger groups of work groups creates the traditional pyramidal structure of formal organizations, as shown in Figure 5.5. The structure exists because of the communication links and because of the aggregation of expectations from the work groups. Monitors of aggregates are often identified as **middle managers**.

The formal organization hierarchy is made real by formalizing information flow as well as authority and accountability through the middle managers. The hierarchy is the designated channel by which expectations are negotiated, exchanging information in both directions until the external needs and governing board strategies are matched by commitments on the part of divisions and individual work groups. It is also the channel for the distribution of performance information, with the reports of actual performance and comparison to expectation reflecting the accountability of each level. A specific measure, such as patient satisfaction scores, can be reported to an individual work group, an aggregate of several similar work groups, and a healthcare system as a whole, as indicated in Figure 5.6. At each level, the routine report gives the individual values and the average of the units directly accountable. The values for the units in the hierarchy below those reporting directly are

FIGURE 5.5 Linking Work Groups into the Accountability Hierarchy

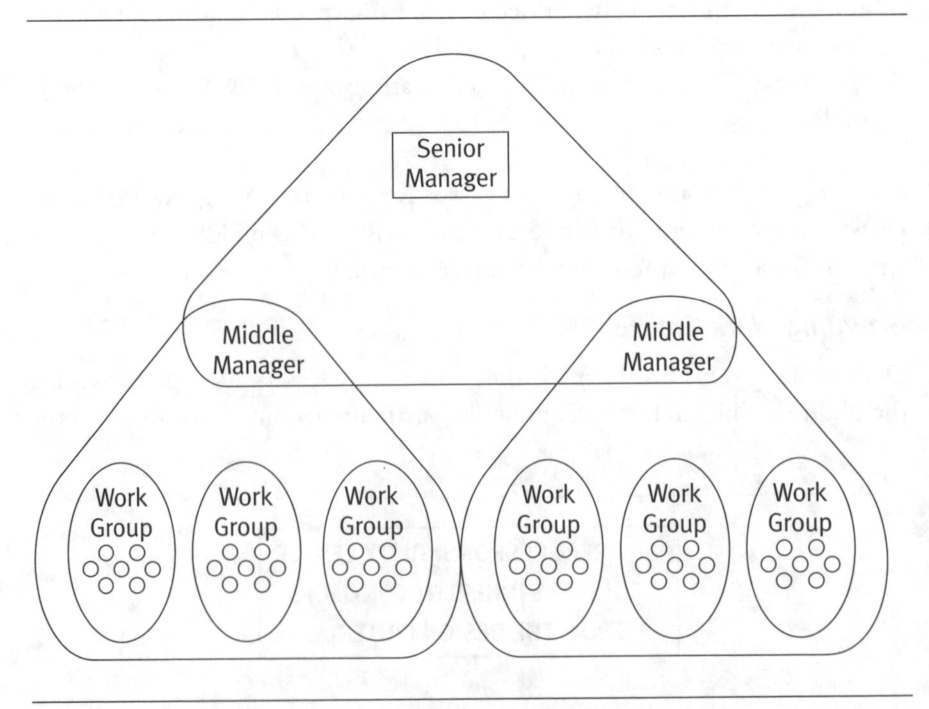

not reported; they are available on request. The process is informally called "rolling up" the information.

As Mintzberg suggests, it is relatively easy to tie elements of the organization horizontally as well as vertically. The information flows for negotiation and monitoring can specify as many ties to the technical and support activities as necessary.[14] Technical and logistic support units can establish specific assignments between their work groups and operational core work groups. Such an association allows the technical and logistic units to subdivide their work according to line clients, developing expertise and encouraging a strong relationship.

The function of middle management is to facilitate the effective performance of the work groups. The agreement with the work groups is one of assurances from the organization and expectations accepted by the group, where the assurances to one group are often the expectation of another. For example, a patient care unit might have an expectation on patient satisfaction. Achieving the expectation would require satisfactory plant services, so that the amenities on the unit (heat, light, appearance, cleanliness) were maintained. The middle manager's linking function includes making sure the plant expectations are achieved. Middle managers often coordinate two or more work groups so that both can achieve their expectations.

The middle managers' first task is to deliver on the assurances. Their second is to assist the work groups in meeting their expectations. They communicate open systems needs downward and subordinates' views upward.

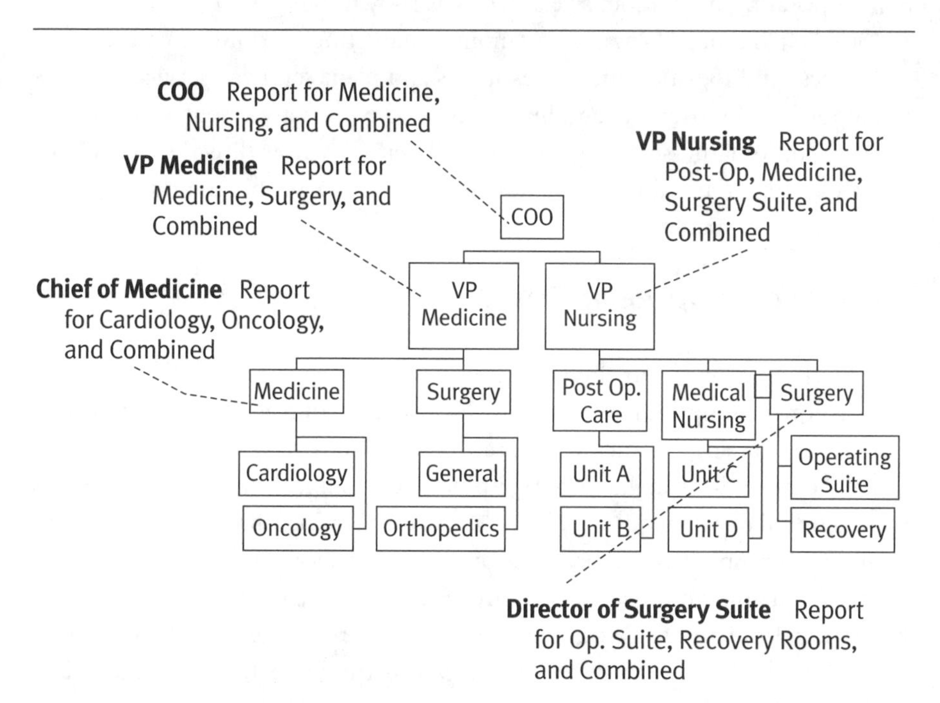

FIGURE 5.6
Vertical Information Flows in a Functional Accountability Hierarchy

They are accountable upward for adherence to agreed-upon expectations, downward for resolving issues their subordinates cannot, and both ways for negotiating the expectations. That is to say, middle managers have an explicit obligation to respond to their subordinates as well as to their superiors. Their contribution is now frequently evaluated by all these people, a process called "360-degree review." This perspective of middle management is contrary to the popular perspective, which views middle managers as "bosses." Substantial training and reinforcement is necessary to imbed the new philosophy.

Mintzberg notes that the parts of the pyramid all have boundary-spanning activities with each other and often with the external environment. Some of the accountability hierarchies serve the central purpose of the organization and are called the **operating core** (traditionally **line units**), while others serve **technical** and **logistic support** activities (traditionally called **staff units**), and still others constitute the **strategic apex**.[15]

Mintzberg's model (Figure 5.7) fits healthcare organizations well. It underlies the three parts of the text.

- *Governance.* The strategic apex of Mintzberg's model, is responsible for external relations, surveillance, and strategic responses.
- *Caring.* The "line" of the healthcare organization delivers service to the ultimate customer or patient. The caring system includes all the professional caregivers. The emergence of the healthcare organization from its predecessor hospitals and independent physician offices is marked by the formal incorporation of physicians, but leading organizations are incorporating comprehensive services as shown in Figure 3.3.
- *Learning.* Technical (finance, planning, marketing, and information services) and logistic (human resources and plant services) services supporting the strategic and line units. These units are essential to the operation of large-scale organizations. Their growth is directly related to the organization's ability to handle more complex problems and to replace smaller enterprises.

Organizing the Operating Core

The functional clinical organization

The work groups within the operating core are formed using the same criteria as for forming individual groups. They are traditionally formed around functional (nursing, medicine, laboratory, etc.) activities, with separate functional organizations at large geographic sites. Clinical care has been given by functional organizations for decades. The operating core of the traditional community hospital as it appeared around 1985 is shown in Figure .8. Clinical services, nursing, and medical staff are separate, and all are organized around professional functions. Two major problems have emerged under the impact of external cost and quality pressures. One is the inflexibility of Figure 5.8. The other is the development of physician accountability.

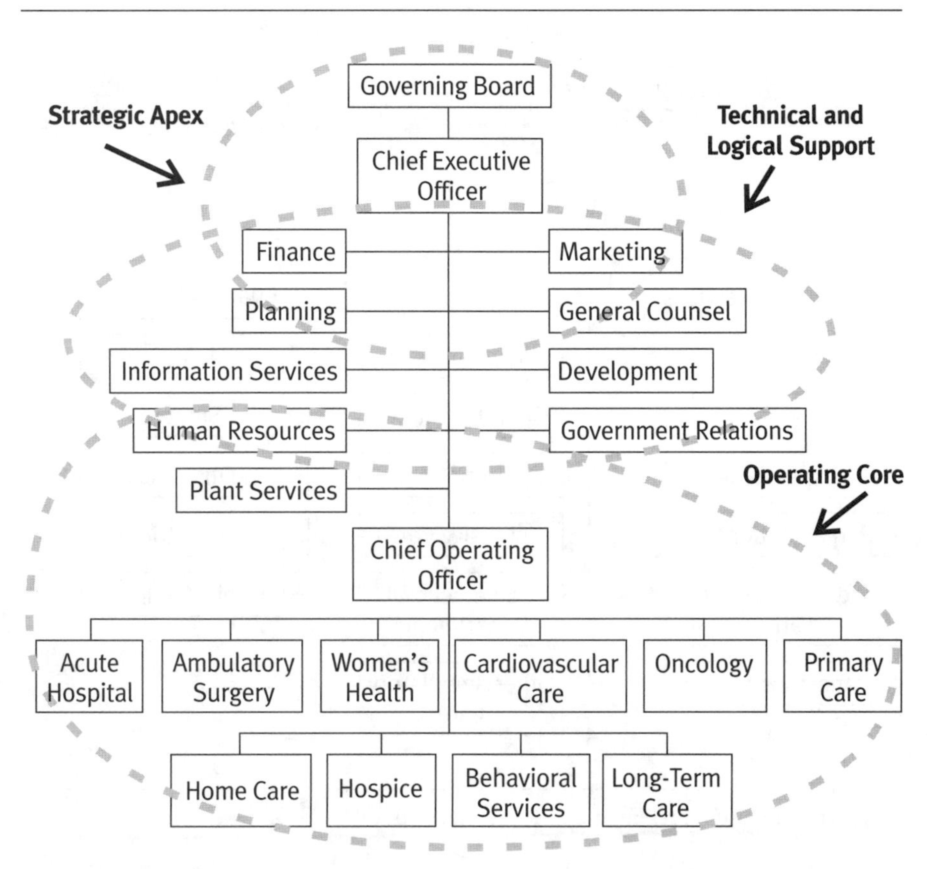

FIGURE 5.7 Accountability Hierarchy of a Large Healthcare Organization, After Mintzberg

Adapted from Mintzberg, *The Structuring of Organizations*, 18–35.

The organization of Figure 5.8 has one great strength, that the hierarchical chains—medicine, nursing, and the clinical support services—have strong professional content. Participants in each group share similar training, usually regulated by licensure or certification. The work groups can make use of their staff's professional knowledge, skills, and socialization to define and control activities. As a result, peers confer about highly technical matters, and consensus about a new practice can be reached quickly, unless it crosses hierarchical lines.

Conversely, the Figure 5.8 organization creates a large number of hierarchies with a tendency to concern themselves with their own objectives rather than the organization's. Disparaging terms, such as "smokestacks" and "silos" have been used. The professional hierarchies all pressure the executive office to give them equal recognition, regardless of their relative contributions. This results in many short hierarchies, such as social services and cardiopulmonology, and a few long and complex ones, such as nursing or laboratory. As a result, middle managers on the same level have vastly different hierarchies reporting to them. The professions seize upon tasks,

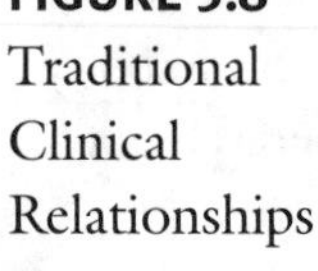

FIGURE 5.8
Traditional Clinical Relationships

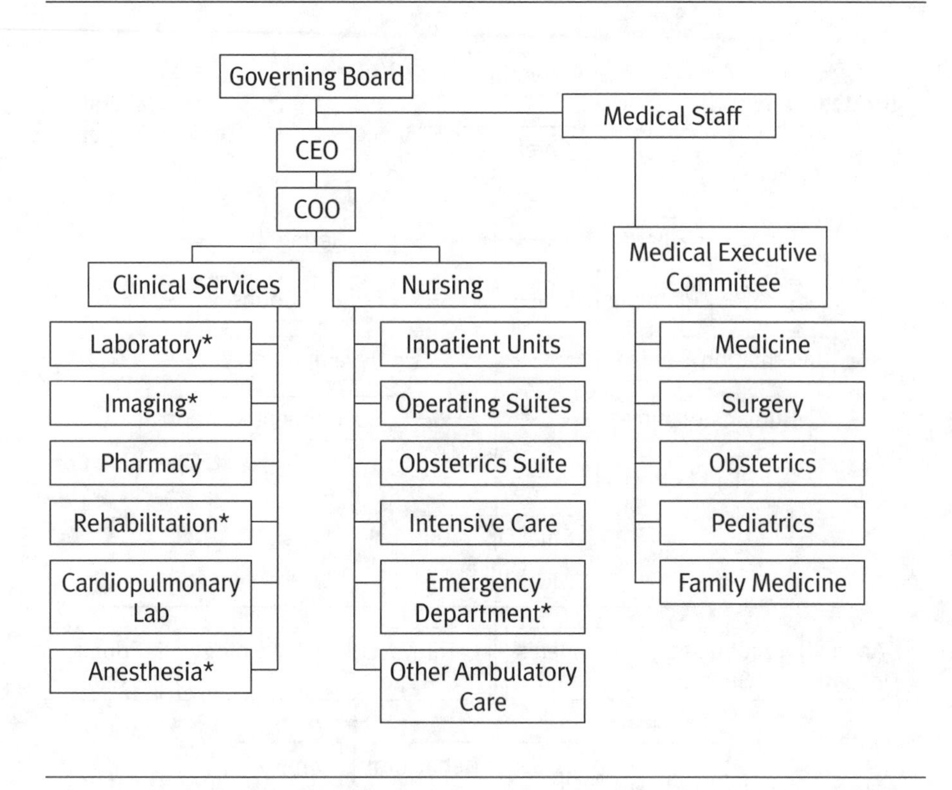

*Departments also represented on the medical staff.

such as drawing a blood specimen or taking an electrocardiogram, and insist that their group is the only one who can train and supervise workers in that task. Finally, and most distressingly, the silos "pass the buck." "It's not our fault," they say, "It's the other silo's fault." The tendency of the professions to proliferate, driven by the increasing specialization of science, has emphasized the weaknesses of the conventional organization. There are more professions, more hierarchies, and more concerns about the weakness of the conventional organization in 1999 than there were in 1960.

Six approaches help overcome the silo phenomenon:

1. Build on the informal organization and the professional commitment of healthcare workers to do a good job. A culture encouraging cooperation and reinforcing the need to succeed as a whole will help people collaborate. Leadership example and formal incentives can help.[16]
2. Deliberately design performance measures, information systems, and incentives to encourage collaboration. If a work group has expectations that can only be met by collaboration, it will collaborate. Conversely, if its expectations cover only things it can do on its own, it will resist collaboration.[17]

3. Use designated "liaison positions" to encourage information transfer.[18] These are particularly useful in relating line to technical and logistic support units. They also appear in routine interfacing tasks such as patient scheduling positions.
4. Rely on the linking function of line managers.[19] The middle manager or executives can be the intermediaries for two or more of the units reporting to them.
5. Use the collateral organization to design expectations and work processes optimizing the whole.[20]
6. Formalize multiple accountabilities in a matrix structure.

Successful healthcare organizations rely constantly on the first four. The fifth, using the collateral organization, and the sixth, matrix structures, are discussed below.

Expanding physician accountability

For many years it was common to indicate the hospital medical staff as a separate and distinct organization. Varieties of reporting relationships were used, many of them deliberately ambiguous, to explain how the medical staff, executive office, and governing board shared responsibilities. There was also a tendency to treat the medical staff organization as a parliamentary body representing the wishes of the staff majority rather than responding to the exchange needs of the organization.

The pressure for improved cost and quality has moved thinking steadily away from this view. Although many are concerned with the need to protect the physician's independent authority in patient care, a medical staff hierarchy under the executive office, similar to that of nursing or finance, is now common. The medical staff hierarchy has long been divided according to clinical specialties. In recent years, as the need for quality, economy, and appropriateness of care has increased, each specialty has begun to accept accountability for episodes of care. Following principles of continuous improvement and the new approaches to accountability shown in Figure 5.2,[21] the members of the specialty reach a prospective consensus on the diagnostic studies, treatment, and acceptable outcomes for groups of similar patients. As discussed in Chapter 8, these agreements are increasingly formalized under the label of patient care protocols or guidelines, thus expanding the accountability commitment of the formal hierarchy. Physician autonomy is protected by allowing each doctor to depart from the guidelines with documentation of the necessity.

The emerging development in clinical organization is disease-oriented organization called patient-focused care. For example, an orthopedic care center focused on fractures, corrective surgery, and joint replacement would include several different functions from Figure 5.8, but the accountability would be to the center, not the functional manager. A women's health center would assume all the birthing functions outright, but would have a similar subset for gynecological surgery, nursing, and imaging. It also might have a focused primary care activity. These examples are shown in Figure 5.9. Organizations that have established patient-focused units report significant improvements in cost, satisfaction, and quality of care.[22]

The service line organization

The ultimate result of patient-focused care would be complete organizational units for each disease group. Market-oriented analyses quickly reveal other categories that can substitute for functional organization.[23] Common examples include segmentation by demography (women's health, children's hospital), disease (oncology, mental health) or treatment resources (home care, nursing home). Organizations of this type are called **service lines** or **business units**. Large healthcare organizations are creating more of them, and some independent organizations are appearing.[24] Service lines can also include non-healthcare activities, such as health insurance.

As Figure 5.9 shows, the typical service line organization is often functional inside. That is, the women's health unit tends to be a smaller copy of the original functional organization. In cases in which patients need services not in the unit itself, the service line organization must contract with a functional organization. Thus, the silo problem is not fully solved. Service lines also may differ radically in their expectations. For example, a long-term care division would have no direct accountability to professional units providing clinical services in an acute inpatient division. As a result, it might depart from the standards of quality expected in the rest of the organization. Conversely, if the traditional clinical organization is followed, nursing and medicine in

FIGURE 5.9 Examples of Patient-Focused Organizations

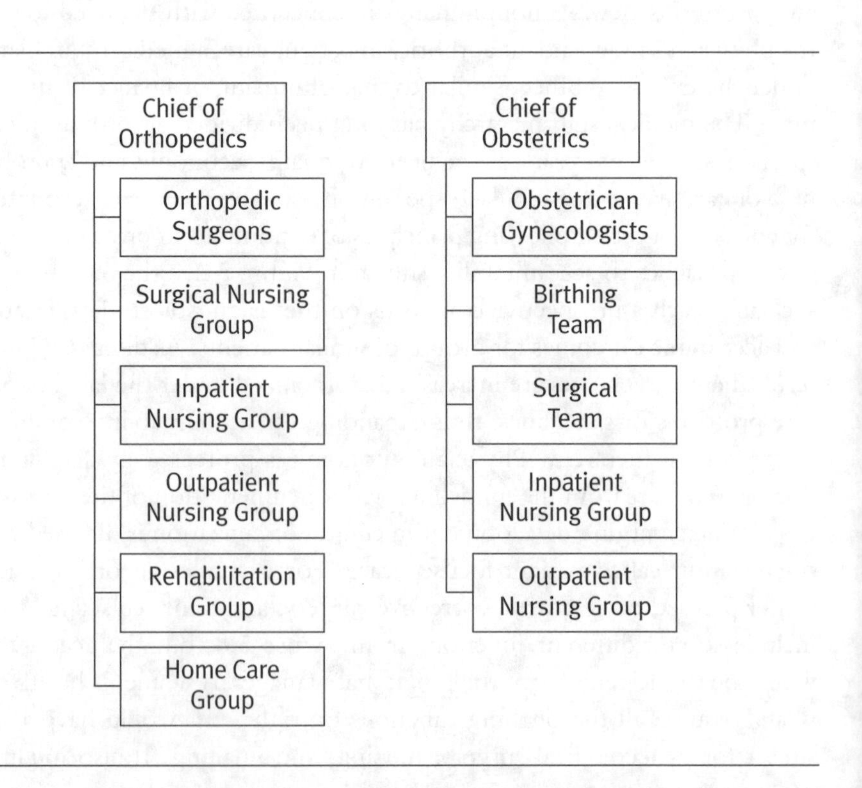

long-term care have no accountability for the cost or quality of overall service provided the long-term care patients. They might give long-term care patients lower priority, or even ignore them. Matrix organization designs, discussed below, attempt to address these problems.

The Collateral Organization, or Decision-Making Structure

Whether patient-focused or traditional, the accountability hierarchy is designed to give care. It starts stopped hearts, replaces organs, cures infections, delivers babies, and carries out thousands of specific tasks in the process. A modern healthcare organization cannot survive by current operations alone, however. It must also set goals, identify alternatives, resolve conflicts, set priorities, and build consensus, and it must do these things in ways that empower its members. Theoretically, no decision that affects a member's rights or abilities should be made without his or her awareness and understanding, and as many decisions as possible should have member consent. The **collateral organization**, a system of task forces, committees, and ad hoc groups is used to bring different perspectives on issues to the table, discuss, and resolve them. It accommodates most of the nonclinical decisions and some important clinical ones.

No real organization could function without an effective collateral organization. Without the means of addressing common problems, such as future agendas and expenditure priorities, and means of relating between the line accountability chains, the conflict, confusion, and tension would soon stop any healthcare organization from functioning. The inventions that permit the growth of large organizations outside of healthcare, like the nineteenth-century railroads and the twentieth-century chemical and automobile industries, are largely in the collateral organization.[25,26]

Collateral organization always involves two or more units of the formal hierarchy. It often spans units in different hierarchies and several different levels of the hierarchy. Most senior and middle managers are involved in several collateral activities. Figure 5.10 gives some common examples. Collateral relationships are either permanent or ad hoc; in general they shift much more often than hierarchical ones. The well-designed organization attempts to move the consensus as quickly as possible into the formal accountability hierarchy where quantitative expectations can be negotiated to encourage efficient responses. Most institutions have several planning committees operating simultaneously at various levels of the organization. Many are formed as issues arise and disbanded after a single decision. A capital budget committee is needed at least annually, and is usually permanent, like the credentials committee of the medical staff. At operational levels, groups such as the pharmacy committee and the medical data committee are permanent resources.

FIGURE 5.10 Examples of the Collateral Organization

Committee Title	Purpose	Membership	Principal Technical Support	Duration
Stratetic Planning	Develop and evaluate strategic options	Board members, CEO, COO, CFO, VP of planning	Planning	Permanent
Programmatic Planning	Develop and evaluate specific programs and implementation options	Managers of units directly involved, planning staff, finance staff	Planning	Ad Hoc (one for each important project)
Pharmacy and Therapeutics	Decide drugs for hospital use; study and improve drug costs	Physicians representing several specialties, nurses, chief pharmacist	Pharmacy	Permanent
Capital Budget Request	Prioritize competing requests for capital funds	Medical staff leaders, executive office, clinical service representatives, CFO	Finance	Annual
Outpatient Scheduling Study	Improve patient service in outpatient areas	Medical, nursing, clinical service managers directly involved	Management Engineering	Ad Hoc
Clinical Protocol Development	Develop care plan for specific diagnosis	Medical leaders from involved specialties, nursing, clinical support services	Medical Records, Information Services, Finance	Ad Hoc

Yet because it does not actually give care, the entire collateral organization is overhead, a cost burden on the line. As the market gets more demanding, decision processes must yield more difficult decisions better and faster, just as the line must learn to give higher quality, more efficient care. The executive group usually develops and manages the collateral organization, with substantial input from others. Improving the collateral organization calls for understanding the kinds of decisions to be made, developing new patterns of delegation, and supporting the decision structure effectively.

Classifying Decisions

As it resolves the problems presented by its stakeholders, develops management strategy, and pursues continuous improvement of operations, any firm or organization must make countless decisions. It must reach these continually and collaboratively among both worker and customer stakeholders, building new consensuses as needs, power relationships, and technologies change.[27,28] The decisions can be grouped into the five categories shown in Figure 5.11: mission or vision (what the business is and why); resource allocation (services, quality, volume, price, and profit); implementation (operating procedures and technology); human resources (recruiting, selecting, training, and motivating

FIGURE 5.11
A Classification of Decision Processes

Type	Level	
	Strategic	Programmatic
Mission/Vision	Environmental assessment	Marketing plans
	Strategic plans	Specific joint ventures
Resource Allocation	Service plan	Facilities plan
		Human resources plan
	Financial plan	Operating budget
		Capital budget
	Technology selection	Equipment selection
Implementation	Personnel selection	Individual credentialing, recruitment, and development
	Human resource policies	Incentive programs
	Process design	Patient care protocols
		Policies and procedures
Organizational	Accountability hierarchy	Information plan
	Management system	Participation in care teams
		Conflict resolution mechanism
		Appeals mechanism

personnel); and organizational design (decision procedures, communication, and authority).[29]

Decisions in each category are similar in information requirements, the nature of the discussion, and the kinds of members who should participate. Many of the most important decisions are parts of sequences that start at the most universal or strategic level of the organization and are worked out in detail among many small groups. This concept is also reflected in Figure 5.11, in the columns "strategic" and "programmatic." Strategic decisions are those affecting the organization as a whole, including setting the rules for programmatic decisions. Programmatic ones are those directed at specific programs or groups. (Admittedly, real life processes are iterative and overlapping compared to the neat categories. Real decisions require substantial checking, both up and down and back and forth across the rows and columns of the figure.)

One way to promote effective decision making is to develop common patterns or practices for each of the categories. Then members of the organization will understand that if they have a concern about a certain issue, the organization will address that issue in a predictable way and offer predictable opportunities to influence the outcome. Mission and vision setting define the organization, rest on environmental assessment, include partnerships with other organizations, and establish directions that guide all the remaining categories. At the programmatic level, they are implemented by specific contracts that are negotiated by teams from the units that will manage the contract. Resource allocation translates the mission and vision into long-range plans of services and finances at the strategic level and shorter term, more specific operating and capital budgets at the programmatic level. Implementation begins with leadership selection at the strategic level and is expanded into detailed operational procedures for each program. Human resources begins with overall policies on selection, training, and rewards and moves to staffing plans and training programs for each unit. Organization design establishes the formal structure of accountability and the roles and membership of standing and ad hoc committees. Policies for information access, conflict resolution, and performance evaluation should support the design. Much of the remaining chapters of the text is devoted to processes to decide the topics identified in the figure. This chapter, for example, addresses the organizational design processes.

Figure 5.11 is not the only way decision processes can be described, but it is a useful summary that parallels actual practice in leading healthcare organizations. Without some such systematic overview of decision processes, the collateral organization loses focus. Small groups of people make decisions that can be well-intentioned and even highly appropriate for their needs, but have disabling consequences for others. Issues affecting all, but not in an immediate or urgent way, get overlooked. Expediency and individual influence direct the organization, rather than carefully developed, broad consensus.

Achieving Effective Delegation

Certain guidelines apply to all categories of decisions in well-managed healthcare organizations. To build consensus, almost all decisions will be made by groups. To be effective, the groups must share common perspectives on the criteria for success, the rights of individual participants and stakeholder groups, and the rules for delegating.

Criteria for effective decisions

Good decisions support continuous improvement of line activities. Improvement involves making economically viable and timely decisions, designing new processes, and getting widespread agreement and support within the empowerment concept. The twin tests of any decision are **realism** in the marketplace and **conviction** among those who must implement it. Realism means the decision will lead to a successful future for the enterprise. It will meet the test of competition. Conviction means that the decision is persuasive; that is, most members of the organization will believe that the decisions are realistic, and they as individuals will have a successful future.

Recognizing stakeholder rights

Modern healthcare organizations operate in an environment in which all stakeholders have opinions and expect their opinions to receive serious attention. Hospitals earlier in the twentieth century were a different environment where traditional treaties assigned authority for decisions and rigidly divided the organization "turf" among the stakeholders.[30] The doctor knew best, the nurse was "his handmaiden," and the patient followed orders rather than participating in care. Trustees felt they handled the business matters and often thought of themselves as beholden to the institution, rather than the constituencies it serves.[31] Managers thought of themselves as the third leg of a (wobbly) three-legged stool with the physicians and the trustees.[32]

Ideas like these fail both realism and conviction tests. (Few will regret their passing; they are beginning to sound sexist and even absurd.) The twenty-first century requires a much more democratic and dynamic structure of decision-making authority. People from a variety of backgrounds must learn to share decisions they once considered their professional prerogatives and also must learn to make decisions outside their professional areas. People will have both cognitive and emotional difficulties with the transition. At a cognitive level, training can overcome ignorance of outsiders' values and lack of technical knowledge. A broader fact base in the presentation of each decision will help people reach beyond their field. The education will be specific rather than general. Successful organizations will teach people how to choose between trans plasminogen activase (TPA) and streptokinase, not how to be cardiologists and health economists. This expanded cognitive requirement is a major force in the growth of information systems, discussed in Chapters 9 and 10.

Coaching, leadership, and practice will help the emotional adjustment to new decision roles. Revising the mission and vision starts a process of reeducation because it focuses all stakeholders' attention on what the organization in fact is—the best device available to the stakeholders to achieve common goals. It is reviewed annually in part to reinforce everybody's adjustment to new ways. The initial years particularly require leadership skills, patience, and sensitivity from healthcare managers. Beyond revisiting the vision, it is important to reinforce the new style with examples and cases showing its advantages. That is, the decision system must advertise its successes. So the first problems attacked are easy ones where most people agree improvement is possible. The capital and operating budget programs evolve over several years as people become comfortable with the accountability involved. Pilot programs test next steps, provide visible examples, and develop coaches. At each step, victories are deliberately identified and celebrated.

Building effective delegation

New rules must replace the old turf domains for delegating decisions. The realism criterion demands continuous improvement of both cost and quality. The conviction criterion must assure all stakeholders that their individual interests will not be subverted by decisions beyond their immediate surveillance.[33] The processes to meet these criteria must integrate complex patient and customer values with extensive technical knowledge from a wide span of professions. The integration should be complete, timely, and efficient. A missing or misstated stakeholder or technical viewpoint may lead to failure. Decisions should be prompt, if only to clear the field for the next problem. Stakeholder gridlock will be fatal. Finally, the decisions should be efficient, optimizing the scarce time of the decision makers.

Dynamic, accountable delegation is used to meet these criteria. "Dynamic" means that the topics are selected by the central governance structure according to stakeholder needs related to the topic itself, rather than unvarying treaties. There are no sacred cows or private domains. "Accountable" protects the right to have one's view heard if necessary. Each stakeholder group understands that it has a reliable mechanism to a fair hearing on any question, at its discretion. Such a mechanism rarely existed under the old treaties. "Delegation" assigns decisions to the stakeholders most important to their implementation. Within accountability limits, delegation is complete. The boundaries of an acceptable decision are established in advance, and decisions within the boundaries are accepted without debate. The decisions are not micromanaged by meddling or ritualistic reviews.

The most widespread model of successful accountable delegation is the medical staff credentialing system, where decisions about individual physicians are made by physicians professionally competent to do so, but the criteria, process, and result are subject to review by a governing board representing a much broader constituency.

Dynamic accountability allows special committees to negotiate specific conflicts or directly represent a minority position, such as placing physicians on governing boards. At the same time, it allows a reversibility the old rules never had. A specific decision or a class of decisions can always be reviewed if some stakeholders feel aggrieved enough. In practice a very small fraction of the delegated decisions is challenged. This is because the delegates understand the guidelines they receive from the other stakeholders and understand that it is in their interest to make the right to review moot by accommodating others' needs in the initial decision.

Under accountable delegation, the governing board sets the mission and vision on behalf of the customer stakeholders, understanding that broad member participation and acceptance are essential. Doctors and employees buy into the mission by making suggestions, but ultimately they do so by signing on. Beyond the mission and vision, the more abstract, global, or central the decision (generally toward the top and left of Figure 5.11), the greater the need for direct customer participation. Trustees focus on the scope of services, long-range financial plan, and budget guidelines. These decisions provide patterns for delegation of the balance of the resource allocation and implementation decisions to insiders.

The larger the contribution of clinical knowledge to the solution (generally toward the bottom and right of Figure 5.11), the more authority to propose solutions is delegated to the inside stakeholders. Most budget detail, care plan, and implementation decisions are delegated to insiders held accountable to the mission and vision and overall cost constraints. Cross-functional teams are also accountable delegation. In the case of clinical guidelines, the delegation is actually from individual physicians to the team. It involves admitting the realism of customer input, accepting the market pressures for cost and quality.

Supporting the Decision System

The executive office takes a direct role in designing the collateral organizations processes as it does for the identification of work groups and the design of the accountability hierarchy. Under the concept of accountable delegation, it carries out these responsibilities with due regard to the needs of the stakeholders. Conversely, other parts of the organization take leading roles for the rest of Figure 5.11. The executive office oversees the process, but generally plays a supporting, rather than a direct, role. (This means that executive managers do not make the mission and vision, resource allocation, operations, and human resource decisions, a critical distinction between modern and traditional bureaucratic perspectives that often surprises students. They see management as captaining the ship, shouting orders over the gale. It's not. It's convincing the largest possible group of people to give the largest possible amount of their resources to organizational success.)

Designing the decision process

There are four parts to designing an effective decision process. First, the rules guiding the process must have recognized authorities.[34] Decision-making rules tend to be easy to forget and even easier to attack when the decision itself is not what the stakeholder hoped for. Conflicts about the rules can disable the entire continuous improvement effort. The bylaws for the board and medical staff constitute the major authorities, documenting agreements that are historically tested and formally recognized. Procedure manuals, memoranda from accountable individuals, and the organization's culture define less important ones. Well-written rules develop authority as they are used. Decisions reached and conflicts resolved become a body of "case law" that is accepted by all. As good rules become accepted, they legitimate the process and diminish conflict.

Second, good design must include appeals mechanisms for both the specific decision and the decision process. Good design strives to eliminate the need for appeals, and, in fact, appeals are rare. However, to meet the conviction criterion, any stakeholder who feels aggrieved enough must be able to appeal either process or result. If the appeal generates a sufficient constituency for change, change can occur. If not, the individual can accept the decision or leave the organization. The decision system can do no more than provide an avenue for prompt and fair hearing, but it must do that much. The board and its major committees will be important as the final appeals bodies.

Third, the rules are supported by appointing and charging committees, setting agendas, establishing timetables, keeping minutes, training people to follow procedures, and supplying information and coaches. Leaders in all parts of the organization must know what the relevant bylaws and procedures say, or how to find out. A beginning doctor, worker, or trustee is not expected to memorize the decision-making rules, but rather to know and trust someone who does. Knowing or finding the answer is properly the role of every first-line supervisor and medical division chief. Training these people in decision making is an obvious step, already incorporated in the continuous improvement programs of well-managed institutions.[35]

Fourth, the decision system must be enforced. A few flagrant departures can destroy it. Exceptions to the rules and special pleadings beyond the appeals process must be strongly and promptly resisted. Enforcement means that behavior is redirected according to the rules. Punishment is not involved. Except in the rare case of deliberately destructive behavior, the individuals are simply shown that following procedures is the effective path.

Figure 5.12 includes some examples of the delegation process. The accountability of the sector to which the decision is delegated is reflected in the charges and the authorities. Ideally, the charge should reflect the limits of the acceptable decisions and the authorities for the rules governing process. In reality, many of these messages are implicit, taken for granted in the organization culture. Others are vague or ambiguous, because the various stakeholders have not fully formulated their own views. As organization members become familiar with delegated decision making, they learn to overcome these difficulties. The enterprise as a whole learns ways to address tough questions fairly and effectively and moves ahead of its competitors as a result.

Using middle management effectively

Middle managers are usually professionally trained people with unique insights into the trends of specific technology. Their responsibilities emphasize being able to communicate across reporting hierarchies, and they are members and leaders of most of the committees, task forces, and work groups that constitute the collateral structure.

In poorly designed organizations, middle managers are so consumed by daily problems that they have no time for the advance planning that the collateral organization must do. A catch-22 is involved: middle managers are overworked, so they are tempted to add more middle managers; but adding more middle managers intensifies the communication problem without necessarily improving productivity or quality. Recent successful approaches have empowered work groups and group leaders to solve their own problems, limited the activities and improved the effectiveness of the collateral organization, and reduced the middle management structure.

To make the improved structures work, middle managers must be effective both in teaching their work groups how to use their empowerment effectively and in participating in collateral organizations. Middle managers often lack training in management because they are promoted from clinical professions. They sometimes come with dysfunctional accountability perspectives learned from community stereotypes. They must be taught skills including problem analysis, coaching, and meeting management. One of the tasks

Decision	Committee	Delegation From	Delegation To	Accountability	Authority
Financial Guidelines	Finance	Governing Board	Finance Committee, Finance, CEO	Strategic and financial plans	Bylaws
New Program Evaluation	Ad Hoc	Executive Office	Caregivers and Managers Directly Involved	Mission, cost, quality	Budget procedure manual
Drug Selection and Use	Pharmacy and Therapeutics	Medical Executive Committee	Designated Physician and Nursing Representatives, Pharmacist	Quality, cost, physician satisfaction	Medical staff bylaws
Outpatient Scheduling	Ad Hoc	Executive Office	Caregivers and Managers Directly Involved	Cost, output, patient and physician satisfaction	Traditionally accepted
Clinical Protocol	Ad Hoc	Medical Staff Department	Involved Specialists, Nurses	Quality, cost, patient, physician, and nurse satisfaction	Medical staff bylaws

FIGURE 5.12 Structuring the Collateral Organization

of senior management is to help middle managers by coaching, by graduated experience opportunities, and by example.

Extending the Formal Hierarchy: The Matrix Organization

Matrix organizations are those in which work groups or middle managers have explicit, permanent, dual accountability. Matrix reporting can be developed around any pair of the potential conflict points: geography, time, skill or profession, task or patient. Figure 5.13 illustrates the underlying concept. In each case, the work group would have only the vertical accountability under the traditional structure; it has a dual accountability under the matrix. The housekeeping work group in the surgical suite, Figure 5.13C, reports both to the head of the housekeeping department and to the supervisor of operating room nurses. The nursing work group for orthopedic patients (5.13D) reports both to the supervisor for surgical nursing and to the orthopedic service of the medical staff.

Most of these relationships are already recognized in the informal or collateral organizations. The matrix organization can be thought of as adding accountability to the collateral relationship as well as the functional one. The practical effect of the matrix organization is to emphasize the most important cross-functional responsibilities by making them permanent and adding them to the expectation setting process and to conventional reporting relationships.

FIGURE 5.13 Elementary Models of Matrix Organizations

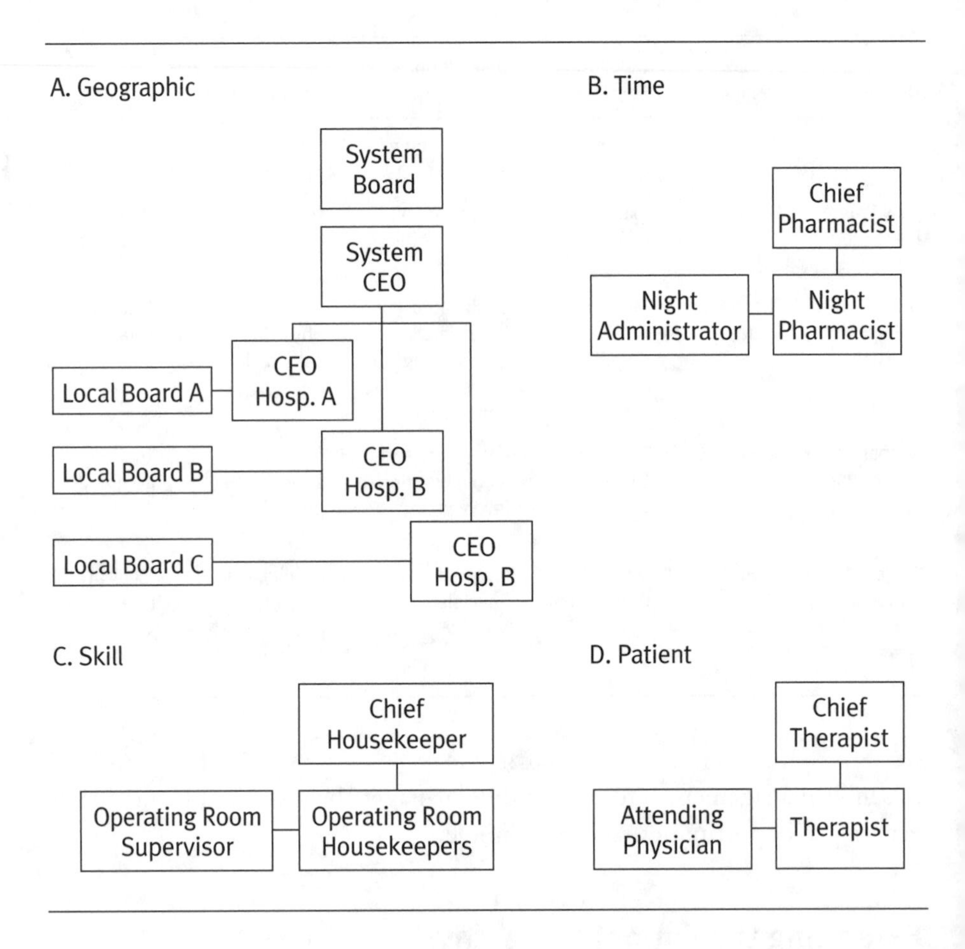

It has intuitive appeal in healthcare organizations because it parallels the informal relationships between the silos that have permitted the formal organization to work as well as it does. Matrix organization explicitly defines the most important obligation outside the group leader's own profession or trade.

The matrix organization concept has had a long history as a tempting device.[36] It has proven more difficult to implement in healthcare than it might at first appear,[37] for two reasons. First, although the silo problems frequently involve several professions or hierarchies, it is difficult to create a multiple reporting matrix. The intrinsic conflicts with the units *not* formalized in the matrix remain; indeed, they can be exacerbated. Second, the dual reporting structure can easily deteriorate into a competitive relationship among three people, the group leader and the two supervisors. (For example, consider the opportunities to form two-on-one adversarial pairs in Figure 5.13 among the orthopedic head nurse, the orthopedists, and a nursing supervisor whose specialty is surgical nursing.)[38]

The first problem has been met by making the second accountability to a cross-functional team, such as an orthopedic service line team. The physical therapists in Figure 5.10 would understand their accountability as to the chief physical therapist and the PT department and to the orthopedics work group.

The second problem is managed by using multidimensional performance measurement and getting all parties to agree to the expectations. This is in fact the device that subordinates the silo to the patients' cross-functional needs. In both cases, the solutions have been made practical by the improved information capabilities of the organization.

The matrix solution explicitly identifies a dual accountability. In contrast, the service line approach uses a single accountability to the service line group and effectively reduces the functional group to a collateral capacity. Matrix organizations between the professional functions of the traditional clinical hierarchy and the market-oriented service lines or business units hold great promise. Other matrix designs balancing relationships that are less directly market-oriented appear to be useful in specific kinds of healthcare organizations.

The matrix concept can also be applied in what are called multidivisional or multi-unit organizations, as shown in Figure 5.13A.[39] Matrix accountability is usually helpful when the subsidiaries reach sufficient size to be competitive on their own. They are held formally accountable to a local governance group and the central organization. The subsidiaries of Henry Ford Health System, Figure 3.12, are an example. Although for-profit systems tend to avoid a matrix structure, not-for-profit systems often decentralize the governance function, centralizing only some elements of strategic planning and finance, and giving at least the subsidiary CEO an explicit dual accountability.[40]

Multi-Unit Organizations

A single healthcare facility might begin as an informal organization of less than a dozen people. By the time it reached 50 people, it would have a formal hierarchy and some established collateral activities. By developing these three parts of the organization, it could grow to a few thousand members, the size of a large hospital or very large clinic. But if it then decided to acquire a second healthcare organization, particularly one in a different geographic or product market, new organizational questions would arise. The healthcare industry has been moving rapidly toward that situation. As noted in Chapter 1, more than half of all hospitals are now in multi-unit organizations. The largest and most structured of these arrangements, integrated healthcare systems, have been thriving. Multi-organizational arrangements tie together formal units capable of independent existence and often having independent competitors. They constitute a new and rapidly evolving level of organization in healthcare. Three issues contribute to understanding the new level: why multi-organization systems are formed, what their components can be, and how they are structured.

Why Multi-Unit Organizations Are Created

Conceptually, from the theories of open systems and strategic management, organizations grow in ways that increase the satisfaction of their stakeholders, and they stop growing when the next increment would represent a net decrease in satisfaction.[41] A certain amount of trial and error and variation around the prevailing level of achievement is predictable. People will try to make an organization too ambitious and fail. Others will delay and be overtaken by successful larger and more innovative models.[42] Success will be widely copied and soon embedded in the prevailing practice. Organizations in general have become larger and more diverse as the management learned skills to make larger units more effective.

Large organizations have several advantages that make them attractive.

1. *Returns to size.* A larger organization of a single limited type is potentially more efficient and more responsive to a specific customer need than a small one. For example, an obstetrical delivery unit as it grows in size almost automatically encounters the following advantages:
   - The demand for services, while always randomly varying, becomes more stable, so that idle periods waiting for patients are reduced and average loads get much closer to peak loads. Thus, caregivers and facilities are more efficient.
   - Volumes of activity permit several skill levels of personnel. Assistants with less training can multiply the services of expensive professionals without impairing quality.
   - The volume of purchases allows the organization to negotiate better prices.
2. *Returns to scope of service.* Larger organizations can afford a wider array of services, making themselves more attractive to the market.
   - The small obstetrical unit might add prenatal care because it helps attract patients, reduces complications of childbirth (and therefore costs), and generates activities that can be done in the slack times when there are no deliveries.
   - It might then add other women's health services and well-child care because its market demanded them.
   - At larger volumes, the unit can support its own educational programs for patients and staff.
   - As it grows, the unit can afford to add specialty services, such as intensive neonatal care and services for high-risk mothers, that are used only rarely.
3. *Improved quality.* Caregiver teams do better with practice. Outcomes from higher volume institutions are superior to those in smaller ones.[43]
4. *Improved control of the environment.* Larger units can be more effective in negotiating prices and conditions, allowing them to attract more patients and personnel.
   - As it grows, the obstetrical unit can attract the attention of powerful organizations that can be convinced to assist in meeting mutual goals. A large unit could approach the school system, the local government,

and local industry to address problems of inadequate prenatal care and teenaged pregnancies.

- Representing a large number of influentials who are also voters, the organization can lobby more effectively and protect itself from adverse law and regulation. Licensure laws, government health insurance coverage, taxation, and employment regulation would all be important to the obstetrical unit.
- Controlling a large share of the market, the organization can affect the price it receives for services. It can lobby for increased Medicaid prices for obstetrical services. It can advertise to support demand at a profitable price. (Controlling the price of services sold is illegal under antitrust law in certain circumstances, but the proscription is not automatic until the seller approaches half of the total provider capability, is deliberately predatory, or colludes with other providers.)

5. *Improved opportunities for capital.* Multiple organization structures open new financial opportunities that expand the available funds or, in some cases, protect existing fund sources from risk or damage. The financial aspects of multiple corporate structures are discussed in Chapter 14.

Conversely, there are two forces that keep organizations from growing:

1. *Market limitations.* Geography, wealth, and taste cause both customers and caregivers to choose other organizations. For the obstetrics unit, there are only a certain number of patients within a reasonable travel time for obstetrical services. A fraction of these women may prefer a smaller competitor. Similarly, doctors and nurses may look on the organization as impersonal, rigid, or out-of-date, and choose other employment.
2. *Organizational limitations.* All organizations are prey to failure in their accountability hierarchy, where the subordinate units substitute their own goals for those of the collective, and in their collateral structures, where decisions get delayed, stalled, or diverted to special interests. In either case, the ability of the organization to satisfy its customers and workers declines. Large organizations represent large consensuses that may be difficult to build and even harder to hold together. The obstetric unit, having added units in several cities, may discover that those units run better by themselves than with a formal relationship.

Forms of Multi-Unit Organizations

There are two major forms of multi-unit organization. **Alliances** are interorganizational relations that are entered into primarily for strategic purposes.[44] They stop short of changing ownership and allow members to disaffiliate relatively easily and quickly. As a result, the central organization must spend considerable energy sustaining the internal relationships. It can undertake only activities that the entire body consents to, even though all members do not participate, thus severely restricting its scope and flexibility. There is reason to think alliances are inherently transient: They either evolve toward more centralized structures or they disappear.[45]

Multicorporate organizations involve separate corporate charters, with control expressed through ownership positions. Although the variations are limitless, three underlying schemes of multicorporate structures can be detected either alone or in combination in specific examples:

1. *Parent subsidiary.* A corporation may establish or acquire a wholly owned subsidiary that is usually dedicated to a specific activity. The most common example may be the creation of separate corporations, usually called *foundations* for managing endowment and frequently also for stimulating teaching and research. The foundation is usually tax exempt; the parent may or may not be. Alternatively, the subsidiary could be for-profit for a particularly risky activity or protection of existing tax advantages. It would either use its for-profit status to reward private investors or it would be engaging in an activity categorized as taxable unrelated income by the IRS.
2. *Holding company.* This common model consists of one parent and a variety of subsidiaries that may differ in tax structure, purpose, location, or other parameters. The holding company model retains certain central control, specified in the reserved powers discussed below, but offers great flexibility in protecting assets and tax advantages, developing partnerships, and expanding sources of capital.
3. *Joint venture.* Two or more parent corporations invest in a subsidiary. The reasons for separate incorporation may include risk in tax, but they are also likely to include the advantages of having additional investors. The most common form of partnership activity is a joint venture partnership. Shared service organizations constitute one form of joint venture. The parents are frequently otherwise competing hospital corporations. Another common form is a joint venture with individuals in the hospital's medical staff or with a corporate structure of the staff itself. The physician hospital organization is a joint venture.

How Components of Multi-Unit Organizations Are Described

Four distinct dimensions describe multi-unit organizations:

1. *Size* is most often measured by dollar volumes flowing through a corporate entity, but it can also be measured by numbers of customers, employees, or affiliated units.
2. *Geography* is the extent to which the units are in the same or different healthcare markets. Two systems equal in size, uniformity, and formality are different if one is concentrated in a single geographic market and the other operates in several markets. (Henry Ford Health System,

concentrated in southeast Michigan, and The Mayo Clinics, operating in Minnesota, Florida, and Arizona, are examples.)

3. *Uniformity* is the extent to which the units produce the same, complementary, or disparate scope of services. Structures that combine similar organizations (a chain of obstetrical delivery units, for example) are said to be horizontally integrated. Those combining complementary organizations (a prenatal care unit; a delivery unit; a well-baby and postpartum unit; and women's, children's, and adolescent primary care services, for example) are said to be vertically integrated. The ultimate vertical integration combines most ambulatory and inpatient acute care services and health insurance (Kaiser-Permanente, for example). **Diversified organizations** are composed of disparate services that are neither complementary nor competing. Diversification is rare in healthcare. A few hospitals own diverse businesses such as food and laundry services, for example.
4. *Formality* is measured by the degree to which the central or parent organization retains control. Structures that retain much control in the parent are said to be **centralized**. Those that allow much power in the subsidiary are **decentralized**.

How Multi-Unit Organizations Are Designed

The design of multi-unit organizations is an extension of the concepts of informal organization, formal hierarchy, collateral organization to a new level of complexity, because each of the units carries out these concepts already. Clearly, design must follow market realities; a focused organization of similar small clinics will not look like Kaiser-Permanente. The design process in use at present tends to accept as given the size, geography, and uniformity of the units and adjusts the formality to get optimal results from that configuration. Given the record to date, it is not surprising that there is no science of multi-organization design.[46]

Size of multi-unit organizations

The average size of comparable healthcare corporations has grown steadily in the past quarter century. Hospitals, nursing home chains, and HMOs all tend to be larger as corporate units. Even physician services, where the smallest possible unit, the solo practitioner, still remains, are organized into bigger units now than they were at the start of Medicare in 1967. The trend is clearly toward oligopolistic competition: A few organizations in each scope of service set compete in a single geographic area.

Geography

Many of the existing multi-unit organizations affiliate units that operate in separate geographic markets. Each unit competes with different corporations, under different laws and health insurance arrangements. Most of the religious hospital chains are examples. Before the 1990s, only a minority of multi-unit organizations pursued a strategy of growth within a single market. Vertically integrated models like Group Health of Puget Sound were relatively rare. Horizontally integrated models became more common as stronger hospitals in most larger cities acquired weaker competitors. There are now examples in most large cities.

U.S. cities differ significantly in many characteristics, including the incidence of disease and the quantities and costs of healthcare. They evolve at different rates and have different market interests at any one time. A central corporation that tries to impose a single approach (the use of HMO physician panels, for example) must find locations receptive to its philosophy. Conversely, an organization like a religious hospital chain that inherits its geographic locations will need more decentralization to succeed. However, a competing model does exist—if the service is narrowly defined and standardized to be optimally efficient, the central organization may compete successfully in many markets. Thus, fancy restaurants tend to be individually owned, but McDonald's sells worldwide. So far, there is no healthcare McDonald's.

Uniformity Although horizontal integration continues at a rapid pace within and across geographic markets, the trend of the 1990s is to vertical integration. The traditional hospital represents a kind of vertical integration, and a number of its components are copied by single service competitors like freestanding laboratories, drug stores, and clinics. In general, healthcare organizations are winning the competition against these entities, but the victory is less than decisive. Organizations integrating physician services are growing rapidly, and many of these are allied with healthcare organizations.[47] Healthcare systems or networks, which generally incorporate hospitals, medical organizations, and insurance intermediaries, have grown steadily since the passage of the HMO Act in 1972, and are growing rapidly at present. The trend suggests that the most common organization of the future will be integrated across all acute care services, will have extensive preventive services through alliances, and will have a substantial chronic care capability. They are likely also to have close ties to health insurance intermediaries, but the form of these ties will vary.

Formality No multi-unit organization is completely centralized or completely decentralized. (The former would be a single organization and the latter would not be an organization at all.) More decentralized, looser affiliations rely on alliances rather than ownership arrangements. Alliances tend to exist among organizations not competing in the same geographic or service market, because direct competition tends to destroy consensus.[48] Alliances among similar hospitals in different geographic markets are common, as noted in Chapter 1. Alliances between competitors in adjacent markets are increasing. Regional affiliations link organizations that compete in adjacent geographic markets. Certain levels of hospital-physician relations, without formal ownership arrangements, can be understood as alliances in adjacent service markets. Contracts between hospitals and long-term care units are similar. These alliances may be interim stages, presaging future centralization by merger or acquisition.

At the same time, overly centralized organizations encounter serious difficulties as well. Particularly when the parent has subsidiaries in several different markets, responding to local needs becomes a problem, and carrying out empowerment concepts becomes more difficult. The successful centralized institutions have followed the model of the U.S. Constitution, centralizing certain decisions, called reserved powers, and deliberately decentralizing all decisions not specifically centralized. Reserved powers tend to be the core elements that define the central corporation—the mission, particular values of the owners, financial security, and the right to acquire or divest units. They are implemented by specific bylaws requirements for central authorization. The following reserved powers are common:

- appointment of the subsidiary governance board and chief executive;
- approval of the strategic plan of the subsidiary;
- approval of the financial plan and annual budget;
- issuance of long-term debt; and
- sale or purchase of any corporation or subsidiary, or the entry into any contract that might impair the authority of the central body in one of the preceding four.

This approach has allowed many for-profit and religious not-for-profit chains to operate in diverse geographic environments. It also is used in large vertically integrated systems, such as Intermountain and Henry Ford Health System.[49] It tends to succeed where a clear and attractive mission can be articulated and the central organization demonstrates its ability to achieve that mission.

Hospitals that are part of geographically diverse systems still look much like their independent competitors. They have better resources in governance, finance, training, information systems, and recruitment that they are still learning to exploit. It can be argued that these central resources give the systems significant advantages, but the only available evidence suggests that decision making has actually been decentralized in response to the severe environmental pressures of the early 1980s.[50]

Examples of multi-unit organization

Figure 5.14 describes four multi-unit organizations: Premier Alliance, Mercy Health Services, Henry Ford Health System, and Columbia HCA, Inc. They are representative examples of the diversity and strength of the concept. One of them, Premier, does not provide healthcare. Its purpose is to support large healthcare systems that are effective in their own markets. Mercy Health Services was one of the first reorganizations of Catholic hospitals. Like many of the Catholic systems, it was founded as a chain of hospitals serving independent

FIGURE 5.14 Representative Multi-Unit Organizations

Organization	Type	History	Services	Size	Structure
VHA	Alliance	Founded in 1979	Education, research, consultation, and purchasing services	more than 1600 member institutions[1]	Decentralized. Affiliates have only a contract relationship.
Mercy Health Services[2,5]	Vertically integrated, geographically diverse, religious chain	Founded in 1976, by Detroit Province, Sisters of Mercy	Hospitals, physician organizations, HMO, PPO, long-term care facilities, home and hospice care	15 acute institutions, plus homecare and specialty sites	Moderately centralized. Mission, plans, CEO, and financial powers reserved, but MHS has been innovative in arrangements to meet local needs.
Henry Ford Heath System[3,4]	Vertically integrated not-for-profit system serving southeast Michigan	Founded in 1917 by Henry Ford as an innovative healthcare organization	Ambulatory care, hospitals, employed and affiliated physician groups, HMO, PPO, some community clinics and long-term care	9 hospitals, 33 outpatient care sites	Centralized. Mission, plans, CEO, financial and acquisition powers reserved. Local units have boards, but their strategic authority is limited.
Columbia HCA[5]	For-profit hospital chain	Restructured in 1998 as a spin-off from another chain	Prinicipally traditional hospital services	336 hospitals	Centralized. Mission, plans, CEO, financial and acquisition powers reserved. Local units have boards, but their strategic authority is limited.

[1]See the VHA website: www.VHA.com
[2]See the Mercy Health Services website: www.mercyhealth.com
[3]See the Henry Ford Health System website: www.henryfordhealth.org
[4]Mercy Health Services and Henry Ford Health System have engaged in several collaborative ventures, including the contract management of 2 facilities and a point-of-service HMO product.
[5]See the Columbia HCA website: www.careermosaic.com/cm/columbia/columbia1

communities. Over almost 20 years, it has grown both vertically and horizontally. Ford started as an integrated health system with salaried physicians. It is now a major force in southeast Michigan, providing comprehensive medical care under all forms of insurance, medical education, and research. Columbia HCA grew to be one of the earliest and most successful chains of for-profit hospitals and other healthcare services. After significant restructuring in 1998, it continues to operate acute facilities in a number of markets.

Suggested Readings

Griffith, J. R., V. K. Sahney, and R. A. Mohr. 1994. *Reengineering Healthcare: Building on Continuous Quality Improvement.* Chicago: Health Administration Press.

Mintzberg, H. 1979. *The Structuring of Organizations: A Synthesis of the Research.* Englewood Cliffs, NJ: Prentice-Hall.

Nadler, D. A., and M. L. Tushman. 1997. *Competing by Design: The Power of Organizational Architecture.* New York: Oxford University Press.

Leatt, P., S. M. Shortell, and J. R. Kimberly. 1997. "Organization Design." In *Essentials of Health Care Management,* edited by S. M. Shortell and A. D. Kaluzny, 256–85. New York: Delmar.

Notes

1. *The New Shorter Oxford English Dictionary on Historic Principles.* Oxford, UK: Clarendon Press, v. 2, p. 2020 (1993)
2. M. Weber, *The Theory of Social and Economic Organizations.* Glencoe, IL: Free Press (1967)
3. H. Mintzberg, *The Structuring of Organizations: A Synthesis of the Research.* Englewood Cliffs, NJ: Prentice-Hall, pp. 46–53 (1979)
4. E. Freidson, *Doctoring Together: A Study of Professional and Social Control.* Chicago: University of Chicago Press (1980)
5. J. K. Stross and W. R. Harlan, "The Dissemination of New Medical Information." *Journal of American Medical Association* 241(24), pp. 2622–24 (June 15, 1979)
6. T. J. Peters and R. H. Waterman, Jr., *In Search of Excellence: Lessons from America's Best-Run Companies.* New York: Harper and Row, Inc (1992)
7. J. R. Griffith, V. K. Sahney, and R. A. Mohr, *Reengineering Healthcare: Building on Continuous Quality Improvement.* Chicago: Health Administration Press (1994)
8. M. M. Melum and M. K. Sinorius, *Total Quality Management: The Health Care Pioneers.* Chicago: American Hospital Association Publishing, Inc (1992)
9. J. R. Griffith, *Designing 21st Century Healthcare: Leadership in Hospitals and Healthcare Sytems.* Chicago: Health Administration Press (1998)
10. N. Machiavelli, *The Prince*, 2nd ed. Oxford: The Clarendon Press (1913)
11. H. Fayol, *General and Industrial Management.* London: Pitman (1949)
12. F. W. Taylor, *Principles of Scientific Management.* New York: Harper and Brothers (1911)
13. T. A. D'Aunno and M. D. Fottler, "Motivating People." *Health Care Management Organization Design and Behavior*, S. M. Shortell and A. D. Kaluzny, eds. Albany, NY: Delmar Publishers, pp. 57–84 (1994); Also see F. J. Roethlisberger and W. J. Dixon, *Management and the Worker: An Account of a Research Program Conducted by the Western Electric Company and Hawthorne Works,* Chicago. Cambridge, MA: Harvard University Press (1939); R. E. Likert, *The Human Organization.* New York: McGraw Hill (1967); E. Katz and R. Kahn, *The Social Psychology of Organizations*, 2nd ed. New York: John Wiley & Sons (1978); J. Pfeffer, *Competitive Advantage Through People: Unleashing the Power of the Work Force*, Boston, MA: Harvard Business School Press (1994)

14. H. Mintzberg, *The Structuring of Organizations: A Synthesis of the Research.* Englewood Cliffs, NJ: Prentice-Hall, pp. 148–60 (1979)
15. *Ibid*, pp. 18–34 (1979)
16. T. J. Peters and R. H. Waterman, Jr., *In Search of Excellence: Lessons from America's Best-Run Companies.* New York: Harper and Row, Inc (1992)
17. H. Mintzberg, *The Structuring of Organizations*, pp. 148–60
18. *Ibid*, 162–63
19. *Ibid*, 165–67
20. P. Leatt, S. M. Shortell and J. R. Kimberly, "Organization Design." *Health Care Management Organization Design and Behavior*, S. M. Shortell and A. D. Kaluzny eds. Albany, NY: Delmar Publishers, pp. 256–58 (1994)
21. J. M. Eisenberg, *The Physician's Practice,* New York: Wiley (1980)
22. J. R. Griffith, *Designing 21st Century Healthcare: Leadership in Hospitals and Healthcare Systems.* Chicago: Health Administration Press pp. 32–6, 119–21, 197–8 (1998)
23. P. Kotler and R. N. Clarke, *Marketing in Health Care Organizations.* Englewood Cliffs, NJ: Prentice-Hall, Inc., pp. 233–51 (1987)
24. R. Herzlinger, *Market-Driven Health Care: Who Wins, Who Loses in the Transformation of America's Largest Service Industry.* Reading, MA: Addison-Wesley Pub. (1997)
25. A. D. Chandler, *The Visible Hand: The Managerial Revolution in American Business.* Cambridge, MA: Belknap Press (1977)
26. A. P. Sloan, *My Years with General Motors.* Garden City, NY: Doubleday (1964)
27. H. A. Simon, *Administrative Behavior; a Study of Decision-Making Process in Administrative Organization*, 3rd ed. New York: Free Press (1976)
28. H. Mintzberg, *The Structuring of Organizations: A Synthesis of the Research.* Englewood Cliffs, NJ: Prentice-Hall, pp. 58–64 (1979)
29. J. R. Griffith, "Reengineering Health Care: Management Systems for Survivors." *Hospitals & Health Services Administration* 39, pp. 451–70 (Winter, 1994)
30. P. Starr, *The Social Transformation of American Medicine.* New York: Basic Books, pp. 145–178 (1982)
31. C. Perrow, "Goals and Power Structures: A Historical Case Study." *Hospital in Modern Society*, E. Freidson, ed. Glencoe, IL: Free Press (1963)
32. R. L. Johnson, "Revisiting the Wobbly Three-Legged Stool." *Health Care Management Review* 4(3), pp. 15–22 (Summer, 1979)
33. A. L. Delbecq and S. L. Gill, "Justice as a Prelude to Teamwork in Medical Centers." *Health Care Management Review* 10(1), pp. 45–51 (Winter, 1985)
34. S. L. Gill, E. W. Springer, and A. L. Delbecq, "Commitment and Discipline in Hospitals: Leadership Protocols and Legal Precedents." *Health Care Management Review* 12(3), pp. 75–82 (Summer, 1987)
35. M. M. Melum and M. K. Sinioris, *Total Quality Management: The Health Care Pioneers.* Chicago: American Hospital Publishing, pp. 93–128 (1992)
36. D. Neuhauser, "The Hospital as a Matrix Organization." *Hospital Administration* 17(3), pp. 8–25 (Fall 1972)
37. L. R. Burns, "Matrix Management in Hospitals: Testing Theories of Matrix Structure and Development." *Administrative Science Quarterly* 34(3), pp. 349–368 (September, 1989)

38. L. F. McMahon, Jr., R. B. Fettler, J. L. Freeman, and J. D. Thompson, "Hospital Matrix Management in DRG-Based Prospective Payment." *Hospital & Health Services Administration* 31(1), pp. 62–74 (January/February, 1986)
39. J. P. Clement, "Vertical Integration and Diversification of Acute Care Hospitals: Conceptual Definitions." *Hospital & Health Services Administration* 33(1), pp. 99–110 (Spring, 1988)
40. Sisters of Mercy Health Corporation, *Integrated Governance and Management Process: Conceptual Design*. Farmington Hills, MI: SMHC (1980)
41. S. S. Mick, "Explaining Vertical Integration in Health Care: An Analysis and Synthesis of Transaction-Cost Economics and Strategic Management Theory." *Innovation in Health Care Delivery: Insights of Organization Theory*, S. S. Mick, ed. San Francisco: Jossey-Bass Publishers, pp. 207–40 (1990)
42. S. M. Shortell, "The Evolution of Hospital Systems: Unfulfilled Promises and Self-Fulfilling Prophecies." *Medical Care Review* 45(2), pp. 177–214 (1988)
43. R. G. Hughes, S. S. Hunt, and H. S. Luft, "Effects of Surgeon Volume and Hospital Volume on Quality of Care in Hospitals." *Medical Care* 25(6): 489–503, (Jun, 1987)
44. B. B. Longest, "Interorganizational Linkages in the Health Care Sector." *Health Care Management Review* 15(1), pp. 17–28 (1990)
45. H. S. Zuckerman and T. D. D'Aunno, "Hospital Alliances: Cooperative Strategy in a Competitive Environment." *Health Care Management Review* 15(2), pp. 21–30 (Spring, 1990)
46. S. M. Shortell, "The Evolution of Hospital Systems: Unfulfilled Promises and Self-Fulfilling Prophecies." *Medical Care Review* 45(2), pp. 177–214 (1988)
47. S. M. Shortell, R. R. Gillies, D. A. Anderson, J. B. Mitchell, and K. L. Morgan, "Creating Organized Delivery Systems: The Barriers and Facilitators." *Hospital & Health Services Administration* 38(4), pp. 447–66 (Winter, 1993)
48. E. J. Zajac and T. D. D'Aunno, "Managing Strategic Alliances." *Health Care Management Organization Design and Behavior*, S. M. Shortell and A. D. Kaluzny, eds. Albany, NY: Delmar Publishers, pp. 274–93 (1994)
49. J. R. Griffith, V. K. Sahney, and R. A. Mohr, *Reengineering Healthcare: Building on Continuous Quality Improvement*. Chicago: Health Administration Press (1994)
50. J. A. Alexander, "Adaptive Changes in Corporate Control Practices." *Academy of Management Journal* 34(1), pp. 162–193 (January, 1991)

CHAPTER

6

MEASURING PERFORMANCE

Well-managed healthcare organizations study their open systems environment, develop community-oriented strategies in response, and continuously improve their operating processes. They have a strong customer focus, an emphasis on mission and vision, and a commitment to empowering their operating core. This philosophy leads them to the activities described so far in this book—a strategically focused governing board, a service-oriented executive group, and a flexible, decentralized organization.

Continuous improvement requires realistic and convincing analysis of opportunities. To meet these criteria, the decision processes of well-managed healthcare organizations rely heavily on the use of quantitative data covering multiple dimensions of activities.[1] Quantitative information begins as simple counts and measures recorded in the course of events. Rarely will these suffice. Definitions and collection routines are required to ensure accuracy. The original measures are useful only in context of other events, requiring adjustments that must be carefully specified and uniformly administered. And random variation clouds analysis; comparison must acknowledge the limits of accuracy on each measure. The ability to define, acquire, store, retrieve, and analyze these data, to maintain a "source of truth" about the various elements of the organization and its environment, becomes a critical resource. Mastery of performance measurement allows the well-managed healthcare organization to gain a competitive advantage.

Simply put, behind the expectations and actuals that generate the Henry Ford spider (Figure 3.14) lie vast databases, analytic skills, and reporting mechanisms. These are as important as the physical and human resources for the organization's success. This chapter explores the use of numbers in healthcare management. It discusses what they are, where they come from, and how they are analyzed. Chapter 15, on information services, describes the implementation of the information strategy.

Purpose of Quantitative Information

The purpose of quantitative information in organizations is to improve the quality of exchanges between the organization and its partners and constituents. Quantitative information allows communication about expectations and performance to be:

- *Explicit.* "High blood pressure" is ambiguous. "Diastolic pressure of 100 mm of mercury" is unambiguous. "High health insurance cost" is ambiguous. "One hundred forty dollars per member per month" is explicit. Removing ambiguity clarifies communication and speeds conclusion of negotiation.

- *Precise.* "Diastolic pressure of 100 +/−5 mm mercury" and "one hundred forty dollars per member per month guaranteed" are statements of precision. Precision is only possible with quantitative information. The notions of expectations and improvement depend on precision; they are unworkable without it.
- *Efficient.* The concept of blood pressure measurement offers a new order of medical control. The graph in Figure 6.1a conveys quantitative information that actually defines the disease of hypertension. A full explanation of Figure 6.1A would be quite lengthy, but any literate person can see the message—"This patient's blood pressure is trending upwards and is already in the dangerous range." Figure 6.1B shows the same graph, but with different dimensions. Its message is "The cost of our services is trending upward and has already exceeded the amount our customer agreed to pay."
- *Timely.* Information that is explicit, precise, and efficient can be conveyed quickly. The message reaches the person or group that can do something about it in time for them to act.

Rapid learning, quick response, and close tolerances demand numbers because words alone are too ambiguous, too inefficient, and too slow.

Kinds of Quantitative Information

The only disadvantage to the use of quantitative information is the cost of collecting the supporting data. Much of this cost is hidden from the accounting system, but it is real. The solution is to make the data collection as efficient as possible, and the keys to efficient data collection are an understanding of data needs, a systematic scheme for collecting data as a routine part of care activities themselves, and an understanding of the levels of precision required.

Dimensions for Quantitative Performance in Organizations

Figure 6.2 shows the dimensions of information required to measure performance of healthcare activities. They provide a comprehensive description of performance for a function or a final product. They apply to any level of organization, from the work group to an integrated system. Three of these dimensions, demand, cost, and output/productivity, are familiar from the conventional accounting system. They are expanded from the traditional accounting view to reflect all of the areas where expectations can be established. The other three, human resources, quality, and customer satisfaction, are more recent additions, reflecting increased market concerns and improved

FIGURE 6.1 Efficiency Possible with Quantitative Information

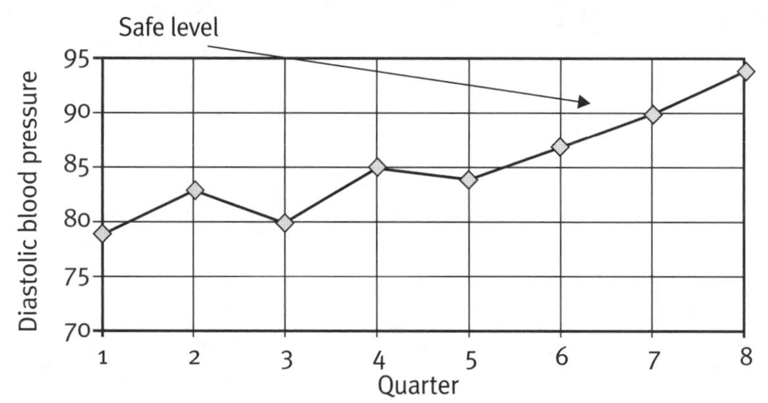

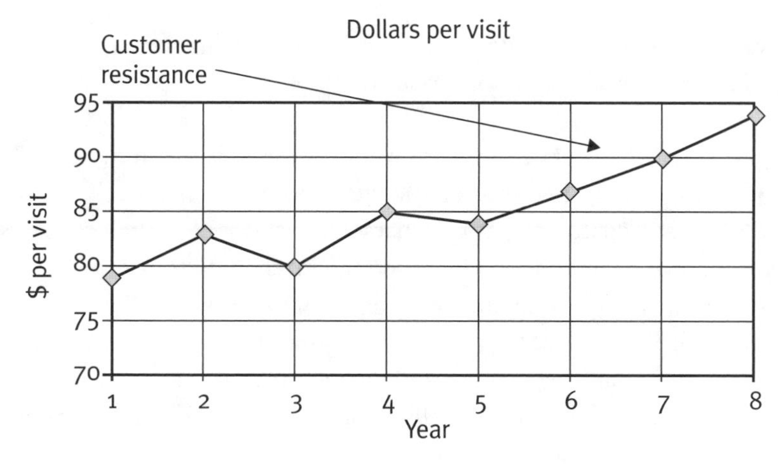

measurement technology. Conceptually at least, the six dimensions apply to any product or service. A manufacturer or a hairdresser would want to know demand, cost, workers available, sales, quality, customer satisfaction, and profit, but as the detail develops, the measures become unique to healthcare. The six are clearly interrelated, often in precise mathematical terms. If all six are managed, the business is likely to succeed; if even one is overlooked, it is likely to fail.

Input-related measures

Three measurement dimensions relate to the starting points of the exchange. There must always be a demand for service, raw materials, and people to perform the work. Several kinds of measures are needed for each dimension, to support the various kinds of decisions that must be made.

FIGURE 6.2
Dimensions of Healthcare Performance

Input-Oriented	Output-Oriented
Demand	Output/Productivity
Requests for service	Treatments or discreet
Market share	Services rendered
Appropriateness of service	Productivity
Logistics of service	(Resources/treatment or service)
Cost/Resources	Quality
Physical counts	Clinical outcomes
Costs	Procedural quality
Resource condition	Structural quality
Human Resources	Customer Satisfaction
Supply	Patient satisfaction
Satisfaction	Referring physician satisfaction
Training	Other customer satisfaction
	Access

Demand

Measures of demand include requests for service, market share, appropriateness of service, and logistics of service.

- *Requests for service.* The simplest level of demand is the number of patients requesting service. Requests are normally counted on a specific time basis and often segregated by patient characteristic as well as the service itself. Demand can be aggregated by function (**intermediate products**) or episodes of care for individual patients (**final products**). For example, demand for imaging service would be counted by type of examination, patient demographics, diagnosis, referring physician, insurance carrier, and time of request and time filled. Final product demand aggregates where imaging is important include trauma, pneumonia, chronic lung disease, and breast cancer. The parameters recorded are necessary for some part of the service, but they also provide a database for analysis of demand processes.
- *Market share.* The percentage of total demand in a market served by the organization is an important indicator of success. Most organizations strive for increasing **market share**. The measurement of market share requires an estimate of the demand going to other suppliers, a number usually purchased or acquired from an independent source. The imaging department would want to know its market share by insurance carrier, referring physician, and kind of examination to develop a strategy protecting and expanding share.
- *Appropriateness of service.* The goal of healthcare is to provide all appropriate service, but only appropriate service. Counting appropriate demand always requires judgment, either in establishing rules applicable to all cases, or in conducting individual review of specific cases. Various

promotional, educational, and management activities are undertaken to minimize inappropriate requests and maximize appropriate ones. Requests received can be counted as appropriate or inappropriate, and strategies devised to discourage inappropriate ones.

Counting requests that were not received but should have been is more complicated. It involves identifying a population at risk and subtracting the number who requested service. The provider organization must undertake special studies to obtain data on the population at risk. For example, breast cancer screening guidelines were established in 1997 after extensive national debate.[2] Mammography in women under 40 is inappropriate; and mammography in women over 50 is appropriate. (Women 40 to 50 have an option.) Counting women over 50 who did not request a mammography requires identifying and measuring a population at risk, probably using some form of census or household survey, rather than the population seeking services, which would serve for a market share estimate.

- *Logistics of service.* Scheduling systems manage both the demand itself and the resources available to meet it. They make a fundamental contribution to productivity. Few healthcare activities are controlled by the caregiver; most depend on demand. For example, an imaging department would schedule patients to minimize waiting in the facility for service. It might use a sophisticated scheduling system to ensure that emergency patients receive priority, non-emergency patients are treated with minimum delay, and staffing levels are balanced to expected demand. Measures of scheduling would include the delay for patients seeking mammography, by women with an identified lump and women seeking routine examinations; delay for reporting back to referring physician; and measures of the productivity of the staff (examinations per person-hour) and the facility (examinations per machine-hour).

Costs and resources

Resources are counted by physical units, costs, and various measures of condition.

- *Physical units* are units of resource such as worker hours, specific supplies, and items of equipment. They are normally organized by type, labor, supplies, equipment, and other. Physical quantities are important in managing production processes; staffing decisions and care decisions are made about physical resources, not dollar amounts. Most counts of physical units are obtained in the accounting process. Examples are "radiologic technician hours worked," "number of films used," "inventory of film available" and "hours of imaging machine operation."
- *Costs* are economic measures of resources. Physical units are multiplied by a market or transfer price to obtain costs. Costs are recorded in the accounting process at the level of individual purchases. They are routinely

aggregated by type and also by characteristic, as variable, semivariable, and fixed, as well as direct and indirect (described more fully in Chapter 14). Costs are recorded and summarized by functional work group and are highly accurate at that level. In the imaging unit, film would be a variable cost, labor a semivariable or fixed one, the equipment fixed. All of these are direct. Resources such as malpractice insurance and support from the executive office are indirect.

Costs for the component intermediate products, for example, chest films, uterine ultrasounds, skull magnetic resonance examinations, can be identified by special study or by establishing the activity as a responsibility center. Because most clinical work groups do a wide range of activities, unit costs of individual services include a number of estimates that reduce the accuracy of unit costs. Costs for final products and service lines are established by reaggregating unit costs, a process called **activity-based costing.**[3] Well-designed accounting systems now produce activity-based costs that are generally reliable, but caution is necessary for highly sensitive analysis.[4] Breast screening patients would be one final product group; breast cancer patients another.

- *Resource condition measures* are important in some processes. "Fluoroscopy machines more than five years old," "percentage of inventory items out of stock," and "percentage of soft tissue dyes out of date" are examples.

Human resources

Supply measures of human resources count numbers of workers available, by skill level or job classification. As healthcare facilities cross-train personnel, counts of workers with specific training within a skill level become important. The supply measure is not identical to the cost measure because pay will be based on actual work as opposed to availability. Examples would be the number of imaging technicians employed, and the number trained to operate ultrasound machines. These counts would be different from the number working on a given day, or paid for a given day.

Satisfaction measures assess worker and physician satisfaction with all aspects of working conditions. It is important to differentiate among various classes of workers because they have different responses and different supply markets. Physicians may or may not be employees, but they cannot be omitted. Satisfaction affects both retention of current workers and recruitment of future ones.

Output-related measures

Three dimensions of output measures are now in common use. They include counts of activity, productivity measures constructed from output counts and resources, quality-of-care measures, and customer satisfaction measures.

Outputs

- *Treatments or services rendered.* Outputs are units of demand filled, as opposed to requested. The same parameters are useful. Outputs must be counted for all but the most trivial services and are usually captured in a patient invoice prepared by the accounting department. Separate counts of requests and output permit rapid identification of unfilled requests and provide data to ensure that the number remains very small. Once captured, output counts can be aggregated by intermediate products (function) or final products (episodes of care). Accurate identification and counts of output are essential to many quality measures. Studies to improve processes often begin with a comparison of outputs to demand at very specific levels. Imaging might analyze data on women scheduled for breast exams who did not arrive; repeat exams, incidences where the original film was flawed and had to be retaken; and cases of women diagnosed as negative who developed breast lumps shortly after examination.

- *Productivity.* **Productivity** is the ratio of inputs (resources) to outputs, or vice versa. Convenience and tradition cause some ratios to be inverted. It does not matter because:

$$\text{inputs}/\text{outputs} = 1/(\text{outputs}/\text{inputs})$$

The term "efficiency" is almost synonymous with productivity, but this text will avoid it when specific measures are referenced. Like resources, productivity is measured in both physical and dollar units. Lab tests/hour worked and lab cost/test are productivity measures. So are length of stay (days of care consumed/patient treated) and cost/case (cost of care/patients treated).

Productivity measures can be calculated for all components of cost (variable, fixed, direct, indirect). Imaging productivity measures include film cost/examination and direct labor cost/examination, facilities cost/exam and indirect cost/exam. Unit costs can also be calculated for marginal costs—the cost that would be incurred if output increased or saved if output declined. Because fixed costs would not change, the marginal cost would be less than the total, or long-run average cost.

Load and occupancy ratios are productivity measures for fixed resources; they compare the resource used (an output) to the resource available (an input). Bed occupancy (number of patient days of care rendered/number of bed days available) is an example.

Productivity measures are essential for strategic management because they can be compared to history, competition, and benchmarks. The actual productivity of imaging, cost/examination or personnel hours/examination, can be compared to price, price or cost information from competitors, and the distribution of similar costs in other, noncompeting institutions. The actual productivity measures are routinely compared to constraints.

Quality

Quality measures include clinical outcomes measures, procedural quality measures, and structural quality measures, each of which has its own advantages and disadvantages.

- *Clinical outcomes measures.* **Outcomes measures** of the quality of the final product assess aspects of the patient's condition on discharge or conclusion of an episode of illness or care, whether the patient lived or died, got better or not, or achieved a specific recovery. Most are in the form of counts or rates (counts divided by the total population at risk) and are treated as attributes measures. "Perinatal mortality," "heart attack survival," and "hip surgery patients walking after six weeks" are examples. There are four approaches to developing measures:

  1. *Negative results or departures from established expectations*, for example, deaths, hospital-acquired infections, complications, and adverse effects. The events can be counted individually or aggregated into a general measure.[5] Unexpected laboratory findings on confirmatory studies such as surgical tissue reports and autopsies also fit this group. It is always possible to state these measures in positive terms (i.e., the number or rate achieving the desired goal). A positive statement is preferable except where the failure rate is very low.
  2. *Placement at termination of care*, whether home, ambulatory care, home care, other hospital, nursing home, or other. The measure is only appropriate when there is a defined end point to the episode of care, such as discharge from the hospital, transfer back to primary care physician, or simply an anniversary in a chronic disease.
  3. *Subjective assessment of condition*, for example, the caregiver's opinion of whether the patient is cured, improved, stable with reduced function, or unstable and deteriorating.
  4. *Objective assessment of condition* using various scales of physiological function, such as scales of laboratory values or scales of ability to perform functions of daily living, and any departure from planned course such as readmission, complication, or deterioration.

  Data often come from medical records, but special surveys are sometimes necessary. Once outcomes measures are generated, they are available at any level of aggregation, from the individual patient to the entire patient population of the hospital. They can be aggregated only by patient or disease groups; there is no such thing as a clinical outcome from functional services. (The outcome must be related to the entire episode of care; it cannot be attributed to any particular component.) Outcomes measures often require collection of data from beyond the episode of care itself. Special surveys are sometimes required to collect the data. For example, cancer survival is usually assessed five years after treatment.

  Using measures of clinical outcomes presents a number of serious problems. Outcomes are difficult to define in some situations, such as terminal care. The measures may not be sensitive, because only very small percentages of patients fail. It is difficult to aggregate diverse measures such as perinatal mortality, orthopedic patients experiencing full recovery, and postoperative infections, into a single index or indicator for an institution. Outcomes depend on many factors, some of which may be beyond the control of the healthcare organization.[6] Perinatal mortality, for example, depends on the health of the mother before and throughout the pregnancy. The number of hip surgery patients walking in six weeks depends on their condition when they requested surgery. Finally, outcomes measures are difficult to relate to potential corrections. For example, if 20 percent of patients fail to walk six weeks after hip surgery, why did they fail? Was it poor surgical technique, poor postoperative care, or factors outside the normal care system, such as inadequate housing or lack of motivation on the patient's part?

Despite their limitations, buyer pressure is strong to use all reasonable outcomes measures in assessing performance.[7,8,9] Some outcomes measures are already required by accreditation agencies, and the number will certainly grow.

- *Procedural quality measures.* These are counts of compliance to accepted clinical practice. "Patients with care plans" and "patients asked to file advance directives" are examples. All functional areas have generally accepted practices and most have established mechanisms to count procedural quality. The measures are often useful in establishing cause of outcomes problems or opportunities for improvement. Statistical analysis can show the relationship between specific process measures and outcomes, identifying the critical elements of a process or function.
- *Structural quality measures.* These are measures of resources present that can be used to infer quality or the lack of it. Many are simple yes/no tallies covering safety equipment, sanitation procedures, and the like. "X-ray machines passing radiation safety examinations" and "presence of certified radiologist" are examples. Some are productivity measures, such as "percentage of examinations by appropriately trained technician." Although structural measures do not guarantee quality, the difficulties of obtaining process and outcomes measures lead most institutions to use all forms.

Customer satisfaction

Satisfaction emphasizes the user viewpoint, rather than the professional one that prevails with clinical outcomes.

- *Patient satisfaction.* Patient satisfaction is a form of outcomes measure. Data on whether the patient was pleased with the care received are normally collected by careful random survey of treated patients and their families.[10] It is routine to use an outside agency, working with a well-developed, standard protocol that permits comparison to other institutions.[11] Topics surveyed include access, amenities, patient information and education, respect for patients' values and emotional needs, and continuity of care. Surveys are often tailored to specific patient groups.[12] Picker Institute, a leading nonprofit survey organization, provides statistical analysis including correlation of items, benchmarks and peer group comparisons, identification of problem areas, and priorities for improvement.[13]

Less rigorous methods, including internally developed protocols and sampling, can be biased, and they cannot be compared to other institutions. The goal of patient satisfaction is to "delight" the patient, achieving a rating of "very satisfied" and a positive response to questions about returning or recommending the organization to friends and acquaintances. Satisfaction data can also be collected from the community population rather than the patient population. Such data are important for marketing.

- *Referring physician satisfaction.* Referring physicians act as agents for their patients and are concerned with clinical outcomes, patient satisfaction, and cost. If they are dissatisfied, they may divert market share. Their opinion is routinely assessed informally. Formal surveys are an important adjunct in larger institutions.
- *Access.* Access measures reveal whether resources are available to meet demand. They are frequently developed from demand and human resources data. "Imaging facilities in primary care locations," "breast screening sites per 1,000 women over 50," and "percentage of population within 30 minutes of a birthing facility" are examples. The standards for access are set by the marketplace. Logistics management measures can also be used access measures. Delays for routine mammography or diagnosis of a breast lump are examples.
- *Other customer satisfaction.* Some customers of work groups are neither doctors nor patients. The technical support units have other organizational units as customers. Development offices have donors and potential donors as customers. The satisfaction of these groups can be measured by survey.

Examples of performance measures

The performance measurement dimensions are applicable to any level of aggregation, from individual task to healthcare organization as a whole. Figure 6.3 gives three examples, a single home health visit by a trained health aide (an intermediate product), an inpatient episode for hip replacement (a final product), and a comprehensive HMO provider (an organization). As the dimensions are applied to more aggregate situations, they fit closely with the balanced scorecard approaches being used to report governing board performance.

Performance Constraint

Continuous improvement requires that a **constraint**, or acceptable level of performance, be established for all measures in all six dimensions. The kinds of constraints include competitive market performance, profit requirements, comparative performance from noncompetitors, and negotiated expectations.

FIGURE 6.3 Examples of Performance Measurement

Dimension	Home Health Visit	Hip Replacement	HMO
Demand	# visits requested, by type	# patients referred	# members, market share
	% of all home health in community	% of all hip replacements to citizens of community	% of all insured persons, or total population, by age
	% appropriate home visits	% appropriate surgeries	% of all costs appropriate
	time schedule for visits	delay for surgery	telephone answer delay
Cost/Resources	nurse hours, supply counts, vehicles, etc.	OR time, hospital days, PT visits, number of prostheses, etc.	hospital days, physicians paid, etc.
	costs of physical resources	costs of physical resources	costs of physical resources
	% equipment defects reported	Age of operating theater and equipment	# accredited hospitals
Human Resources	# RNs, aides, etc.	# orthopedic surgeons	# primary care practitioners
	% workers "recommend to others"	% workers "recommend to others"	% workers "recommend to others"
	% aides trained in CPR	% aides trained in exercise	% workers trained in two functions
Outputs/	# visits completed	# procedures	# member months
Productivity	visits/employee day	cases/surgeon	FTE/member month
	$ per visit	$ per case	$ per member month
Quality	% sustain activity level	% walking at 6 weeks	% immunized at 2 years
	% visit protocol met	% care protocol met	patients with appropriate preventive care
	Ratio RNs/aides	Accredited hospital facility	State insurance approval
Satisfaction	% patients "recommend to others"	% patients "recommend to others"	% members "recommend to others"
	% referring physicians "recommend to others"	% referring physicians "recommend to others"	% primary physicians "recommend to others"
	# of insurer panel contracts	# of insurer panel contracts	# of employers offering to employees
	Communities covered	Delay for new patient evaluation	# primary physicians in panel

Market performance

The performance actually accepted by the customer in competitive settings is the clearest and most rigorous constraint known. It creates the acid test of operations wherever it can be applied. If others operate at a certain net revenue, or price paid, any activity that exceeds that price is suspect. (Gross revenue—the price the institution charged or would like to receive—is irrelevant to performance measurement.) Similarly, if competitors can convince patients that their quality, access, or amenities are superior, their achievements must be matched.

Many measures of market performance are simply unavailable, and substitutes must be found. Global payment mechanisms, such as payment per day of care, or per hospitalization, or capitation (payment per member month), are excellent market statements in themselves, but they severely limit the use of price or net revenue as a measure of performance in components below the pricing level. Under these payment mechanisms, for example, no revenue is assigned to any functional unit contributing to the care. As a result, price and profit are not available as indicators of market constraint.

Market performance can be evaluated at a function or final product level if a vendor is willing to accept a contract specifying the six dimensions. Many functional services can be purchased as an alternative to producing them within the organization. When performance is fully specified, the possibility of **outsourcing** or purchasing the function becomes realistic. Many organizations outsource portions of their technical and logistic support services, for example. At least conceptually, a market exists for alternative sources of clinical functions such as imaging, laboratory, home care, and specialist physician services. Specialized independent functional services can sell to integrated organizations. Healthcare organizations can also be vendors, selling services to other organizations. Commercial vendors offer outsourcing for most learning services and for the executive function (contract management). The bids offered by external sources are useful comparisons. If equivalent service can be purchased for a certain price, quality, and satisfaction, the internal function must operate at the same level. If the external vendor offers to meet all imaging demand for $2.5 million per year, the internal department should operate at that cost or less. If equivalent breast screening examinations are offered to the organization for $150 each by an independent imaging company, the internal cost should not exceed $150. (Equivalency is often difficult to judge, but the concept should be clear.)

Profit

With rare exceptions, any organization that expects to survive and grow must earn a profit overall. (Long-range financial planning, the procedure for establishing the necessary profit, is discussed in Chapter 14.) Profit can be calculated only where net revenue is actually available. Many functional units sell some portions of their service for net prices and can make profit calculations if they can isolate the costs of those services.

Benchmarks

Data on performance of other, similar aggregates are used to establish acceptable performance ranges, in place of or in supplement to direct market tests. Such data usually come from noncompetitors. Healthcare organizations in other communities are happy to exchange comparative information. Organized efforts are necessary to establish definitions and make adjustments necessary to ensure comparability, and alliances have been established for the exchange of comparative data on many performance elements. Competitors protect their performance data, so they are not often known. Various governmental requirements and voluntary agreements open specific measures to comparison.[14] California and Pennsylvania require extensive disclosure, for example. Much data about Medicare are available, and commercial consultants organize them for convenient access.[15]

Benchmarks, or best practices from such comparisons, are used as a guide and long-range target; it is often wise to identify how the organization compares with nonbenchmark organizations as well. The benchmark establishes the long-term goal; the relative rank determines the priority of reaching it. A certain standing in a frequency distribution can be a short term goal or can justify a lower goal while higher priority needs are pursued.

Negotiated constraints

Even in the absence of competitive and comparative data, organizations negotiate performance expectations. Once agreed upon, these are important constraints, with significant rewards and penalties for individual managers. Historical values are important in the negotiations. Improvement can be negotiated; it would be unwise to accept last year's performance as satisfactory for next year. Market price, comparative data, and competitor data are ways to improve the negotiation.

Figure 6.4 shows the kinds of constraint measurement and examples of their application drawn from the three applications shown in Figure 6.3.

Using Performance Management Data

Performance measures are generated as a part of the work itself. Each activity is recorded, either electronically or on paper, in specified forms that generate the data. With six dimensions for each RC and final product, multiple measures

FIGURE 6.4 Kinds of Constraint Measurement and Examples

Performance Constraint	Home Health Visit	Hip Replacement	HMO
Competitive	Competitor price, quality, access to patient	Medicare price per case, quality standards	Competitor premium, patient satisfaction
Competitive	Competitor outsourcing bid to insurer or owner	Competitor outsourcing bid to insurer or referring physicians	Offer for merger or acquisition
Profit Requirement	% profit margin	% profit margin on cases paid directly	% profit margin
Benchmark	Best known price/visit, quality, satisfaction	Best known price per case, quality, satisfaction	Lowest comparable premium, highest satisfaction
Negotiated	Historic trend in demand	"Halfway to benchmark"	Planned physician panel expansion

for most dimensions, several dozen important final products, and 50 to 100 work groups, the volume of data that must be processed is very large, running thousands of items per day. To fulfill its purposes, information must be accurate. But there is obviously a limit to the amount of resources that can be expended on data collection. The issue is to design ways of collecting data that are accurate, convenient, and cheap, and the answer is the computer.

Advantages of automation

Computers contribute to efficient data collection in several ways. These advantages are summarized in Figure 6.5.

- Input can be speeded and controlled by programs that prompt for completeness and audit for consistency. Omissions, spelling, and inconsistencies can be corrected immediately, eliminating errors and confusion. For example, the entry "William Smith, Social Security # 187-27-0887, admitted for pediatric asthma" looks reasonable, but checked against an electronic database several questions would arise:
  - Is this William G. Smithe, aged 40, Soc. Sec. # 187-27-0877?
  - If yes, is pediatric asthma the correct diagnosis, or is it adult asthma?
  - If no, what are the middle initial and age?
- Automation makes it possible to eliminate repeated entry. For example, most patient orders must have at least two means of identifying the patient. Electronic identification substitutes an audit of the request for laborious copying of names and numbers. The laboratory will not receive Smithe's specimen and report it as Smith's.
- Automation can change many patient care decisions from recall to recognition by prompting for the clinically indicated next step. Recognition is faster and more accurate than recall. Expectations translate to checklists and prompts that, in themselves, improve performance. If a specific test or procedure is mandatory for a certain condition, a prompt will appear in the automated ordering sequence whenever the doctor identifies the condition.
- By using agreed on care plans, a variety of clinical situations can be programmed to prevent accidental error. For example, the following can be prevented by expanding the audit functions to include clinical guidelines:
  - some accidental misstatements and omissions
  - inappropriate therapy selections (as with drugs of similar name but different uses)
  - conflicts with prior orders
  - absence of supporting diagnostic tests or values
  - interactions between drugs
  - failure to obtain consultation or supervision
- Output can be speeded and organized. When the laboratory does Smithe's tests, the report will be available to the physician immediately, together with the history of Smithe's prior tests. The precision of the laboratory test value

and the range of values in a comparable normal population can be added to assist in interpreting the tests.

- Calculations can be made rapidly and cheaply. Smithe's laboratory results can instantaneously update the mean and standard deviation of each test. They can be cross-referenced by his final product, adult asthma. The tests can be entered on his patient ledger, priced, and added to the laboratory daily output statistics.
- An accessible archive is created. The data can be retrieved for Smithe, for the test, for the laboratory, for the insurance intermediary, and for adult asthma. Statistical databases combine Smithe's data with other in each class.

Major data systems

The principal data systems that generate the six dimensions of information are shown in Figure 6.6. Although the groupings can be revised, about 12 systems are necessary to support the information needs of a modern health-care organization. The systems can be conveniently grouped into those that emphasize capture of data, those that support the background record keeping and analysis, and those that directly support decisions by caregivers and others in the provider organization. Although considerable amounts of data are still processed manually at some stages of their collection, enormous strides have been made in automation in recent years, and even larger ones are likely for the near future. The drawback to computerization is that the systems to do it cost tens or hundreds of millions of dollars and take years to develop. The payback is considerably larger than the investment, however. Even the smallest healthcare organizations are developing computer capability, and it is unlikely that organizations that do not automate most of each of the 12 principal data systems will survive. The activities and status of each system are as follows.

FIGURE 6.5 Contributions of Automated Data Systems

Contribution	Example
1. Rapid, audited input	Automatic check for name, identity, spelling, vital statistics
2. No repeat input	All users access central registration file for patient ID and medical condition
3. Recognition for clinical tasks	Protocol suggests normally indicated treatment, prompts for order or explanation before proceeding
4. Verification and cross check of orders	Drugs checked for patient sensitivity, interactions
5. Prompt result reporting	Instantaneous transmission of diagnostic test findings
6. Statistical and accounting calculations	Charges to date, variance, or range of history of laboratory values
7. Accessible archive	Comparison to similar patients or protocol

FIGURE 6.6
Relationship of Major Data-Processing Systems

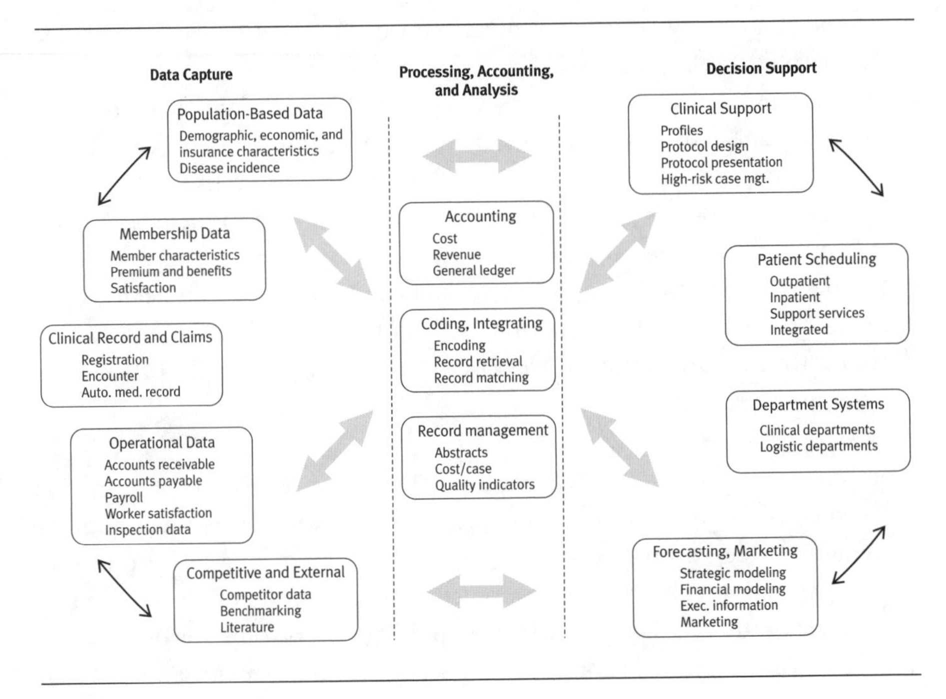

I. **Systems Designed to Capture Data**

A. *Population assessment systems.* These capture the underlying demographic, economic, and epidemiologic character of the organization's potential market. Current data and trends of geographic distributions, age, child-bearing habits, employment, health insurance, disease patterns, and risk factors are used to evaluate population needs, market share, and market opportunities. The data for these systems come from a variety of sources, but purchase of electronic census and related data is spreading rapidly.

B. *Membership systems.* These record details of health insurance coverage, including dependents, and utilization for individual subscribers, and group, benefits, premium, and account status for groups. The records are essential for insurance operations, but also supply data for clinical support activities. The systems are almost completely automated.

C. *Clinical transaction and claims systems.* These record the name, vital statistics, and details of care for each patient. They also capture records used for payment of providers. Each patient is assigned a unique lifetime number and the systems include elaborate mechanisms to identify patients quickly and correctly. The data from the systems drive much of the processing and accounting activity and are essential for all the decision support systems on the right side of Figure 6.6. Patient registration, order entry, and results reporting are highly automated, and automation is increasing rapidly.

D. *Operational systems.* These record the day-to-day business of the providers, including initial accounting transactions such as payables and payroll. They also record process quality data and worker satisfaction data. The system is essential for provider operation, but it also supports analysis of work processes and worker morale. Many of the accounting transactions are automated, but much of the quality and satisfaction data is manually collected and entered for automated storage and retrieval.

E. *Competitor analysis systems.* These capture data about local competitors and also benchmark and best practice data about similar operations elsewhere. The data come from a wide variety of sources and are frequently estimated or inferred. They are essential for forecasting and marketing activities. The systems are rarely automated.

II. **Processing, Accounting, and Analysis**

A. *Accounting systems.* These tally individual transactions from clinical and operational systems and produce detailed reports of receivables, payables, payrolls, employment benefits, inventories, and equipment depreciation. They generate cost and constraint reports at all levels of aggregation, and much of the general financial reports for the firm as a whole. They perform a variety of cost accounting and financial analyses used by all the operating core, technological, and logistics support activities. They model the long-range financial plan, allowing evaluation of alternative planning scenarios. The systems are highly automated.

B. *Coding and integrating systems.* These systems allow aggregation of accounting and medical record data by disease, patient characteristic, or site of care. They include the various patient classification systems. They are essential to translate individual patient and provider records to aggregates useful for decision support. The systems are almost completely automated.

C. *Record management systems.* These aggregate individual patient care transactions by patient to form the medical record or history. The medical record itself is a critical part of care management. Aggregated by various patient characteristics of interest through the coding system, the information generated is used in all decision support systems. Record systems are partly automated, and major investments are being made to complete automation. It is likely that for inpatient care and major ambulatory treatment, all but a few relatively rare transactions will be automated within the next few years. Office care will be more difficult.

III. **Systems Supporting Decisions**

A. *Clinical support systems.* These generate statistical analyses and profiles that are used to identify patient care improvement opportunities. They also include care protocols and other agreements on clinical procedures and expectations. The systems are largely manual at the present time, but automation will spread with automation of medical record systems.

B. *Patient scheduling systems.* These use historic data on demand and accounting data on availability and cost to schedule patient care transactions. They are partially automated and are growing more sophisticated.

C. *Departmental service and reporting systems.* These govern the internal activities of departments, including many aspects of detailed productivity and quality control. They include personnel scheduling, materials management, work processes, quality inspections, and a variety of internal records. Automation varies by department, but specially designed systems are available for the larger clinical departments and most technical and logistic support activities.

D. *Planning and marketing data systems.* These translate data from all other systems to scenarios and forecasts of future events and are used to evaluate strategies and record strategic decisions. They include financial planning models, models of market development and competitor analysis, and planning databases for facilities, human resources, and information development. Data capture and reporting are increasingly automated through executive information systems. Major strides have been made in the automation of modeling, although the decision processes are supported, rather than directed by the models.

In addition to these sources for routine, ongoing data collection, special nonrecurring studies are also useful. Using research techniques, measurements can be as reliable and valid as desired, within the limits of current technology. Special studies are useful for a variety of purposes, including verifying assumptions about improvement in performance, evaluating new methods or new measures, or collecting very expensive performance measures. Surveys of doctor, patient, and community attitudes, now routine, can be expanded to address particular issues in depth. Processes can be studied in detail, and proposed improvements can be evaluated by special analyses or field trials. Marginal and variable costs can be evaluated in depth. Proposals for new routine measures can be pretested. Investigations of medical and nursing care for specific kinds of cases can be conducted, including formal trials of new methods.

Approaches to Quantification

Measuring health and healthcare is a science in itself. Many elements are simply counted by the accounting system. Patients, workers, visits, tests, surgeries, and dollars are examples. Gender, age, address, insurance coverage, worker training, and other characteristics are relatively easy to quantify. The only issues are completeness and uniformity of recording. But to use the six dimensions for continuous improvement, one must address three separate but equally serious problems:

1. *The need to scale performance,* that is, to capture characteristics that otherwise would be only descriptive and subjective. While some important

elements are easily counted or measured, others present challenges. Unmet demand, for example, is far more difficult to measure than demand translated to output. Pain is as serious a measurement problem as it is a medical one.

2. *The need for reliability and validity.* It is not enough to measure blood pressure; the value reported must be both reproducible and reflective of the patient's true condition. When these criteria are applied to complex phenomena, multiple dimensions must be considered. The concept of a satisfactory surgery is represented by a checklist of measures, and so is that of a healthy baby.
3. *The need to gain uniformity for fair comparison.* No two patients or treatments are ever alike, but inescapably comparisons must be made between similar groups. What patients are acceptably "similar"? "Healthy newborns" certainly, but identifying comparable groups of impaired newborns is not so obvious. What time period is reasonable? An episode of pregnancy is clear enough, but when is a fracture healed? Many diseases continue over long periods of time without discrete stopping points.

Quantifying the six dimensions is a matter of continually searching for measures that evolve from subjective, almost intuitive beginnings. The measures themselves can be understood as estimations that improve in precision as they evolve. Similarly, the measurement systems grow and mature. Design and improvement of measures involves scaling, specification of populations, and adjustments to compare diverse populations.

Scaling

The process for translating real activities and characteristics to numbers is called scaling. There are four measurement categories, or scales. Which category is used in a given situation will depend on cost and value, and scaling may evolve through several levels over time. Figure 67 summarizes scaling.

1. *Nominal scales.* These identify categories that are useful in accommodating the differences in patients, such as gender, race, or specific diagnoses. Classifications for diseases, procedures, and prescription drugs are all nominal scales underpinning healthcare measurement. The International Classification of Diseases is a nominal scale now used almost universally to describe the illnesses leading to hospitalization. It became the foundation for another famous nominal scale, DRGs. Other nominal scales are useful in differentiating personnel and activities.

   Nominal scales generate **attributes measures**, that is, a binary (yes or no) value for each case. The principal statistic for an attributes measure is the portion passing a certain threshold:

   portion passing = number yesses/total number examined

FIGURE 6.7 Scales for Quantifying Information

Scale	Description	Examples	Uses	Limitations
Nominal	Scale without rank or comparability	Men/women; DRGs	Identifying different populations	No comparison between groups
Ordinal	Ordered scale, intervals not even in size or importance	Patient satisfaction scores, infant Apgar scores	Classifying complex events by desirability or action required	Improvement moving between intervals differs
Interval	Even, uniform intervals,but no absolute end point	Temperature, blood pressure	Finer classification by desirability or action required	Improvement moving between intervals is constant, but relative improvement is unknown
Ratio	Ordered scale with even or predictable categories and an absolute end point	Height, percentile standing, dollars	Comparison between and within group, calculation of variance and means	Strongest scale; relative change in scale is equal to relative change in objective achievement

The hip replacement walking measure is a nominal scale, number walking/number of procedures.

2. *Ordinal scales.* These identify categories that move reliably in a uniform direction, so higher numbers represent consistently different situations from lower ones. (Nominal scales are assigned arbitrarily so that high numbers have no intrinsic meaning.) The five numerical classes of Pap smears, for example, indicate progressively more serious disease as the numbers get higher. Burns, cancers, respiratory distress, infant distress, and several other clinical characteristics are quantified by ordinal scales. For example, intensive care units use an ordinal scale to determine patient condition and necessity for admission.[16] Individual patients' daily nursing requirements are often assessed with ordinal scales.[17] Satisfaction questionnaires use ordinal scales. Ordinal scales are usually treated as attributes measures. Often two or more ordinal categories are grouped together to form the portion passing.
3. *Interval scales.* These are ordinal scales that have uniform values between entries, but an arbitrary end point or starting point. Temperature is an easily recognized interval scale, because two popular scales, Celsius and Fahrenheit, both have uniform ordinal steps (degrees), but they have two different, equally arbitrary zero points. As a result, it is impossible to make relative comparisons. A fever of 100° F is not 1.4 percent worse than normal; the same condition expressed in Celsius is 37.78° C, 2 percent

worse than the Celsius normal of 37.0°. Blood pressure is an interval scale. The starting point, atmospheric pressure, is not only variable, it bears no intrinsic relation to the disease of hypertension. A diastolic pressure of 100 mm mercury is not 25 percent worse than 80 mm mercury. Interval scales generate **variables measures**; that is, a continuous measure that can take any value over a range.

4. *Ratio scales.* A ratio scale fulfills all the requirements of interval measures but has, in addition, a non-arbitrary zero value. This permits the use of percentages. Height, weight, and percentile standing on comparative distributions are all ratio scales. In accounting, dollars are a ratio scale. Ratios of actual to expected values, such as used in spider diagrams, are ratio scales, even if the underlying measure is not. Percentage of patients walking after hip replacement is a nominal scale, but the actual percentage divided by the expected percentage is a ratio scale. Ratio scales generate variables measures.

Healthcare organizations routinely use all four scaling approaches. While ratio scales have certain advantages, the other approaches are useful in continuous improvement programs as well. Improvement of measures and measurement systems may involve moving from nominal to ordinal or ratio scales.

Evaluating and Improving Measures

Measures are judged by the extent to which their use allows the organization to improve mission achievement. To be valuable, measures must be valid, reliable and timely.

Validity

A performance measure is valid if the reported values of cases are associated with the exchange objectives (e.g., if patients with higher scores are healthier, if cases with lower values cost less). If an invalid measure is used, energy can be directed toward achieving high scores on that measure rather than achieving the true goals. The result may be a disabling distortion of intended activity. An anecdote may be the best way to illustrate the importance of validity. A factory produced nails, and someone wished to improve performance by setting output goals for the employees. So a goal was set at a certain *number* of nails per hour. After a short time, the goal was exceeded, but the factory was producing mostly tacks. So the goal was changed to a certain number of *pounds* of nails per hour. Again the goal was exceeded, but this time the factory was producing spikes. The moral is that validity of measurements depends on what the goals are. If one wants a variety of nails, one's measures and expectations must reflect that.

Often an elaborate, expensive measurement system is used to establish the validity of a much cheaper one. The ultimate standard for length is an optical measurement system used by the National Bureau of Standards. The validity of the common desk ruler is traceable through several substitutes that are progressively cheaper and less accurate. A measure can be perfectly reliable, but still invalid. Using a ruler that is too short, everyone can agree the distance between two points is almost exactly ten centimeters. A valid ruler would show that it is almost exactly nine centimeters.

In healthcare, validity is usually associated with an objective of health. Thus, if the objective of hip replacement surgery is the full recovery of functioning, an independent panel examining the patient's functioning in his or her life setting several months after surgery would be the ultimate validity, comparable to the optical standard for length. It might be applied in selected situations, to evaluate a less expensive measure, or when new hip replacement processes are considered. Self-reported functioning would be one substitute for the ultimate, much cheaper but potentially subject to bias, like the too-short ruler. The ability to walk a specified distance at a specified postsurgical time would be a second substitute. One or both substitutes might be used to evaluate the annual results for a hip replacement program.

Reliability A measure is reliable if repeated application to an identical situation yields the same value. The standard deviation of the reported values is the measure of reliability. Lack of reliability impairs precision of measurement. If the average of several measurements is ten centimeters, but the standard deviation of individual measures is one millimeter, the measure is reliable to plus or minus three standard deviations 99 percent of the time, and four standard deviations roughly all but once in a thousand trials.

Reliability is frequently assessed across differing measurement conditions. Time trends in the measure and its standard deviation are common. Testing and retesting against the same population, comparison of different observers, and split sample calculations are common. Reliability is enhanced by clear definitions, good measuring tools, audits, and training of observers. The hip replacement program might check the reliability of its self-assessed function measure over time, by patient categories such as age and the presence of other disease, and against the percentage of nonrespondents. It might review trends, individual observer values, and values by day of the week to identify reliability issues.

Timeliness There are two important criteria of timeliness: frequency and delay. Delay is the interval between measurement and report. The measurement system that reports too late for the monitor to respond is useless. (In the worst case, efforts to correct a reported problem that no longer exists may destabilize the system.) Reports that are too infrequent allow correctable conditions to exist longer than necessary. Reports that come too often waste the monitor's time. There is a response cycle, a finite time required to respond to a measure. Reporting more frequently than once per response cycle is not useful. In some of the complex issues of quality and productivity, the response cycles are quite long. It may take months to evaluate and redesign the hip replacement process, for example. Weekly reports of outcomes make no contribution; quarterly ones would be more appropriate.

Specification and Adjustment

Most performance measures are dependent both upon the process being measured and the characteristics of the population involved. It is important to separate the two; serious errors result if a difference attributable to a population is taken as reflecting a process. Any comparison of performance measures requires understanding of the difference in population; comparing across similar populations. Two approaches are used: specification and adjustment.

Specification

Specification defines subpopulations with similar characteristics within a larger, more heterogeneous population. Specification is necessary whenever a difference in performance exists between two population subgroups. The characteristic used for specification can be nominal or ordinal. Ratio or interval scales can be converted to specification by grouping them into categories. One might identify similar patient populations by gender, education, an interval scaled condition such as blood pressure, or a ratio scale such as age. If necessary, one could develop specified subpopulations for combinations of characteristics, such as women, over age 50, college graduates, with previous history of diastolic blood pressure over 90 mm mercury. Hip replacement recovery rates might be specified by the degree of loss of function prior to surgery and age. Common taxonomies for patient care performance are shown in Figure 6.8.

Adjustment

Adjusted rates recalculate the whole population rate from the specific rates, standardizing heterogeneous populations to a uniform structure. They are most useful when comparing several different populations, such as the mortality rates for states, which are usually adjusted for age to the age distribution of the United States as a whole. The age-adjusted rate for each state is the mortality rate it would have if its population had the same age distribution as the nation.

Figure 6.9 shows the crude, specific, and age-adjusted death rates for Utah and Florida. Are Floridians more likely to die than Utahns, as the crude rates suggest? Yes, they are if they are under 65, but not among Florida's large retired population. And overall, an age-adjusted comparison shows the Florida rate to be 20 percent lower than Utah, not 73 percent higher as the crude rates indicate. Each adjustment requires additional data and calculations, but the misleading character of the crude rate is clearly shown.

Population characteristics, including mortality and morbidity rates, are often adjusted for age, sex, race, and socioeconomic status, and specific rates are frequently used for specific diseases. Fertility rates are specific to the

FIGURE 6.8 Common Patient-Specification Taxonomies

Category	Classifications
Demographic	Age Sex Race Education
Economic	Income Employment Social class
Geographic	Zip code of residence Census tract Political subdivision
Healthcare Finance	Managed versus traditional insurance Private versus government insurance
Diagnosis	Disease classification Procedure Diagnosis-related group (DRG) Ambulatory visit group
Risk	Health behavior attribute Preexisting condition Chronic or high-cost disease

number of fertile women, and rates of diseases such as cancers and heart disease are expressed for the population over 45.

Severity adjustment

Healthcare organizations frequently adjust performance measures for the severity of illness of their patients. There are two basic approaches. One uses the Medicare DRG payment system as a basis. DRGs are assigned based on discharge diagnosis, grouping clinically similar diagnoses that are also similar in cost. Every Medicare inpatient must be assigned a DRG, and HCFA has assigned a weight to each DRG based on national surveys of the cost of care of those patients. Then for each of the *i* patient groups:

$$\Sigma\,(\text{patient}_i * \text{DRG weight}_I) \,/\, \Sigma\,(\text{patient}_i) = \text{average DRG weight, or severity index}$$

and

$$\Sigma\,(\text{cost/patient}_i) \,/\, \Sigma\,(\text{DRG weight}_I) = \text{weighted cost/patient}$$

The weighted cost/patient (or other performance measure, such as length of stay or clinical outcomes) can more accurately be compared between institutions.

Although the DRG weight is universal and cheap, it has several limitations. The weight explains less than half the variation between cases. The

Age Category	Utah			Florida		
	Deaths	Population	Death Rate	Deaths	Population	Death Rate
0–14	450	538	8.4	2,742	2,412	11.4
15–44	804	789	10.2	11,822	5,595	21.1
45–64	1,446	245	56.0	19,367	2,548	76.0
65–75	2,894	90	321.6	30,618	1,369	223.7
> 75	4,624	62	754.8	68,168	1,059	643.7
All ages	10,218	1,742	56.3	122,077	12,983	94.0
Crude death rate			56.3			94.0
Utah death rate standardized to Florida population						113.0

FIGURE 6.9 Age-Specific, Crude, and Adjusted Rates, Utah versus Florida

unexplained variation tends to occur among very high cost patients, but these patients are in several DRGs. The assignment process and the weights are focused on the Medicare recipients, almost all over 65 years of age. Younger users of the hospital can be assigned DRGs, but the values are not necessarily correct. One large category of hospitalization, obstetrics, occurs very rarely in the Medicare population, so the basis for assigning the weight is particularly suspect.

Some commercial systems improve on the DRG algorithm. They either create new groups and calculate new weights for them, or expand the existing groups to identify the sicker patients in them. Similar approaches have been developed for outpatient care, but their use is not widespread. Many use the diagnoses and the reported care given, which is reported to insurers using **current procedural terminology (CPT)** groups.[18]

The second severity-weighting approach uses patient conditions other than diagnosis.

Acuity approaches use binary or simple ordinal scales indicating departure from normal function in several physiological and psychological factors known to influence resource use.[19] They are popular for estimating nursing time.[20] Items evaluated include therapeutic and diagnostic needs as well as those involving eating, dressing, and elimination; the emotional state; and the amount of observation ordered by the doctor. Scales are now tailored to the clinical area. Representative acuity variations for obstetrical labor and delivery care are shown in Figure 6.10. For nurse staffing, values for each patient are reported by the head nurse. Computerized systems calculate acuity, assign staffing requirements to individual patients, and add up the nursing personnel required on each floor.

FIGURE 6.10
Patient Acuity Variation

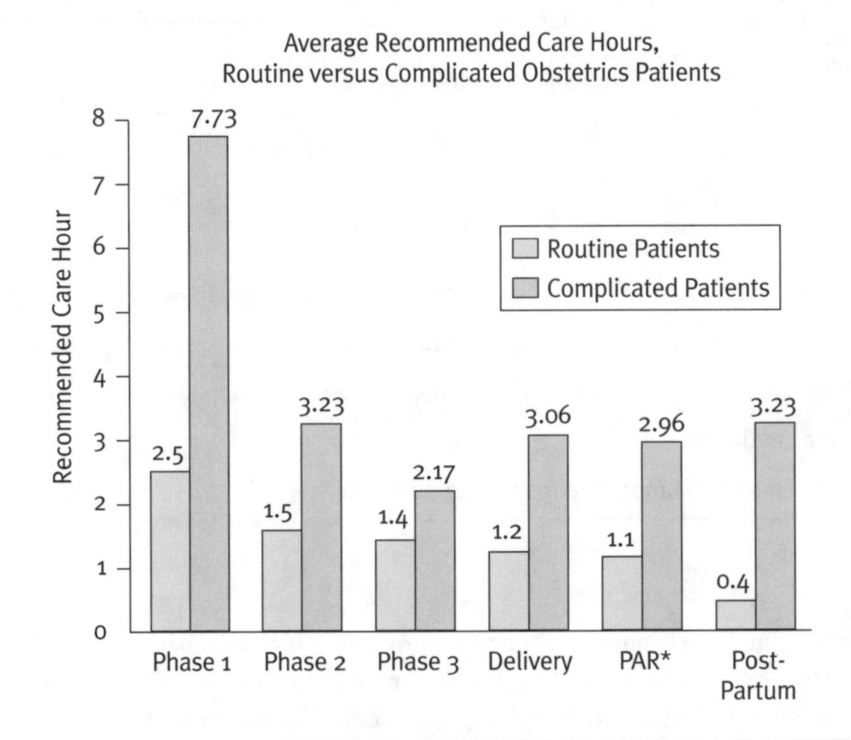

RUGS, a severity grouping system based on functional capability, is widely used in nursing homes.[21] Patients are assigned to category by their ability to eat, dress, toilet, walk, and similar activities, and the weights are established by studies of the nursing time they require.

APACHE is a physiologically-based acuity system, using laboratory values for critical blood chemistry. It was developed in intensive care units and is particularly useful with very ill patients.[22] However, larger scale studies indicate that the contribution of the APACHE approach may be insufficient.[23]

Although severity adjustments are popular, their real value is questionable. An adjustment is useful when it successfully isolates factors approached by radically different mechanisms, such as preventive activity as opposed to care. Formal studies evaluating this capability suggest that most currently available adjustments are of limited value.[24,25] A better approach to the underlying problem of heterogeneity in patient mix is summarized in the following steps:

1. *Finely subdividing the complaints, diagnoses, and procedures* improves the homogeneity of groups. Often a combination of demographic and clinical characteristics identifies acceptably homogeneous groups. Segregating births by mother's age, presence of prenatal care, and Apgar score is an example. Regression analysis helps identify the important variables to use.
2. *Comparing over time, rather than between institutions.* While patient characteristics certainly change over time, the differences at a single

institution are much less than those between institutions operating in radically different environments, such as inner city or suburban.
3. *Selecting external comparisons from similar sites.* Results for suburban institutions can be compared to other suburban institutions.
4. *Conducting special studies of situations that still show important variations after the first three steps.* This is a normal part of the Shewhart cycle, but the improvement team can be alert to the possibility that some exogenous factor is causing the problem they address.
5. *Emphasizing continuous improvement rather than identification of error.* It is fear of blame, in the form of reduced reputation, loss of income, or potential tort liability that underlies much concern with acuity adjustment. These elements are deliberately de-emphasized in continuous improvement approaches. Many forms of incentive payment actually exaggerate the problem; that is one reason why they are avoided.

A Strategy for Improving Measurement

A strategy for designing measures attempts not only to maximize the value of the measures in improving control, but also to minimize the cost of measurement itself. Rather than addressing specific measures, successful strategies set out classes of measures like Figure 6.2 and address how to obtain large numbers of measures in a coordinated program. Sound strategy also incorporates information improvement into process improvement; each major change in the process should generate better information as well as better results. A change in the protocols for hip replacement should search for new performance measures as well as better clinical results.

Generally, although not universally, the processes that improve measures increase the cost of measurement. Information investments are conceptually weighed in terms of their contribution to value and their cost, assigning priority to those with the highest value/cost ratio. In reality, the data for the comparisons are difficult to obtain, and a number of simplifying assumptions are often necessary. Many healthcare organizations have designated a portion of their investments to information improvement on the belief that a general campaign will pay off. Then information requests are prioritized against each other, but not in competition with other investments.

Cost

The cost of a measurement system is a combination of two elements: first, the resources consumed in obtaining, processing, reporting, and setting expectations for it and second, the costs of incorrect reports. It is convenient to label the first group accounting costs and the second hidden costs. Thoughtful measurement design must always address both.

Accounting costs are frequently buried in other activities. The cost of the data entry to order a test, administer a drug, or take an x-ray are lumped together with other parts of the activity. They can only be identified by special study. Marginal costs of individual new measures are low, but a systematic expansion of data processing capability may cost tens of millions. It may permit hundreds of additional measurements, making the true cost of each unmeasurable. Not only hardware and software is involved in the expansion cost; measurement definitions, scaling, tests of validity, and training of personnel are all initial investment costs.

Accounting costs tend to increase with improvements in reliability, validity, and timeliness, but automation has greatly reduced accounting costs and simultaneously increased the accuracy and timeliness of cost, revenue, output, and productivity information. The same basic data collection and processing system can be used to generate a large number of accurate measures. Careful attention to system design allows improvements in accuracy and timeliness of the information at modest increase in cost.

Hidden costs occur because of two possible incorrect interpretations of the data. *False negatives* occur when a correctable condition is not reported to the monitors, and, therefore, the monitors achieve less performance than they might. *False positives* occur when the measurement system reports a correctable situation when in fact none exists. Both are costly. The first results in suboptimal performance, and the second leads to costly, disruptive, and futile investigations. Hidden costs decrease with improved reliability, validity, and timeliness.

Value

The value of information is measured by the improvement in mission achievement. If a measure contributes cost saving of $5,000, that is its value. A measure that is viewed as essential by a stakeholder is enormously valuable for that reason. A measure that avoids serious error—the compass or the altimeter on an airplane—is essential. A measure nobody refers to is valueless. A measure that misleads has negative value.

While the concept is clear, its assessment is usually a matter of judgment. It is rarely possible to isolate the contribution of a specific measure or even a measurement system. The value of information is frequently confounded by other forces causing behavioral change. For example, market pressures may have pushed the organization to redesign the payroll process. The new process costs less to collect more detailed data. Its reports are expanded and more reliable. They give summary indicators both clearer and faster. And in designing the new process, the group saw some minor changes in other processes that they implemented. When the new process is installed, costs are $5,000 lower, and satisfaction and quality measures are the same to slightly higher. What caused the change? Was it (a) the market pressure that initiated the activity? or (b) the new payroll process? or (c) the improved understanding the work group gained from the study? Isolating the contribution of the new measures from the market pressures and the redesigned process is impossible.

The association between value and reliability, validity, and timeliness is similarly complex. Generally speaking, the more reliable, valid, and timely the measure is, the greater its value will be, but there are two important exceptions. First, when a crude measure is introduced it may cause dramatic changes in performance, the so-called sentinel effect. Second, improvements in measures are only useful up to the point at which the monitor can no longer change actual performance.

In a world where neither costs nor values can be easily assessed, it is difficult to justify expenditure on programs to improve measurement. There does seem to be a clear association between good measurement and success, however. Most well-managed organizations inside and outside of healthcare use measures heavily and are increasing their investment in them. The theory that good management depends on precise, quantitative understanding is compelling and has a number of articulate advocates. (It is inseparable from continuous improvement approaches.) And the performance of companies outside the healthcare field that have pursued information aggressively has substantially exceeded the performance of companies in general.[26]

Well-managed organizations solve the problem by developing a specific information strategy. The strategy has two important elements: a commitment to a continuing investment in information improvement and a plan to move in the directions with the greatest apparent value first. Developing and supporting this strategy is one of the functions of information services and is discussed in Chapter 15. The commitment of leading organizations is quite strong and specific. It extends over a minimum of five years and amounts to 0.25 to 0.5 percent of their net revenue, or 5 to 10 percent of their net profit.[27] Funds are earmarked in the capital budget for information services and are thus protected from the general competitive review described in Chapter 12.

Using Measures to Improve Performance

Information is data processed in ways that help people make decisions. The effective translation of data to information is as important as the quality of the data themselves. It occurs in three different but related ways: analysis of the past to help identify opportunities for improvement, forecasting to the future to help evaluate competing opportunities, and reporting of current performance to help control.

Analyzing Historic Data

Even a partially automated information system quickly builds up a large archive of data that can be systematically mined to understand processes better. The archive, a critical resource for the organization, is carefully managed as part of Information Services (Chapter 15).

An issue is identified, questions are posed of the archive, and the answers to the question suggest the directions fruitful for improvement. Figure 6.11

provides a simple illustration; one way to discover improvement opportunities is to search for specific correctable weaknesses, a "special cause" as opposed to a "common cause" in continuous improvement jargon.[28] A series of statistical tests is necessary to rule out various special causes. Any special causes that are found are pursued with their own Shewhart "Plan Do Check Act" cycle.[29] An ongoing dialogue between the operators and the database, identifying special causes, is part of the improvement process.

Seven tools of continuous quality improvement

Advocates of continuous improvement have emphasized a set of seven tools for analyzing problems like the satisfaction shortfall.[30] These can be taught directly to operating teams to assist them in improving processes.

FIGURE 6.11 Investigating a Satisfaction Shortfall: Searching for Improvement by Identifying Correctable Weaknesses

I. The issue: Patient satisfaction scores have dropped substantially below expectation.

II. The analysis: Search for specialized responses.

Responses	*Analysis*	*Result*
1. Statistically significant?	test mean and variance of most recent sample against previous samples	yes—proceed with analysis no—reevaluate need to proceed
2. Related to certain market segments?	test means of segments	yes—pursue segment specific strategy no—pursue general strategy
3. Related to certain treatment teams?	test means of teams	yes—review with team no—pursue general strategy
4. Related to certain diagnoses?	test means of diagnoses	yes—study those diagnoses no—pursue general strategy
5. Related to certain staffing levels?	test association of source with average staffing level at time of treatment	yes—consider additional staffing no—pursue general strategy

III. General Strategy:

Plan: Develop focus groups of patients and caregivers to identify correctable reasons for low scores.

Do: Devise process changes to address these.

Check: Test changes.

Act: Adopt permanently if improvement results and other dimensions are within acceptable limits.

1. **Flow process charts** show the steps in a process in the order in which they must be performed, with the criteria and results for various alternatives, or branches. Figure 6.12 shows a simple example. Several flow process charts appear elsewhere in the book. Various kinds of actions, such as evaluations, inspections, and direct services are often shown in different shapes to help follow the process.
2. **Fishbone,** or **cause and effect, diagrams** show relationships between complex flows and allow the team to identify components, test them as specific causes, and focus their investigation. Figure 6.13 illustrates a fishbone diagram that might analyze causes of low staffing, if the test of patient satisfaction scores showed it to be important.

FIGURE 6.12 Flow Process Chart

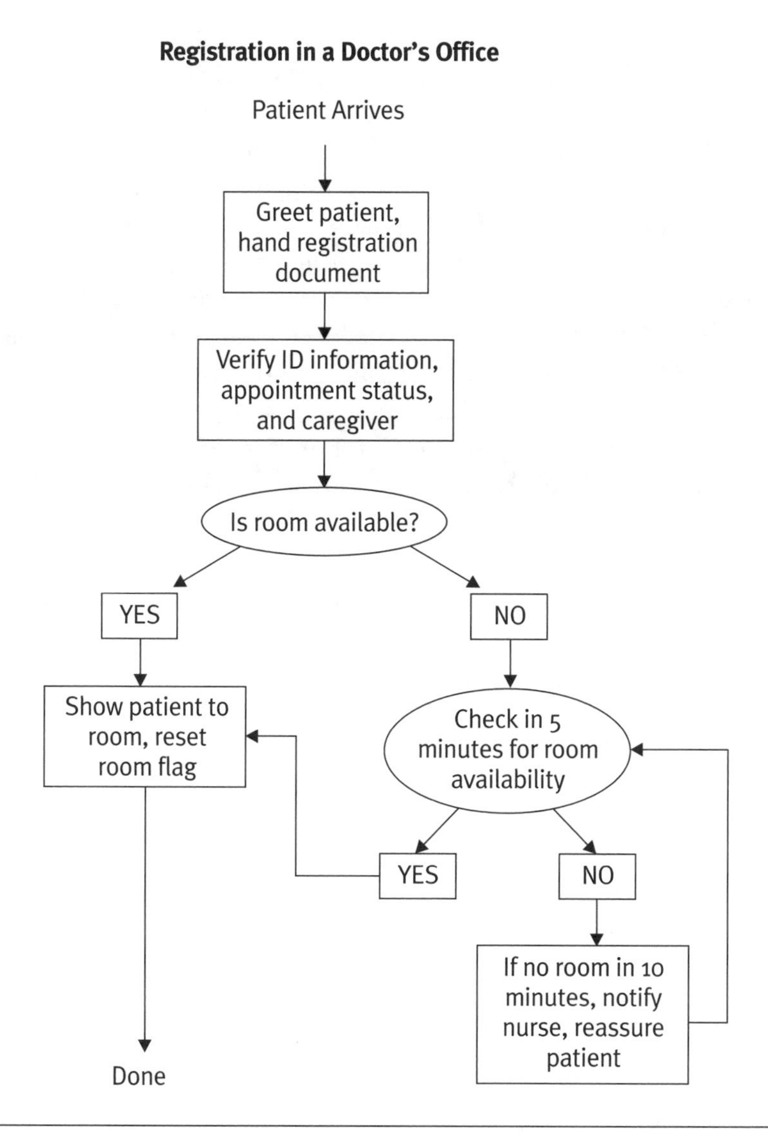

FIGURE 6.13 Fishbone Diagram

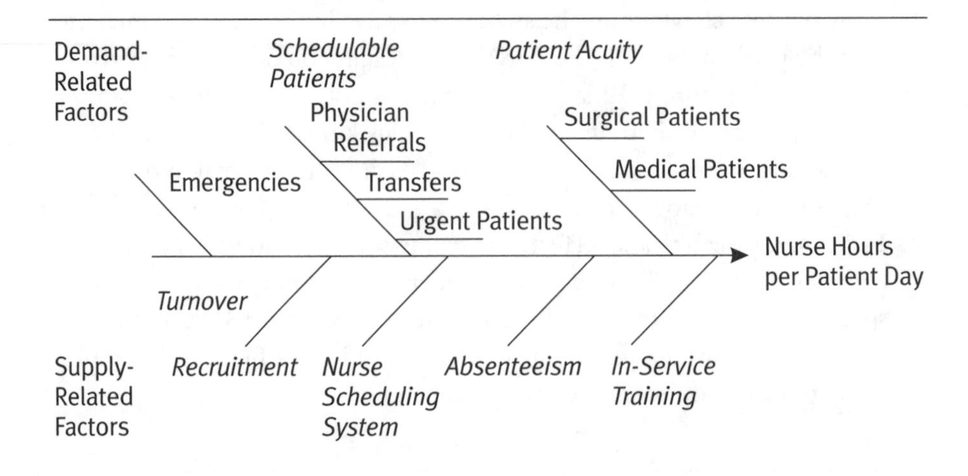

3. The **scatter diagram** is a graphic device for showing association between two measures. Figure 6.14 shows occupancy, a productivity measure, versus bed size for hospitals in southeast Michigan. The relationship indicated by the diagram can be tested using regression analysis. In the case of Figure 6.14, the apparent relationship is significant.
4. The **bar chart** is a display of differing values by some useful dimension, such as day of week, operator, site, or patient group. It is useful for revealing special causes that are related to resources, and correctable by process changes, equipment replacement, and personnel training. For example, the bar chart shown in Figure 6.15 shows varying lengths of stay for surgeons doing cholecystectomies. It reflects considerable variation. **Pareto analysis** simply examines the components of a problem in terms

FIGURE 6.14 Scatter Diagram: Hospital Occupancy by Bed Size (Data from Southeast Michigan, 1990)

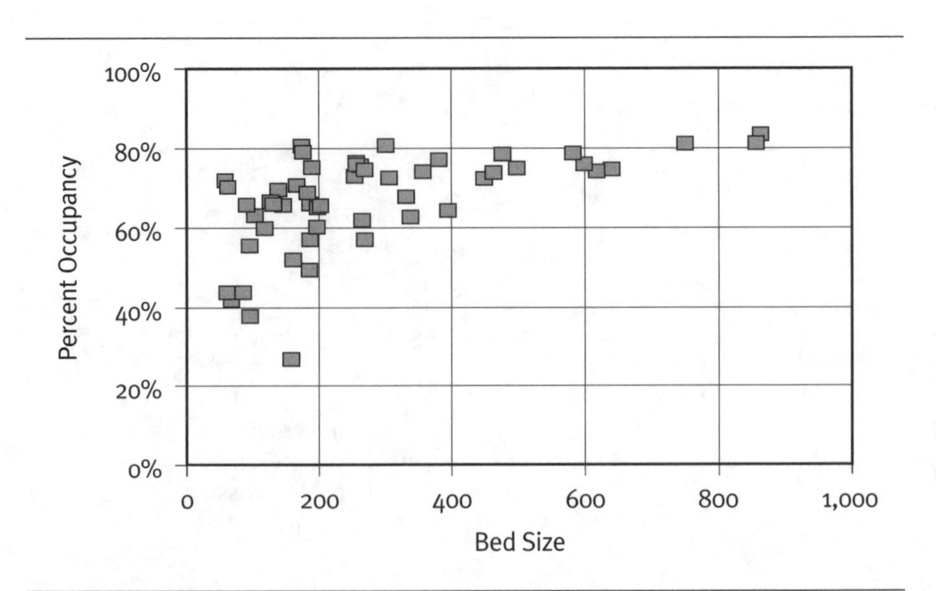

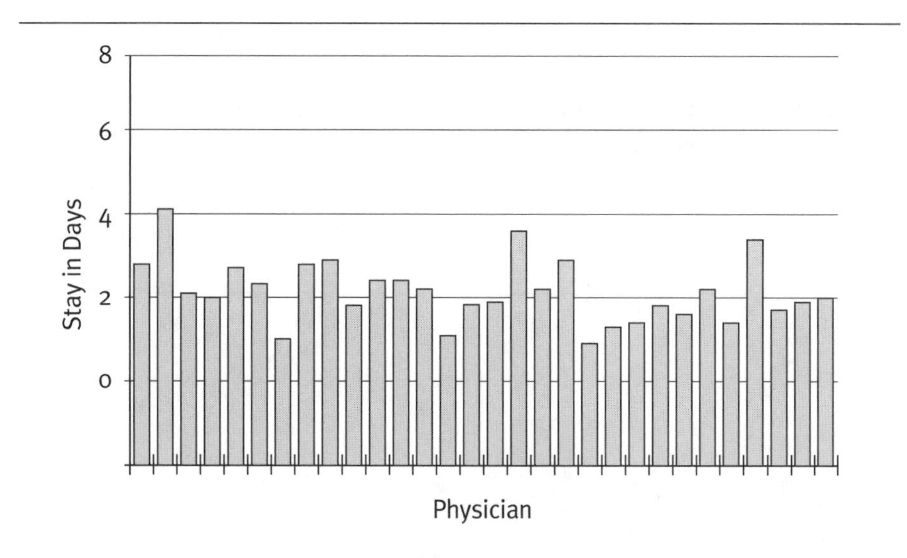

FIGURE 6.15 Bar Chart: Average Length of Stay by Attending Physician, Uncomplicated Cholecystectomy

of their contribution to it. It is a bar chart format, with the items rank ordered on a dependent variable such as cost, profit, or satisfaction. The "Pareto Rule" is that in general a few components will include a large part of the problem. Focusing on the biggest contributors allows the team to find solutions that may not work for every case, but that work well enough overall to be valuable. Figure 6.16 is the same subject as Figure 6.15. The expected length of stay from Medicare data has been subtracted from the actual lengths of stay for each patient and the difference has been totaled to create an excess days per physician statistic. The values are ranked in the table and, predictably, a few physicians contribute to the increased stay.

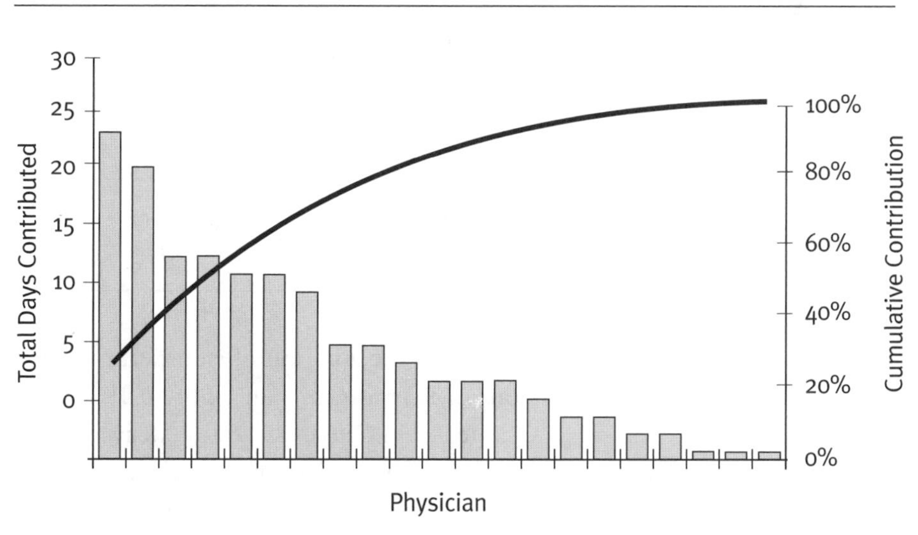

FIGURE 6.16 Pareto Diagram: Contribution of Days Over Medicare Average, by Physician

5. The **histogram** is built from the bar chart data. It groups individual values and shows the relative frequency of each group. An example is shown in Figure 6.17, again using the cholecystectomy length of stay. This time, individual patient values were grouped by frequency, yielding the display shown in the figure. The few patients who stay a long time contribute to the long tail to the right.

FIGURE 6.17
Histogram

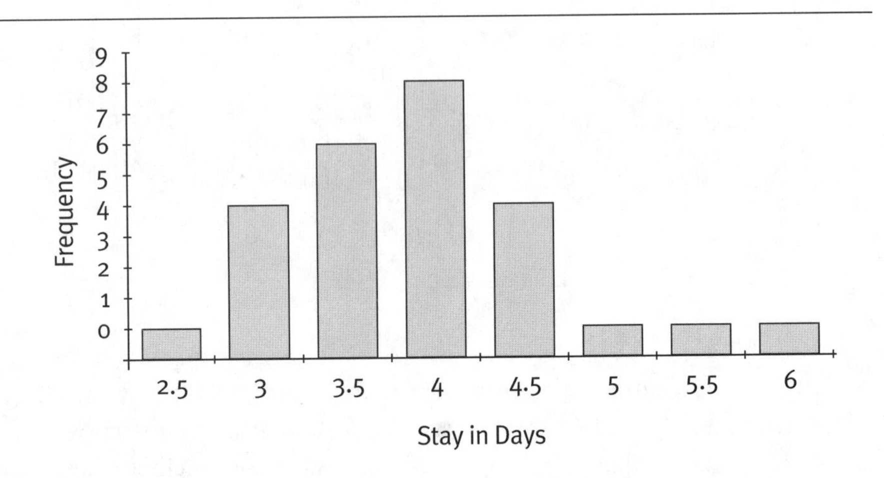

6. The **run chart** displays data over time and allows a visual perception of trends. Figure 6.18 shows a run chart with decreasing demand over several months.

FIGURE 6.18
Run Chart (Office Visits by Day of Week)

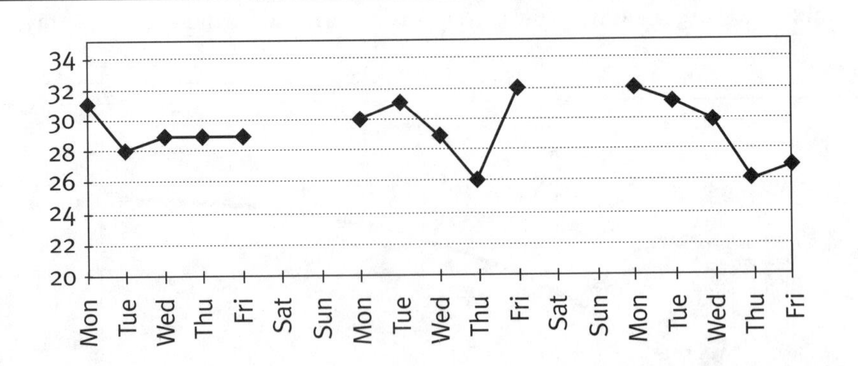

7. The **control chart** is a run chart with the addition of statistical quality control limits. One form of control chart is shown in Figure 6.19. Figure 6.19 shows a success story, a reduction in Caesarean section deliveries that occurred around month 21. It also shows the control limits that would trigger a reinvestigation of Caesarean sections. More complex examples are shown in Figure 6.25 below.

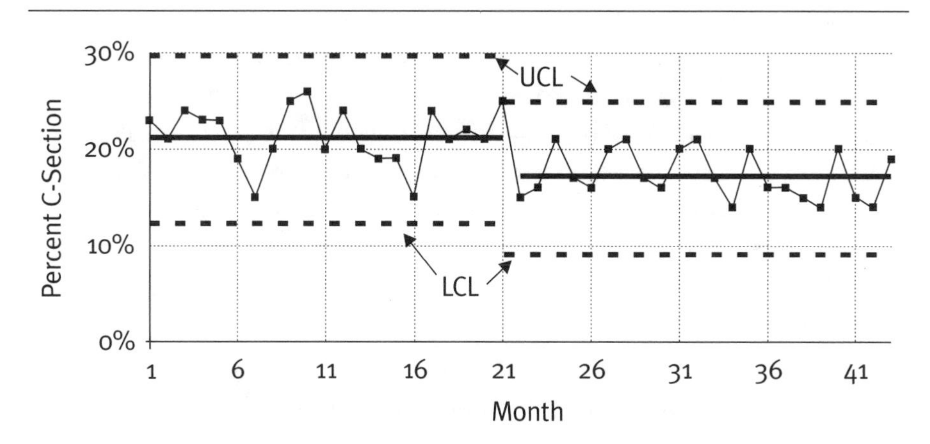

FIGURE 6.19 Attributes Control Chart (Caesarean Section Percentage by Month)

The seven tools can be taught successfully to healthcare workers and are included in elementary continuous improvement training programs. The statistical analyses and graphics can be prepared with common spreadsheet software.[31] Thus a team pursuing the general strategy to overcome the patient satisfaction shortfall of Figure 6.11 could easily prepare the examples shown here, and the tools would probably help them understand how to improve the care processes and patient satisfaction.

Advanced analytic tools

The seven tools may have their greatest value in teaching people how to think analytically. As tools, their utility is soon exhausted. Notably, they do not allow an untrained team to complete any of the statistical analyses listed in Figure 6.11. An analyst with a knowledge of the data and a graduate degree could answer the questions faster and more reliably. Similarly, they do not address the intricacies of cost analysis. Well-managed institutions provide internal consultants who can support and go beyond the seven tools. The work groups and final product teams at any level can call upon skilled planners, marketers, cost analysts, and management engineers to assist a team at any stage of its efforts. The kinds of analysis they can add include:

- *Advanced graphic displays.* These are often helpful in conveying quantitative information and appear constantly in analyses and proposals. A wide variety of graphs are available on common spreadsheet packages. Selection of the proper graph is important, and an experienced analyst can improve the accuracy and efficiency of information transfer.[32]
- *Univariate statistical analysis.* Arithmetic means, standard deviations, and standard errors are applicable to a great many situations, guiding the team to select topics that are likely to be fruitful. Some statistics—for example, low frequency events—require other tests that are more efficient.
- *Multivariate statistical analysis.* Regression and analysis of variance techniques have expanded dramatically over the past 20 years. A

statistician familiar with the different approaches can develop answers faster, and can guard against dangers of using the wrong test or violating conditions for interpreting results.

- *Cost analysis.* Most economic decisions hinge on unit costs and, as Chapter 14 indicates, accurate estimates are often problematic. A cost analyst familiar with available data and its limitations can produce the most accurate estimate possible in each specific situation.

Regression Forecasts

Forecasts predict future operating environments. Demand for service and prices of purchased resources are routinely forecast as part of the budget process. The budget office collaborates with planning and marketing to develop forecasts for the most global demand events, such as new patients, hospital admissions, and outpatient visits, broken down into major market segments. Price forecasting is usually developed by market survey or from commercial forecasters who sell opinions.

Global demand and demand for many specific care episodes such as DRGs can be forecast from institutional history, usually by regression analysis.[33] Regression based forecasts are often called *ceteris paribus* forecasts, because they assume that "all other things are equal," particularly that the expressed relationship will continue in the future. Several regression-based techniques are available to develop forecasts from internal historical data. In addition, commercial databases allow forecast of demand by disease episode based on national statistics and population characteristics. Population itself is measured and forecast for political units by a system of federal and state cooperation.[34] Some data are available from commercial sources for small geographic areas, such as zip codes. Thus, most final product teams have two forecasts for future demand:

1. Time series regression analysis of the form
   $\text{Demand} = \beta\,(\text{year}) \pm \varepsilon$
2. Epidemiologic analysis of the form
   $\text{Demand} = \beta_1\,(\text{population}) + \beta_2\,(\text{age}) + \beta_3\,(\text{sex}) + \beta_4\,(\text{income}) + C \pm \varepsilon$

Demand for specific intermediate products is forecast from regression analysis of the historic relation of the service to more global measures. For example, several recent years' data on the number of laboratory tests is regressed against the number of inpatient admissions, clinic visits, and year. A regression model such as:

$$\text{Lab tests} = \beta_1\,(\text{admissions}) + \beta_2\,(\text{visits}) + \beta_3\,(\text{year}) + C \pm \varepsilon$$

can be used for the initial forecast, where the forecast year and values for admissions and visits are inserted into the regression equation.

Further refinements can be introduced. Cyclic variation for seasons or days of the week can be accommodated. The demand can be segmented and forecast by segment at whatever level the data and statistical significance will support. The *ceteris paribus* forecasts can be almost fully automated. Well-managed organizations have sophisticated forecasting systems including several forecasting models and a database of agreed-upon forecasts of major measures.

Ceteris paribus forecasts are rarely adequate in themselves. Historically based forecasts are impossible when new services are developed because there is no history to use. "Other things being equal" rarely prevails even in existing services. The opinions and evidence from planning and marketing are used to refine the global forecasts. Line operators can adjust forecasts for areas under their authority, based on their judgment. Line operators are recognized to have excellent judgment about short-term forecasts. Planning and marketing personnel can spot variations from the *ceteris paribus* assumption and make adjustments not possible from computerized models.

Benchmarking Forecasts

Benchmarking is a form of quantitative goal identification establishing the desired forecast, as opposed to the most likely one developed by regression forecasting. A benchmark is the best known value for a specific measure, from any source. Benchmarks are obtained by constructing comparative data sets and ranking them. The benchmark can be a powerful tool to guide process improvement. Related to the benchmark is the process used to generate it, called **best practice**. If both are available, a team might decide to emulate best practice (explicitly abandoning the *ceteris paribus* assumption) and, allowing for implementation delays and learning time, achieve best practice over a few budget cycles. Its forecasts for each cycle would be based on performance relative to the benchmark.

An example of benchmarking and its use is in infant mortality, a complex problem where American healthcare does not do well. Nations with better maternal and infant healthcare are generally below ten deaths per 1,000 births. The best nations achieve less than five, although they are often small, economically advanced, well-educated and ethnically homogeneous populations. Healthcare organizations in American inner cities have a hard time matching these numbers, and it is known that the problems involved include reducing unwanted pregnancies, eliminating mothers' substance abuse and improving their nutrition, providing early prenatal care, and improving care at birth. Not all of these problems are under the control of the healthcare system. Collaboration with other social agencies would be required. Additional funding will be necessary, even though the outcome could reduce overall expenditures. An improved process is thus a multiyear project. A typical inner-city hospital might face forecasts and benchmarks like the ones shown in Figure 6.20. A

FIGURE 6.20
Forecasts and Benchmarks Compared to Create a Process-Improvement Strategy

Problem:
High-risk mothers and babies drive infant mortality rates up.

Benchmarks:

World	Japan	4.6/1,000 births
United States	Maine	6.9/1,000 births
Comparable cities		14.2/1,000 births

Strategies	**Time to Visible Result**	**Anticipated change in mortality**
Encourage prenatal care Within three months, open new care center with focus on teen activities, healthcare for teen girls.	12 months	Year 1: 0% Year 2: 10% Year 3: 20%
Expand use of contraceptives Offer contraceptives and counseling to teen girls and boys.	12 months	Year 1: 0% Year 2: 05% Year 3: 10%
Drug use prevention and education Work with high schools, police, and social services on drug abatement.	24 months	Year 1: 0% Year 2: 0% Year: 3 05%

Budget Expectations

Calculation	*Value*
Year 1: No change	21/1,000 births
Year 2: Initial value decreased by 5% for reduced pregnancies 10% for prenatal care	18/1,000 births
Year 3: Initial value decreased by 10% for reduced pregnancies, 20% for prenatal care, 5% for drug abatement	14.4/1,000 births

deliberate program to improve performance might identify an interim goal of nine, and start programs to achieve it in three years.

Performance Modeling

Models are simplified representations of reality that can be manipulated to test various hypotheses about the future. Real-world trials are rarely the best way to begin to evaluate a complex proposal. Models are easier to adjust and less costly if something goes wrong. Modeling recognizes that performance depends on both **exogenous events**, those largely outside the control of the line operator, and **endogenous events**, those largely within the control of the operator. Models require an **objective function**, that is, a quantitative statement of the relationship between events and desired results, and constraints, limits on the range of acceptable operating conditions.

The modeler can then modify the endogenous assumptions and test the relationship between them and performance, eventually finding an optimal performance within the constraints. Next, in a process called **sensitivity**

analysis, the modeler modifies the exogenous events, usually developing most favorable, expected, and least favorable scenarios. These show the robustness of the proposal and indicate the degree of risk involved. Several forms of models are used by well-managed healthcare organizations to evaluate proposals.

The planning department routinely produces short-run and long-run forecasts for a number of important demand measures. It maintains a database that allows generations of forecasts for almost any service demand on request. These are used in strategic positioning, the development of facility and service plans, and the construction of expectations for the next budget year. The reliability of the forecasts, the advice available from the planning department, and the speed with which the request can be serviced are critical elements in long-term success of the organization. The data for incidence rates, advice on segmentation of the population, and ranges of current practice on use are frequently available from national consulting services. Calculation and presentation software are also available to make construction of forecasts, sensitivity analysis, and exploration of alternative scenarios quickly and easy.

Business plans

Models that deal with future events as fixed numbers, rather than as random events subject to a predictable variance, are called **deterministic models**. The most common are business plans, but several others are useful in specific situations.

Business plans are the most universally used model. They describe an operating proposal, identify exogenous and endogenous conditions, and forecast demand, output, revenue, costs, and profit or cost savings over several years. They may use regression or benchmark modeling to forecast components. Demand and prices are usually taken as exogenous, and quality concerns are handled as a constraint. (For example, examining only alternatives that appear likely to give the same or better quality scores.) Business plans are used to justify new programs and capital expenditure, evaluate make-or-buy alternatives, show returns on improved processes, and estimate break-even conditions and earnings associated with increasing demand. The long-range financial plan used by the board (Figures 3.6 and 3.7) is a sophisticated business plan. Scenarios evaluating alternative exogenous and endogenous assumptions are frequently useful for strategy selection.[35]

Business plans assume deterministic conditions, that is, they accept the forecasts without error terms or allowance for random variation. They examine alternative exogenous scenarios using sensitivity analysis. Although they are conceptually algebraic models, they are prepared on computer spreadsheets and presented as year-by-year forecasts. The algebra is buried in the spreadsheet design. Spreadsheet capabilities make graphic summaries easy, and they are widely used and expected.

Many line teams will have members who can prepare elementary business plans. Consultation from technical personnel in planning, marketing, and finance is useful both in the model design and in evaluating the assumptions.

The neatness and precision of the spreadsheets and graphs and concealment of the underlying algebra can be misleading. The key questions about business plans deal with the assumptions, such as the sources of forecasts, the realism of alternative scenarios, time allowances made for implementation and learning, and the operating conditions necessary to reach the performance level used in the analysis. As more complex problems are addressed, the spreadsheets themselves get quite elaborate, and the model builder must have extensive experience.[36]

Community-based epidemiologic planning

Healthcare systems now identify geographic communities, or markets, whose healthcare needs they will meet. The demographic, economic, and epidemiological characteristics of these communities are a fundamental data set for planning decisions of all kinds. The general model to estimate local demand for a given service is an equation:

$$\left\{\begin{matrix}\text{Demand for}\\ \text{a service}\end{matrix}\right\} = \left\{\begin{matrix}\text{Population}\\ \text{at risk}\end{matrix}\right\} \times \left\{\begin{matrix}\text{Incidence}\\ \text{rate}\end{matrix}\right\} \times \left\{\begin{matrix}\text{Average}\\ \text{use per}\\ \text{incidence}\end{matrix}\right\} \times \left\{\begin{matrix}\text{Market}\\ \text{share}\end{matrix}\right\}$$

It can be applied to either intermediate services or final products. It is usually calculated for specific risk groups to accommodate the fact that most conditions for which people seek healthcare differ by age, sex, income, and other factors.[37] The individual terms must themselves be forecast, using regression analysis, benchmarking, or other techniques. State agencies now prepare detailed population forecasts that are more reliable than any other sources, except for very small geographic areas. Sensitivity analyses evaluate alternative forecasts, greatly improving the final decision process.

Examples of the use of the model are shown in Figure 6.21. Obstetrics is the easiest to understand. It also has the best supporting data, allowing great refinement in the estimate. Obstetrical deliveries occur only to young women. The population at risk and the anticipated fertility rates are frequently available for each year of age. The use per incident for deliveries is essentially one. Market share can be measured from history because births are recorded both by the mother's address and the site of delivery. All of these data must be forecast into the future. The fertility rates and market share can be forecast from history or by survey of child-bearing intentions.

The remaining examples of Figure 6.21 show the application of the model in other areas. Post-partum care days in obstetrics resemble the forecast for deliveries, but each mother uses about two days, a number that differs by locale. Well-baby visits are planned events important to provide immunizations, instruction to the mother, and early detection of developmental problems. The population at risk is all babies born in the last year; the incidence and the number of visits per baby are set by policy; and the market share is closely related to the obstetrics share. The forecast would be used not only to estimate

FIGURE 6.21 Applications of the Epidemiologic Planning Model

Example	Population at Risk	Incidence Rate	Use per Incident	Market Share
Obstetrics deliveries	Fertile women	Births/fertile woman-year	1 deliveries/ woman	% of all births to women in community
Post-partum care	Delivered women	Births/fertile woman-year	2.0 days/ delivery	% of all births to women in community
Well-baby visits	Infants < 1 year	Births/fertile woman-year	4.0 visits/ year	% of all well-baby visits in community
Emergency department visits	Economic, geographic subsets of population	ED visits/ person for each subset	1.0 visits/ arrival	% of community visits seeking this ED
Hip replacements	Population aged 50–65, over 65	Hip replacement/ person for each subset	1.0 surgeries/ patient	% of candidates seeking this institution

demand, but as a quality standard—a well-managed health insurance program will strive to achieve 100 percent of scheduled visits.

Emergency department visits are expensive, and managed care strategies call for minimizing them. They are a function of availability of health insurance, other primary care sources, and lifestyle. As a result, the population at risk would be segregated economically or geographically to identify different incidence rates. For many purposes, it would also be necessary to adjust for time of day and day of week. This would be done by using several different incidence rates. The use term could be set at one, yielding a forecast of visits, or the average number of hours of use, yielding an estimate of use of facilities. Hip replacement surgery occurs almost exclusively among the elderly, and the use term can be adjusted to forecast either procedures or expected days of inpatient stay.

Using the incidence of diseases, the model can forecast many final product episodes. Epidemiologic studies have developed the incidence of most common and expensive illness and analyzed the population characteristics associated with it. Data are available from the Centers for Disease Control and Prevention[38] and commercial sources. Estimates can be compared to actual values for diseases reducible by prevention or management, such as cancer, heart disease, and AIDS, to reveal unique risks or treatment practices in the community. These are useful in identifying cost-improvement possibilities. A simple example is births to very young single mothers. These are associated with high-cost problems in infant care. Programs to reduce these births by discouraging teenaged pregnancy are cost-effective. Programs to reach young mothers early in their pregnancies reduce the risk and cost of problems. Under capitation insurance contracts, these gains work directly to reduce overall cost of care.

Other deterministic models

Other algebraic models can be developed as needed. They show the relationship between exogenous characteristics and desired endogenous ones, such as the relation between demand and staffing, and are useful for illustrating assumptions and gaining improved understanding of operating possibilities.[39]

PERT (project evaluation and review technique) charts are programs for analyzing construction projects and similar sets of complex, time-dependent, interrelated activities. The value of PERT charts lies in their ability to identify critical paths, the sequences and timetables of events that will delay the overall project if they are not met. PERT charting is routine for major construction projects and renovations. It is also useful for complex new program development. Commercial software supports the analysis, but the inputs require substantial knowledge of change processes. PERT charting is generally done by one or two people in the organization who are experienced with it.

A variety of programming models are used in commercial applications, including linear programming and forms of dynamic programming. These models differ from the business plan in their ability to find the optimum set of endogenous conditions. They have found limited use in healthcare, although linear programming is theoretically applicable to personnel staffing and inventory management. The few applications that have occurred have been incorporated in specific software for departmental operation. A technique called data envelopment analysis allows estimation of optimal operational efficiency in certain multidimensional problems.[40] Development of programming models is demanding. Special coursework is essential, along with extensive experience in other modeling forms.

Stochastic models

Some situations cannot be effectively modeled by deterministic techniques. They are usually those where the exogenous conditions cannot be predicted easily in advance, but still have an important effect on the outcomes. Stochastic means subject to chance variation. **Stochastic models** incorporate chance variation in the analysis and evaluation of the solutions. The traditional example of a stochastic problem is the arrival of women for obstetric delivery. Each event is unpredictable even a few hours in advance, yet it is so important that the healthcare organization must have adequate staff and facilities to serve the patient when she arrives. A model will be constructed showing how often the staff and facilities will be overtaxed for a given level of average demand. Because the demand is random with wide variation from hour to hour, a deterministic model based on the average demand would be disastrously unsatisfactory.

Figure 6.22 shows the results of a model to determine obstetric birthing rooms and staffing. (The model is simplified to illustrate the issues involved.) On the average, women arriving for delivery will require two rooms and staff groups. Just under 2,200 women deliver each year, and they require on the average about eight hours of service. But because of the stochastic demand, they will keep two rooms and staff occupied most of the time, need a third about 20 percent of the time, a fourth about 10 percent, a fifth less than 5 percent. Only about once a year will six units be required. Quality and patient satisfaction require that some provision be made for the five-unit and six-unit situations, but because of the cost, the solution will not be to routinely staff for five units, nor to build six units.[41]

Stochastic models are usually constructed around **Monte Carlo simulation**, a computerized test of a model situation by repeated trial. Although advanced spreadsheet software has the capability of doing Monte Carlo simulation, the most important parts of the model are its design and the measurement of the parameters. The birthing room example in Figure 6.22 requires not only forecasts of mean values but reliable distributions of arrival times, service times, and staffing requirements. The final evaluation will weigh probabilities of rare events and the extent to which they violate constraints against the cost of meeting them.

Simulation can also be adapted to expand sensitivity analysis of deterministic models. Exogenous variables must be given realistic distributions of possible values, and the impact of variation can be explored to reveal changes required in endogenous variables and resulting values of the objective function. A range of scenarios, rather than just a few extremes, can be evaluated.[42] Advanced software is usually necessary to do this and is offered by several vendors. These systems allow financial planning in a stochastic mode and are called **decision support systems** (DSS). To date, they have found limited

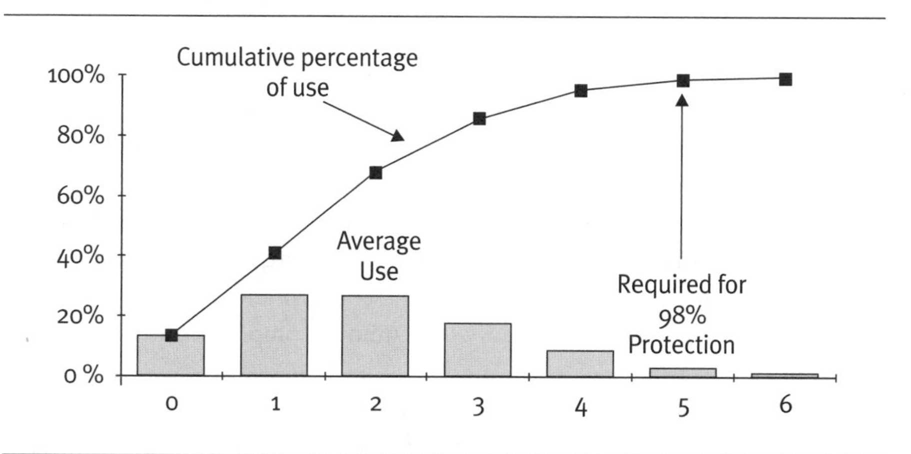

FIGURE 6.22 Stochastic Analysis of Birthing Room Requirements (% of time rooms in use)

application in healthcare, probably because they require very large, reliable databases.[43] New program analysis has been reported in a proposed health promotion center[44] and a pharmacy.[45] As healthcare organizations improve their automated data archives, DSS applications will grow. At least theoretically, a sophisticated DSS model could be used with a process improvement team in real time, allowing the team to experiment with various changes to endogenous events and see the impact on constraints and objective function almost immediately.[46]

Experimentation

Many improvement possibilities require more than an abstract model evaluation. Relationships between exogenous and endogenous events and final objectives are not always easy to state or even understand. All models are simplifications of reality; one of the most common simplifications is omission of interactions between various events. As a result, real world trials do not always behave as the model indicated. In addition, trials offer opportunities to demonstrate, convince, and teach. The model site can be the teaching site to roll out the results to the larger organization. For these reasons, the "check" step of PDCA frequently includes a field trial.[47]

Quantitative information contributes to the field trial in several ways. It allows the improvement team to analyze relationships between various events and design the improvement itself. It supports simple models that rule out unpromising experiments and reveal correctable weaknesses in promising ones. Models also show the kinds of data required for evaluation and the length of trial necessary to achieve reliable results. They often suggest potential difficulties with the trial or its interpretation that can be accommodated in design or analysis to strengthen the conclusions.

The most rigorous form of experiments are random controlled trials carefully designed and controlled to yield results appropriate to a large, uncontrolled population or market, such as the United States or all developed countries. They are supported by research funds from large corporations or government. Design and publication are both subject to rigorous critical review. Many healthcare organizations participate in alliances or networks formed for the purpose of research. Most clinical research developing and testing new methods of diagnosis and treatment is done this way.

Experiments on operations are difficult to do at the same level of rigor. Trials are often pre/post, using historical data as a control, or pre/post with a control. The results are superior to no trial at all and are usually strong enough to support decisions. Technically, a single organization can represent only itself. Transferability from one organization to another may be limited; indeed the objective may be to develop a unique competitive advantage for a single firm.

The level of rigor is only one of the considerations in the trial design. The cost of the trial, including potential dangers to patients or employees, and other benefits such as building consensus or serving as a training site must also be considered. A good field trial is one that:

- presents no increased danger to patients or staff;
- is free of avoidable distortion or bias;
- is conducted over enough patients or events to yield statistically significant results;
- evaluates an improvement worth several times the accounting cost of conducting the trial; and
- can be modified in course to yield the greatest possible overall improvement.

These standards are considerably less rigorous than those for formal research. The loss of rigor increases the chance that the result may be caused by something other than the experimental modification, and the chance that a second trial will not yield the same results. The so-called **Hawthorne effect** is a frequent issue. A famous series of experiments showed that the fact of experimentation and the attention it drew could improve performance, independent of the experiment itself.[48] Organization field trials often approach the problem of rigor by making allowance for the Hawthorne effect and related risks in judging the results, and by approaching the experiment sequentially. Thus, very strong initial results lead to continuation of the trial; weaker ones to consideration of improvements in the proposal; and disappointing ones to discontinuation. If feasible, the continuation can be undertaken on a second site, where pride of authorship is less likely to enhance the results.

A field trial should have the following components:

1. A hypothesis or proposal expressing the relationship between an endogenous event, process, or method, and an objective function, such as "If we change Process A in a certain defined way, we will achieve better outcomes as measured by cost, profit, and quality."
2. Justification from literature or analysis of operational data suggesting that the hypothesis is plausible, that the answer is not obvious, and that a trial is likely to yield improvements worth many times its cost.
3. A method of implementing the change in a real field setting, including site, initial investment in equipment and training, safety factors, and time schedules.
4. A method of measuring the changes in outcomes and any other variables important to the decision.
5. An estimation of the length or size of the trial necessary to demonstrate the improvement.
6. A review of the moral and practical implications for patients and employees involved in the trial.

7. A critical analysis of the reliability, validity, and value of the expected results, including a review of confounding factors that should be considered.

While the steps seem onerous, a field trial involves a disruption of an ongoing process and the danger of doing harm is always present. The steps can be simplified in undemanding situations; operating teams try new approaches constantly as part of their learning. But a trial involving more than a few people in direct personal communication deserves at least a review of all seven items.

Well-managed institutions establish mechanisms facilitating review of field trials. The support includes consultants trained in experimental design and analysis and ad hoc work groups to gain consensus on methods, explore implications, and provide a critical analysis. A **human subjects committee** can contribute unbiased review of potential dangers to patients and employees. It is required by most funding bodies for formal research, but it clearly has a role whenever a process change involves patient care or risks to employees. Similarly, large-scale trials can be given critical review by formal committees from outside the area in question, emulating the research review process.

Monitoring and Controlling

Control, the ability to achieve desired future events, is the essence of all economic activity and the central justification for the organization.[49] Control implies both predictability and uniformity. Variation is a measure of the lack of control, and monitoring is the measurement of variation. Control is actually achieved by individuals and organizations through a series of human interactions where the quantitative measurement of relevant factors is only a supplement to more powerful and less precise processes. As activities and organizations grow more complex, the role of quantification becomes more central, but it never replaces the underlying human factors.

Continuous improvement theory emphasizes that control is built in, not monitored, and certainly not imposed. Control begins with the design of service and process. The right process, training, tools and supplies, and demand levels lead to control; failures in these cannot be replaced by incentives or statistical systems. A monitoring process, statistical systems, and incentives are necessary to maintain the system after it is designed. Even if it was perfectly designed at the outset, an unmonitored system will deteriorate as a function of environmental changes, wear, and fatigue. Monitoring detects the need for maintenance and the opportunity for improvement.

Cybernetic Systems

The concept of monitoring begins with a cybernetic system, the addition of a separate, new activity to a process. A process translates inputs—including demand and resources—to outputs—goods or services sold for revenue and profit. It can be represented as shown in Figure 6.23A. The monitor shown in Figure 6.23B is added to evaluate the performance, identify necessary corrections, and make them. The monitor relies on the same measures of performance as shown in Figure 6.2. The word **cybernetic** comes from the ancient Greek *cybernos*, or helmsman, the monitor who kept the ship on course. Monitors of some systems are purely mechanical; the thermostat on the heating system is an example. Most human activities are monitored by the person doing them.

Figure 6.23B applies to any process, from a nurse giving patient care to a complete healthcare organization. The monitor in direct contact with the process is called the primary monitor. It is possible to monitor monitors, thus establishing a nest of sequential monitoring functions. The accountability hierarchy is such a nest; each level monitors not the underlying activities, but the performance of the level immediately below it. The governing board can be understood as the primary monitor for the organization as a whole.

The monitor, whether it is the nurse, the governing board, or anyone in between, proceeds by comparing the performance information (technically the signal) against the expectation. If the two are not identical, an error signal is generated and the monitor acts upon it. This does not automatically require quantification; the nurse will be working with a wide variety of verbal, visual, and sensory data that is not quantified at all. Quantification is necessary when the direct contact is lost.

As an example of an activity beyond the individual worker, consider a nursing station shown in Figure 6.24. The head nurse is the monitor; nurses

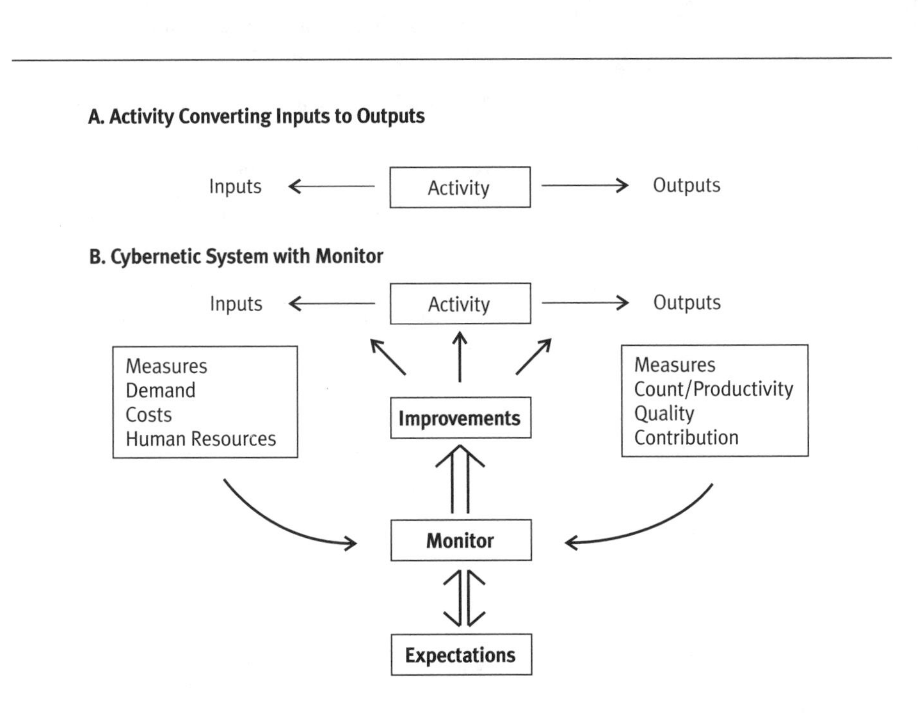

FIGURE 6.23 Cybernetic System

and other nursing personnel are the major resources; arriving patients are the demands; and treated patients are the outputs. The budget for a nursing unit will specify quantitative expectations for all six performance dimensions, and measures of achievement will reach the head nurse regularly on these and many other indicators. (Some will be by direct observation and will not be quantitative.) The head nurse will compare signals to expectations. He or she will expect no error signals, and in a well-managed institution will rarely see them. The failures that do occur should always be studied for ways to eliminate them in the future, by changing the process. The head nurse's main effort will turn to possibilities for further improvement, which can be evaluated and implemented in future years' expectations.

Spider Charts

Ratio-scaled performance can be reported on spider charts, like Figure 3.14, at any level of the organization from the work group up. The Henry Ford Health System does this, interlocking the performance measures and representing all the quadrants (cost, quality, satisfaction, and market share). The charts themselves are easily created from spreadsheet software, but careful attention must be paid to defining the performance measures, expectations, and data collection processes to insure reliable and valid reports. The charts provide a quick, graphic summary of performance on up to 16 variables.

FIGURE 6.24 Examples of Monitor Function on a Nursing RC

Dimension	Measures	Possible Improvements
Demand	Number of patients	Patient satisfaction, physician satisfaction, scheduling, case management
Costs	Labor costs	Personnel scheduling, cross-training, new processes
	Supplies costs	New processes, clinical protocols
Human Resources	Employee satisfaction	Personnel scheduling, supervisory training, new job requirements
Output/ Productivity	Cost per visit or per day	Change processes to reduce variable costs, increase demand to reduce fixed costs
	Cost per member month	Change processes to reduce variable costs, decrease demand, reduce fixed costs by elimination
Quality	Recovery rates	Personnel training, clinical protocols, new processes
	Patient satisfaction	Personnel training, clinical protocols, new processes
	Procedure	Personnel training, clinical protocols, new processes
Contribution	Profit or cost target	Search for improvable inputs, outputs, and processes

Statistical Quality Control

Statistical quality control will be necessary to identify variations that are significant or likely to be correctable.[50] Significant variations can be called special cause variation or error signals. Nonsignificant variations can be called random variation, common cause variation, or noise. Significance can be tested by standard statistical techniques, and statistical quality control is now frequently automated and graphically reported.[51] Measures for a specific time period are taken for a sample or for all activity during the period. Each measurement is called a lot, and lots are collected sequentially. Values and control limits for both the mean and the variance covering sequential time periods can be plotted for variables statistics (those arising from interval and ratio scales), as shown in Figure 6.25. The more common attributes measures can be expressed as a percentage passing (or failing) the threshold for each time period and plotted over time as shown in Figure 6.19. All three of these graphs are control charts. They can be reviewed over time for trends or changes, using statistical techniques to identify the special cause or statistically significant variation.

Several alternatives and improvements can make the statistical tests more sensitive in specific situations. For further discussion at an elementary level, see Gitlow, *Planning for Quality, Productivity, and Competitive Position*, and at an advanced level Feigenbaum's *Total Quality Control* under Suggested Readings below.

Control charts allow monitors to scan large numbers of measures and quickly identify where further improvements are likely.[52] However, there are a number of ways in which the analysis can be misused. Misuse will waste resources, and it may be destructive because it diverts us from important alternatives or results in insupportable accusations and loss of morale. Here are some of the principal problems:

1. The lots must be from the same process. Many uncontrollable events change medical care processes over time, such as changes in the condition of arriving patients. Runs of uncommon patients and other factors affecting the lots must always be ruled out before "outliers" are acknowledged.
2. No inference of good or poor quality can ever be made about a lot until special causes have been identified or ruled out. It is useful to use 99 percent confidence limits (three times the standard deviation) to identify outliers. This reduces the number of outliers identified and raises the probability that a correctable cause can be found.
3. No inference of good or poor quality can ever be made about individual cases in the lot using this approach (or about the practitioners treating the patients in the lot). Many outliers are actually random events.

FIGURE 6.25
Process Control Charts for Variables Measures

A. Control Chart for the Mean

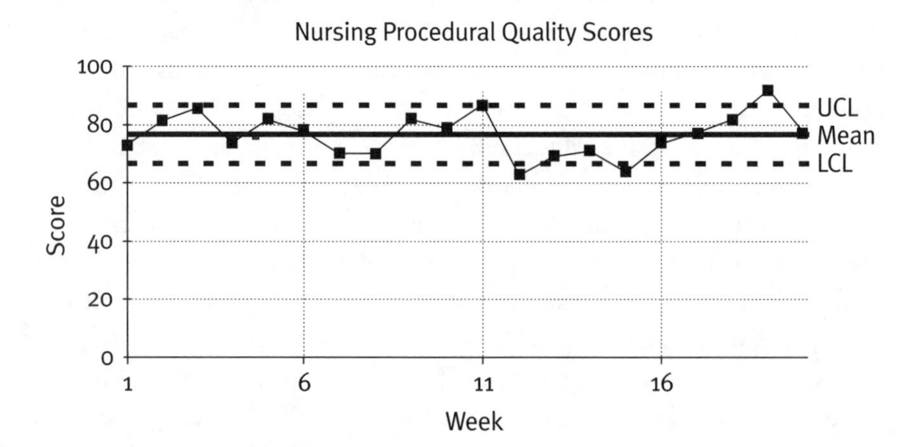

B. Control Chart for Variation

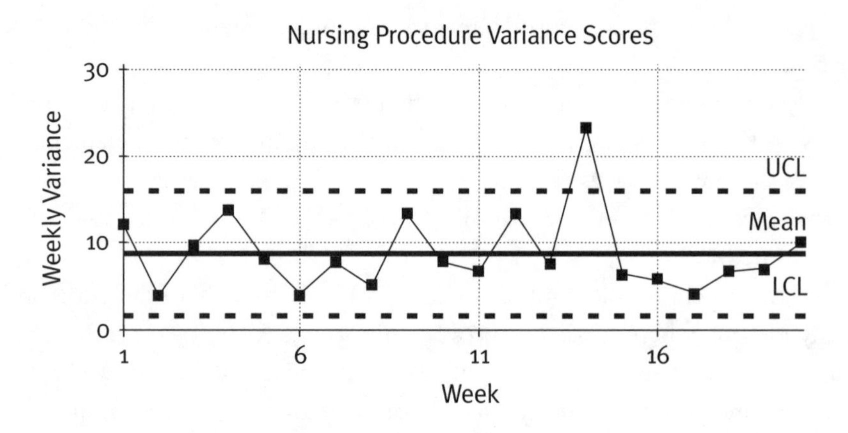

Suggested Readings

Austin, C. J., and S. B. Boxerman. 1995. *Quantitative Analysis for Health Services Administration*. Chicago: Health Administration Press.

Deming, W. E. 1986. *Out of the Crisis*. Boston: Massachusetts Institute of Technology Center for Advanced Engineering Study.

Feigenbaum, A. V. 1991. *Total Quality Control*, 3rd ed. (rev.). New York: McGraw-Hill.

Flood, A. B., S. M. Shortell, and W. R. Scott. 1997. "Organizational Performance: Managing for Efficiency and Effectiveness." In *Essentials of Health Care Management*, edited by S. Shortell and A. D. Kaluzny, 381–429. New York: Delmar.

Krowinski, W. J., and S. R. Steiber. 1996. *Measuring and Managing Patient Satisfaction*, 2nd ed. Chicago: American Hospital Publishing.

Mendenhall, W., and R. J. Beaver. 1994. *Introduction to Probability and Statistics,* 9th ed. Belmont, CA: Duxbury Press.

Montgomery, D. C., L. A. Johnson, and J. S. Gardiner. 1990. *Forecasting and Time Series Analysis,* 2nd ed. New York: McGraw-Hill.

Notes

1. K. Castaneda-Mendez, K. Mangan, and A. M. Lavery, "The Role and Application of the Balanced Scorecard in Healthcare Quality Management." *Journal for Healthcare Quality* 20(1), pp. 10–13 (January–February, 1998)
2. P. Eastman, "NCI Adopts New Mammography Screening Guidelines for Women." *Journal of the National Cancer Institute* 89(8), pp. 538–39 (April 16, 1997); Anonymous, "NIH Consensus Statement. Breast Cancer Screening for Women Ages 40–49." *NIH Consensus Statement* 15(1), pp. 1–35 (January 21–23, 1997)
3. R. S. Kaplan and R. Cooper, *Cost & Effect: Using Integrated Cost Systems to Drive Profitability and Performance.* Boston: Harvard Business School Press (1998)
4. J. J. Baker, "Activity-Based Costing for Integrated Delivery Systems." *Journal of Health Care Finance* 22(2), pp. 57–61 (Winter, 1995)
5. D. J. Brailer, E. Kroch, M. V. Pauly, and J. Huang, "Comorbidity-Adjusted Complication Risk: A New Outcome Quality Measure." *Medical Care* 34(5), pp. 490–505 (May, 1996)
6. T. P. Hofer, S. J. Bernstein, R. A. Hayward, and S. DeMonner, "Validating Quality Indicators for Hospital Care." *Joint Commission Journal on Quality Improvement* 23(9), pp. 455–67 (September, 1997)
7. M. L. Millenson, *Demanding Medical Excellence: Doctors and Accountability in the Information Age.* Chicago: University of Chicago Press (1997)
8. ———, "Perspective on Measurement." *Health Affairs* 17(4): 7–41
9. M. Johantgen, A. Elixhauser, J. K. Bali, M. Goldfarb, and D. R. Harris, "Quality Indicators Using Hospital Discharge Data: State and National Applications." *Joint Commission Journal on Quality Improvement* 24(2), pp. 88–105 (February, 1998)
10. J. H. Seibert, J. M. Strohmeyer and R. G. Carey, "Evaluating the Physician Office Visit: In Pursuit of a Valid and Reliable Measure of Quality Improvement Efforts." *Journal of Ambulatory Care Management* 19(1), pp. 17–37 (January, 1996)
11. R. C. Ford, S. A. Bach and M. D. Fottler, "Methods of Measuring Patient Satisfaction in Health Care Organizations." *Health Care Management Review* 22(2), pp. 74–89 (Spring, 1997)
12. W. J. Krowinski, S. R. Steiber, *Measuring and Managing Patient Satisfaction,* 2nd Ed. Chicago: American Hospital Publishing (1996)
13. Pickert Institute home page: www.pickert.org (October 28, 1998 version)
14. R. Hodges, L. Kelley, and A. Wilkes, "Benchmarking and Networking Through Collaborative Groups." *Journal for Healthcare Quality* 18(1), pp. 26–31 (January–February, 1996)

15. See, for example, publications and services of the Medstat Corporation: www.medstat.com; Sachs Group: www.sach.com; and HCIA, Inc.: www.hcia.com (October 27, 1998)
16. W. A. Knause, E. A. Draper, and D. P. Wagner, "The Use of Intensive Care: New Research Initiatives and Their Application for National Health Policy," *Milbank Memorial Fund Quarterly* 61, pp. 561–583 (Fall, 1983)
17. R. C. Jelinek, "An Operational Analysis of the Patient Care Function," *Inquiry* 6(2), pp. 53–58 (June, 1969)
18. J. P. Weiner, B. H. Starfield, D. M. Steinwachs, and L. M. Mumford, "Development and Application of a Population-Oriented Measure of Ambulatory Care Case-Mix." *Medical Care* 29(5), pp. 452–72 (May, 1991); B. Starfield, J. Weiner, L. Mumford, and D. Steinwachs, "Ambulatory Care Groups: A Categorization of Diagnoses for Research and Management." *Health Services Research* 26(1), pp. 53–74 (April, 1991)
19. P. A. Gross, "Practical Healthcare Epidemiology: Basics of Stratifying for Severity of Illness." *Infection Control & Hospital Epidemiology* 17(10), pp. 675–86 (1996)
20. C. Y. Phillips, A. Castorr, P. A. Prescott, and K, Soeken, "Nursing Intensity: Going Beyond Patient Classification." *Journal of Nursing Administration* 22(4), pp. 46–52 (April, 1992)
21. B. E. Fries, D. P. Schneider, W. J. Foley, and M, Dowling, "Case-Mix Classification of Medicare Residents in Skilled Nursing Facilities: Resource Utilization Groups (RUG-T18)." *Medical Care* 27(9), pp. 843–58 (September, 1989)
22. V. J. Gooder, B. R. Farr, and M. P. Young, "Accuracy and Efficiency of an Automated System for Calculating APACHE II Scores in an Intensive Care Unit." *Proceedings/AMIA Annual Fall Symposium*, pp. 131–5 (1997); T. A. Mackenzie, A. Greenaway-Coates, M. S. Djurfeldt, and W. M. Hopman, "Use of Severity of Illness to Evaluate Quality of Care." *International Journal for Quality in Health Care* 8(2), pp. 125–30 (April, 1996)
23. L. I. Iezzoni, A. S. Ash, M. Shwartz, J. Daley, J. S. Hughes, and Y. D. Mackiernan, "Judging Hospitals by Severity-Adjusted Mortality Rates: The Influence of the Severity-Adjustment Method." *American Journal of Public Health* 86(10), pp. 1379–87 (October, 1996)
24. L. I. Iezzoni, "The Risks of Risk Adjustment." *Journal of the American Medical Association* 278(19), pp. 1600–7 (November, 19 1997); L. I. Iezzoni, A. S. Ash, M. Shwartz, J. Daley, J. S. Hughes, and Y. D. Mackiernan, "Judging Hospitals by Severity-Adjusted Mortality Rates: The Influence of the Severity-Adjustment Method." *American Journal of Public Health* 86(10), pp.1379–87 (October, 1996)
25. J. W. Thomas and M. L. Ashcraft, "Measuring Severity of Illness: Six Severity Systems and Their Ability to Explain Cost Variations." *Inquiry* 28(1), pp. 39–55 (1991)
26. The Malcom Baldrige National Quality Award home page: www.quality.nist.gov (October 27, 1998)
27. J. R. Griffith, V. K. Sahney, and R. A. Mohr, *Reengineering Healthcare: Building*

on Continuous Quality Improvement. Chicago: Health Administration Press (1995)

28. W. E. Deming, *Out of the Crisis.* Boston: Massachusetts Institute of Technology, Center for Advanced Engineering Study, pp. 309–371 (1986)
29. *Ibid*, p. 39 (1986)
30. Joint Commission on Accreditation of Healthcare Organizations, *Six Hospitals in Search of Quality, Striving Towards Improvement.* Oakbrook Terrace, IL: JCAHO, pp. 255–259 (1992)
31. D. C. Kibbe and R. P. Scoville, "Computer Software for Healthcare CQI," and "Tutorial: Using Microsoft Excel for Healthcare CQI." *Quality Management In Healthcare* 1(4), pp. 50–58 (Summer, 1993) and 2(1), pp. 63–71 (Fall, 1993)
32. S. L. Jarvenpaa and G. W. Dickson, "Graphics and Managerial Decision Making: Research Based Guidelines." *Communications of the ACM* 31(6), pp. 764–74 (1988)
33. T. W. Weiss, C. M. Ashton, and N. P. Wray, "Forecasting Areawide Hospital Utilization: A Comparison of Five Univariate Time Series Techniques." *Health Services Management Research* 6(3), pp. 178–190 (August, 1993)
34. U.S. Bureau of the Census, *Current Population Reports: Cooperative Program for Federal-State Population Estimates*, Series P-26. Washington DC: U.S. Department of Commerce, Bureau of the Census.
35. R. D. Zentner and B. D. Gelb, "Scenarios: A Planning Tool for Healthcare Organizations." *Hospital & Health Services Administration* 36(2), pp. 211–22 (Summer 1991)
36. P. Kokol, "Structured Spreadsheet Modeling in Medical Decision Making and Research." *Journal of Medical Systems* 14(3), pp. 107–17 (1990)
37. J. R. Griffith, W. M. Hancock, and F. C. Munson, *Cost Control in Hospitals.* Chicago: Health Administration Press, pp. 23–89 (1976)
38. Centers for Disease Control, US Dept. of Health and Human Services, home page: www.cdc.gov (October 27, 1998)
39. M. Kim and W. M. Hancock, "Applications of Staffing, Scheduling and Budgeting Methods to Hospital Ancillary Units." *Journal of Medical Systems* 13(1), pp. 37–47 (1989)
40. Y. L. Huang, "An Application of Data Envelopment Analysis: Measuring the Relative Performance of Florida General Hospitals." *Journal of Medical Systems* 14(4), pp. 191–6 (1990)
41. J. D. Thompson, "Predicting Requirements for Maternity Facilities." *Hospitals* (Feb. 16, 1963)
42. L. C. Gapenski, "Using Monte Carlo Simulation to Make Better Capital Investment Decisions." *Hospital & Health Services Administration* 35(2), pp. 207–19 (Summer, 1990)
43. M. E. Hatcher and C. Connelly, "A Case Mix Simulation Decision Support System Model for Negotiating Hospital Rates." *Journal of Medical Systems* 12(6), pp. 341–63 (1988)
44. M. E. Hatcher and N. Rao, " A Simulation Based Decision Support System for a Health Promotion Center." *Journal of Medical Systems* 12(1), pp. 11–29 (1988)
45. A. S. Zaki, "Developing a DSS for a Distribution Facility: An Application in the Healthcare Industry." *Journal of Medical Systems* 13(6), pp. 331–46 (1989)

46. M. E. Hatcher, "Uniqueness of Group Decision Support Systems (GDSS) in Medical and Health Applications," *Journal of Medical Systems* 14(6), pp. 351–34 (1990)
47. C. H. Moore, "Experimental Design in Healthcare." *Quality Management in Healthcare* 2(2), pp. 13–26 (Winter, 1994)
48. F. J. Roethlisberger and W. J. Dickson, *Management and the Worker: An Account of a Research Program Conducted by the Western Electric Company, Hawthorne Works, Chicago*. Cambridge, MA: Harvard University Press (1939)
49. A. D. Chandler, *The Visible Hand: The Managerial Revolution in American Business*. Cambridge, MA: Belknap Press (1977)
50. P. E. Pisek, "Tutorial: Introduction to Control Charts." *Quality Management in Healthcare* 1(1), pp. 65–74 (Fall, 1992)
51. H. Gitlow, S. Gitlow, A. Oppenheim, and R. Oppenheim, *Tools and Methods for the Improvement of Quality*. Homewood, IL: Irwin, pp. 78–110 (1989)
52. L. J. Finison, K. S. Finison, "Applying Control Charts to Quality Improvement." *Journal for Healthcare Quality* 18(6): 32–41 (Nov–Dec, 1996)

PART

II

Caring: Building Quality of Clinical Service

The central function of the healthcare organization is the health of its community. Two major but overlapping streams of healthcare organization activity contribute to community health. The first and larger is healthcare delivered to the satisfaction of the patient and the buyer. The second, but most rapidly evolving and growing in importance, is outreach and prevention, the set of activities the organization supports to eliminate and reduce disease and to contribute to quality of life beyond the traditional bounds of healthcare. Part II discusses both.

Modern healthcare is more than a team effort; it is an effort of teams of teams. The teams apply their particular technology to the patient's total needs. They often work in isolated locations, sometimes at odd hours and with minimal communication outside their own group. Their job, which they routinely do quite well, is always to assess the patient's condition from their unique perspective, identify potential improvements, select the most beneficial course of action, and either carry it out or arrange for other teams to do so. These steps—assessment, diagnosis, therapeutic selection, and therapy—are shown in Figure II.1. They are carried out again and again, repeated on each patient until the assessment shows no further opportunities for improvement.

Modern healthcare relies on several structures to implement the conceptual model as well as it does. The oldest, and still most important, is professional training, inculcating knowledge, skills, and values into each practitioner until he or she knows almost instinctively what to do in most situations. The implication of professional training is specialization. Given that no human being can learn it all, each selects an area of expertise and masters it. The result is the legion of clinical professions that make up any healthcare organization.

The organization supports professionalization in two related ways. The informal organization places each practitioner among peers, in a culture that encourages quality. The formal organization provides the logistical support and communications the individual practitioners need. Communications includes the planning and monitoring of performance that allow the practitioners to improve, particularly addressing integration of the many professions. The chapters of Part II are organized around the major groups of professions, beginning with an overview of the clinical process itself, in Chapter 7, and continuing to the organizational structures for medicine, nursing, other clinical professions, and extended care activities.

FIGURE II.1
Conceptual Model of Clinical Care

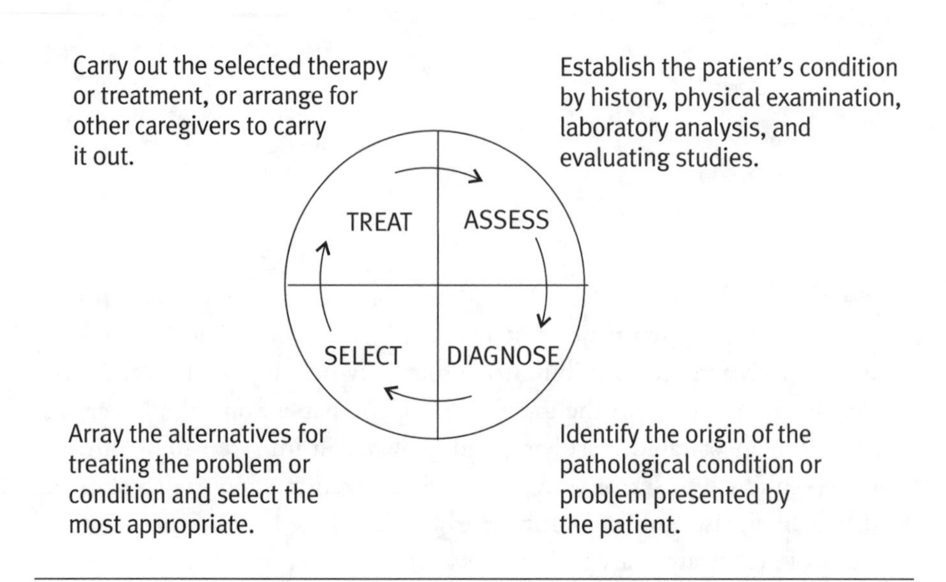

Outreach and prevention recognize that many factors beyond healthcare contribute to health. Healthcare organizations can both contribute and benefit beyond their traditional functions. Activities that eliminate the need for healthcare by improving the environment or changing behavior contribute to health. Healthcare organizations are often able to support those activities, ranging from childhood immunizations to social centers for senior citizens. Under capitation risk sharing, healthcare organizations benefit from the success of prevention and outreach activities. As capitation has become more widespread, commitment to prevention and outreach has grown. It is likely to become the major distinction of successful community healthcare organizations.

CHAPTER

7

IMPROVING QUALITY AND ECONOMY IN PATIENT CARE

Quality and Economy as the Mission of Healthcare Organizations

In the twenty-first century, the first-line healthcare organization, whether it is a comprehensive healthcare system, a clinic, hospital, or home care organization, will improve cost and quality as its core strategy for long run success. The marketplace demands no less.[1,2] The strategy will include continuous improvement of clinical performance and deliberate outreach and prevention activities. In adopting this strategy, healthcare organizations have followed the lead of many other enterprises. Educational institutions, banks, manufacturers, and retailers face comparable pressures from the marketplace, and many of the most successful are making a similar commitment to continuous improvement in cost and quality.[3]

The concept of using the healthcare organization for continuous improvement is not new. It is imbedded in the history of actions by leading practitioners and managers, and of organizations like the American College of Surgeons and the JCAHO. What is new is a more aggressive pursuit, broader application incorporating office and home care as well as inpatient, a shift away from professional and toward consumer criteria, more attention to the prevention and consequences of disease, more collaboration with non-healthcare organizations, and a more realistic recognition of the inevitable economic limits.

The broad outline for continuous improvement is also clear. It is based on **evidence-based medicine**, the concept that ideal medical treatment is supported by careful and systematic evaluation emphasizing rigorous controlled trials. A group sponsored by the American Medical Association developed the evidence-based medicine concept beginning in 1992. It rapidly became the central criterion of guideline design and a core value for medicine in the United States and many other countries. The working group developed an extensive procedure for designing guidelines around the systematic analysis of scientific literature evaluating clinical outcomes.[4]

The successful approach consists of four components: (1) a mechanism to develop a local, evidence-based consensus on care, (2) well-designed processes to provide those responses, (3) a deliberate program of outreach to the community on disease prevention and health promotion, and (4) a system to review actual performance and identify future improvements. The approach has been tested both in the best-managed community hospitals[5,6,7] and leading HMOs.[8,9,10,11] Healthcare management for the next generation will expand and improve the four components.

Definitions

The vision must be achieved without resolving the exact definitions of what "quality" and "economy" of healthcare are. In fact, the control systems themselves—and the gap between superior performance and average—stimulate our thinking on these two central characteristics of healthcare. The two concepts are intertwined. Although it is often useful to think of an ideal quality of care, reality means that quality must always be imperfectly understood and judged in comparison to economic limits. (That is, caregivers never have complete knowledge or unlimited resources.) A starting point on the practical question of building systems to control cost and quality is to accept the consensus definitions developed by the Institute of Medicine (IOM):[12]

> **Quality of Care.** The degree to which health services for individuals and populations increase the likelihood of desired health outcomes and are consistent with current professional knowledge.
>
> **Appropriate Care.** Care for which expected health benefits exceed negative consequences.[13]
>
> **Efficiency.** Maximization of the quality of a comparable unit of healthcare delivered for a given unit of health resources used.[14]

Quality, appropriateness, and efficiency are interrelated. (Quality care must be appropriate, and inefficiency reduces the opportunity for quality at a given level of resources.) But one can be expensive without being inefficient or inappropriate; the cost issue is related to the overall level of health expenditures in light of the other needs of the community.

> **Economy.** The total level of expenditure for healthcare, given realistic performance on quality and efficiency and a realistic assessment of available resources.

Abstract or universal answers to the determination of quality and economy are matters that go well beyond the skills and views of physicians and healthcare professionals. (The Institute of Medicine's discussion papers provide a useful summary of the thorny issues involved.[15]) Specific cases are another matter. Despite the complexities, the questions of economy and quality are answered every day in every community in the nation. The actions taken, or not taken, for each patient determine the answers. The evidence is clear that the task is not uniformly well done. Quality of care,[16,17,18,19] utilization of services,[20,21] and patient satisfaction[22] vary substantially between communities, organizations, and physician specialties.

Premises

Three premises underpin processes to control cost and quality in healthcare:

1. The community at large must establish the desired level of economy. It does so through market decisions, such as the demand for health insurance at various price levels, and political actions, such as the governmental budgets for healthcare programs and institutional budgets for operations and capital. A central function of the governing board is to monitor and contribute to the consensus setting process.
2. Community decisions cannot be intelligently made without extensive input and advice from healthcare professionals. Although physicians are the leading spokespersons of the professional team because of their scientific and technical education, the process must include all clinical activities and the viewpoints of all clinical professionals.
3. The control of cost and quality depends on the entire institutional infrastructure. The governance, caring, and learning systems form the foundation for quality control activities of healthcare professionals, and the effectiveness of quality control is limited by the effectiveness of these systems.

That is to say, the content of this chapter presumes the other 16 chapters. One cannot achieve the necessary levels of control of cost and quality without a clear mission, governing board review of the medical staff, a well-designed structure for making and implementing decisions, a competent planning function, a sound finance system, and modern information systems. Further, the technology of quality control is built on an organization of several of the clinical professions. Each must have a recruitment plan that meets competitive economic needs, a process for selection and removal of clinicians based on demonstrated competence, and education to maintain and improve that competence. These in turn demand effective human resources and plant support. Conversely, all this can be present, but without an ongoing system to study and improve clinical performance it will not be enough. A comprehensive program of quality improvement must integrate these elements into a whole that is increasingly effective.

Plan for the Chapter

This thesis is expanded in the remainder of this chapter, as follows:

- *The clinical quality improvement program.* An overview of the theory that guides medical decision making; implications of the theory; quality improvement of individual patient care decisions and expectations; a system to achieve them; and a formal process of assessment.

- *Role of clinical expectations.* Kinds of guidelines; how guidelines contribute to quality and economy; sources and criteria for guidelines; limitations of guidelines.
- *Strategic clinical improvement.* Prioritizing guideline development; establishing accountability for guideline programs; supporting effective guideline use.
- *Preventing illness and promoting health.* Primary, secondary, and tertiary prevention; addressing prevention in clinical expectations; cost effectiveness of prevention; outreach and health promotion.
- *Measures and information systems.* Sources of measures for monitoring quality and economy; information processing and display requirements; monitoring individual performance and using rewards and sanctions.

The Clinical Quality Improvement Program

Other things being equal, well-intentioned, well-trained, well-supported clinical professionals will deliver good quality, but highly variable, cost of care. Much of the variation will come not from the efficiency of individual caregivers but from the array of activities selected for the patient. Evidence from well-managed institutions suggests that quality can be improved and cost stabilized by deliberate action to develop consensus among the caregivers about the many decisions that go into a course of treatment.[23,24] A clinical improvement program is an organized effort to build and implement consensus providing each patient with optimal treatment.[25] To understand such a program, it is wise to begin with an analysis of the care decisions made by individual practitioners about individual patients.

Decision Theory and Case Management

A simple decision theory model guiding clinical behavior

Conceptually, quality care must be appropriate; care that omits appropriate elements or includes inappropriate elements cannot be of the highest quality. Care is appropriate when the marginal cost of service is exactly equal to the marginal benefit; that is, when the last service ordered contributed more value through improved outcome than it cost, and the next service that might be ordered will contribute less than it costs.[26] Real medical care proceeds in multiple and interacting cycles of the care process shown in Figure II.1, but each considered step is a simple binary decision, to be answered either yes or no. There are thousands of such decisions, mostly answered no, in a given episode of care. Many considerations recur. That is, a laboratory test may be considered today and again tomorrow. The recurrence is often independent of the decision; whether or not the service was ordered today, it can be reconsidered tomorrow. Each binary decision is reached by the doctor's (or other caregiver's) internal calculus, an amalgam of training and experience. Obviously, given the number of decisions and the difficulty of measuring the costs and benefits, that calculus must be fast, reliable, and robust.

Costs and benefits must usually be evaluated for both alternatives. There are only a few easy decisions, those in which one side heavily outweighs the other. For example, immunizations are almost always appropriate. For patients with severe diabetes, insulin is required. For most realistic problems, decisions are complex and numerous, and time is part of the problem. When the possible costs include death or disability and the decisions must be made quickly, the skills of the physician are most tested.

Doctors' evaluations center on probabilities, because few things in medicine are certain. Thus, doctors treating patients with pain in the abdomen weigh first the probability that it is self-limiting, knowing that most afflictions, in fact, cure themselves in a few hours or days. Next, they consider alternative intervention paths: direct treatment versus further investigation to refine the diagnosis. Finally, they weigh specific alternatives on the chosen path: drugs versus surgery on the treatment path, laboratory tests, imaging, or optical scope on the investigatory path. The doctors' decision-making processes can be modeled as decision theory, although the actions of real doctors are considerably more complicated than the theory.[27] Taking the most drastic of the interventions, surgery, the possibilities look something like the list in Figure 7.1.

The figure shows that the decision depends on the probability that the patient has appendicitis or a disease treatable with the same surgery and on the values placed on the costs of surgery and the costs of waiting. The question can be readdressed hourly until the patient either improves or is operated on. For a given set of symptoms, the doctor assumes a certain probability of appendicitis and certain values for the costs of doing and not doing surgery. The decision the doctor faces is not fatal. If the patient does not have appendicitis, and

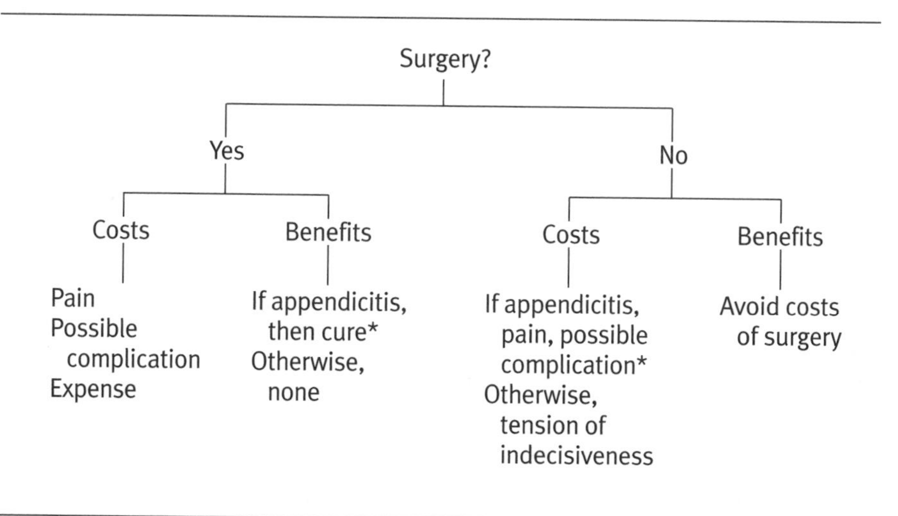

FIGURE 7.1 Decision Tree for Evaluating Surgical Treatment for Appendicitis

*A few other diseases might also be corrected by the same procedure, with the diagnosis made after surgery is begun.

no surgery is performed, he or she will recover (or a new diagnosis can be established). If the patient does have appendicitis and no surgery is performed, he or she will get worse. Surgery can be done then, with full but possibly slower and more costly recovery. The cost of acting now is weighed against the cost of waiting. As patients' agents, physicians are indifferent to surgery when

$$\text{Cost of having surgery} = \text{Cost of not having surgery}$$

but because surgery will be wasted if the patient does not have appendicitis, the cost of having surgery is

$$(\text{Probability of not appendicitis})\ (\text{Costs of surgery})$$

but because the question can be revisited later if surgery is not done, the cost of not having surgery is

$$(\text{Probability of appendicitis})\ (\text{Costs of delay})$$

If we let

$$\begin{aligned} p &= \text{Probability of appendicitis at the point of indifference} \\ (1 - p) &= \text{Probability not appendicitis} \\ C &= \text{Cost of surgery} \\ D &= \text{Cost of delay} \end{aligned}$$

$$(C \text{ and } D \text{ will always be less than } 0),$$

then the equation is

$$C(1 - p) = Dp$$

$$p = C/(D + C).$$

It may be helpful to assign some arbitrary dollar values to these concepts. Using negative signs for costs, let us assume that surgery is worth −$5,000, and delay is worth −$1,000. Then

$$\begin{aligned} &(\text{Indifference Probability of Appendicitis}) \\ &= (-\$5{,}000)/(-\$5{,}000 - \$1{,}000) \\ &= (\$5{,}000)/(\$6{,}000) \\ &= .83 \end{aligned}$$

or a 5 in 6 chance of appendicitis. The doctor must be approximately 80 percent sure the patient has appendicitis to order surgery. A higher cost of delay and lower cost of intervention would lead to a lower probability of appendicitis required to justify surgery. If the cost of surgery were cut in half, relative to the cost of delay, then the indifference probability would be $2,500/$3,500, or about 70 percent. More surgery would be done, and more of it would be unnecessary, but it would still be optimum care. Conversely, if the costs of surgery were twice as great, the indifference probability would rise to $10,000/$11,000, or 91 percent. Fewer operations would be done, and almost all would be necessary.

Like most models, this one simplifies reality and is not entirely accurate. Few doctors consciously review probabilities in the way the model suggests, and even fewer would attempt to estimate and solve an equation or draw a diagram such as that presented in Figure 7.1. Evidence suggests, however, that even the simple form shown here predicts real behavior. For a very low-cost intervention, say a $5 laboratory test, there is a strong predisposition to do the test. Very high-cost interventions are approached more slowly. When the cost of delay for surgery is reduced, doctors actually do less surgery.[28] Emergencies can be defined as situations in which the cost of delay is very high. In such cases, the mathematics of this simple formula suggest that action be taken on any hint that the patient actually needs the intervention being contemplated. In life-threatening emergencies (essentially situations in which delay costs are infinite), that is what occurs.

Use of decision theory to improve patient quality of care

Decision theory suggests three routes to improving the contribution of medicine to health, that is, to improving the quality of care:

1. Increasing the value of intervention
   a. improving the results of therapeutic intervention, improving the outcome for each patient, or increasing the variety of cases for which an intervention is appropriate
   b. improving the discriminatory power of diagnostic tests, that is, the ability to detect whether the patient has a certain disease or condition
2. Reducing the cost of intervention
   a. reducing the danger of harm to the patient
   b. reducing the resources consumed by the intervention
   c. reducing conflict between interventions
   d. reducing the pain or discomfort associated with an intervention
3. Reducing the cost of delay
   a. improving the ability to predict the patient's course, as with an improved diagnostic test or new understanding of the implications of specific signs and symptoms
   b. reducing delays between orders and intervention
   c. reducing intervention failures and repetitions

In general, therapeutic services improve the quality of care when they add a new intervention; increase the effectiveness of an existing one; or reduce the dangers, expenses, or discomfort associated with treatment. Diagnostic services improve the quality of care when they add new knowledge about the case and when they make acquiring the knowledge faster, cheaper, or more convenient.

Building Continuous Improvement on Professional Foundations

Professional self-direction is a hallmark of the successful healthcare organization. The organization builds on the professional training and culture, empowering caregivers to make the complex decisions of patient care and take professional pride in them. When effective logistics, measurement of performance, and the organization culture support self-direction, it encourages clinicians to do their best and minimizes costly and painful problems of enforcement. Logistics provides the proper training and tools to do each job. Performance measurement keeps caregivers' attention on customer needs. The culture emphasizes the value of each worker's contribution, encourages questions and ensures that they are answered. It creates open channels of communication and processes of decision making, so no worker needs to feel excluded. The culture is based on success and rewards. Expectations are set so that they are routinely achieved. Their achievement proves their practicality and establishes social norms encouraging achievement. Expectations that prove too difficult are withdrawn for further study. Financial incentives are designed to complement the professional ones.

Figure 7.2 shows the major elements of a continuous improvement process based on professionalism.[29] The process is a compound application of the cybernetic process described in Chapter 6. Stimulus for change comes from the upper part of the figure, where new technology is reviewed, ideas conceived, and actual performance compared against expectations and benchmarks. A Shewhart cycle goes on in the middle of the figure; clinical changes must be thoroughly planned and tested before installation. Changes are embedded into practice by revised work processes, including equipment and supplies, training in new methods, and various incentives for adapting. These lead to the ultimate goal of improved clinical goals and changed caregiver behavior. The new perspective and revised processes interact with the indications for change, making the process continuous.

For example, an effort to raise mammogram rates among middle-aged women might be stimulated by buyer emphasis on the importance of this secondary prevention activity. A thorough study of current practices might reveal several possible changes such as direct incentives to patients, improved scheduling and access, and more explanation and encouragement by primary care nurses. These would be pilot tested to make sure they all contribute to the goal, and then "rolled out" to the primary care sites of a large system through a specific training program, possibly combined with revisions to reporting forms or scheduling procedures. Incentives such as recognition or small prizes might be offered to nurses, based on improvement in their patient populations. Actual improvement would be monitored through medical records entries or insurance claims.

Participation and empowerment are critical components of the process. The primary care nurses and breast examination center personnel must play a

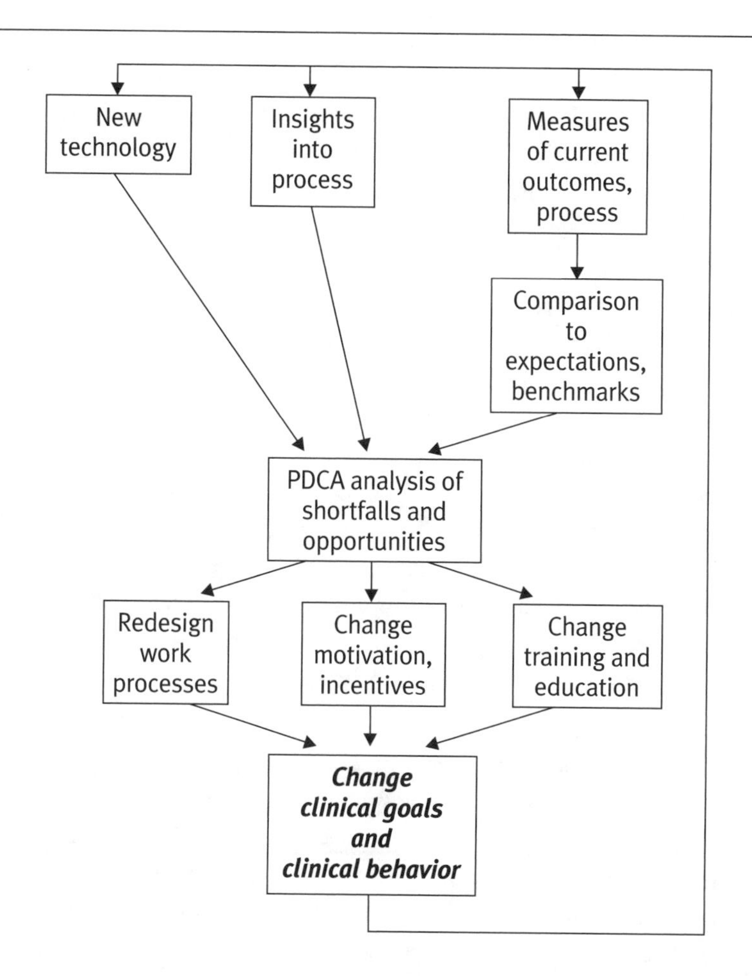

FIGURE 7.2 Continuous Improvement of Care Processes

SOURCE: Modified from Donabedian, A. "Reflections on the Effectiveness of Quality Assurance" in R. H. Palmer, A. Donabedian, G. J. Povar, *Striving for Quality in Health Care: An Inquiry into Policy and Practice*, p. 65–66.

major role in the entire process of Figure 7.2 for it to succeed. Not only their knowledge of the details is essential; participation in designing the solution and understanding the monitoring and reward systems is also necessary to make the new process both realistic and convincing to the people who must make them work. Other caregivers participate in proportion to their contribution to the selected goal. Primary care physicians and breast radiologists must understand the changes and be supportive of them.

The concepts of Figure 7.2 are not new. A number of efforts have been made to implement them, beginning with Codman's efforts before World War I.[30,31] Many successful applications have been reported.[32,33,34] Five major elements distinguish the continuous improvement approach from the earlier efforts:[35]

1. Continuous improvement assumes no upper limit, but rather that any performance of a complex system is improvable. In other words, there is

no "good enough." Earlier efforts emphasized departure from a standard that was accepted as good enough.

2. Continuous improvement explores broadly for its revisions, deliberately considering not only elements of care outside the direct control of the doctor but also the interaction of elements in a complex system. Earlier efforts frequently emphasized the identification of individual performance, at the level of the case or the practitioner.
3. Continuous improvement assumes that the customer's perspective is dominant. Earlier efforts tended to focus heavily on professional values, sometimes to the point of ignoring the patient's perceptions.
4. Continuous improvement focuses on the improvement of overall or group performance rather than the identification and correction of outliers. Earlier approaches tended not only to isolate poor performers, but also to focus on punishment more than improvement.
5. Continuous improvement emphasizes the necessity of organizationwide commitment, from the governing board and CEO level to the individual caregiver. Earlier efforts tended to isolate the review activity in a narrow set of medical staff committees.

The continuous improvement concept not only has had impressive success in other industries and widespread endorsement in healthcare, it also is consistent with human relations theory and offers an avenue to integrate the various care activities more closely in a patient or customer-oriented framework. Professionals are self-directed under continuous improvement, but their direction is kept consistent with customer needs for quality and economy.[36,37]

The Organization's Contribution to Clinical Improvement

Routine implementation of Figure 7.2 is often espoused, but difficult to achieve.[38] Behind successful applications lies a basic technical capability: accounting and laboratory and nursing must be well-run in a technical sense; governance must understand the virtues of the environment being built; and so on. Planning and marketing are particularly important: adjusting to a changing external environment without disrupting a supportive corporate environment is difficult. Sound strategies and maximum lead time are often the keys.

The healthcare organizations leading the development of continuous improvement have an underlying commitment to patient care and humanitarian values, as summarized in Figure 7.3:[39]

- Each member of the organization understands that his or her work is on behalf of patients and that excellence will be rewarded.
- Expectations encourage individual judgment to meet particular patient needs and unusual circumstances. They specify situations in which

judgment is particularly appropriate and provide a practical procedure to follow when protocols should be overridden.

- Each caregiver understands that he or she is privileged to provide optimum care and to represent his or her patients' needs vigorously.
- The expectation-setting process emphasizes scientific sources and is approached as a stimulating intellectual challenge. That is, it is approached as a rewarding rather than a burdensome event.
- All workers and managers understand the importance of respect for each individual's contribution, open exchange of information, and prompt response to questions.
- Participation in the development of expectations is widespread. An effort is made to ensure that no one is surprised by an unanticipated demand for change.
- The climate encourages change, while also reassuring members of their personal security. The major components of reassurance include consistent procedures and processes; well-understood avenues for comment and prompt, sensitive response; avoidance of imposed consensus; and recognition of the importance of dissent.
- Compliance with expectations for the process of management (e.g., scheduling, documentation, timeliness, and courtesy) is accepted as essential. Violations are discouraged with measured sanctions promptly applied. For example, the penalty for incomplete medical records (usually a temporary loss of privileges) is quickly and routinely applied. As a result, well-run organizations have few incomplete records.
- A spirit of fairness and helpfulness characterizes discussion of departures from the expectations about the care itself. The fact that such departures are rare permits extensive investigation. Sanctions are used reluctantly but predictably in the case of repeated unjustifiable practice.
- The values of the organization are advertised. Recruitment emphasizes the philosophy of the organization so it attracts doctors and employees who are congenial to its orientation.

Role of Clinical Expectations

Clinical activities are not random or haphazard, but rather formalized, often scientific responses to specific patient stimuli. Every time nurses give an injection, they make several specific checks on the site, the drug, skin preparation, and equipment. Every time surgeons start an operation, the anticipated equipment is prepared in advance. Every time patients tell a symptom to doctors, the doctors' responses are predictable for that symptom, considering other information at their command. This predictability is essential to implement quality assurance. It allows the identification of "expectations" in clinical behavior in exactly the same sense as the term is introduced in Chapter 3 and applied in other hospital systems.

FIGURE 7.3
Core Values of Leading Continuous Improvement Organizations

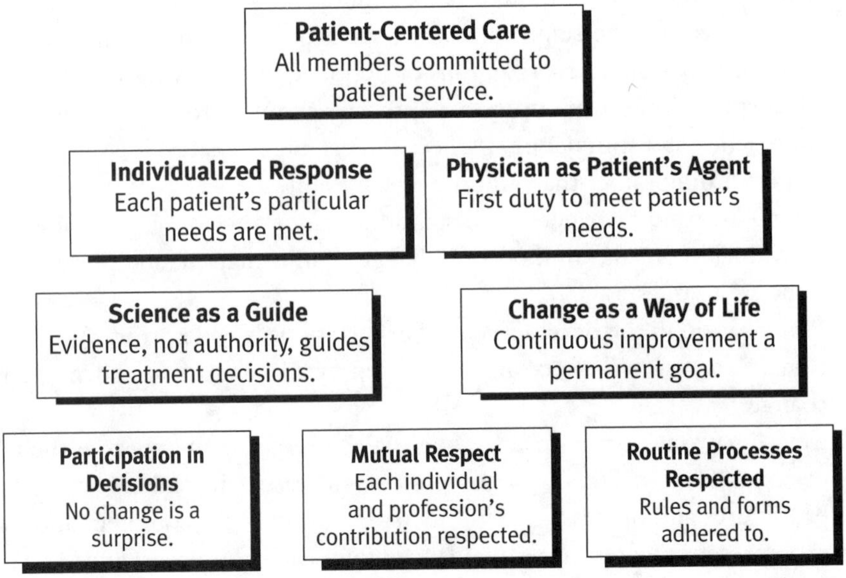

Definition of Clinical Expectations

The consensuses reflected in these everyday events constitute **clinical expectations** about the process of care. One can define the term for management purposes by emphasizing its application to the activities of professionals, the recurring nature of the situation addressed, and the need for a consensus rather than an individual professional's opinion or patient's need. Clinical expectations are the consensuses reached regarding the correct professional response to specific, recurring situations in patient care.

Clinical expectations make cooperation among different individuals and professions possible. They are necessary to allow any level of sophisticated teamwork to exist in healthcare. Reflecting this necessity, clinical expectations are developed by the professions themselves. Secondarily, they provide the basis for assessing or monitoring clinical performance. Third, they have become a convenient statement of contracts with patients and insurers. The courts and the marketplace have reinforced the right of consumers to have their care conform to clinical expectations developed by professionals.

Types of Clinical Expectations

Clinical expectations can be divided into three types, depending on the level of application. The terms "expectation," "guideline," and "protocol" are used interchangeably.

- **Intermediate product protocols** determine how functional elements of care are carried out. They cover tasks of care accomplished by individuals, such as giving an injection or taking a chest x-ray, and sets of activities for team procedures, such as surgical operations, rehabilitation programs, or multistep diagnostic activities. They are usually written, but are often carried out from memory. They are established and maintained by the individual professions and the functional accountability hierarchy of the organization.
- **Care plans** constitute expectations for the care of individual patients based on evaluation of individual needs. Care plans can be understood as lengthy aggregates of intermediate product protocols, the set of examinations, tests, and treatments that best meets the specific patient's needs. Care plans are often developed by the treating doctor or nurse, but can also be developed by cross-functional care teams. They can be either written or not, and in simple cases are often documented only by the medical record, after the fact.
- **Patient management protocols** (also called "final product protocols" and "care guidelines") define normal care of a common group of patients, such as uncomplicated pregnancies or acute anginal pain. They specify the intermediate products and outcomes quality goals for care, and by implication, the cost. They are organized around episodes of patient care, usually classified by disease or condition. They are developed by cross-functional teams and are written so that they can be easily communicated among the caregiving professions.

The formal statement of both intermediate and patient management protocols represents consensus on the best practice for the typical or uncomplicated patient. Because many patients are not typical, and have complications, part of the professional role is always considering the modification of the expectation to individual patient needs.

Intermediate product protocols

Figure 7.4 is an example of an intermediate product protocol. The profession most directly involved usually establishes intermediate protocols, and they are codified in textbooks for the profession. Modification may be necessary to accommodate the equipment and facilities or the patient population of a specific site. In many cases, the profession involved can accomplish this without assistance. Other applications will require review by other professionals to ensure coordination.

Intermediate product protocols exist in large numbers. They determine that the activity will have the desired outcome (the wound dressing will protect the wound, the laboratory value will be correct) and that the record will reveal exactly what was done. Good intermediate product protocols have the following components:

FIGURE 7.4 Example of an Intermediate Product Protocol

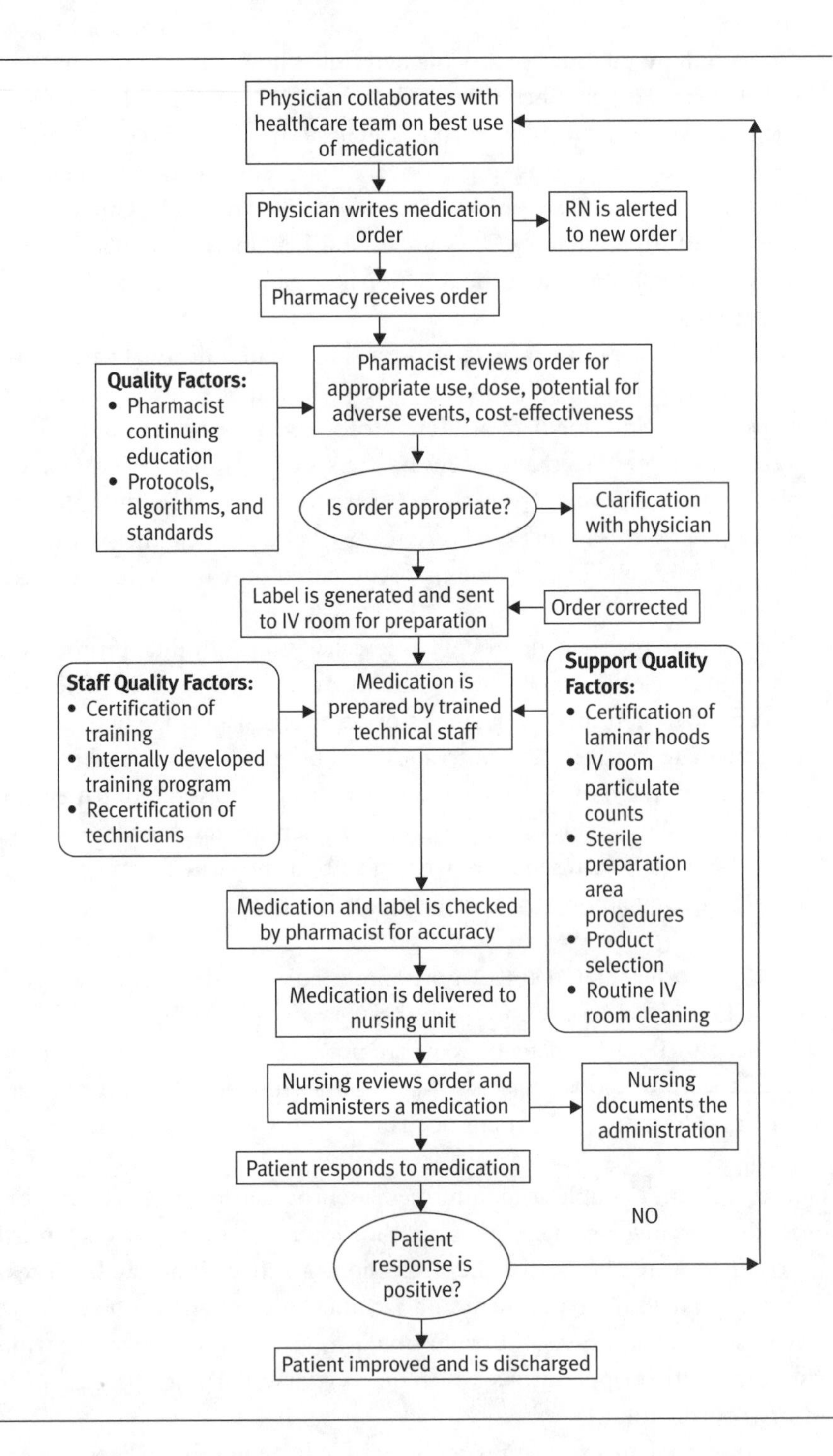

1. *Authorization*—statement of who may order the procedure
2. *Indication*—statement clarifying clinical conditions that support its appropriate use
3. *Counter indications*—conditions where the procedure must be modified, replaced, or avoided

4. *Required supplies, equipment, and conditions*—all special requirements and the sources that meet them
5. *Actions*—clear, step-by-step statements of what must be done
6. *Recording*—instructions for recording the procedure and observation of the patient's reaction
7. *Follow-up*—subsequent actions including checks on the patient's response, measures of effectiveness, indications for repeating the procedure, and disposal or clean-up of supplies

Intermediate product protocols tend to be stable over time and between patients and institutions, but they can be modified to improve quality and efficiency. An important source of improvement is eliminating unnecessary or inappropriate procedures by making the indications or authorizations more restrictive. For example, elaborate diagnostic tests and expensive drugs can reference failure of simpler approaches as indications. Some very expensive procedures can require prior approval or a formal second opinion. The activities themselves can be modified to be safer or less expensive; changes in equipment and supplies often require such adjustments. Follow-up specifications can improve patients' reactions by describing specific signs or symptoms and the appropriate response and can reduce environmental dangers by improving clean-up. A dramatic example of procedure improvement is the development of automated unit dose drug administration used in inpatient care. The new system has better controls to guard against prescribing the wrong drug, administering the wrong dose, or recording the dose incorrectly. The result is both lower cost and higher quality.[40]

Sets of interrelated intermediate protocols will become more commonplace. Surgical care provides several examples. Preoperative care includes obtaining informed consent, instructing the patient, obtaining final diagnostic values from lab and x-ray, completing the pre-anesthesia examination, and administering preoperative medications. To perform surgery without delay, each activity must be orchestrated to occur at the earliest possible time, and in the proper order. The preoperative care process requires advance agreement on the tasks and their order among several clinical support and medical professions. Many of these agreements are independent of the patient's specific disease. While the protocols could be incorporated in the patient management protocols of each of the several hundred surgical procedures, it is probably easier to develop them around the clinical services, making them intermediate products.

Care plans

Individualized patient care plans are almost universal. They are not replaced by patient management protocols; every patient's individual needs should be evaluated to make sure the protocol will meet them. A care plan is developed prospectively, based on the patient's presenting needs or symptoms. The physician or other caregiver reviews the usual options, often as reflected in the management protocol, and selects the most appropriate in light of the patient's condition.

Formal care plans are used to manage complex problems where management protocols do not fit, such as multiple concurrent conditions and expensive chronic diseases like AIDS and multiple sclerosis. In the most complex cases, the care plan may be a written consensus of professional viewpoints, closely monitored to gain the best possible results while minimizing cost.[41,42] A good plan will address all the following elements:

1. *Assessment and treatment goals.* Justification of the procedures selected, identification of specific risks, and a statement of clinical goals, such as "restore ability to dress and feed self."
2. *Component activities.* A list, often selected from relevant care guidelines and intermediate protocols, of procedures desired for the patient.
3. *Recording.* A formal routine for recording what was done and reporting it to others caring for the case.
4. *Measures of progress and a time schedule for improvement.* Where possible, measures of improvement should be used, and they should parallel the goals developed in the assessment.
5. *Danger signals and counter indications.* Specific events indicating a need to reconsider the plan.

Patient management protocols

Patient management protocols are built around the fact that most patients with similar needs or symptoms will have similar plans and can expect to follow similar courses. They are an expression of consensus about the most desirable care plan for the modal, or uncomplicated patient. The Institute of Medicine identifies several types for different purposes: "appropriateness guidelines," used to judge insurance benefit coverage; "management criteria sets," used prospectively to guide care; and "care evaluation guidelines," used retrospectively to evaluate care.[43] These distinctions are of limited use in a continuous improvement context. It is clear that the optimal plan of treatment should be the same prospectively and retrospectively, and also that the best way to improve quality and economy is to gain agreement on the plan in advance.

Several hundred diseases now have established nationally promulgated guidelines that serve as a basis for local review and implementation. Most inpatient institutions have protocols in place for several dozen of their most common conditions.

A number of sources for obtaining guidelines of this kind are operated as public services or part of professional association services. The federal Agency for Health Care Policy and Research established a National Guideline Clearinghouse on the Internet in 1998.[44] It will assist in developing 12 evidence-based practice centers in the United States and Canada to systematically assess evidence for clinical procedures.[45] The Primary Care Guideline Service of the University of California–San Francisco offers about 100 different categories of guidelines, with several examples in most categories.[46] The site also has a brief bibliography on guideline development and links to two sets of criteria for posting guidelines on the web. Figure 7.5 outlines the guidelines for managing acute myocardial infarction (AMI, or heart attack) developed by the American College of Cardiology and the American Heart Association, and promulgated by them, reflecting their belief:

> It is important that the medical profession play a significant role in critically evaluating the use of diagnostic procedures and therapies in the management or prevention of disease. Rigorous and expert analysis of the available data documenting relative benefits and risks of those procedures and therapies can produce helpful guidelines that improve the effectiveness of care, optimize patient outcomes, and impact the overall cost of care favorably by focusing resources on the most effective strategies.[47]

Consistent with that belief, the AMI guideline is widely available at nominal charge.

Part I of the figure documents the scope of the full guideline, from which Parts II and III are brief portions. The complete guideline is a comprehensive discussion of cardiac care from primary preventive measures through to tertiary prevention or rehabilitation; it is 75,000 words long (about six times the length of this chapter). To identify and resolve the alternative approaches, it was constructed with the help of more than 20 participants. To maintain an evidence-based approach, the discussion is supported by 787 footnotes mostly citing clinical research.

Part II describes the clinical problem addressed at the very beginning of the guideline: a symptom, severe chest pain, rather than a diagnosis. The possible causes of the symptom are numerous, but the guideline begins with triage, a rapid evaluation to identify pains likely to be ischemic, or circulatory system, related. Taking the incidence of 900,000 AMI per year as a guideline, something over one million patients will appear at emergency departments with this symptom, averaging about five times a week for all the departments in the nation. Those who have an AMI are in a life-threatening situation. The evidence from the literature reveals an interesting fact. Treatments begun within an hour of arrival will save twice as many lives as those that are delayed for several hours.[48] The authors of the guideline are emphatic about the need for prompt care.

> . . . [T]he benefit of reperfusion therapy [definitive treatment for AMI] is greatest if therapy is initiated early. The initial evaluation of the patient ideally should be accomplished within 10 minutes of his or her arrival in the ED; certainly no more than 20 minutes should elapse before an assessment is made.[49]

This wording is strong enough to suggest a legal standard of care—emergency departments failing to meet it are at risk of malpractice liability.

FIGURE 7.5
Managing Patients with Acute Myocardial Infarction

Part I: Scope of the Guidelines

1. Topics Covered
   A. Prehospital issues
   B. Initial recognition and management in the emergency department
   C. Hospital management
   D. Rationale and approach to pharmacotherapy
   E. Preparation for discharge from the hospital
   F. Long-term management
2. Participation
   A. Sponsorship—American College of Cardiology and American Heart Association
   B. Contributors—committee of 13 and task force of 9
3. Content and Distribution
   A. Length of approximately 75,000 words, 800 citations, 12 tables, 10 figures
   B. Publication—*Journal of the American College of Cardiology,* Circulation
   C. Internet distribution through www.acc.org/clinical/guidelines/nov96/index.html
4. Purpose and Applicability
   A. Purpose—"These guidelines are intended for physicians, nurses, and allied healthcare personnel who care for patients with suspected or established acute myocardial infarction (MI)." (p. 1333)
   B. Applicability—"Each year 900,000 people in the United States experience acute myocardial infaraction (MI). Of these, roughly 225,000 die, including 125,000 who die 'in the field' before obtaining medical care." (p. 1333)

Part II: The Initial Treatment Activities

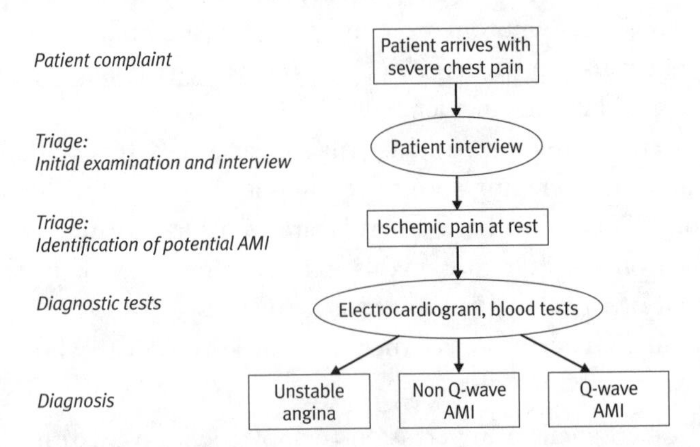

Goal: Establish the triage identification within 10 minutes and the diagnosis within 30 minutes.

SOURCE: Adapted from Ryan TJ, Anderson JL, Antman EM, Braniff BA, Broonks NH, Califf RM, Hillis LD, Hiratzka LF, Rapaport E, Riegel BJ, Russell RO, Smith EE III, Weaver WD. ACC/AHA Guidelines for the Management of Patients with Acute Myocardial Infarction: A Report of the American College of Cardiology/American Heart Association Task Force on Practice Guidelines (Committee on Management of Acute Myocardial Infarction). *J Am Coll Cardiol* 1996; 28: 1323–1428.

FIGURE 7.5 Managing Patients with Acute Myocardial Infarction (continued)

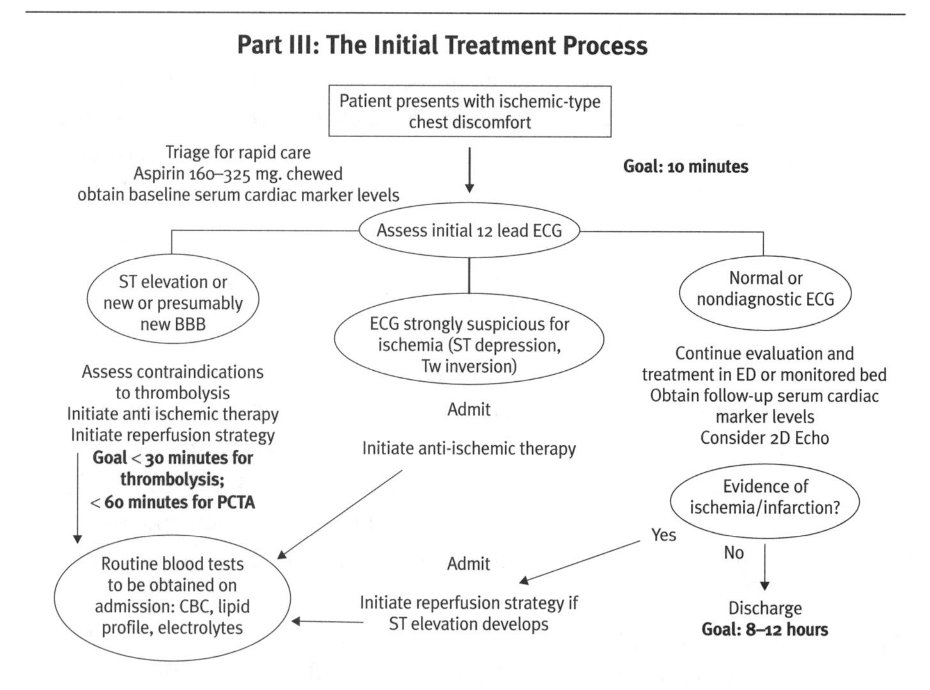

Notes to Part III

- 2D Echo—Echocardiogram
- BBB—Bundle branch block
- ECG—Electrocardiograph
- ED—Emergency department
- PTCA—percutaneous transluminal coronary angioplasty
- ST—Diagnostic segment of the ECG tracing
- TW—Diagnostic segment of the ECG tracing

SOURCE: Adapted from Antman EM, Braunwald E. Acute Myocardial Infarction. In: Braunwald EB, ed. *Heart Disease: A Textbook of Cardiovascular Medicine*, 1996, Philadelphia, PA: WB Saunders.

Thus, the first critical element of the guideline is not about clinical judgement or care plans, but about organization and teamwork. It will take a deliberate effort to get the AMI patient to definitive treatment early.

Part III of Figure 7.5 shows the steps that must follow the triage of a potential AMI in the emergency department. These include early treatment and further tests to establish a more detailed and more reliable diagnosis. The treatment includes oxygen, nitroglycerin, and pain relief. It also includes chewed aspirin, a recent addition that has reduced mortality. The tests include a battery of blood chemistries and an electrocardiogram. Again, the guideline is rigorous. It recommends:

> Emergency department acute MI protocol that yields a targeted clinical examination and a 12-lead ECG within 10 minutes and a door-to-needle [for reperfusion] time that is less than 30 minutes.

And it notes that the results of these must be interpreted by a skilled clinician:

> Initial errors in ECG interpretation can result in up to 12% of patients being categorized inappropriately (ST elevation versus no elevation), demonstrating a potential benefit of accurate computer-interpreted electrocardiography and facsimile transmission to an expert.[50]

From a management perspective, the guideline is challenging. Here is what must happen to ensure compliance:

- Emergency physicians, other emergency caregivers, cardiologists, and primary care physicians must reach consensus accepting or modifying the guidelines for local use. This will involve a local review team and a publicized opportunity for those not on the team to comment.
- A triage nurse for each shift must be trained to identify ischemic pain, or a triage physician designated. (Potential AMI patients arrive without notice, on any shift.)
- Sufficient ECG equipment must be made readily available in the ED. For larger departments, this may be two or three dedicated machines.
- Several people on each shift must be trained in administering the 12-lead ECG, so that a person is available when needed.
- All ER nurses must be trained in the initial treatment, so that they start it without a written order when the triage person indicates it. The nurses or designated technicians must also draw blood for the laboratory analysis.
- The laboratory must respond with blood chemistry analyses within about ten minutes.
- Arrangements must be made for skilled interpretation, by training of emergency physicians, acquiring interpretation software, or arranging for fax to a cardiologist. The laboratory data help in determining the patient's exact condition and the best reperfusion approach.
- Consensus must be reached in advance on the criteria for selecting among the reperfusion options, which vary substantially in cost, effectiveness, and risk of complications depending on the patient's exact condition.
- Provision must be made for thrombolysis reperfusion and, if available, percutaneous transluminal coronary angioplasty (PCTA) within 30 to 60 minutes. A team outside the ED usually completes these treatments.
- Informed consent to PCTA must be obtained from the patient if possible and necessary.

Taken as a whole, steps on the list represent a new level of performance for most EDs. Consensus building, training, advance preparation, and practice are the keys to success. In addition to these "mission critical" steps, the patient's family should get explanations and reassurance. After the 30-minute interval, arrangements must be made for completion of the medical record, billing, and transfer to inpatient care.

Figure 7.6 shows the further management of AMI, after the patient has been admitted to inpatient care. A day-to-day checklist for nursing personnel covering all the major elements of care has replaced the flow process presentation. The 12 activity groups cover all aspects of the uncomplicated stroke patient's needs, including discharge planning and family support, in a cryptic form. The condensed format helps caregivers scan the form quickly and, if desired, indicate compliance by checking off each requirement. The branching logic of care is de-emphasized but still present, reflected in phrases like "consider," "per CRS team," and "check w."

Using Clinical Expectations

How protocols change the delivery of care

The evidence to date suggests the use of protocols contributes to performance; few serious objections to the approach remain. From the point of view of the caregiver, protocols provide resolution of elements previously uncertain or imperfectly understood, a convenient, easily learned template, improved reliability of specific services, and a method of self-assessment. These benefits come from the codification of formerly unwritten or unorganized activities, the identification and resolution of differing opinions or approaches, the education involved in the review process, and the development of support systems to deliver the necessary steps correctly, promptly, and economically. Beyond that, the protocol is available as a prompt (it is more often internalized than referred to directly) and as a basis for measuring departures and comparing outcomes.

The goal is to make the patient management guideline the accepted professional behavior and a reward in itself. To the extent that this is successful, five things happen:

1. The guideline is widely used and becomes habitual.
2. The several professions can use it to anticipate care events.
3. Doctors can use it as a shorthand or outline to guide their decisions and their communications to others. The individual plan becomes the exception to the guideline.
4. The logistics for delivering the guideline components are convenient and reliable. Intermediate products in the guideline must be readily available and delivered uniformly in terms of quality and timeliness.
5. The guideline defines the measures of performance and incorporates information collection that can be used for its evaluation and improvement. The individualized plans also contribute information for guideline revision.

Protocols improve performance by several different mechanisms:

- Elimination of unnecessary or redundant tasks. These often appear when two functional groups compare their intermediate protocols or usual practices.

FIGURE 7.6 Inpatient Management Protocol for Acute Myocardial Infarction

Time Frame	Day 1	Day 2	Day 3	Day 4	Day 5
Problems	Interm. Goals	Interm. Goals	Interm. Goals	Interm. Goals	Interm. Goals
1. Neuro deficit	1. Stable neuro status	1. Continue	1. Continue	1. Continue	1. No further evaluation
2. Knowledge deficit	2. Pt. and/or family V/U room and unit routines	2. Pt. and/or family V/U neuro deficits	2. Continue	2. Pt. and/or family D/U safety	2. Continue
3. Immobility	3. Pt. and/or family V/U restricted activity AROM and PROM	3. Pt. and/or family V/U PT/OT	3. Continue	3. Pt. and/or family D/U or therapy and appliances	3. Self-care as much as possible
4. Nutrition	4. Prevent aspiration	4. Pt. and/or family V/U or diet	4. Adequate nutrition	4. Continue	4. Continue
1. Consults/ Assess-ments/ Indicators	Dr. H&P-Assessment to determine embolic or thrombolytic. Consider ECHO. Consider CRS. Consider Neuro and other consults. Nursing HYP v.s. q4º (Glasgow coma). All to consider swallow eval.	Continue routine assessments. VS w/neuro's q4º if stable.	Continue routine assessments. VS w/Neuro's q6º if stable. Assess need for home or nrsg. home, appliances, and follow-up	Continue routine assessments. VS q.i.d.	Continue routine assessments. VS q.i.d.
2. Tests	CT of Brain Carotid–U.S. Doppler Chest X-Ray EKG Consider ECHO Consider MRI CBC w/Diff., MCP, PT, PTT, UA	Daily: Pt, PTT if indicated. Follow-up Day 1 lab abnormalities.	Consider repeat CT of head for Day 4–order is indicated. Follow-up Day 2 lab abnormalities.	CT of head if indicated (could be done as out-patient if necessary). Follow-up Day 3 lab abnormalities.	Follow-up Day 4 lab abnormalities.
3. Treatments	I&O Medical problems–evaluated and treated. Assess managed deficits. Implement CRS recommenda-tions.	I&O Continue progressive treatment per CRS team.	I&O Continue same progressive.	I&O Continue same progressive.	I&O Continue same progressive.

Continued

FIGURE 7.6 Inpatient Management Protocol for Acute Myocardial Infarction (continued)

Time Frame / Problems	Day 1 Interm. Goals	Day 2 Interm. Goals	Day 3 Interm. Goals	Day 4 Interm. Goals	Day 5 Interm. Goals
4. Meds/IV's	IV to maintain hydration. Medical therapy a necessary.	Maintain hydration. Continue IV if necessary. Heplock if intake good. Continue medical therapy as ordered.	Continue same.	Continue same. DC Heplock if still in place.	Continue same.
5. Nutrition	NPO until initial assessment. Step 1 Dysphasia diet (no thin liquid).	Progressive diet per S.T. (Maintenance) and assistant as needed.	Continue same.	Continue same.	Continue same.
6. Activity	PT or nurse assisted.	Cont. w/progressive activity per CRS team and nursing.	Continue w/progression.	Continue w/progression. Encouraging self-care as much as possible.	Continue w/progression. Self-care as much as possible.
7. PT and Family Education/ Counseling	Orient to room, unit, and routines. Review meds. Family education regarding DX, tests, ancillary specialist, physician specialist, disposition options, and course of care.	Continue teaching. Coping w/changes and safety.	Reinforce teaching.	Reinforce teaching. Instruct PT and/or family on appliance, meds, diet, and follow-up.	Reinforce teaching. Discharge teaching on follow-up. Written instructions for meds., diets, follow-up, activity, appointments given.
8. Discharge Planning	Social services Psych/social assessment (Family and caregiver assessment)	Continue	Check w/attending physician re: discharge date and disposition	Written order for anticipated discharge in AM.	Discharge w/home health notified or transportation to SNF.

- Emphasis on tasks previously overlooked or omitted. These often improve quality, by ensuring the optimal outcome or preventing a complication.
- Standardization of supplies, with resulting savings in inventory, training costs, and opportunities to negotiate volume discounts on purchases.
- Scheduling or resequencing to reduce errors or delays. These frequently have implications for quality, cost, and satisfaction.
- Substitution of lower cost personnel for specific services. These often require retraining and sometimes expanded intermediate protocols.
- Reengineering, or the invention of new approaches to the care process. These often combine several of the preceding opportunities. The new

process may require substantial investment but delivers a better product overall.

Most institutions evolve through these opportunities, reaching the last few only after several rounds of study and implementation. Protocols have supported major changes in the use of less expensive sites for care, such as rehabilitation hospitals, same-day surgery programs, and hospices, and the development of alternatives to expensive and dangerous treatments such as spinal fusions for back pain.

Sources and criteria for expectations

The criteria for guidelines have evolved rapidly.[51,52] Individual institutions develop guidelines by review and revision of published sources. Development de novo is unnecessary in most situations. No guideline developed elsewhere should ever be implemented without careful review of the implications of using it in a specific institution. The development process has at least three components. It opens the debatable issues, and encourages discussion and consensus. It allows the caregivers time to learn new approaches.[53] The proposed guidelines can be checked against current practice and pilot-tested to identify areas where new supplies, tools, or training will be required. As guidelines evolve, they reveal entire new approaches to care, and with them changes in staffing and physical facilities.[54]

The problem of writing clinical expectations is that much of what is important in medicine is ambiguous, debatable, or conditional. Expectations that overstate the real limits of clarity and validity create a danger of overspecification, of standardizing what should be left conditional. There are two important ways to achieve the necessary flexibility and adaptability:

1. The expectation can be set separately on smaller, well-defined groups, where the indicated actions are less ambiguous. Patient demographics (age, sex, living conditions) or diseases (type, severity, or comorbidity) can be used to specify alternative treatments. For example, a low-cost antibiotic might be specified for a certain infection, unless the patient has an allergy to it.

   This approach leads to conditional expectations, a branching logic to allow the guidelines to fit a larger set of real patients. Conditional expectations require more data, both for setting the expectation and for monitoring it. As data capture becomes more common and data processing less expensive, conditional expectations become more practical and more commonplace.
2. Rather than specifying alternatives, the expectations can include provisions for the attending physician to justify exceptions. Where there is no scientific consensus on the correct action, any evidence indicating that the doctor is aware of the expectation and is departing from it in good faith is acceptable. The general approach can often be expanded by:

- Specifying the optional or conditional possibilities. Continuing the antibiotic example, the guideline might say, "A low-cost antibiotic is the treatment of choice. Expensive antibiotics should be considered if the response is unsatisfactory after two days."
- Establishing a statistical estimate of the frequency of exceptions. For example, the management guideline might state, "Expensive antibiotics have been found necessary in 13 to 18 percent of cases." Applying the guideline becomes impossible in any specific case, but a judgment about performance can be made based on a relatively small number of cases.

Achieving compliance with protocols

A successful protocol strategy rests on an organizational culture that emphasizes candor, collegiality, a commitment to patients, and a commitment to evidence-based medicine. The elements of the culture are shown in Figure 7.3. Protocols are not taught; in fact, formal education approaches "have little direct impact on improving professional practices."[55] Rather, they are internalized, both into the fabric of the institution and into the minds of caregivers.[56,57] The continuous improvement process is started by justifying the need. Profiles of current practice, compared if possible to benchmarks, almost always show striking variation between physicians for ostensibly similar patients and large opportunities for improvement on major measures of cost and outcomes.[58]

Compliance may require revising support systems, changing supplies and physical arrangements, or improving information flows. Economic incentives may be necessary to gain widespread compliance, although the exact design of incentives is unclear.[59] Compliance should never be complete; a relatively large fraction of patients will not fit the unmodified protocol. Statistics on compliance such as the percentage of departures by cause can help improve the protocols themselves and motivate better compliance.

The governance system must stimulate such far-reaching changes. It does so by establishing a supportive culture; putting the necessary planning, budgeting, and information systems in place; and using its annual environmental assessment exercise to establish the desirability of the approach. As the program continues, these activities themselves expand and are revised, but they continue to be a critical infrastructure.

Designing patient management protocols can be a divisive process. It is the responsibility of the executive management group to avoid unnecessary conflict by selecting areas in which agreement appears obtainable and by resolving or, if necessary, allowing both sides to proceed in major controversies. Many arguments are better avoided; time changes all perspectives, and in the interim allowing alternative management guidelines can end the debate.

Limitations of protocols

While protocols have proven to be a powerful device for improving care, they have important limitations.

1. The correct protocol must be used. If a patient is misdiagnosed, applying the wrong protocol could be fatal.
2. Even within the group of correctly diagnosed patients, protocols do not fit all patients. About one-third of patients, depending on the condition involved, will have complications that make the complete use of the protocol inadvisable or impossible.
3. Protocols must be kept up-to-date; significant effort is required for annual reviews and revisions.
4. Protocols are difficult to apply in some settings, particularly outpatient and primary care.

The first problem, accurate diagnoses, is attacked by selection of competent caregivers and the provision of adequate consultative services. Doctors and most other professionals not only have rights, but also responsibilities to tailor care to the individual. To overcome the second problem, patients whose disease does not fit the modal pattern, the attending physician is encouraged to depart from the protocol when in his or her judgment, a revised care plan is in the patient's best interest. Extensive departures are supported by using case management, developing explicit individual care plans to complement the attending physician's judgment on complex cases. The physician's role will focus on two questions: What is the correct protocol for this patient? and Is there a need to depart from the protocol to accommodate this patient's unique characteristics?

The third problem, keeping protocols current, requires routine programs of annual review, including check of outside guideline sources and clinical literature.

The fourth, incorporating protocol information into primary office practice, is a frontier. Specialists working with a pre-selected group of patients with generally similar disease and relatively expensive interventions are likely to have only a dozen or two protocols, of which only a few are used routinely. They can master their protocol set within a few weeks, referring to the rarer ones on paper when necessary. Computerized support for the protocol is easier to build and helps orient the entire treatment team. Primary care doctors, seeing an unfiltered population, face hundreds of different conditions and routinely require dozens of very different protocols. With only a few minutes per patient, retrieving and reading protocols, even from computer screens or printouts, is not always practical.

Campaigns are mounted to change primary care behavior on a single important disease at a time. Some success has been reported using encounter forms that prompt for the correct information. The caregiver with the encounter form on a clip board can be prompted for the protocol steps and record their completion simultaneously. The technical problem, of course, is to get the right form in the clipboard. In a busy office where a routine pregnancy is followed by an acutely ill infant, and then by middle-aged hypertensive within a space of 20 minutes, that problem is not easily solved.

Strategic Clinical Improvement

A comprehensive strategy of continuous improvement using clinical expectations will eventually involve all clinical services and will become the focal point for policy of all kinds. Clinical expectations will drive the operating budget, the capital budget, and large sections of the planning process. The institution will find its recruitment and staffing decisions, equipment selection, and information systems design heavily influenced by the clinical guidelines. The organizational structure will change, putting more emphasis on cross-functional committees that set expectations and reducing the activity of the traditional hierarchy. As the cross-functional teams are held to explicit expectations, a matrix organization is created. Individual caregivers are accountable both to the team and to their functional unit.

Improving Intermediate Protocols

A successful clinical improvement program begins with a strategy for continuous improvement of the cost and quality of intermediate products. Improvements are implemented as part of the annual budget process. They are recorded in procedure manuals and incorporated into orientation and training routines.

Even at the simplest activity level, it can be necessary to coordinate the changes with patient management protocols. The key to success is an organization in which individual professions can relate quickly and professionally to physicians responsible for overall patient management. The physical therapists must have routine access to the orthopedic surgeons, neurosurgeons, and primary care practitioners who refer their cases. Inpatient nurses must have access to specialist physicians; outpatient nurses either to specialist or primary physicians. The dialogue allows intermediate and final protocols to develop collaterally.

Cross-functional teams can collaborate on intermediate protocols. For example, a team to develop the pre-operative care plan for outpatient surgery would include surgeons, operating room nurses, surgical care nurses, and representatives from anesthesiology, pathology, and radiology. A particularly successful example in many healthcare systems is the "Formulary and Therapeutics Committee." The committee evaluates specific drugs in terms of their appropriateness to various diagnoses, the possibilities of lower cost substitutes, and the need to inventory at the institution. It also reviews safety factors in drug administration and the overall quality of pharmaceutical service. Well-managed committees go beyond this to the interaction of pharmacy and other clinical services, including special training required for nursing and medicine in administration techniques, contra-indications, and symptoms of adverse reactions.

Continuous Improvement of Patient Management Guidelines

Having protocols is not enough; there must be a strategy to use them to meet external economic and quality demands, to keep them current, and to integrate them with each other.[60] The traditional accountability hierarchy is no longer adequate, and new structures are emerging.

As Figure 7.2 suggests, four kinds of information suggest avenues for improvement:

1. *Data on adverse effects, untoward outcomes, incidents, complaints and malpractice.* These measures of quality failures need to be kept at or very near benchmark levels.
2. *Patient and family satisfaction survey.* The criterion now widely used is "would return" or "would recommend service to others." Simple satisfaction may not be sufficient to retain and increase market share.
3. *Total costs per patient or per episode.* Provider files may be incomplete to recover this information. Insurance claims files are a better source. Costs of the institutional portion of care are frequently used while more comprehensive data are developed.
4. *Clinical literature, best practices, and the subjective opinion of respected clinicians.* Consistent with the evidence-based approach, clinical trials and the experience of other institutions frequently suggest improvement opportunities.

It is impossible to attack all the opportunities raised by review of these four sources. The continuous improvement strategy identifies those with the highest value to the institution and initiates improvement activities to achieve them. Value in this context is related principally to three factors: patient satisfaction, the maintenance of optimal health, and cost.

Improvement strategies focus first on unsatisfactory outcomes, including patient dissatisfaction, high cost, and poor quality. In situations in which market forces set the price, most episodes of care must cost less than they earn in revenue. The loss per episode is a common criterion for prioritizing conditions for study. The study of quality issues frequently reveals dollar-saving opportunities as a by-product. It is also true that continuing poor quality is likely to drive costs up, through malpractice settlements or the eventual loss of market share and volume. The variability of satisfaction, cost, and quality measures is an indicator of potential improvement. Internal benchmarks and protocols can be developed from the best local practice. Once the institution has stable compliance with internal benchmarks, attention can be turned to benchmarks from other markets.

Figure 7.7 shows the flow chart for designing patient management protocols, with the group holding the major accountability indicated in italics. A high-ranking management committee or leadership team guides the process of expectation setting in most institutions. Its membership includes representatives of the medical executive committee or physician association and other important clinical leaders from the functional hierarchy. The management committee should include spokespersons for the governing board and the executive, for primary care physicians, for specialist physicians, and for critical functional groups such as nursing. The committee selects the priority conditions to address and appoints cross-functional teams. The management committee also supports the improvement process by encouraging the participation of all the people who are materially affected, setting timelines, and negotiating controversy.

The cross-functional teams charged with developing patient management guidelines should involve all relevant professional skills. Figure 7.8 gives examples of patient management development teams. The teams usually include both primary care and the modal treating specialty for the disease or condition. Conditions usually treated by primary care providers have representatives from all relevant primary care professions. Leadership should go to the group or specialty that will use the protocol most. Active roles for nursing and other clinical support services should be formally recognized in committee appointments. Nursing may lead in the development of many guidelines. It is almost always essential to development and implementation of intermediate product protocols guidelines, and these must be integrated with the final product.[61] Other functional groups, such as pharmacy or rehabilitation therapies, are important to some teams, but not to all.

Each cross-functional team should have an annual review of progress and selection of new participants, preferably timed to precede the annual budget cycle. Often these teams work sequentially within their area, attacking the most promising diseases or conditions first and proceeding to others as they gain experience. Committee or task force membership and agendas are selected simultaneously with new priorities. Good leadership frequently reminds team members that professional self-improvement and the ability to respond to shared economic pressures are the rewards of the process. It reinforces this belief in selecting the team leaders and subcommittee chairs. Expected timetables for reports are set at the time of assignment, and foreseeable needs for technical consultation are also identified.

Including both primary and referral specialist members on cross functional teams recognizes their dual role in most conditions. Their perspectives differ because they see the patients at different stages of the disease, and the question of when consultation and referral are appropriate is part of the guideline development. The conflicts that arise constitute a population-based version of the individual clinical decisions presented in Figure 7.1, and they must inevitably be resolved. If clear criteria can be written for meeting

FIGURE 7.7 Patient Management Protocol Development and Accountability

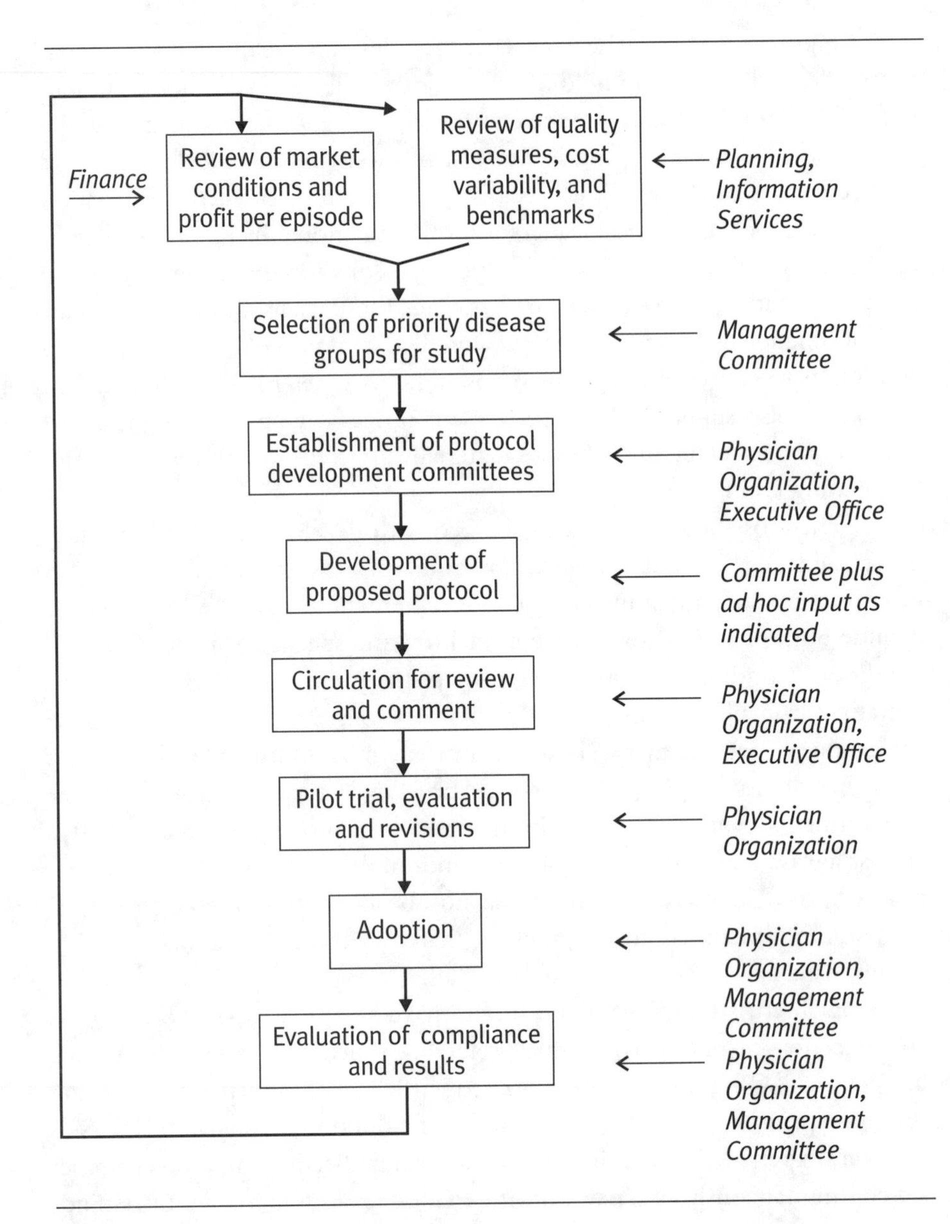

patient needs in primary care settings, quality can often be improved and cost reduced. Chronic patients' needs are often more holistic than intensive. That is, a diabetic, a hypertensive, or even a patient with AIDS or multiple sclerosis may be better served by a primary practitioner backed by specialist referral and consultation than either complete primary or complete specialist care.

Prevention and Health Promotion

A guidelines strategy sets several clinical teams in continuous improvement, but the guidelines by design address only those who become patients. Prevention and health promotion for citizens before they become patients or in a

FIGURE 7.8
Representative Patient Management Teams

Clinical Area	Typical Payment Aggregate or Patient Group	Team Members*	Typical Disease or Treatment Analysis
Trauma	Emergency department visit Trauma DRGs Trauma cost PMPM**	Emergency physicians Trauma surgeons Pediatricians Health educators	Pediatric and adult trauma care and prevention
Stroke	Stroke DRGs Rehabilitation per diem Stroke cost PMPM	Neurologists Gerontologists Rehabilitation therapists Nurses	Acute and rehabilitation care for cerebrovascular accidents
Obstetrics	Normal delivery DRG Caesarean section DRG Obstetric cost PMPM	Obstetricians Family practitioners Midwives Obstetrical nurses	Prenatal care, normal delivery, Caesarean section, postnatal care

* Each team would call in other specialists as indicated.
** PMPM: per member per month

different manner from the caregiving relationship are also important. Healthcare organizations provide prevention and health promotion for three reasons. First, prevention opportunities arise from the same scientific knowledge as treatment opportunities. Second, healthcare professionals are respected authority figures and their advice is given at times when the patient is receptive. Finally, under managed care, healthcare organizations can be rewarded for prevention; each episode of illness prevented translates eventually to reductions in cost of care. The first two reasons are not new. Healthcare professionals and institutions have responded to them with preventive activities for generations. The introduction of managed care has brought a new emphasis to preventive activities and intensified the response.

Prevention is generally considered to be direct interventions to avoid or reduce disease or disability. Preventive activities are undertaken by caregivers and by civic agencies for preventive services such as pure water, criminal justice, and legislation on firearms and dangerous substances. **Health promotion** includes all activities to change patient or customer behavior. It is undertaken by caregivers and by civic agencies such as public health departments, education systems, and voluntary associations. Both prevention and promotion can be categorized as primary, secondary, or tertiary. **Primary prevention** activities are those that take place before the disease occurs and eliminate or reduce its occurrence. Immunization, seat belts, condoms, sewage treatment, and restrictions on alcohol sale are examples. **Secondary prevention** reduces the consequences of disease, often by early detection and treatment. Self-examinations for cancer, routine dental inspections, mammographies, sigmoidoscopies, and management of chronic diseases like diabetes, hypertension, and asthma are examples. **Tertiary prevention** is the avoidance of complications or sequellae. Early physical therapy for strokes, retraining in activities of daily living, and respite services to help family caregivers are examples. Secondary and tertiary prevention are done mainly by caregivers and the patients themselves.

Intermediate protocols and clinical guidelines should incorporate all categories of prevention and health promotion. The protocol for well-baby visits should include immunizations, a check for potential developmental disabilities, and education for the mother on nutrition, home safety, and domestic violence. Diabetic and hypertension protocols should include selection of the optimal pharmacological treatment and guidance to the patient in life-style and nutrition. Home care visit protocols should include inspection for hazards and discussion of patient needs and symptoms with family members.

Cost Effectiveness of Prevention and Health Promotion

Many prevention opportunities are most effective before people consider themselves patients and require deliberate outreach into the community. Outreach efforts involve expense, and a sound prevention strategy directs the efforts to the highest possible payoff. The model for understanding the cost effectiveness of preventive outreach is a decision theory model paralleling the individual treatment decision, but it is applied to populations rather than individuals. The costs for preventive activity include the resources consumed in administering the activity and also the costs of any adverse consequence. Thus, the costs of immunization, the preventive activity generally felt to have the highest cost effectiveness, are:

Promotional/educational costs + Costs of immunization +
Cost of adverse reactions

or, if the first two terms are summarized as "Intervention costs"

Intervention costs + Cost of adverse reactions

and the costs of common secondary prevention such as cancer screening are:

Intervention costs + Cost of follow up for false positives

The benefits in both cases are the costs of disease or treatment avoided. The cost effectiveness ratio is usually expressed as the ratio of benefits to costs:

Costs of disease or treatment avoided/Total cost of preventive activity

An inexpensive, very safe vaccine such as diphtheria or measles can have very high benefit cost ratios. A relatively expensive secondary preventive activity that generates a high rate of false positives such as mammography can have higher costs than benefits and therefore a benefit cost ratio less than one. Thus, while the prevention of disease is always desirable, it is not always cost effective, and optimization of preventive activity involves finding the most cost-effective projects.

Cost effectiveness can be improved by reducing the intervention costs or the adverse consequences costs, or by increasing the effectiveness of the preventive intervention. If a population N is subject to the preventive intervention, n_1 recipients will avoid the disease who would previously have had it, n_2 will suffer the adverse reaction, and n_3 will have neither consequence. If N women have mammographies, n_1 women will be detected with early stage cancer and can get inexpensive treatment, n_2 will have false positives and get further testing and treatment that is unnecessary because they did not have cancer, and n_3 will receive a negative report but get no benefit except reassurance because they did not have cancer. Then, using the unit costs, the benefit cost ratio is:

$$\frac{n_1\ (\textit{Unit cost of treatment avoided})}{N\ (\textit{Mammography cost per person + promotional costs}) + N_2\ (\textit{False positive follow-up})}$$

Assuming that the cost of treatment avoided remains constant, the ratio can be increased by any of the following actions:

1. Decreasing any of the cost terms in the denominator: test cost, promotional cost, or cost of false positive follow-up.
2. Decreasing the number of false positives, n_2. That is, any improvement in the accuracy of the test that reduces the percentage of false positives will increase the benefit cost ratio.
3. Increase the ratio of cases prevented to the population screened, n_1/N. The ratio n_1/N is related to the incidence of the disease in the population screened. Any action that focuses the screening on populations at higher risk improves the benefit cost ratio.

For example, if breast cancer mammography is the preventive activity, the benefit cost ratio can be improved by a cheaper test, a way to tie the promotion to other necessary communications and reduce promotion cost, or a less expensive way to detect false from true positives. So will a new test with a lower rate of false positives. And finally, so will a preliminary screen that rules out the women least likely to have true positives and focuses on the groups or segments at highest risk. Race, age, and genetic history are known to affect the risk, and focused efforts to reach the correct populations become part of a sound prevention strategy. Several kinds of preventive activity become high-priority targets only when they are focused on populations at particular risk. These are often older and disadvantaged populations and occasionally specific ethnic or geographic groups.

Developing Prevention and Health Promotion Strategies

The traditional healthcare organization encouraged prevention in the context of the care process. A stronger, more effective strategy to gain the greatest benefit from prevention and health promotion will have several additional characteristics.[62] It will:

1. Identify primary or secondary prevention opportunities and rank order in terms of the cost benefit ratio. Many of the benefits are subjective. The proper people to evaluate the benefits are those who might receive them. Thus effective strategy deliberately involves representatives of high-risk groups in the ranking process.
2. Focus on problems where primary or secondary prevention has a high cost benefit. One consequence is that more costly or less effective preventive activities take a lower priority; cheap, easy prevention has a high priority. Another consequence is that prevention among the young has a high priority; the potential savings are higher.
3. Focus on those patient groups most at risk for those consequences. The consequence is that preventive interventions are concentrated among disadvantaged populations because these populations have the highest risks.
4. Seek ways to cut the cost of promotion, the preventive activity itself, or the follow-up of false positives. Innovative approaches tie the preventive activity to other contacts with the population at risk, such as education, employment, welfare, and private social contacts such as churches and private charities. The consequence is that the healthcare organization undertakes promotion as a collaborative effort with other community groups.

HMOs and fiscal intermediaries can assist with data for step 1.[63] Gaining help from other groups in the community is effective both in step 3 and step 4. Community groups can publicize prevention opportunities, and they often have channels of communication that are less costly and better targeted. Alliances with school boards, public health agencies, and private agencies such as United Way, the Urban League, and the Urban Ministry are productive.[64,65] It often pays to accept citizens' priorities, rather than professional ones, because the priorities reflect areas important to the population, and thus are easier to reach with promotional material. Domestic violence, teen pregnancy, illegal substance abuse, and access to care are important topics that arise in this way.[66] While a clinical approach might emphasize tobacco and immunizations more heavily, the final list will represent a consensus acceptable to all.

Measures and Information Systems for Clinical Performance

Quantitative performance measurement drives improvement in clinical performance. The information system that supports a successful program must accumulate all six dimensions of data, plus external or comparative information on constraints. It processes these data for four separate purposes:

1. *Caregiving.* Prompting users to prevent oversight or error; for example, using computer assistance or designing an encounter form to prompt the appropriate action. The information used for caregiving is almost entirely specific to individual patients and is required in very short time frames. However, this information provides the basic data for most other purposes.
2. *Education.* Providing visual aids that summarize arguments for existing or proposed expectations
3. *Expectation design and improvement.* Presenting analyses that support revision of existing expectations or the formulation of new ones
4. *Monitoring.* Accumulating a historical record for identifying improvement opportunities and evaluating alternative strategies

To fulfill the purposes, measures should be available for both functional and disease-oriented applications. The technology to meet such a broad agenda is emerging, but it is not likely to be complete within the next decade. The best information systems are themselves improving both by investing in automation of the medical record and by improving the analysis and retrieval of data.

The profile of what is available by dimension is shown in Figures 7.9 and 7.10. It is clear from these figures that both functional and disease applications require substantial expansion beyond traditional data systems.

Demand and Output

As Figure 7.10 shows, functional clinical units can generally rely on historic demand and output data and accounting data for most of what they need in those three areas. Measures of market share and appropriateness of demand require special surveys or other external data. Market share must be based on estimates of how many potential users went to competing sources. For example, the laboratory volumes might be compared to estimates of volumes of all competing laboratories. Disease group market share can be estimated by pooling data from competitors through a third-party agency (some states collect hospital admission data, for example), from a community household survey (covering all citizens, not just users of the institution in question), or from the epidemiological model, estimating total local demand from analytic models based on patient characteristics (often available from consulting firms).

Cost and Productivity

As noted in Chapter 6, costs are accumulated by type of resource according to the functional hierarchy. This allows estimates of the average cost for global aggregates of service, but the usual accounting system does not collect

FIGURE 7.9 Profile of Clinical Measurement for Functional Units

Input-Oriented	Output-Oriented
Demand	**Output/Productivity**
Available from historic records of unit	*Available from historic records of unit*
Requests for service	Services rendered
Logistics of service	Global productivity
Requiring special survey or estimation	*Requiring special survey or estimation*
Market share	Productivity of individual services
Appropriateness of service	
Cost/Resources	**Quality**
Available from accounting records	*Available from existing records*
Physical counts	Structural quality
Costs	*Requiring special survey*
Requiring special survey or estimation	Procedural quality
Unit costs of individual services	*Not available*
Resource condition	Clinical outcomes
Human Resources	**Customer Satisfaction**
Available from existing records	*Requiring special survey or estimation*
Supply	Patient satisfaction
Training	Referring physician satisfaction
Requiring special survey or estimation	Other customer satisfaction
Employee satisfaction	Access

information at a level that will support estimates of particular intermediate activities. That is to say, the costs of operating the laboratory are readily available, along with a count of tests of all kinds. The average cost per laboratory test is the ratio of the two. The cost of a specific test, such as a test for high-density lipids (HDLs) in the blood, is not known. The test is performed on automated equipment, usually simultaneously with several other tests. The labor and the equipment costs cannot be exactly distributed between the various tests done by the same equipment. Whatever biases or errors are in the estimated cost will be distributed to various disease groups. The overall fraction of the cost involved in such errors is often substantial.

This shortfall of the traditional information quickly becomes critical to improvement teams working with final products in cross-functional disease groups. Several strategies exist to deal with the problem.

1. *Expanding the number of functional accounts and responsibility centers.* The problem is improved if the costs can be aggregated by "automated hematology" rather than by "hematology" or "clinical laboratory."
2. *Using the Pareto Rule (Chapter 6) and concentrating on the largest components of the final product cost.* HDL cost errors are probably trivial;

FIGURE 7.10 Profile of Clinical Measurement for Disease-Oriented Units

Input-Oriented	Output-Oriented
Demand	**Output/Productivity**
Available from historic records	*Available from historic records*
Requests for care	Patients treated
	Global productivity
Requiring special survey or estimation	*Requiring special survey or estimation*
Market share	Productivity of individual services
Appropriateness of service	
Logistics of service	
Cost/Resources	**Quality**
Available from existing records	*Available from existing records*
Total costs per patient	Clinical outcomes (part)
Requiring special survey or estimation	*Requiring special survey*
Unit costs and marginal costs of individual services	Clinical outcomes (part)
Human Resources	**Customer Satisfaction**
Available from existing records	*Requiring special survey or estimation*
Supply	Patient satisfaction
Training	Referring physician satisfaction
Requiring special survey or estimation	Other customer satisfaction
Employee satisfaction	Access

magnetic resonance cost errors can be critical. Accuracy of estimate is increased where necessary.

3. *Use of relative value scales and other adjusters to improve the estimates.* Published studies indicate the relative cost of HDL tests compared to the other output of automated hematology. While these may not be exact in the local situation, they are useful guides. Relative value scales (RVS) exist for laboratory, x-ray, and physician activities.
4. *Amplifying the cost accounting system with special studies.* If HDL costs are important and subjective estimates or RVS are inadequate, detailed analysis of the test process can establish more precise ones. The level of precision is limited mainly by the cost of the study.

Quality and Satisfaction

Functional units generally have both structural and procedural measures of quality, relying on more or less formal audits to ensure uniformity of services. As noted, outcomes measures are not appropriate to individual components of care. The opposite is true for disease group measures. Some outcomes measures (for example, infections and mortality) are routinely recorded in the medical record. Others (for example, follow-up survival and function status measures) require special surveys. Although these surveys are relatively expensive, the technology for doing them is clearly understood. Disease groups generally rely on functional units for structural and procedural measures.

Figure 7.11 shows the sources and strategy for augmenting quality and satisfaction data. Satisfaction data for all purposes is collected by survey (described more fully in Chapter 6). Patients are surveyed formally, and specific questions can address the larger functional services such as nursing and rehabilitation therapies. The response to the functional services is often critical to the overall patient satisfaction. Respondents are identified by disease group, allowing easy tallying for cross-functional teams. Specialist physicians are generally associated with specific disease groups; the cross-functional teams can easily access their opinions and comments. It is common to supplement surveys with focus groups or discussions with specific physicians to identify opportunities for improvement. Primary or referring physicians can be surveyed, but a direct approach to high volume referrers and selective discussions with those not referring as frequently can be revealing.

Employee satisfaction survey data are usually collected anonymously by functional unit. Translation to the cross-functional team is rarely possible without violating confidentiality requirements. However, the cross-functional team should be able to rely on generally high satisfaction scores in all its functional components. Continued low scores within any functional unit are a matter of serious concern and should be promptly addressed.

FIGURE 7.11 Strategy for Quality and Satisfaction Measurement

Element	Source	Rule for Inclusion	Comment
Patient/family satisfaction	Survey	Always desirable	Universal patient surveys may be required
Outcomes successes	Medical record, possibly survey	Seek measures central to recovery	Benchmark to identify potential; report statistical significance
Functional status and placement	Medical record or special measurement effort	Relate to realistic lifestyle	Same as outcomes
Process measures	Special measurement or analysis	Seek processes related to outcomes and satisfaction	Avoid process measures that lack clear association with outcomes

In summary, usable data are available for most clinical applications, both functional and cross-functional, but by relying on a patchwork of estimates and alternative data sources. The steps, assumptions, and definitions involved in providing the various kinds of information are complicated enough to require specific management. An office of information management is common among leading institutions. It becomes the "source of truth" on what the estimate is, and what its limitations are.

Suggested Readings

Eddy, D. M. 1996. *Clinical Decision Making: From Theory to Practice: A Collection of Essays from the Journal of the American Medical Association.* Sudbury, MS: Jones and Barlett Publishers.

Gray, J. A. M. 1997. *Evidence-Based Healthcare.* New York: Churchill-Livingstone.

Ransom, S. R., and W. W. Pinsky, (eds.). 1999. *Clinical Resource and Quality Management.* Tampa, FL: American College of Physician Executives.

Spath, P. L. (ed.). 1997. *Beyond Clinical Paths: Advanced Tools for Outcomes Management.* Chicago: American Hospital Publishing.

Wagner, E. H., B. T. Austin, and M. Von Korff. 1996. "Organizing Care for Patients with Chronic Illness." *Milbank Quarterly* 74 (4): 511–44.

Weinstein, M. C., and H. V. Feinberg. 1980. *Clinical Decision Analysis.* New York: Saunders.

Notes

1. R. Stevens, "In Sickness and in Wealth." *American Hospitals in the Twentieth Century.* New York: Basic Books, pp. 351–366 (1989)
2. A. C. Enthoven and C. B. Vorhaus, "A Vision of Quality in Health Care Delivery." *Health Affairs* 16(3), pp. 44–57 (May–June 1997)
3. American Society for Quality: www.asq.org (October 19, 1998)
4. G. Ellrodt, D. J. Cook, J. Lee, M. Cho, D. Hunt, and S. Weingarten, "Evidence-Based Disease Management." *Journal of the American Medical Association* 278(20), pp. 1687–92 (Nov 26, 1997)
5. S. M. Shortell, *Effective Hospital-Physician Relationships.* Chicago: Health Administration Press (1991)
6. K. B. Bayley, D. J. Lansky, M. R. London, L. A. Skokan, and K. B. Eden, "Clinical Practice Evaluation at Providence Health System." *Quality Management in Health Care* 4(4), pp. 21–9 (Summer, 1996)
7. J. R. Griffith, *Designing 21st Century Healthcare: Leadership in Hospitals and Healthcare Organizations.* Chicago: Health Administration Press (1998)
8. W. G. Manning, A. Liebowitz, G. A. Goldberg, et al. "A Controlled Trial of the Effect of Prepaid Group Practice on Use of Service." *The New England Journal of Medicine* 310, pp. 1505–10 (June 7, 1984)
9. E. Freidson, "The Reorganization of the Medical Profession." *Medical Care Review* 42, pp. 11–36 (Spring, 1985)

10. D. M. Berwick, M. W. Baker, and E. Kramer, "The State of Quality Management in HMOs." *HMO Practice* 6(1), pp. 26–32 (March 6, 1992)
11. M. R. Handley, and M. E. Stuart, "An Evidence-Based Approach to Evaluating and Improving Clinical Practice: Guideline Development." *HMO Practice* 8(1), pp. 10–19 (March, 1994)
12. Institute of Medicine, *Medicare: A Strategy for Quality Assurance*, Vol. 1, K. N. Lohr, ed. Washington, DC: National Academy Press, pp. 20–25 (1990)
13. R. H. Palmer, A. Donabedian, and G. J. Povar, *Striving for Quality in Health Care: An Inquiry into Policy and Practice*. Chicago: Health Administration Press, p. 54 (1991)
14. *Ibid*, 55
15. Institute of Medicine, *Medicare: A Strategy for Quality Assurance*, Vol. 2, K. N. Lohr, ed. Washington, DC: National Academy Press (1990)
16. T. A. Brennan, L. L. Leape, N. M. Laird, L. Hebert, A. R. Localio, et al, "Incidence of Adverse Events and Negligence in Hospitalized Patients: Results of the Harvard Medical Practice Study I." *New England Journal of Medicine* 324(6), pp. 370–6 (Feb 7, 1991)
17. E. B. Keeler, L. V. Rubenstein, K. L. Kahn, D. Draper, E. R. Harrison, et al, "Hospital Characteristics and Quality Of Care." *Journal of the American Medical Association* 268(13), pp. 1709–14 (October 7, 1992)
18. D. G. Safran, A. R. Tarlov, and W. H. Rogers, "Primary Care Performance in Fee-for-Service and Prepaid Health Care Systems: Results from the Medical Outcomes Study." *Journal of the American Medical Association* 271(20), pp. 1579–86 (May 25,1994)
19. S. Greenfield, E. C. Nelson, M. Zubkoff, W. Manning, W. Rogers, et al, "Variations in Resource Utilization Among Medical Specialties and Systems of Care: Results from the Medical Outcomes Study." *Journal of the American Medical Association* 267(12), pp. 1624–30 (March 25, 1992)
20. R. L. Kravitz, S. Greenfield, W. Rogers, W. G. Manning, Jr., M. Zubkoff, et al, "Differences in the Mix of Patients Among Medical Specialties and Systems of Care. Results from the Medical Outcomes Study." *Journal of the American Medical Association* 267(12), pp. 1617–23 (March 25, 1992)
21. Dartmouth Medical School, Center for the Evaluative Clinical Sciences. *Dartmouth Atlas of Healthcare*. Chicago: American Hospital Publishing (1998)
22. H. R. Rubin, B. Gandek, W. H. Rogers, M. Kosinski, C. A. McHorney, and J. E. Ware, Jr., "Patients' Ratings of Outpatient Visits in Different Practice Settings: Results from the Medical Outcomes Study." *Journal of the American Medical Association* 270(7), pp. 835–40 (August 18, 1993)
23. B. C. James, "Implementing Practice Guidelines Through Clinical Quality Improvement." *Frontiers of Health Services Management* 10(1), pp. 3–37 (Fall, 1993)
24. P. P. Harteloh and F. W. Verheggen, "Quality Assurance in Health Care From a Traditional Towards a Modern Approach." *Health Policy* 27(3), pp. 261–70 (March,1994)
25. P. B. Batalden, E. C. Nelson, and J. S. Roberts, "Linking Outcomes Measurement to Continual Improvement: The Serial 'V' Way of Thinking About Improving

Clinical Care." *Joint Commission Journal On Quality Improvement* 20(4), pp. 167–80 (April, 1994)

26. A. D. Donabedian, J. R. C. Wheeler, and L. Wyszewianski, "Quality Cost and Health: An Integrative Model." *Medical Care* 20, pp. 975–992 (October, 1982)
27. M. C. Weinstein and H. V. Fineberg, *Clinical Decision Analysis.* New York: Saunders (1980)
28. R. R. Neutra, "Appendicitis: Decreasing Normal Removals Without Increasing Perforations." *Medical Care* 16(11), pp. 956–61 (November, 1978)
29. A. D. Donabedian, "Reflections on the Effectiveness of Quality Assurance." in *Striving for Quality in Health Care*, Palmer et al, eds., pg. 86 (1991)
30. E. A. Codman, *A Study in Hospital Efficiency: The First Five Years, Boston.* Boston: Thomas Todd (1916)
31. A. D. Donabedian, "Reflections on the Effectiveness of Quality Assurance." In *Striving for Quality in Health Care*, Palmer et al, eds. (1991)
32. D. M. Berwick, "Sounding Board. Continuous Improvement as an Ideal in Health Care." *New England Journal of Medicine* 320(1), pp. 53–56 (1989)
33. M. R. Handley and M. E. Stuart, "An Evidence-Based Approach to Evaluating and Improving Clinical Practice: Guideline Development." *HMO Practice* 8(1), pp. 10–19 (March, 1994)
34. R. E. Ward, and J. E. Lafata, "Clinical Effectiveness: An Emerging Discipline" Ch. 4 in S.R. Ransom and W.W. Pinsky, eds., *Clinical Resource and Quality Management.* Tampa, Florida: American College of Physician Executives, pp. 89–115 (1999)
35. Institute of Medicine, *Medicare*, Vol. 1, pp. 62–63
36. D. Mechanic, "Physicians and Patients in Transition." *The Hastings Center Report*, pp. 9–12 (December, 1985)
37. B. C. James, "Implementing Practice Guidelines Through Clinical Quality Improvement." *Frontiers of Health Services Management* 10(1), pp. 3–37, discussion pp. 54–56 (Fall, 1993)
38. E. H. Wagner, B. T. Austin, and M. Von Korff, "Organizing Care for Patients with Chronic Illness." *Milbank Quarterly* 74(4), pp. 511–44 (1996)
39. S. M. Shortell, *Effective Hospital-Physician Relationships.* Chicago: Health Administration Press, pp. 245–63 (1991)
40. C. E. Hynniman, "Drug Product Distribution Systems and Departmental Operations." *American Journal of Hospital Pharmacy* 48(10), pp. 524–35 (October, 1991)
41. J. B. Christianson, L. H. Warrick, F. E. Netting, F. G. Williams, W. Read, and J. Murphy, "Hospital Case Management: Bridging Acute and Long-Term Care." *Health Affairs* 10(2), pp. 173–84 (1991)
42. F. G. Williams, L. H. Warrick, J. B. Christianson, and F. E. Netting, "Critical Factors for Successful Hospital-Based Case Management." *Health Care Management Review* 18(1), pp. 63–70 (Winter, 1993)
43. Institute of Medicine, *Medicare*, Vol. 1, pp. 304–306
44. Agency for Health Care Policy and Research. Internet home page: www.ahcpr.gov/clinic
45. C. Marwick, "Proponents Gather to Discuss Practicing Evidence-Based

Medicine." *Journal of the American Medical Association* 278(7), pp. 531–532 (August 20, 1997)

46. Website of the University of California San Francisco: itsa.ucsf.edu/petsam/#7 (October 12, 1998)
47. T. J. Ryan, J. L. Anderson, E. M. Antman, B. A. Braniff, N. H. Brooks, et al, "ACC/AHA Guidelines for the Management of Patients with Acute Myocardial Infarction: A Report of the American College of Cardiology/American Heart Association Task Force on Practice Guidelines (Committee on Management of Acute Myocardial Infarction)." *Journal of the American College of Cardiology* 28:1328–1428, p.1331 (1996)
48. T. J. Ryan, J. L. Anderson, E. M. Antman, et al., p. 1331
49. *Ibid*, p. 1331
50. *Ibid*, p. 1340
51. D. M. Eddy, "Guidelines—How Should They Be Designed?" *Clinical Decision Making: From Theory to Practice*. Sudbury, MA: Jones and Bartlett, pp. 34–40 (1996)
52. D. L. Sackett, et al. *Evidence-Based Medicine: How to Practice and Teach EBM*. New York: Churchill Livingstone. (1997) On-line update to book, Centre for Evidence-Based Medicine, Oxford University.
53. P. B. Batalden and J. J. Mohr, "Building Knowledge of Health Care as a System." *Quality Management in Health Care* 5(3), pp. 1–12 (Spring, 1997)
54. P. L. Spath (ed.), *Beyond Clinical Paths: Advanced Tools for Outcomes Management*. Chicago: American Hospital Publishing (1997)
55. D. A. Davis, M. A. Thomson, A. D. Oxman, and R. B. Haynes, "Changing Physician Performance. A Systematic Review of the Effect of Continuing Medical Education Strategies." *Journal of the American Medical Association* 274(23), pp. 1836–7 (Dec 20, 1995)
56. D. E. Pathman, T. R. Konrad, G. L. Freed, V. A. Freeman, and G. G. Koch, "The Awareness-to-Adherence Model of the Steps to Clinical Guideline." *Medical Care* 34(9), pp. 873–89 (September, 1996)
57. E. J. Proenca, "Why Outcomes Management Doesn't (Always) Work: An Organizational Perspective." *Quality Management in Health Care* 3(4), pp. 1–9 (Summer, 1995)
58. J. H. Evans, III, Y. Hwang, and N. Nagarajan, "Physicians' Response to Length-of-Stay Profiling." *Medical Care* 33(11), pp. 1106–19 (November, 1995)
59. J. R. Griffith, *Designing 21st Century Healthcare: Leadership in Hospitals and Healthcare Organizations*, Chapter 5, pp. 247–65. Chicago: Health Administration Press (1998)
60. P. B. Batalden and J. J. Mohr, "Building Knowledge of Health Care as a System." *Quality Management in Health Care* 5(3), pp. 1–12 (Spring, 1997)
61. K. Zander, "Nursing Care Management: Resolving the DRG Paradox." *Nursing Clinics of North America* 23(3), pp. 503–519 (September, 1988)
62. J. Showstack, N. Lurie, S. Leatherman, E. Fisher, and T. Inui, "Health of the Public: The Private Sector Challenge." *Journal of the American Medical Association* 276(13), pp. 1071–4 (Oct 2, 1996)
63. R. S. Thompson, "What Have HMOs Learned About Clinical Prevention

Services? An Examination of the Experience at Group Health Cooperative of Puget Sound." *Milbank Quarterly* 74(4), pp. 469–509 (1996)

64. T. G. Rundall, "The Integration of Public Health and Medicine." *Frontiers of Health Services Management* 10(4), pp. 3–24 (Summer, 1994)
65. W. E. Welton, T. A. Kantner, and S. M. Katz, "Developing Tomorrow's Integrated Community Health Systems: A Leadership Challenge for Public Health and Primary Care." *Milbank Quarterly* 75(2), pp. 261–88 (1997)
66. J. R. Griffith, *Designing 21st Century Health Care.* Chicago: Health Administration Press, pp. 57–66, 132–5, 231–6 (1998)

CHAPTER

8

ORGANIZED PHYSICIAN SERVICES

Introduction: Models of Physician Organization

Doctors have been ascribed magical powers, granted extraordinary privileges and confidences, and expected to assume extra moral obligations since the dawn of human existence. The twentieth century saw a revolution in this social contract. The magical powers became reality through scientific advance. The privileges and confidences originally vested in one individual were divided among many specialists concerned with particular organ systems or methods of treatment. Nonphysician caregivers became more popular and gained authority in specific clinical situations. The anticipation of moral obligation was blemished by the suspicion and retribution of malpractice litigation. Still, the doctor remains the leader of the clinical team and the principal agent for the patient, perhaps simply because it is difficult to imagine any other structure.

Thus, the core of any substantial healthcare organization is a group or several groups of physicians. The success of the organization is dependent upon their collective performance, but that performance remains the sum of individual encounters between patients and physicians. The link between the organization and the physician is symbiotic; without physicians it is impossible to give more than elementary healthcare, and without healthcare organizations, most physicians cannot practice modern medicine. The paradox is the tension between the independence of the physicians' daily work and collective nature of modern care. Both elements are essential and must be preserved. A physician with too little independence will fail to meet patients' varying needs. One with too little accountability will have difficulty adapting to the teamwork of modern technology, and will deliver highly variable, suboptimal care.[1]

There is typically one physician for every thousand persons or so in the organization's market share. Larger organizations have several hundred physicians representing a wide variety of specialties and growing numbers of nonmedical practitioners. Technology and economics have increased the differences among them. About half are in primary care; they work mostly in office settings and see a broad range of illness and affliction. The balance are in referral or specialty practice. Specialists work mostly in institutional settings and by definition see a limited range of conditions in which they are expert. Both groups are supported by nonmedical practitioners, but the relationship of primary physicians to nurse practitioners and midwives is different from the relationship of specialists to their supporting team.

The economic relationship is also varied. Historically, individual physicians earned their income from their patients' fees, but collective compensation mechanisms became necessary as the complexity of care and finance increased. Specialists have found single specialty groups useful. Primary doctors have been slower to form groups, but recently many have become employees of the healthcare organization. Managed care contracts are often offered to multispecialty groups, and complex income sharing arrangements result.[2] Individual doctors usually work under several financial arrangements during their careers, often combining traditional fee-for-service with one or more managed care contracts at the same time. These complex patterns are likely to continue for the foreseeable future.

Although the change in technology has been relatively steady over the last 50 years, its impact is cumulative. The change in economics is recent and abrupt, concentrated in the last decade, and a briefer interval in many communities. The result is that the culture and structure of physician organization are an unfinished work in progress. Two historical models were the starting points, but they have demonstrated weaknesses. A variety of innovations have emerged, but none has shown a dominant advantage.

In most communities, the historical starting point was the traditional hospital medical staff. The medical staff organization provided a review of competence, a mechanism for participation in collective decisions, and a vehicle for quality review and education.[3] Most physicians required hospital admitting privileges, so that participation was widespread. Well-managed institutions were able to use the mechanism to ensure quality of inpatient care. However, the traditional staff organization has a number of weaknesses in the context of comprehensive health insurance and economic limitations. The organization applied only to institutional practice; it did not apply to the physician's office practice. Partly because the importance of hospital practice varied among specialties, the level of participation in the organization varied. Referral specialists tended to dominate the organization, to the disadvantage of primary care physicians. The emphasis was strictly on quality of care, to the exclusion of economic issues. Because hospital staff membership involved no direct economic commitment by individual physicians and small physician groups, any discussion of fees raised the possibility of collusion in restraint of trade, an antitrust violation. Although the hospital had the obligation to limit staff membership in specialties to its capacity, and the right to plan the size of its staff by specialty, mechanisms to do this were unwieldy and unpopular.

The second historical model was the employed medical staff. Federal hospitals, many academic medical centers, and several large multispecialty groups, such as the Permanente groups of Kaiser Permanente, and the Henry Ford Health System employed physicians. The structure of other large groups such as Mayo and Cleveland Clinics was a pooled fee arrangement with distribution via an executive committee, similar to that of law and accounting firms. For the individual doctor, the result was closer to employment than to fee-for-service. Many hospitals employed primary care physicians and placed them in areas of low access or market share as the demand for comprehensive insurance rose, adding employment models to their fee-for-service medical staffs.

Experience with employed staffs has revealed two serious limitations. First, employment of physicians is a long-term investment that is effectively a fixed cost for the institution. Capital funds go for the purchase of existing practices, construction of facilities, and long-term commitments necessary to attract physicians. The funds represent a drain on limited resources that is avoided in independent practice models, where the individual physician is responsible for the investment. They also limit flexibility. Once extensive investments have been made, it is difficult to redirect them to new market needs. Second, experience strongly suggests that employed physicians are not as responsive to patient needs. They do not offer as flexible hours, or see as many patients, or pay attention to patient perceptions as well as fee-for-service physicians.[4]

As the weaknesses of these approaches became clear, many innovative solutions were developed. Most of these establish a cadre of physicians appropriate to comprehensive care as an independent organization, capable of accepting contracts for large patient populations and managing their healthcare needs. The names of these organizations and their structures differ substantially. Independent physician associations (IPAs), medical foundations, networks, medical service organizations (MSOs), and physician-hospital organizations (PHOs) are the most common names. Their organizations tend to be various models of democratic cooperatives; the leadership is elected and strategic management is vested in elected councils. Most of these organizations allow their members to continue traditional practice, and they do not immediately change geographic coverage. As a result, they are often called **"groups without walls"** or **"virtually integrated groups."**

Open systems theory suggests that the success of these organizations is determined by their ability to fulfill the desires of their constituents, in this case the patients, the payors, the institutions essential to care, and the doctors who participate. A physician organization will succeed not only because it supplies healthcare at attractive quality and cost, but also because it offers physicians an economically and professionally rewarding lifestyle. While the final structure of the twenty-first century physician organization remains uncertain, some basic elements are widely accepted:[5]

- Organization will prevail over independence. The final structure will increase the accountability of the individual practitioner.
- The alliance between the practitioners and the institution will become stronger. The physician organization will be closely linked to the institutional organization.

- Doctors will retain substantial influence over the institutional organization through the physician organization. More skillful management will be required to integrate a broader set of stakeholder needs at both the institutional and the physician organization levels.

The functions the emerging organization must perform will define the eventual structure. Those functions are much clearer than the future structure.

Plan for the Chapter

The remainder of the chapter covers the purpose and functions of the physician organization, including a description of the privilege relationship, the unique contract that establishes the ground rules for collaboration. It reviews the existing economic and organizational relationships between physicians and healthcare organizations and concludes with a review of measures of physician and physician organization performance.

Purposes

Purposes of the Physician Organization

Following open systems concept of meeting major stakeholder needs, one may group the purposes of the conjoint medical staff under three headings:

1. *The provision of high-quality, cost-effective care to the community*
    - to provide the maximum scope of services consistent with community healthcare needs and economic capability;
    - to promote health and prevent disease as a basic goal of customer stakeholders and an essential element of economical care;
    - to support a variety of healthcare financing arrangements, permitting customer choice and allowing the largest possible market share;
    - to support a system of recruiting, selecting, and promoting physicians whose capabilities most closely reflect the desires of the community; and
    - to achieve continuous improvement in the cost and quality of patient care.
2. *The support of rewarding professional life*
    - to provide each physician with a competitive livelihood and a satisfying opportunity to practice quality medicine;
    - to promote the clinical knowledge and skill of individual members; and
    - to provide equal opportunity for all qualified members of the organization and to ensure their rights by due process.
3. *The maintenance of the organization itself*
    - to maintain communications between members of the organization and community decision-making bodies in a manner that promotes

full understanding, responsiveness, and fairness in matters affecting the work environment;
- to ensure an adequate financial base; and
- to aid in the resolution of conflicting desires between its customers, its owners, and its members.

Functions

The physician organization must complete six major functions to achieve the purposes:

1. Improvement of clinical quality and cost expectations
2. Credentialing and privileging of physicians
3. Staff planning and recruitment
4. Continuing education for physicians and other clinical professionals
5. Representation, communication, and resolution of conflicts
6. Negotiation and maintenance of collective compensation arrangements

These functions are summarized in Figure 8.1.

FIGURE 8.1 Functions of Physician Organizations

Function	Purpose	Activities
Improvement of clinical quality and cost expectations	Provide high-quality cost-effective healthcare	Continuous improvement of care through clinical protocols, case management, and prevention
Review of privileges and credentials	Ensure continued effectiveness of individual staff members	Recruitment and selection of new members, renewal of privileges
Physician supply planning and recruitment	Ensure an adequate supply of well-trained physicians	Physician needs planning, recruitment
Continuing education of physicians and other clinical services	Ensure a well-trained body of caregivers	Case reviews, protocol development, scientific programs, and graduate medical education
Representation and communication	Bring clinical viewpoint to all activities of the organization	Governing board, strategic planning, budgeting participation
Maintenance of collective compensation agreements	Allow customer access to a full range of healthcare financing opportunities	Negotiation and implementation of risk-sharing contracts with payors and intermediaries

Improvement of Clinical Quality and Cost Expectations

As indicated in Chapter 7, protocols and guidelines are the accepted device for continuous clinical quality improvement. Physicians play an active role in establishing priorities for protocol development, in designing and implementing protocols, in selecting and using measures of clinical performance, and in promoting health among active patients and the community at large. Figure 7.8 indicates the extensive physician roles in protocol design and use.

Most final product protocols are established by a medically dominated committee. A good final product panel will include active representation from all the specialties involved in treatment. Leadership of the committee is usually assigned to the **modal specialists**, the specialists who treat the largest percentage of patients with the disease or condition. The trend in protocols has been to extend them to encompass treatment before the central episode to emphasize prevention and follow-up to maximize recovery. With this comes an expansion of team membership, incorporating primary care physicians as well as specialists. The **hospital-based specialties**—laboratory, imaging, anesthesia, and emergency care—contribute to care of many diseases. Ambulatory care protocols are normally led by primary care physicians, but continuing specialist input is valuable. Some conditions are treated by different practitioners depending on their severity. Obstetrics and newborn care, for example, can be successfully managed by midwives, pediatric nurse practitioners, family practice physicians, obstetricians, and pediatricians. A large number of cardiovascular diseases are managed by nurse practitioners, family practice physicians, general internists, cardiologists, and cardiovascular surgeons depending on their severity. All of these groups must be involved in protocol design. Several protocols may result, and the criteria for assigning patients must be uniform across the set.

Intermediate protocols are generally the product of a clinical support service or a single medical specialty, but the attending physicians are customers for the product. They order it and use it in the patient's care. Well-designed intermediate protocols are reviewed by user panels, and the panel's suggestions are incorporated in the improvements. The opportunity to comment on any protocol should be open to all physicians.

The role of the physician organization is to see that the right clinical expertise is available for each of these tasks and to integrate the results of protocol design into the other five functions. This will require a hierarchical organization to identify participants at various levels, funnel comments to a central point for resolution and communicate decisions back to participants, integrate credentialing, planning, education, and compensation activities with protocols. To be effective, the organization would need to include all the major modal specialists, the hospital-based specialists, and the primary care physicians. It would have to provide ongoing communication between all these groups and the institutional organization as priorities were set, proposals developed and evaluated, and incentives coordinated. Given the complexity and seriousness of the issues involved, conflicts would be inevitable and a robust mechanism for resolving them a fundamental part of the organization.

The most important applications of case management are in complex chronic cases that almost by definition involve several different physician specialties as well as a battery of functional units of the institutional organization. Establishing the authority of the case manager, agreeing on the individual plan, and evaluating progress are activities that require the physician organization and the institutional organization.

Preventive activity occurs in the physicians' offices and in outreach sites remote from healthcare. The message must be consistent to be optimally effective, and referrals from the outreach activity must receive satisfactory and appropriate service. The physician organization is part of the alliance between the institution and community organizations providing outreach.

Review of Privileges and Credentials

The task of ensuring quality and cost effectiveness in medical practice is based on a simple premise, that well-trained doctors in a supportive surrounding will provide their patients with excellent care. In accordance with the process outlined in Figure 8.2, each doctor is formally granted the privilege of participating in the physician group and of providing treatment within her or his training and experience. In continuous improvement terms, each doctor is empowered to practice good medicine. Credentialing is a fundamental quality assurance activity. Both JCAHO and NCQA require that it be done rigorously.

Elements of privilege

The privilege agreement is nationally standardized by the accrediting organizations, NCQA and JCAHO, and by various court decisions. It is a contract with four critical elements:

1. *Bylaws.* The doctors collectively establish mutually acceptable rules and regulations. These define the doctors' rights to participate in the organization and provide care as part of the organization, the obligation to ensure quality and economy of care to their own patients, and the obligation to participate in educational and quality improvement activities. They may also define rules for compensation. The bylaws also define how the physician organization makes decisions, including its accountability hierarchy and how the rules may be amended. Given the complexity of most of these issues, the bylaws themselves are supplemented by various procedural statements included by reference. Because of the importance of credentialing, and because the privileges give access to the community owned resources of the institution, the bylaws are approved both by its physician members and by the institutional governing board.
   The bylaws are the principal source of due process protection. They establish all procedural elements, including application requirements,

FIGURE 8.2
Flow Chart of Physician Credentialing

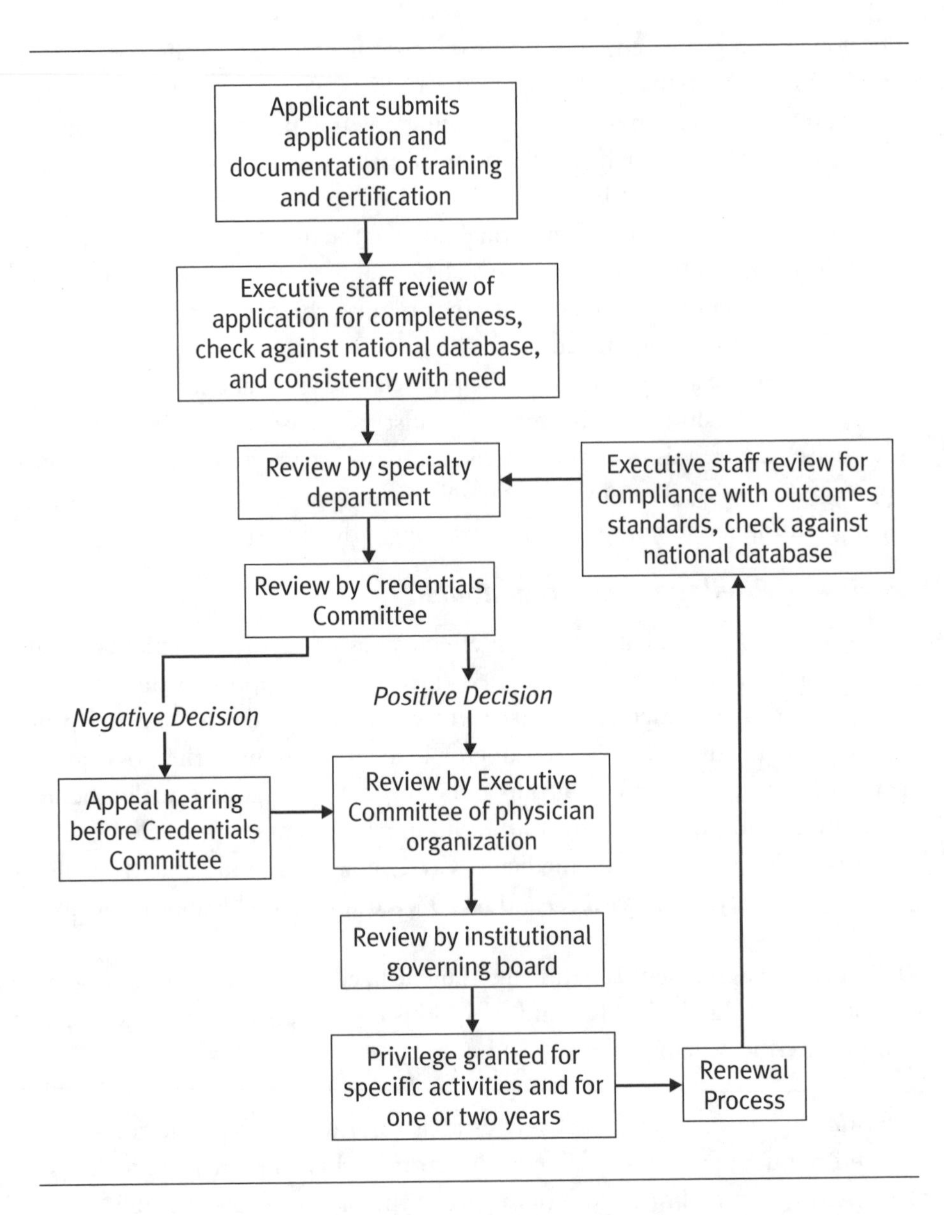

timing, review processes, confidentiality, committees and participants, methods of establishing expectations, sources of data, and appeals procedures. Regular review and updating of bylaws is important.

2. *Privileges.* The organization extends the privilege of membership to each doctor willing to accept the bylaws and judged competent to participate. The privilege is extended for specific kinds of patient care matching the physician's training, specialty certification, and demonstrated capability. It is limited to one or two years and is renewed based on peer review of actual clinical performance.[6] The review process leading to privileges is frequently called credentialing. Those privileged to practice in the hospital

were traditionally called **attending physicians**. Hospital privileges are subject to the final review of the institutional governing board. Because each doctor accepts responsibility for his or her own patients and the obligation to participate in peer review, only doctors need judge other doctors on medical matters. In larger organizations the group of peers is physicians with similar specialization. This concept of peer review is a central element of professional autonomy. It is highly prized by most doctors, and they invest much time and energy in carrying out their obligations.

3. *Independent doctor-patient relationship*. Each doctor establishes her or his own relationship to each patient and is expected to pursue diligently the obligations of that relationship. That is, the contract recognizes that the doctor has explicit obligations to his or her patients as individuals.
4. *Continuous quality improvement and peer review.* Doctors receiving privileges are expected to participate in the ongoing activities of the organization, including development of protocols, and assistance to other clinical professions. They are also expected to participate in review of the quality of care of their peers and be the subject of such review. Privileges will be curtailed should the clinical performance of the physician fail to meet the expectations of peers.

The contractual consideration on the part of the institution is access to its resources, sometimes including health insurance contracts or other monetary compensation, and that for the doctor is willingness to practice good medicine and accept the obligations. As a contract, privilege is subject to all the legal provisions normally pertaining to business contracts.[7]

Trends in the concept of privilege

The privilege system has robust flexibility. It can cover care in various settings, be tailored to unique geographic needs or special markets, and adapt to any insurance or physician payment system. It accommodates other professionals giving medical care (for example, dentists, psychologists, nurse anesthetists, and chiropractors). Among other examples of its flexibility, the system permits but does not require tangible compensation as part of the consideration.

The origins of the privileging and peer review system lie in actions taken in the late 1920s by the American College of Surgeons to improve the quality of surgical practice in hospitals.[8] Its development since has been influenced by legal decisions.[9] In the 1950s, the legal doctrines of charitable and governmental immunity protecting hospitals from suit were overturned. National accreditation recognizing peer review was transferred to the Joint Commission on Accreditation of Hospitals (now Healthcare Organizations) in 1953. The obligation of the institution to ensure quality practice by physicians on its staff was substantially strengthened by the Darling decision of 1965, holding the hospital explicitly liable for failure to ensure a qualified medical staff.[10]

In the 1970s the courts and legislatures also turned their attention to the rights of individual physicians. Under theories of nondiscrimination and antitrust, the concept of privilege was expanded to include due process, equal opportunity, and the avoidance of restraint of trade. These actions were consistent with major improvements in civil rights and a broadened application of free market concepts in U.S. society generally.

In the 1980s the role of the medical staff was again broadened, this time to incorporate concepts of control of costs as well as quality. Prospective per case payment required that hospitals deliver care through their medical staffs at fixed prices. HMOs and PPOs extended the concept of control of cost beyond the case or hospital stay to the care of the patient over the contract period. Also in the 1980s, the courts required organizations to guard against restriction of trade; the privileging process cannot be used to exclude competing doctors.[11] By 1990, the elements of the privilege relationship had been elaborated to include scientific quality, customer responsiveness, nondiscrimination, due process, antitrust, and cost control.

This somewhat ponderous mechanism differs from the usual employment relation between an organization and its members principally in providing more adequate protection to the doctor. The CEO and the management staff, for example, serve at the pleasure of the governing board and can be discharged at any legally constituted meeting for any grounds not discriminatory or libelous. Only civil service, some union contracts, and the tenure system of professors provide individuals rights similar to credentialing.

Privilege review process

Committee membership

The decision to grant privileges is made by a credentials committee and is subject to several levels of subsequent review. The ideal member of the credentials committee possesses the attributes of a good judge: He or she is patient, consistent, thorough, factual, and considerate. Clearly, clinical knowledge and skill are required, but detailed clinical knowledge is more valuable in expectation setting than in evaluating credentials. Committee members should be widely respected. Physicians with other important leadership tasks should not serve simultaneously on the credentials committee, and membership should rotate fairly frequently. An executive officer should staff the committee, both to assist in the workload and to ensure compliance with the bylaws.

Operation of the credentials committee

The bylaws specify both the processes through which credentialing occurs and the structure that supports those processes. The process calls for initial review of training, experience, and moral character; extension of privileges for specific procedures, diseases, or venues (such as outpatient or intensive care); and subsequent annual or biennial renewal. Failure to do so in one case but not in another is potentially discriminatory. General failure to follow the bylaws is capricious.[12]

The institutional organization is liable for failure to provide due process, failure to remove incompetent doctors, and failure to establish appropriate standards of practice. The individuals participating in the process are liable for arbitrary, capricious, or discriminatory behavior.[13]

The executive staff member to the committee implements all procedures under the bylaws and the direction of the chair. Formal procedures for advance notice, agenda, attendance, minutes, and appeal mechanisms are mandatory. Doctors under review should have the opportunity to see the information compiled about them and to comment on it. Because the committee should function at a secondary level, evaluating the sum of the year's activities rather than actual patient care, the need for new direct testimony is minimized. When it is necessary, the statements should be carefully identified and recorded. The summary of the individual's activities should be compiled in writing and documented. It may include formal evaluation by peers.[14] Review of procedures by legal counsel is desirable, and counsel should attend any appeals session. The doctor is also entitled to counsel. The well-managed organization protects committee members and others in the credentialing chain with insurance, legal counsel, and, above all, prevention of lawsuits through the maintenance of due process and sound evidence in support of the committee's decisions. Properly run, the credentials process will not be negatively viewed by the medical staff.[15]

The federal Health Care Quality Improvement Act, Title IV of P.L. 100-177 of 1986, mandates reporting of loss of credentials or other disciplinary action to a federal information bank. The purpose of the act is to reduce the chance of an incompetent physician moving to a new location and misrepresenting his or her skills. Specifically the act requires healthcare organizations

- to notify the National Practitioner Data Bank of
    - any physician's or dentist's loss of credentials for any period greater than 30 days;
    - any voluntary surrender of privileges to avoid investigation;
    - any requirement for medical proctoring or supervision imposed as a result of peer review;
    - any malpractice settlement against any member of the medical staff or "other health practitioner" as defined in the act; and
- to check the information bank prior to initial privileging.

The act also protects any person reporting to or working for a professional review body such as an accredited organization's credentialing committee from legal action by the individual disciplined, by raising the standard of proof.[16]

The act could easily have a negative effect on the quality of care, because it can discourage disciplinary action where it is indicated. It should not and need not. The well-managed institution can probably avoid this by continuing annual privileges review and using a system of routine measurement and corrective education. Both the institutional and the physician organizations must support the activities of this committee with a variety of records and data, but the key evaluations must be made by physicians. The opinion of peer specialists must be sought when appropriate. Many larger organizations use the credentials committee as a coordinating body, with initial review in the specialty departments.

Standards for granting and renewing privileges

Medical quality control is moving to the use of prospectively accepted protocols and measured performance, as discussed in Chapter 7. These simplify the credentialing review to four questions:

1. Does the physician comply with general requirements for continuing education, maintaining certification, and meeting minimum levels of activity?
2. Does the physician correctly perform the procedures that are his or her direct responsibility?
3. Does the physician achieve outcomes consistent with the expectations of the community, with due consideration of differences in the population being treated?
4. Has the physician avoided all activity that directly threatens the rights or safety of patients or colleagues?

The committee seeks evidence that negative answers to these questions are rare and unlikely to be repeated. It grants or renews privileges whenever that evidence is convincing. In initial reviews, the first and the last are verified directly, and references are sought as evidence on the others. In subsequent reviews, emphasis is placed on the physician's recent actual performance. The best credentials process limits its review to only these questions. Other issues of quality, patient satisfaction, and cost effectiveness are handled by the quality improvement activities of the medical departments. The credentialing activity is deliberately separated from protocol setting and monitoring to permit fuller exploration of clinical issues in a scientific rather than a judgmental environment. The use of protocols as a referent ensures that the physician will not be held to a unique standard and makes it possible for the committee to evaluate physicians from all specialties. The vast majority of physicians will pass review without difficulty.

Right of the institution to deny privileges

A not-for-profit community healthcare organization may deny or discontinue the right of a physician to use its facilities and personnel in the care of patients on either of two grounds. One is quality, failure to comply with properly established criteria governing quality of care and good character, discussed above. The second is economic, that the doctor overtaxes the facilities available for the kinds of care he or she expects to give, or provides a service that is not supported by the institution as a whole. Thus, a hospital is not obligated to accept a cardiac surgeon if it has no cardiologist, or if it has no cardiopulmonary laboratory, or if it feels it has enough cardiac surgeons already. Similarly, a physician organization is not obligated to accept a pediatric hematologist if it routinely refers pediatric hematology, has no laboratory facilities for pediatric hematology, and is satisfied that the existing arrangements are in the best interests of its members.

Information and data support

The record required by the credentials committee has two major components. Initial reviews require the credentials themselves, documents and references testifying to the education, licensure, certification, experience, and character of applicants. The applicant is often charged with collecting the documents, although these must be scrutinized and verified by the organization. Renewals require information on the clinical performance of current staff members. Two groups—the hierarchy of the physicians organization and institutional employees supporting the quality review, utilization review, and risk management processes—monitor clinical activity and prepare reports during the year on serious examples of negative performance.[17] Processes of these groups include opportunities for the physician to review the cases and justify his or her actions. The executive staff member supporting the committee collects and verifies the factual case from these reports to reduce the burdens on the committee. His or her role includes soliciting references and verifying educational credentials. In complex cases, the committee may seek additional information, using a formal hearing process to protect the rights of the physician.

Privileges and specialty certification

It is increasingly common to insist on full certification in a specialty as a condition of membership or, in the case of young doctors still completing their training, a specific program and timetable for earning certification. Thus, the prototype for specification of privileges is that set of activities normally included in the specialty. Well-run organizations have several additional constraints on the specific activities for which privileges are granted:

- Maintenance of specialty certification. Many specialties have continuing education requirements.
- Restrictions based on the capability of the hospital and the supporting medical specialists. (An individual doctor may be qualified to receive a certain privilege, but the hospital may lack the necessary equipment, facilities, and complementary staff.)
- Maintenance of a minimum number of cases treated annually to ensure that the skills of both the physician and the hospital support team remain up-to-date.
- For new or expanded privileges, evidence of successful treatment of a number of cases under supervision at an acceptable training facility.

The judgments of national specialty boards cannot be the sole criterion for assigning a specific privilege to a given specialty or specialties. First, the issue of quality is not as simple as it first looks. Family practitioners and general internists argue that they can handle a great many uncomplicated cases without referral, while obstetricians, pediatricians, and medical subspecialists argue that their specialized skills are more likely to promote quality. There are two parts to resolving these arguments. The first is correctly identifying the needs of each patient. The identification of the patient's total needs is as important a part of the quality of medical care as the excellence of a specific treatment. It may be wise to sacrifice some elegance in the treatment of a specific disease to improve the patient's total medical condition. The higher the value placed on comprehensive care, the stronger the generalists' argument. Many thoughtful analysts believe that comprehensiveness is undervalued in American healthcare and that the balance has shifted too far toward specialization.

The second problem arising from excessive limitation of privileges is its effect on doctors' incomes. The specialties sometimes conflict with one another or reflect self-interest. A decision to limit obstetrics to obstetricians and newborn care to pediatricians transfers income. It may reduce the income of family practitioners and the availability of doctors throughout the community. It also will increase the fees charged per delivery. The traditional fee structure tends to reward procedures more than diagnosis and specialization more than comprehensiveness and continuity. The result has been relatively low incomes for family practitioners, general internists, and pediatricians. The disparity has generated some sensitivity, and an organization that limits privileges excessively may find itself unable to recruit or retain these specialties. Limitations should be monitored carefully by the executive office, acting on behalf of the institutional board, for compliance with the mission and all aspects of its long-range plan.

Impaired physicians

The credentials committee faces certain predictable problems, among them the impaired physician. Doctors, like other human beings, can be disabled by age, physical or emotional disease, personal trauma, and substance abuse. The prevalence of these difficulties among practicing physicians is hard to estimate, but it is generally conceded to be between 5 and 15 percent. Thus, a medium-sized healthcare organization could have a dozen doctors either impaired or in danger of impairment at any given time. The response of the credentials committee should be tailored to the kind of problem at hand. Aging and uncorrectable physical disability must force reduction of privileges. Alcoholism, abuse of addictive drugs, and depression may be more common among physicians than among the general public. Treatment for depression and substance abuse is clearly indicated, and programs designed especially for doctors can be reached through state medical societies. Arrangements can be made to assist impaired doctors with their practices during the period of recovery, thus assuring that patients receive acceptable care without unduly disrupting the doctor-patient relationship or the doctors' incomes. Larger organizations often have a committee or group set up specifically to deal with this problem. Although it usually keeps affected physicians' identities secret, its activities must be coordinated with those of the credentials committee. While every reasonable effort at rehabilitation should be made, the credentials committee is ultimately accountable for the suspension or removal of privileges.

Medical Staff Planning and Recruitment

A successful physician organization should be properly sized to the community it serves. If it is too large, individual physician income and professional satisfaction goals will not be met, skills may be lost through lack of practice, and doctors may face strong temptations to pursue unnecessary treatment.[18] If it is too small, patients will be unable to get timely service and an adequate choice of practitioners. Doctors may be overworked, endangering quality and the satisfaction of both practitioners and patients. The advent of managed care and continuous improvement has generated major changes in the demand for physicians, with some specialties facing increased demand and others diminished.[19] The solution is to plan the staff size as part of the strategic and long-range planning of the institution.

Modeling future need for physicians

The conceptual model for planning is an extension of the general epidemiological planning model from Chapter 6. It is applied to each specialty of the physician organization.

Model 1

$$\left\{\begin{matrix}\text{Number of}\\ \text{physicians}\\ \text{needed}\end{matrix}\right\} = \left\{\begin{matrix}\text{Population}\\ \text{at risk}\end{matrix}\right\} \times \left\{\begin{matrix}\text{Incidence of}\\ \text{disease/procedure}\end{matrix}\right\} \div \left\{\begin{matrix}\text{Procedures per}\\ \text{physician year}\end{matrix}\right\}$$

$$\left\{\begin{matrix}\text{Number of}\\ \text{recruitments}\end{matrix}\right\} = \left\{\begin{matrix}\text{Number of}\\ \text{physicians}\\ \text{needed}\end{matrix}\right\} - \left\{\begin{matrix}\text{Number of}\\ \text{physicians}\\ \text{available}\end{matrix}\right\}$$

The number of physicians available is adjusted for anticipated retirements. At some point, the number of recruits needed must be adjusted for market share. It is easiest to apply the model to the entire community and then decide on a strategy for the number of recruits for a specific physician organization based on anticipated market share.

The problem with Model 1 is the difficulty of forecasting the Incidence of the Disease or Procedure term and the Procedures per Physician term. New technology, prevention and improved protocols change the incidence, the kind of response, and the specialty required. A forecast of incidence based on local history is usually obtained through the cross-functional teams and the specialties involved. One based on national data should also be used, with due regard to benchmarks and published scientific opinion. Managed care has led to the transfer of some activity from referral specialists to primary care physicians and from physicians to other caregivers, but the marketplace acceptance of the shift is unclear.[20] There appears to be a strong underlying demand for specialist care, so that conservative forecasts retain a relatively high specialist population.

While the model works well with major clinical events like neurosurgery and advanced cancer, it is impractical for primary care and the more general specialties. A simpler model, based on the aggregate experience of existing health systems and communities, has been used.[21,22]

Model 2

$$\left\{\begin{matrix}\text{Number of}\\ \text{physicians}\\ \text{needed}\end{matrix}\right\} = \left\{\begin{matrix}\text{Population}\\ \text{at risk}\end{matrix}\right\} \times \left\{\begin{matrix}\text{Standard physicians}\\ \text{per population,}\\ \text{by specialty}\end{matrix}\right\}$$

$$\left\{\begin{matrix}\text{Number of}\\ \text{recruitments}\end{matrix}\right\} = \left\{\begin{matrix}\text{Number of}\\ \text{physicians}\\ \text{needed}\end{matrix}\right\} - \left\{\begin{matrix}\text{Number of}\\ \text{physicians}\\ \text{available}\end{matrix}\right\}$$

The problem with Model 2 is in forecasting the second term of the first equation. Proposals for the use of standards from staff model HMOs[23] have been severely criticized as understating specialist demand and overstating primary care demand.[24] An analysis of actual physician suggests that most communities now have higher numbers of both primary care and specialist physicians than traditional HMOs, and that there is wide variation in current levels.[25] It is not clear how much care will actually shift to primary practitioners, so that a conservative forecast favors continuation of relatively high specialist use.

Developing a physician supply plan

Good practice calls for a careful analysis of the present situation and anticipated changes using both models. High volume specialties should be individually forecast. Primary care specialties should be considered in the aggregate with careful attention to the individual specialties. Other referral specialties should also be forecast in aggregate and considered at individual levels. Several referents, such as values for staff model HMOs, benchmarks among similar sized cities, and means adjusted for anticipated insurance trends, should be considered to evaluate current levels and show the implications for physician supply. Discussion of the results may prompt early retirements or other changes in the number of physicians available. Strategic judgments are necessary about indications of undersupply and severe oversupply.

In primary care, the analysis must be carried to very small geographic areas because easy access to primary care physicians appears to be important in patient satisfaction. Nurse practitioners, midwives, family practitioners, internists, psychiatrists, obstetricians, pediatricians, and emergency physicians are all prominent primary care providers. Too many primary providers will reduce individual income or increase community costs; too few will cause caregivers to be overworked and patients to be dissatisfied. A recruitment strategy (few communities have a surplus of primary care providers) must specify the type of provider and location, and then consider incentives necessary to attract qualified applicants. A sound approach will promote discussion of the issue among all affected groups, leading to recommendations from the physician organization and final acceptance by the institutional board.

The issues in planning referral specialties center around the existence of sufficient local demand to justify their cost. In general, highly specialized treatment of disease incurs high fixed costs that must be spread over large populations to be cost effective. The income expectations of the specialists themselves are high, and substantial clinical support is necessary. Unit cost falls rapidly as volume increases. It is also true that treatment teams caring for higher volumes of patients will have better quality results.[26] As Figure 8.3 shows, for any given treatment there is an increasing quality structure, a declining cost structure, and increasing specialist incomes as volume increases. There are also competitive standards for all three. If competitive standards are not met, patients and payors will select other sources, after allowing for any inconvenience such as travel to a remote site. The standards dictate a critical volume, V_c. A healthcare organization that operates a specialty below its critical volumes faces both losses and poor quality.

Cardiovascular surgery provides a useful example. The need is dependent on the population of the community, its age and health habits. The United States averaged 2,125 operations per million persons in 1991 and the volume of surgery per site is 700 per year.[27] A community of approximately 350,000 persons is necessary to provide average volumes. The institution that cannot attract that much demand faces unit costs higher than the competitive standard. The surgeon who works in that institution faces lower than average income. Both face the problem that outcomes may be below achievable levels because the team does not get enough practice.

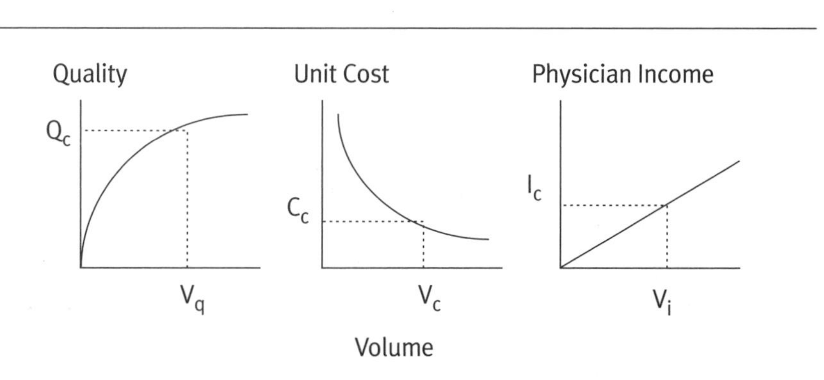

FIGURE 8.3 Critical Volumes for Specialty Services

Integrating the physician recruitment plan with other institutional plans

Community healthcare institutions support an employed team and all of the facilities for inpatient care and referral services like surgery. They also invest in facilities and information systems for primary care practitioners. Thus, capital investment is at stake in recruitment of physicians. In most cases, the decisions are part of the strategic or long-range plan of the institution. As indicated in Chapter 12, decisions are made first on the question of scope of service, "Should we have a cardiovascular surgery program?" and second on the actual facilities and number of physicians required. As illustrated in Figure 8.4, the physician recruitment plan is an extension of these decisions.

Three problems must be resolved in the physician recruitment planning approach.

1. *Uncertainty about the demand.* Prevention, clinical improvement, population aging, and attitudes toward sources of care all change both the overall demand for care and the demand for specific services and specialties.
2. *Uncertainty about the supply.* The activity levels of doctors currently on the staff may change in the future. Incentives may be offered to encourage certain changes, such as recruitment to a less desirable location or early retirement from an oversupplied specialty.
3. *Conflicts over the allocation of demand to specialty.* The expectations of one specialty may not coincide with those of others or of the community

FIGURE 8.4
Cardiac Surgery as an Example of Combined Strategic, Service, and Physician Planning

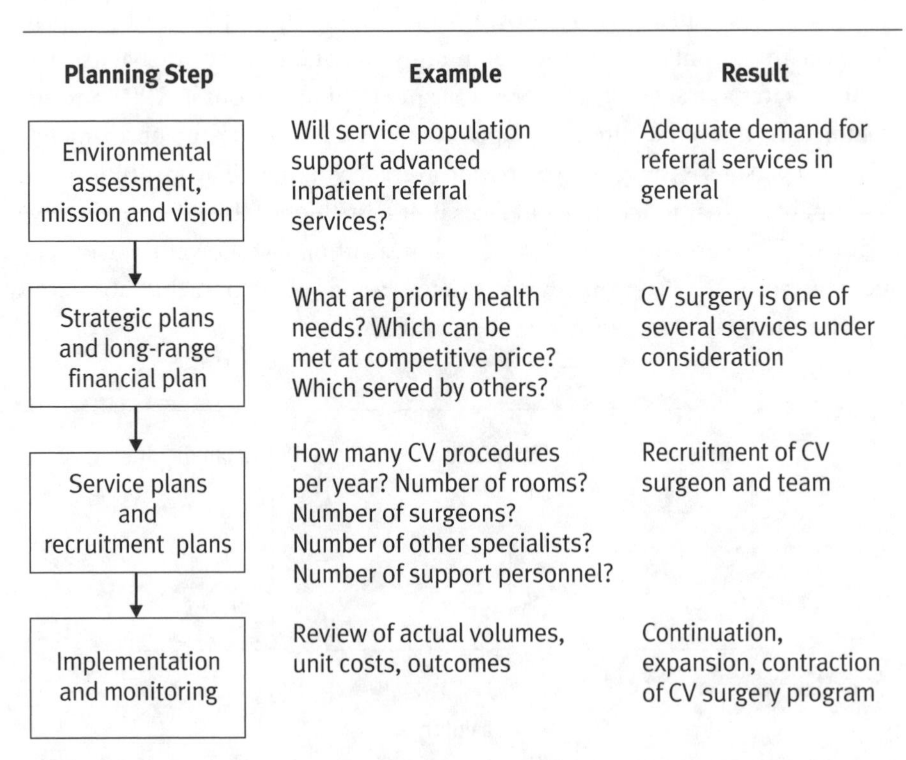

representatives. The specialty level—endocrinologist or cardiologist versus family physician, obstetrician versus midwife—is decided both on issues of outcomes quality and patient satisfaction.

The well-managed healthcare organization will address these problems through discussion and will share the risks and rewards that result with the physicians. Communities using the models to guide the discussion will reach more realistic and convincing plans, and as a result will attract better doctors. The use of planning models remains controversial, however. The forecasts are imprecise, and the questions to be weighed are both intellectually challenging and for many physicians emotionally and financially threatening. The advantages of formal planning are summarized in Figure 8.5. For physicians, the advantages are advanced knowledge and assistance in meeting problems that otherwise might arise unnoticed and be met unaided. Independent physicians cannot meet solely for the purpose of planning supply; it is a per se violation of the Sherman Antitrust Act. Membership in an organization with other purposes is essential. The institution benefits by getting physician input and acceptance, reducing the risk of the its decisions. The joint recruitment effort that results is likely to attract better physicians, and the planning process should help keep them competitive in income, skill, and professional satisfaction.

Recruitment

Good doctors have their choice of practice locations, and they are actively recruited, even in times of relative surplus. A recruitment offer frequently includes arrangements for office facilities and services, income guarantees, malpractice coverage, membership in a medical partnership or group, and introductions to referring physicians or available specialists. As HMO or PPO groups become more common, participation in these is also part of

FIGURE 8.5 Advantages of Physician Supply Planning

Advantage	Physician Benefit	Institution Benefit
1. Shared information and cooperative analysis allow more accurate forecasts	See future sooner and more clearly; have more time to react	Improve safety, return, market attractiveness of investments
2. Facility and employee needs integrated with physician needs	Support available when needed	Volumes adequate to keep costs and quality competitive
3. Better management of physician supply	Facilitate potentially painful transitions	Meet community demand for access; reduce pressure for inappropriate treatment
4. Better management of insurance contracts	More options for insurance contracts; more income stability; more market share	Broader array of options for customers; more market share

the recruiting offer. Home financing, club membership, and other social and family issues are frequently important.[28] A substantial capital resource is necessary to assemble these elements. At the same time, doctors want to work where their colleagues are friendly, complex offers require early assurance that medical credentials are acceptable, and selecting the right candidate involves assessment of clinical skills.

Recruitment has become a relatively well-codified activity, carried out by a search committee of the physician organization. It includes the following components:

- Establishment of criteria for the position and the person sought
- Establishment of compensation and incentives
- Advertising and solicitation of candidates
- Initial selection
- Interviews and visits
- Final selection and negotiation

Because access to the institution is important to almost all physicians, because the institutional board retains the right to approve physician credentials, and because the institution often supplies much of the capital required, recruitment is commonly a collaborative activity. The institution's support contributes to success.

Educational Activities of the Physician Organization

The physician organization has at least two educational functions; larger organizations have three. All staffs are responsible for promoting the continuing education of their own members and for assisting in the clinical education of other members of the institution. Larger organizations have responsibilities for postgraduate and occasionally undergraduate (i.e., candidates for the MD degree) medical education as well.

The interrelation of education with continuous improvement and the development of consensus protocols should not be overlooked. Analysis of past performance, benchmarking, the design of new processes, and the preparation of protocols are educational activities in themselves, affecting all three formal functions. Their educational role is likely to become more central as organizations mature in their use. It is likely that many formal educational programs will arise from needs identified in the continuous improvement process.

Continuing education for attending physicians

Continuing education for doctors is now strongly encouraged as part of licensure and specialty certifications. A variety of educational programs is offered outside the organization; these do not substitute for the continued study of the organization's own patients. Much of this now occurs in the cross functional groups that are charged with improving care for specific diseases. Using educational approaches helps ensure that every doctor fully understands the guidelines, develops group pressure to encourage compliance, and, by changing behavior beforehand, eliminates personal confrontations over failures.

Continuing education need not be limited to clinical subjects. Programs to help doctors understand the corporate approach to decision making, to gain skills in organized activities, and to learn fundamentals of technologies such as quality control and cost accounting are also important.

How much to invest in staff education is a difficult judgment. Programs are often expensive to mount, but they are more expensive to attend. The opportunity cost of doctors' time is very high, and educational time must be judged in the context of other demands from family, practice, and, particularly, other organization demands on the doctors' time. Education outside the hospital is often as useful, but availability differs by community. Subjectively, and according to JCAHO philosophy, every doctor should have access to sufficient educational opportunity to keep themselves current. This requires, and JCAHO specifies, at least monthly educational meetings with required attendance. Beyond this minimum, it is probably wise to decentralize decisions about staff education to the lowest feasible unit of the staff and to accommodate the programs they suggest when attendance figures indicate cost-effective investments. It is worth noting that large successful organizations like Kaiser-Permanente, Henry Ford Health System, and Intermountain Health Care invest heavily in education. They use their size to assemble programs that might not be cost effective for smaller institutions, but they often make the programs themselves available to others.

Education of other hospital members

By tradition, preparation, and law, the doctor is leader of the healthcare team. With this leadership comes an obligation to educate others, not only other clinical professionals, but also trustees, executives, and other management personnel. A particularly important part of this education deals with new clinical developments. New approaches to care frequently require retraining for personnel at several levels, and physicians should participate in that education. In addition, trustees and planners rely on the medical staff to identify new opportunities for care and to make clinical implications clear in terms that promote effective decisions. Many of these educational requirements are met through participation on various committees and day-to-day associations.

Postgraduate medical education

Medicine has acknowledged its obligation to train new doctors since Hippocrates. Clinical training of medical students occurs in a limited number of institutions that incorporate such training in their mission. In 1997, about 20 percent of community hospitals offered training positions for **house officers**, licensed doctors pursuing postgraduate education. Many of these sites were in vertically integrated healthcare organizations, but the majority of training opportunities were in university medical centers.[29]

The content of this education is controlled through certification by individual specialty boards and is coordinated through the AMA. House officers are paid stipends during their training because they provide important direct service, because hospitals feel they are a valuable source of recruits, and because their presence has long been thought to improve overall quality of care. An important benefit to both the community and the attending staff is that house officers are expected to cover patient needs at times when attending doctors are not present. In addition, many of the programs suitable for house officers are appropriate continuing education for attending physicians, and educating house officers is educational in itself.

House officers are generally heavy users of costly services. One avenue for saving costs is the development of better care protocols, emphasizing to the house officer and the attending physician alike legitimate opportunities for economy. Presentation of financial data along with clinical data promotes consideration of the cost-effectiveness of specific diagnoses and treatment steps. Under managed care, economies are translatable to larger profits for the institution. These, in turn, may support a larger or more attractive educational program.

Recent concerns with the relative supply of primary care and referral specialties are likely to lead to extensive revisions of postgraduate training. It is likely that many programs for primary care will be expanded, and that training opportunities will emphasize outpatient as well as inpatient care. Programs for referral specialties seem likely to contract and to move even more tightly to university centers. The result of these changes may cause a restructuring of inpatient care. The direct patient service may be supplied by physicians employed by the hospital or the medical group.

Representation, Communication, and Resolution of Conflicts

Under the theory of the well-managed healthcare organization described in Chapter 2, the only limits to medical staff participation are the need to keep both the content and the timeliness of the decisions consistent with customer demands and the need to recognize the rights of other provider partners. A sound physician organization implements the theory by establishing formal physician participation in all decisions, including the mission and vision, resource allocation, implementation, and institutional organization. The most serious limit on participation is likely to be the shortage of physician time. Participation itself takes time away from patient care, and many physicians resent the hours devoted to it even while recognizing its importance.

The goal of physician representation and communication is to assure all physicians that they are empowered to influence decisions affecting their practices. This means not only that physicians are represented at critical decisions, but that avenues exist to identify issues, discuss implications, and resolve conflicts. The link between the practitioner and the representative is as important as the representation itself.[30] Success requires a robust communications mechanism that identifies issues promptly, solicits and organizes opinion about them, and resolves them fairly.[31] Leading institutions deliberately survey physicians about issues important to them; the physician priorities are incorporated in selecting improvement projects.[32] The dual criteria for organization decisions generally, realism and conviction (Chapter 5), apply here as well. Ideally, all physicians should be convinced that they have heard the issue, that they have had a fair opportunity to be heard about the issue, and that the final decision optimizes market realities, without having had to waste unnecessary time on either step.

Infrastructure of physician representation

The organization's bylaws provide the basis for representation. The bylaws specify not simply the rights and obligations of each party, but also the methods by which communication is encouraged and disagreements are resolved. The bylaws specify the roles of each office and standing committee of the medical staff. They include provision for ad hoc committee formation. They should emphasize the role of the clinical department or section chair to hear, report, and represent the needs of the unit. Most doctors learn the bylaws by experience. Reviews of process at the start of major discussions are helpful. The goal is to have influential physicians throughout the organization, including some who do not hold formal office, familiar with the processes. Then all doctors are close to someone whom they respect who can explain them.

Well-run organizations use both the hierarchical and the collateral organization to develop consensus and reconcile differences within the physician organization (many potential conflicts are between medical specialties) and between the physicians and the rest of the organization. The time burden can often be reduced by sensitive design and administration. Doctors can be welcomed to committees, work groups, and task forces where they make a specific contribution and can be excused from meetings where nonmedical issues are addressed. Meetings can be arranged when necessary rather than periodically. Agendas can be developed with an understanding of the need to save time. Advance preparation and distribution of relevant background material make a noticeable difference, as does proper preparation of the chair.

Where communication and trust are supported by a strong formal communication system, informal devices can be used to great advantage. If all staff members are confident that they will know of decisions important to them in time to react and that they have an avenue to make their views known quickly, much time spent in formal communications can be eliminated. In well-run healthcare organizations, nonmedical managers make a deliberate effort to maintain informal communications with the medical staff. Many successful CEOs and COOs undertake the monitoring function personally. More than one successful CEO says, "I try to stop by the doctors' lounge at least five times a week."[33]

Board membership for the medical staff

The practice of providing seats on the board for the medical staff has become almost universal and is an important advantage of community-based healthcare organizations. Exceptions are mainly limited to those institutions whose corporate charters or enabling legislation preclude such participation. In many organizations, doctors are nominated for these seats by the physician organization. Other doctors may also serve on the board, although they are presumably selected for their personal, rather than their professional, abilities. The board majority should remain nonphysicians; rarely do doctors constitute a substantial minority.

These few individuals, representing only a fraction of the specialties, ages, and financial arrangements of the staff as a whole, must fulfill the complex representation needs of all doctors. Like other board members, they are expected to vote for the best interests of the corporation, rather than any short-term advantage to themselves or to the physicians. They serve the medical staff more by their general clinical and procedural knowledge than by advocating specific decisions. Their board membership allows them to make sure the doctors' opinions are fully and fairly heard.

Formal participation in ongoing decisions

Because only a few physicians can serve on the governing board, the major substantive representation of medical staff viewpoints and needs is provided by direct and extensive participation in the development of improvements before the final proposal is presented to the board. Figure 8.6 shows the usual means for each of the decision processes discussed in Chapter 5.

Mission, vision, and environmental assessment

Doctors participate in substantial numbers in the annual review of the environment and any revision of the mission and vision. Members of the physician executive committee are included in the annual review. Doctors who are respected as leaders by their peers, those who are known to represent particular positions, and doctors who are considered as potential officers are also often invited. The review should encourage doctors' comments on the economic impact of the mission and strategic opportunities on members of the medical staff. Participation enhances the factual base for decision making and eliminates unnecessary conflict between the hospital and the medical staff over income generating services.

Strategic plan

Physicians should participate actively in reviewing the strategic plan. The scope of services must be designed so that the institution and its medical staff together can provide quality care and gain a competitive reward for doing so. Physician input is essential to finding that balance and the balance between the medical specialties. Individual specialties advocating scientific advances in their areas can overstate the promise of much new technology. Two arguments with strong emotional appeal can be anticipated. They have explicit rational tests that should be met before they are accepted. "Lifesaving" is only applicable to those few conditions in which the patient cannot be moved to another facility.

FIGURE 8.6 Physician Representation on Decision Processes

Decision Type	Example	Physician Participation
Mission/ Vision	Environment assessment; strategic plans	Governing board membership; leaders participate in annual review
Resource Allocation	Services plan; financial plan	Membership on board planning and finance committees
	Facilities and human resources plans	Representation on committee and consultation of services directly involved
	Physician recruitment plan	Advice from each specialty unit; opportunity for individual comment
	Budgeting	Participation between line units and services particularly involved
	Capital budgeting	Major voice in ranking all clinical equipment; participate in general ranking
Implementation	Personnel selection	Credentialing of all physicians; participation on executive search committees
	Process design	Participation by services in all final product protocol development; review of intermediate protocols
Organizational	Information plan	Participation in plan and trials
	Conflict resolution	Membership in mediation efforts and appeals panels

To be "essential for recruiting the best people," the item must be available at a visible fraction—say, 20 or 30 percent—of truly competing institutions and in the immediate plans of a majority. Physicians from other specialties are well equipped to mount these challenges.

By the same token, plans and investments that make modest contributions to large groups are sometimes overlooked because they lack persuasive advocates. Doctors in primary care, public health, and preventive medicine can redress this imbalance.

Operating expectations

The medical staff begins contributing to resource allocation by participating in the setting of clinical protocols as described in Chapter 7. Protocols establish the clinical support service resources required for each patient. It is a short jump from them to the service unit's annual operating budget. The leading indicator for necessary budget improvements is frequently demand that fails to meet expectations. Doctor or patient concern with quality, access, amenities, or satisfaction is a cause of deteriorating demand. Soliciting doctors' opinions helps both to identify the problems and to stimulate correction of them.

Doctors should participate in the improvement process and the development of the annual budget for clinical support services. The major services have standing committees for this purpose. The pharmacy and therapeutics committee and the operating room committee are examples where many institutions have had success. Similar opportunities exist for the diagnostic and rehabilitation services. Usually the service works closely with only a few specialties, but an outside clinical view may help identify important new perspectives.

Capital and new programs budget

At the capital budgeting level, doctors' most important contribution is their understanding of clinical implications and the economic impacts on various practicing physicians. Projects where doctors' opinions are irrelevant are rare. All programmatic clinical proposals should include medical review of their scientific merit, demand estimates, procedures and equipment contemplated, likely benefits to patients, risks to patients and staff, and implications for physician income. In cases in which the specialty involved may be biased by its economic concerns, independent evaluations may be solicited. Serious disputes on these technical matters are themselves an indicator of project risk and should be presented as such.

The extent of the review can be tailored to the size and scope of the proposal. All important projects should be given independent review by every relevant specialty group. Differences of opinion between specialty groups arising from independent review should be resolved via the physician organization. That is, projects advocated by the surgical subspecialties should be collectively ranked by surgeons directly involved, then by surgeons of all kinds, and that ranking should be integrated with similar ones from medicine and other specialties by the executive committee. The ranking for all clinical proposals should then be integrated with other proposals by a broader committee including governance and executive as well as physician representation.

Marketing and promotional efforts

Individual physicians can accept uninsured payments from patients directly and sign individual participation contracts with intermediaries. The contracts specify terms of participation including fee schedules and quality and appropriateness criteria. The physician organization allows individual contracting, but it negotiates many contracts collectively for the institution and its members. This approach allows the group to accept risk for the total cost of care on either a **global fee** structure (where the institution receives a single payment that it must then distribute to itself and its physician partners) or capitation.

Physician organizations must have rules for individual participation in risk-sharing contracts. The trend is toward increasing ability to act as agents for members and the institution under previously established guidelines and sign "single signature" contracts whenever the guidelines are met, without individual review. Individual physicians relinquish some autonomy; the reward is a faster and presumably more effective response to intermediary markets.

Physician supply plan

As noted above, physicians participate extensively in the preparation of the medical staff plan.

Facilities, information, and human resources plans

Physician participation on these detailed plans is also important. Most facility proposals are developed by ad hoc task forces that include substantial representation from interested specialties. Physician participation on the Information Services Advisory Committee (Chapter 15) is important. All trials of clinical hardware and software should include review of physician user satisfaction.

Medical staff leadership

While physicians are notably independent in their professional style, there are recognized informal organizations of physicians and means of detecting physician leaders. Physicians tend to follow the lead of clinicians they respect in clinical matters, and of physicians who gain their respect in other professional matters. Clinical leaders are important in gaining consensus on protocols, credentialing, and other matters relating directly to the cost and quality of patient care. Professional leaders are important in winning support for organizational procedures, budgets, insurance contracts, and services arrangements. Leaders are not difficult to identify. They emerge naturally in informal discussions, and most physicians will simply state their leadership candidates. There is surprising consensus.

Well-managed organizations routinely identify and rely on medical leaders. They form the backbone of the medical staff organization, filling the key positions. A sound program identifies leaders early in their careers and begins assigning activities appropriate to their skills. As the doctors mature, their experience deepens and their assignments become more complex. There is a set of doctors moving through the ranks, toward the critical executive positions, board membership, and committee assignments.

Conflict resolution

The intent of physician organization is to identify potential conflicts in advance, analyze and understand them, and respond in a way that is constructive for all parties. The extensive participation outlined above identifies, contains, and resolves many issues, but the process is much more contentious than it appears. Substantial conflicts will still arise and painful sacrifices will be involved in settling them.

The approach implies a fundamental change in the doctor's obligation to act as agent for the patient.[34] Doctors are less independent because of the partnership with each other. They must affiliate more closely with the institution and carry out agency responsibilities within it. That is, faced with a less than satisfactory condition, attending physicians must work within the physician organization and the institutional organization to correct the deficiency. They have a moral obligation not to sacrifice patients' needs to either their own or the organizations'.[35] Conflicts also arise between specialties, between clinical support services and physicians, and between individuals. The well-managed healthcare organization attempts to resolve these as the nation does, by being a society of laws. The following guidelines seem to be helpful:

- The processes for decision making and conflict resolution are respected above the decisions themselves. A strenuous effort is made to follow the processes. This means that the processes themselves must be convenient and flexible to minimize the burden involved. It also means that deliberate circumvention of process is one of the most serious offenses that can occur. Repeated violation of process calls for removal.
- Patient care protocols at all levels encourage professional intervention on behalf of the individual patient. No caregiver should ever feel forced to give or withhold treatment to an individual patient because of the organization's collective position.
- An ethics committee and similar devices exist to evaluate the processes themselves and to assist in individual interpretations. In addition to the usual committee that focuses on clinical issues, there are other bodies with explicit ethical responsibilities, such as committees on human subjects, confidentiality of personal data, sexual harassment, and equal opportunity.
- Conflicts between individuals and groups other than patients are resolved with an emphasis on fairness and long-run benefit. The contribution of each individual to the success of the whole is recognized. Decisions are evaluated on contribution to the good of the whole, more than the power of the advocate. The rules and criteria are consistently applied, giving each individual greater security.
- Appeals mechanisms exist appropriate to the level of the dispute. Ideally, almost any decision can be appealed someplace. A supervisor's decision may be appealed to a higher level of the accountability hierarchy. A capital budget decision may be appealed to the next higher review panel. A credentialing decision may be appealed to the governing board. The

appeals mechanism makes a deliberate effort to conduct an unbiased review.

These guidelines are essentially the same as exist for other members of the well-managed organization. Their application to the physician organization is a deliberate effort to make it more attractive to competent and well-intentioned physicians than the competing forms.

Collective Compensation Agreements

The economic organization of medical practice itself is in flux, as payment moves from direct to insured fees, negotiated fees, global fees, and capitation. Not surprisingly, the transition has generated high levels of anxiety among physicians and an array of entrepreneurial responses by for-profit and not-for-profit organizations. As noted above, the models that will emerge as stable competitors in the marketplace are now unclear.

Economic relations between the organization and its physicians

Many variations of compensation are being tried around the country. Observers differ on the classification. Many foresaw evolution toward a highly integrated endpoint model.[36] Burns and Thorpe, for example, identified four basic types, culminating in an "Integrated Health Organization" where all physicians are salaried.[37] The salaried physician model has a long and distinguished history,[38] but marketplace and political resistance to managed care suggest that this model will not be the sole successful one anytime soon.[39]

The successful physician organization must make a competitive advantage of its ability to accept a full range of individual economic relationships with its physicians. Physicians accepting basic membership would then be free to participate in one or more economic compensation models, subject to the additional requirements of that model. As shown in Figure 8.7, the possible relationships include the traditional one of economic independence, several variants of salaried compensation, and several variants of shared risk or contractual relationships.

Five types of transactions underlie the arrangements in Figure 8.7:

1. *Salary arrangements,* permitting the physician to be a full-time or part-time employee of a corporation, appeal to recent graduates and primary care specialties.
2. *Collective contracts with insurance intermediaries,* offering physicians increased access or more advantageous terms in managed care markets.
3. *Contracts providing office management,* allowing physicians to escape overhead costs and managerial obligations. Almost any office service can be involved, from the facility itself to office employees, supplies, and malpractice insurance.
4. *Sale of existing practices,* allowing physicians to seek early retirement or liquidate a fee-for-service practice in favor of a salaried one. Practices are also sold by the organization to new physicians.

FIGURE 8.7 Compensation Relationships Between Healthcare Organizations and Individual Physicians

Relationship	Type	Example
Independence	Traditional	Physician arranges own payments and contracts.
Salaried for clinical services	Employment	Physician spends full or part time providing medical care at site operated by institution, in return for a salary.
Salaried for management services	Employment	Physician spends full or part time providing administrative services for the organization, in return for a salary.
Purchase of service	Service contract	Physician leases office, personnel services, or information services from the institution.
Joint sales agreement	Preferred provider panels	Physicians and institution agree to participate for separate fees.
Shared risk contracts	Capitation or fee-based risk sharing	Physicians and institution agree to a payment arrangement and share risk for appropriate utilization.
Shared ownership	Joint ownership	Physician and institution hold joint ownership in real property.
Shared equity	Joint venture	Physicians and institution hold joint ownership in a business venture.

NOTE: Many physicians will have several kinds of relationships simultaneously.

5. *Joint investment ventures*, offering physicians the opportunity to make an equity investment with the anticipation of return and a salable asset.[40] These are the most problematic relationships, raising tax, inurement, and fraud issues that must be carefully avoided. They also present some management problems, as when ownership becomes frozen to a limited group of physicians, or when the value of the asset falls and it becomes illiquid.

Each contract under these arrangements must forward the mission of the community healthcare organization, meet certain tests to protect tax exemption, comply with antitrust regulations, and avoid fraud and abuse regulations.[41] In general, the tax requirements call for avoidance of inurement and are met either by maintaining community dominance of the investment and exchanging all goods and services at fair market prices,[42] or by establishing a for-profit corporate structure, usually a limited liability corporation, and paying the tax. The latter strategy protects the tax exemption of the institution. Antitrust requirements are more important when the organization or its physicians have a dominant market position. They are met by demonstrating ability to compete on price and quality and by permitting any qualified physician to participate. Fraud and abuse arise from arrangements intended to benefit providers at customer expense, such as incentives to increase admissions or referrals. Specific regulations have been established in the Medicare program.[43] In general, programs that are attractive to all insurance approaches, and that emphasize improvement of cost and quality meet these requirements. The complexity and extent of specifics on tax, antitrust, and fraud issues indicate the need for qualified legal counsel.

Presumably most organizations will offer multiple economic arrangements. The kinds of models and their relative size will be driven by local markets and can be expected to differ widely between communities. Over several years or decades, it is likely that some variants will prove more attractive to customers and physicians than others and will prevail.

Economic arrangements with insurers

One of the major devices used by HMOs and PPOs is the "panel" of participating physicians. Care is available to the member only through the panel. Although panels can be constructed from individual physicians, there are advantages to negotiation with a physician organization representing a number of physicians or a physician hospital organization including an institutional component. The simplest contracts simply establish fees for various procedures. More complex ones transfer some or all of the disease management risk to the physicians. The major possibilities are shown in Figure 8.8.

Traditional insurance, PPOs, and Medicare use fee-based compensation plans. Physicians enroll individually or through organizations and enter their specific services in a coding taxonomy, Common Procedure Terminology (CPT). The elements of CPT are weighted by a system of relative values, usually the Medicare Resource Based Relative Value Scale (RBRVS). It is possible to accept the physician's fee unquestioned, to establish statistical limits for each procedure called "usual reasonable and customary limits," or to attach an agreed upon multiplier to the RBRVS value.

Medicare promulgates a multiplier each year that is adjusted for geographic location. PPOs, Medicaid, and HMOs using this approach establish their own multiplier, which can be compared to the Medicare standard. Actual multipliers in the late 1990s ranged from about three quarters of the Medicare multiplier to about five quarters. The multipliers change frequently in individual plans. The physicians' contract prohibits charging more than the agreed upon fee. Payments for employed physicians go to the employer; the physician's compensation is negotiated separately, although incentives can be offered based on earnings.

Two incentive modifications can be made to the fee schedule. The simplest is cash for tasks not included in CPT. Thus, incentives can be offered for achieving quality and satisfaction targets or prevention targets. The second is the use of a withhold. Under the withhold contract a predetermined fraction (usually around 20 percent) of the payment is withheld and deposited in a trust account. Performance on cost versus expectations is compared at the end of the year. If costs exceed expectations, the physicians forfeit up to the entire withhold. The plan can be combined with an additional incentive: if costs

FIGURE 8.8
Types of Physician Compensation Arrangements

Type	Application	Description
Fee-Based Compensation		
Unrestricted fees	Traditional insurance	Physician sets fee for each service. No control of cost or utilization.
Limited fees	Medicare, traditional insurance	Physician sets fee for each service within statistical limits. No control of cost or utilization.
Negotiated fees	PPOs, HMOs, Medicare after 1990	Physician accepts fee schedule. Price is controlled but not utilization.
Withhold of fees	HMOs	Percentage of fee is withheld subject to meeting cost goals. Limits intermediary risk for both price and utilization.
Cash incentives	HMOs, PPOs	Cash bonus for attaining specific targets
Combinations	HMOs	e.g., "Negotiated + Withhold + Incentive"
Capitation-Based Compensation		
Global capitation	HMOs	Primary care physicians accept full risk for all costs.
Shared capitation	HMOs	Physician organization and institution accept full risk.
Primary capitation	HMOs	Primary care physicians accept risk for non-specialist, non-institutional care.
Specialist capitation	HMOs	Specialists accept a fixed annual payment for each referred patient.
Combinations	HMOs	e.g., "Primary withhold + specialist capitation + institutional negotiated fee"
"Carveout"	HMOs, PPOs, Medicare	Specific services can be "carved out" of the general arrangement and paid on a separate basis.

are less than expectations, a portion of the surplus can be distributed to the participants. The "risk pool" for the comparison can be structured any of several ways. It can be established for specialists or primary physicians separately for specialists and primary, or holding the primary physician accountable for both primary and specialty care. It can include institutional costs, putting the physician at risk for services that are ordered. The pool can include a large number of doctors or a smaller set with presumably more similar practices. Individual risk pools are generally statistically unsound.

Capitation is a non-fee approach to compensation. It is based on the number of patients the physician is accountable for, on a member selection basis for primary care or a set of referrals for referral specialists. The payment remains fixed no matter how much care the patients use. Capitation can be global, assigning one physician the economic result for all care, professional care only (excluding the institutional costs), specialty care only (with or without associated institutional costs), or primary care only. Separate capitation can be established for each group (institutional, primary, and referral) or some groups can be put on fee-based systems. The physician organization is at risk for actual costs, and payments to its members are based solely on performance. It is possible for the physician organization or the physician hospital organization to accept capitation and to compensate its members with fee-based plans.

Finally, any specific service can be "carved out," that is, excluded from the general arrangement and paid for some other way. Medicare has carved out mental health care and rehabilitation. HMOs carve out drugs, very expensive patients, mental health, and substance abuse. The underlying reason for carve outs is difficulty in controlling costs; either the provider or the insurer is uncomfortable with the risk involved.

The approaches have different consequences in terms of power to control costs and improve quality. Although some models seem to be falling into disfavor, there is no clear consensus and a great deal of experimentation. The goal is to develop a balanced incentive system under which all physicians have an opportunity to earn rewards for truly improved care, and overall compensation attracts physicians to each specialty in proportion to its need. The experiments have become more and more complex, involving mixed capitation and fee models and multiple distributions of surplus and withhold pools.

Designing the Physician Organization

Traditional Clinical Organization

The clinical organizations of hospitals followed the structure of medical specialties. As the functions of clinical improvement, credentialing, and education became more complex, healthcare institutions steadily strengthened that hierarchy. As the economic elements, particularly in the functions of recruitment, representation, and collective contracting, have become more complex, the physician organization is emerging as a second formal organization. All physicians are members of the clinical organization. Their roles in the physician organization depend on their economic arrangements.

As shown in Figure 8.9, the clinical hierarchy can be subdivided to any level indicated by the size or type of staff. A very large healthcare organization might have a dozen departments, several divisions under some departments, and sections or even subsections under some divisions. Each level would have an appointed leader who is accountable for clinical performance. The leaders of larger units are now salaried. A medical executive committee would coordinate their activities and review quality functions.[44] The chief medical officer (CMO) would normally chair the medical executive committee and have a major role as an executive officer. The staff necessary to support the clinical organization functions would be under the CMO's direction.

FIGURE 8.9
Institutional Clinical Organization Structure

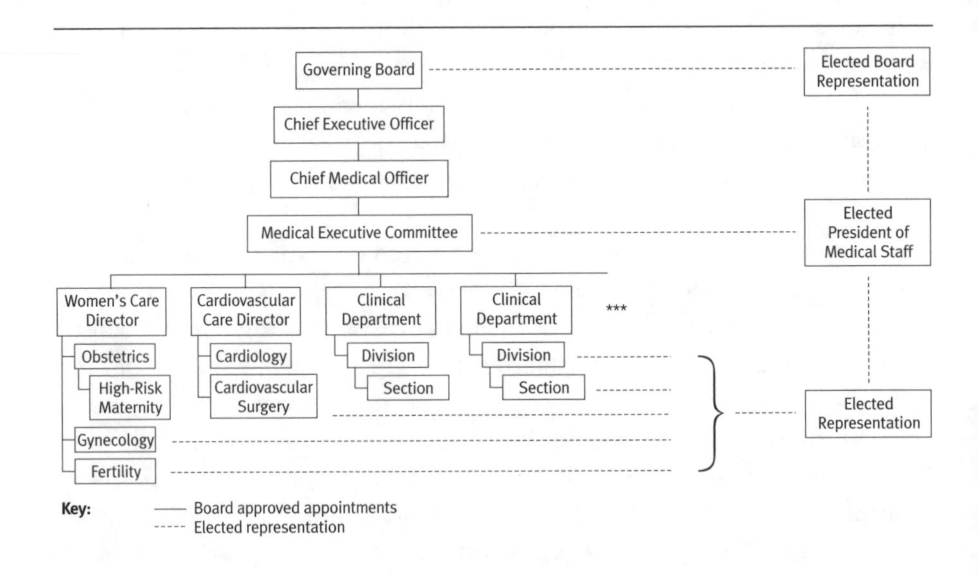

***Numbers of service units, departments, divisions, and sections depends on size of organization. Departments with primary responsibility for service units are accountable through the service unit.

All the units of the clinical organization review relevant budgets and rank capital budget requests. As outcomes measures and final product protocols develop, formally negotiated expectations will become more common. As indicated in Chapter 7, many clinical units participate actively in cross-functional teams setting protocols. The units play prominent roles in education as resident experts in their specialty. In organizations with postgraduate education, the section, division, or department leader is responsible for the quality and effectiveness of the residency program. Many larger organizations have a director of medical education who coordinates all educational activity, particularly postgraduate medical education. The post is usually subordinate to the CMO.

Many institutional organizations also provide for elected representation of the medical staff. Individual physicians elect a president, who usually sits on the medical executive committee, and other representatives to the governing board.

Figure 8.9 has evolved from the traditional hospital organization by the development of service units. These are revised departmental or division structures, given greater authority and multidimensional accountability for a specific set of interrelated patient needs. Leading institutions have established service units for women's services, cardiology, orthopedics, neurological disease including stroke, oncology, behavioral services, and trauma, thus covering most of the expensive medical needs of the population.[45] These units appear to be effective and are likely to be part of most large healthcare organizations in the future.

Three problems emerge. A large set of referral specialists are left without a unit, or with obligations beyond one unit. General surgeons, surgical specialties other than orthopedics, and medical specialties other than oncology, neurology, and cardiology are in this group. So are the hospital-based specialties, imaging, pathology, anesthesia, and rehabilitation. Presumably an "Other Surgery" unit will emerge, accommodating the rest of the surgeons, and the hospital-based specialists will continue as very strong functional units supporting all referral and most primary care. It is not clear what happens to the remaining internists.

Second, primary care tends to be fractionated under this model. Psychiatrists, emergency physicians, and obstetricians join their service units, and the units become uniquely structured organizations with both referral and primary functions. Family physicians, general internists, and pediatricians are left with only their department or section home. These specialties have the least ties to the institution, practicing principally in their offices. Traditionally, their influence in the medical executive committee has been limited, with the intervention-oriented specialties commanding more resources and a bigger say in the decisions.

Third, the model has no vehicle for resolving issues of concern to all specialties other than the medical executive committee. The executive committee is usually structured with one vote for each department, leading to political arguments over the departmental definitions and wide differences in real influence between the members. The committee deals reasonably with credentialing, clinical improvement, and educational issues, and ranks the items in the capital budget (Chapter 14). The combined problems of promoting single signature insurance contracts, administering physician compensation packages, and expanding primary care are usually viewed as exceeding the capability of the committee. A second physician organization is emerging to accomplish these tasks.

The Emerging Physician Organization

Physician organizations are a creation of the last decade and their design is in flux.[46] The emerging organization will be a partner, rather than a component of the institutional organization. It will have a representational decision-making structure relying on two major councils, one representing primary care and the other referral specialists collectively. It will have opportunities to represent various subsidiary organizations such as salaried physicians, incorporated group practices, and networked or virtual groups of individuals, as well as service unit members within its councils. The subsidiary units will collaborate closely with the institutional units and will accept accountability through their institutional ties. Figure 8.10 shows the emerging structure.

The primary care council will give strong voice to family practice, pediatrics, and general internists. Psychiatry and the behavioral service unit will probably make their major input through this council, as behavioral care moves more to an office-based activity. The trauma service has important primary care opportunities, but it also requires extensive collaboration across specialties and

FIGURE 8.10 Emerging Physician Organization Structure

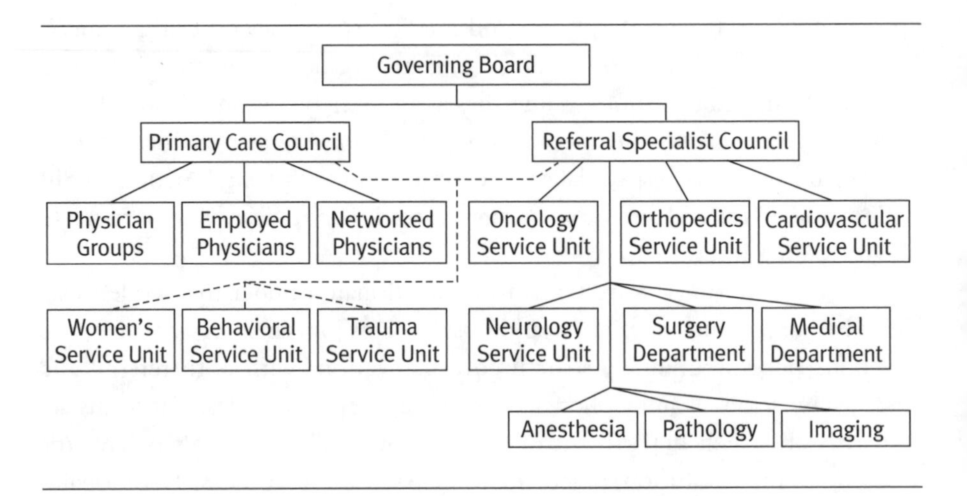

access to many institutional functions. It and women's services, which include both obstetrics and gynecological surgery, will require representation in both councils. The remaining clinical units are clearly part of the referral specialty council. The referral specialty council could fill the JCAHO requirements for the hospital medical executive committee.

The physician organization is usually a private for-profit corporation structured to minimize double taxation by passing its proceeds directly to its members. To gain not-for-profit status, it must have a community dominated board, which would be contrary to its intent. The two councils will rarely have equal numbers of doctors.[47] The referral specialty council will have more members and control a larger dollar volume, but their influence will be offset by the primary council's gatekeeper role. Relatively few patients seek these specialties directly, and managed care plans discourage such contact.

Several elements are necessary to meet market demands for healthcare. Institutional and physician services are obvious. Beyond these, providers must have marketing power to arrange insurance contracts, clinical discipline to ensure cost and quality, and an information system to support prompt communication and monitoring performance. The capital requirements for the package are much higher than most people realize, on the order of several million dollars per practicing physician.[48] Most of this capital is in place, owned largely by the not-for-profit hospital organizations. Necessary maintenance and expansion is on the order of $10,000 per physician per year, and is tax exempt when moved through the not-for-profit structure. Few physicians are interested in an additional annual investment of that magnitude, and almost none could contemplate buying out the institution. It is this capital requirement that insures a strong community role in any eventual healthcare organization.[49] (A different but similar mechanism, access to public equity funds, protects the for-profit organizations.)

Two approaches to integrating the physician organization and the institutional organization are shown in Figure 8.11. The first (a) is a separate organization melding the interests of the community and its physicians. As of 1995, it was the most common type of integration.[50] Now called the physician-hospital organization (PHO), it has equal or near equal representation of community and physician directors. Assuming that it has the appropriate legal structures and approvals, the PHO can accept insurance risk for the hospital and the physicians, hire physicians, operate support activities, and buy practices. Depending on its charter, it can borrow money and issue stock. By combining these activities, it can operate any kind of facility and even operate as an insurance intermediary. The PHO normally assumes the existence of a physicians' organization for their representation. The physician organization and many of its members can legally do all the activities of the PHO, but the PHO includes the hospital as a partner, increasing both institutional resources and community participation. The dual structure allows the physician organization access to institutional capital, and allows the community representation to protect its investments.

An alternative model shown in Figure 8.11B is a community-owned not-for-profit foundation that has both the PHO and the institutional com-

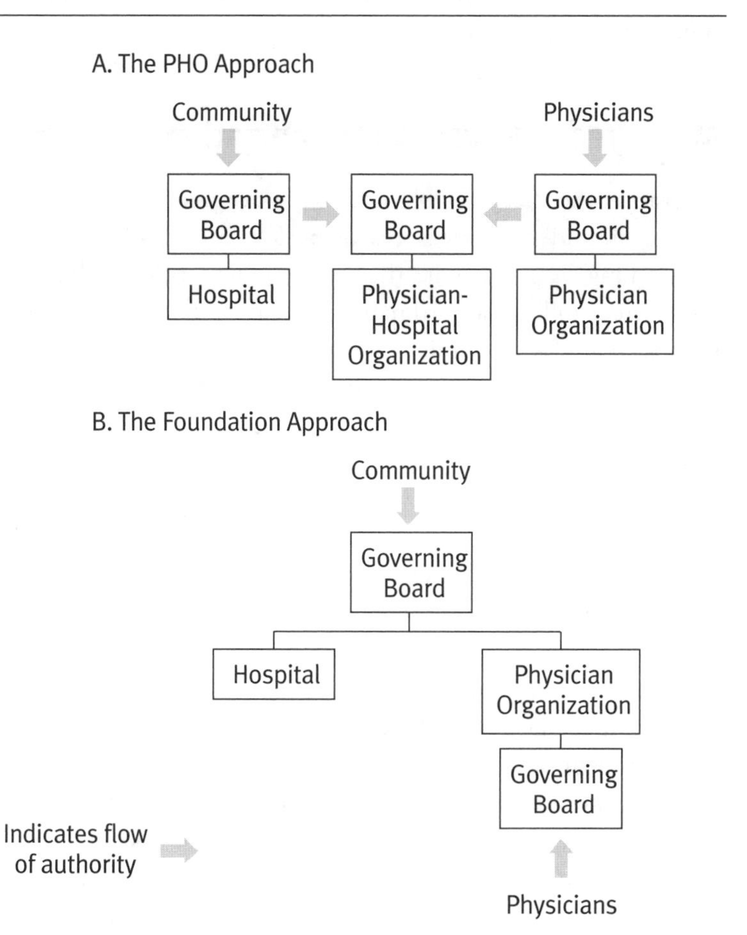

FIGURE 8.11 Models Integrating the Physician Organization

ponent as subsidiaries. A number of famous clinics operate in this manner. The Permanente Foundation is the medical group for Kaiser Permanente. Successful examples, such as Virginia Mason Medical Center[51] and Henry Ford Health System,[52] have strong physician representation throughout their governance and management decision processes. The physician organization may or may not be a separate corporation, but it can implement all the necessary economic and representational arrangements between the integrated organization and the individual physician. This alternative, or something like it, might easily emerge in the future. It has one fewer board than the PHO model, allowing a simplified strategy development process. It can and presumably will subordinate institutional functions to clinical ones. The test will be its ability to meet physician needs for income, autonomy, and service.

A third concept, the independent physicians association, was prominent in the 1980s. It envisioned the physician organization as dominant, contracting directly with insurers or operating its own insurance function and purchasing hospital services. The model did not thrive. IPAs were forced to partner with hospitals controlling the cost of care and gain access to capital and markets. They remain a vehicle for associating several physician organizations to cover a large geographic market, and they still exist as physician organizations in PHOs.[53]

Measures of Physician Organization Performance

Like any other accountable unit of the organization, the physician organizations should have measures of performance and formal expectations for the coming year. That is, the chief medical officer, the medical executive committee, and the subordinate units shown in Figure 8.9, and the governing boards, councils and units of Figure 8.10 should be accountable for multidimensional expectations about their own performance, separate from the measures of clinical performance discussed in Chapter 7. Figure 8.12 suggests some examples.

The physician organization has a commitment to the maximization of appropriate demand that must be measured by market share and access measures. Counts of practices open to new patients and delays for various kinds of scheduled appointments are used. Out-of-staff referrals is a measure of patients selecting the organization but needing or choosing services the organization does not provide.

The medical staff office and the physician organization are accountable for their own operating cost budgets. Physician member satisfaction is now routinely monitored. Samples should be adequate to reflect attitudes by several categories of age and specialty. Success in filling open positions is also important. Payments made to physicians per member month is a measure of the community's economic competitiveness in physician recruitment. Measures

Dimension	Measurement Intent	Example
Demand	Response to community demand for care	Market share Available primary care practitioners Appointment delays Out-of-staff referrals Number and variety of payment contracts available
Costs	Costs of medical staff and physician services operations	Cost budgets for medical staff office, PHO, and physician organization
Physician Resources	Recruitment and retention of physicians	Member satisfaction Payments/physician-month Percentage of positions filled with first choice Measures of staff diversity

FIGURE 8.12 Measures of Physician Organization Performance

of staff diversity are important in primary care, where patients seek particular backgrounds, and also in recruitment.[54]

The popularity of various contractual arrangements in the eyes of the physicians is important in guiding future arrangements. The cost of administration of managed care contracts and the cost of medical staff operation per member physician are indicators of internal efficiency that can be benchmarked against other organizations.

Global measure of clinical outcomes have not proven sensitive, but many measures for specific diseases are useful. An index of these reflects improvements achieved by the physician organizations. Malpractice settlements are a measure of major failures in care. The number of physician complaints or appeals about the medical staff activities and specific satisfaction data reveal trouble spots.

Finally, there are a number of measures of patient and other customer satisfaction, including surveys of physicians to identify weak points in referral processes. Many patient appeals reflect on physician practice. Formal and informal survey of the satisfaction of payors and intermediaries protects market share and opens opportunities for expansion. Profitability is an important index of the health of the enterprise as a whole.

Suggested Readings

Boland, P. 1996. *The Capitation Sourcebook: A Practical Guide to Managing At-Risk Arrangements.* Berkeley: Boland Healthcare Inc.

Connors, R. B. (ed.). 1997. *Integrating the Practice of Medicine: A Decision-Maker's Guide to Organizing and Managing Physician Services.* Chicago: American Hospital Publishing.

Cromwell, J., et al. 1997. *Hospital and Physician Rate-Setting Systems: A Reference Manual for Developing and Implementing Rate Structures.* Chicago: Irwin Professional Pub.

Freidson, E. 1980. *Doctoring Together: A Study of Professional Social Control.* Chicago: University of Chicago Press.

Joint Commission on Accreditation of Healthcare Organizations. *Accreditation Manual for Hospitals.* Chicago: JCAHO. (Issued annually)

Krohn, R. 1998. *Physician Networks: Strategy, Start-Up, and Operation.* Chicago: Health Administration Press.

LeTourneau, B., and W. Curry, eds. 1998. *In Search of Physician Leadership.* Chicago: Health Administration Press.

Penner, M. J. 1997. *Capitation in California: A Study of Physician Organizations Managing Risk.* Chicago: Health Administration Press.

Rolfe, L. K., and P. Wehner. 1995. *Making the Physician Network Work: Leadership, Design, Incentives.* Chicago: American Hospital Publishing.

Rozovsky, F. A. 1994. *Medical Staff Credentialling: A Practical Guide.* Chicago: American Hospital Publishing.

Starr, P. 1982. *The Social Transformation of American Medicine.* New York: Basic Books, Part I, Chapter 6, pp. 198–232; Part II, Chapter 5, pp. 420–49.

Todd, M. K. 1997. *IPA, PHO, and MSO Developmental Strategies: Building Successful Provider Alliances.* New York: Healthcare Financial Management Association/McGraw-Hill.

van Amerongen, D. 1998. *Networks and the Future of Medical Practice.* Chicago: Health Administration Press.

White, C. H. 1997. *The* Hospital *Medical Staff.* New York, Delmar Publishers.

Notes

1. R. H. Palmer, E. A. Wright, E. J. Orav, J. L. Hargraves, and T. A. Louis, "Consistency in Performance Among Primary Care Practitioners." *Medical Care* 34(9 Suppl), pp. SS52–66 (September, 1996)
2. M. R. Gold, R. Hurley, T. Lake, T. Ensor, and R. Berenson, "A National Survey of the Arrangements Managed Care Plans Make with Physicians." *New England Journal of Medicine* 333(25), pp. 1678–83 (Dec 21, 1995)
3. J. R. Griffith, *Well-Managed Health Care Organization*, 3rd ed. Chicago: Health Administration Press, pp. 515–58 (1995)
4. J. R. Griffith, *Designing 21st Century Healthcare.* Chicago: Health Administration Press p. 199 (1998)
5. J. D. Blair, M. D. Fottler, A. R. Paolino, and T. M. Rotarious, *Medical Group Practices Face the Uncertain Future: Challenges, Opportunities, and Strategies.* Englewood, CO: Center for Research in Ambulatory Health Care Administration (1995)
6. Joint Commission on Accreditation of Hospitals, "Standards for Medical Staff—Requirements for Membership and Privileges." *Accreditation Manual for Hospitals.* Chicago: Joint Commission on Accreditation of Hospitals, p. 89 (1984)

7. A. F. Southwick, *The Law of Hospital and Health Care Administration,* 2nd. ed. Chicago: Health Administration Press, pp. 585–622 (1988)
8. P. A. Lembcke, "Evolution of the Medical Audit." *Journal of the American Medical Association* 199, pp. 543–50 (1967)
9. A. F. Southwick, *The Law of Hospital and Health Care Administration,* 2nd. ed. Chicago: Health Administration Press, pp. 589–91 (1988)
10. A. F. Southwick, *The Law of Hospital and Health Care Administration,* 2nd. ed. Chicago: Health Administration Press, p. 341 (1988)
11. *Patrick v Burget, 486* U.S. 94 (1988)
12. A. F. Southwick, *The Law of Hospital and Health Care Administration,* 2nd. ed. Chicago: Health Administration Press, pp. 588, 592–96, 599, 604, 607, 610, 616–17 (1988)
13. A. F. Southwick, *The Law of Hospital and Health Care Administration,* 2nd. ed. Chicago: Health Administration Press, pp. 601–22 (1988)
14. P. G. Ramsey, M. D. Wenrich, J. D. Carline, T. S. Inui, E. B. Larson, and J. P. LoGerfo, "Use of Peer Ratings to Evaluate Physician Performance." *Journal of the American Medical Association* 269(13), pp. 1655–60 (April 7, 1993); G. R. Norman, D. A. Davis, S. Lamb, E. Hanna, P. Caulford, and T. Kaigas, "Competency Assessment of Primary Care Physicians as Part of a Peer Review Program." *Journal of the American Medical Association* 270(9), pp. 1046–51 (September 1, 1993)
15. J. L. Hargraves, R. H. Palmer, E. J. Orav, and E. A. Wright, "Are Differences in Practitioners' Acceptance of a Quality Assurance Intervention Related to Their Performance?" *Medical Care* 34(9 Suppl), pp. SS77–86 (September, 1996)
16. *Health Care Quality Improvement Act PL 99-177* (1986) Rockville, MD: U.S. Department of Health and Human Services, Health Resources and Services Administration, Division of Quality Assurance and Liability Management. (Undated)
17. C. A. Sullivan, "Competency Assessment and Performance Improvement for Health Care Providers." *Journal for Health Care Quality* 16(4), p. 14 (July–August, 1994)
18. T. H. Rice and R. J. Labelle, "Do Physicians Induce Demand for Medical Services." *Journal of Health Politics, Policy, and Law* 14(3), pp. 587–600 (1989)
19. J. P. Weiner, "Forecasting the Effects of Health Reform on U.S. Physician Workforce Requirement. Evidence from HMO Staffing Patterns." *Journal of the American Medical Association* 272(3), pp. 222–30 (July 20, 1994)
20. H. Krakauer, I. Jacoby, M. Millman, and J. E. Lukomnik, "Physician Impact on Hospital Admission and on Mortality Rates in the Medicare Population." *Health Services Research* 31(2), pp. 191–211 (June, 1996)
21. U. E. Reinhardt, "The Supply of Physicians." In *Integrating the Practice of Medicine,* R. B. Conners, ed. Chicago: American Hospital Publishing Inc., pp. 11–36 (1997)
22. T. H. Dial, S. E. Palsbo, C. Bergsten, J. R. Gabel, and J. Weiner, "Clinical Staffing in Staff and Group Model HMOs." *Health Affairs* 14(2), pp. 168–80 (Summer, 1995)
23. L. Greenberg and J. M. Cultice, "Forecasting the Need for Physicians in the United States: The Health Resources and Services Administration's Physician

Requirements Model." *Health Services Research* 31(6), pp. 723–37 (February, 1997)

24. L. G. Hart, E. Wagner, S. Pirzada, A. F. Nelson, and R. A. Rosenblatt. "Physician Staffing Ratios in Staff-Model HMOs: A Cautionary Tale." *Health Affairs* 16(1), pp. 5–70 (January–February, 1997)
25. D. C. Goodman, E. S. Fisher, T. A. Bubolz, J. E. Mohr, J. F. Poage, and J. E. Wennberg, "Benchmarking the U.S. Physician Workforce. An Alternative to Needs-Based or Demand-Based Planning." *Journal of the American Medical Association* 276(22), pp. 1811–7 (December 11, 1996)
26. H. S. Luft, D. W. Garnick, D. H. Mark, and S. J. McPhee, *Hospital Volume, Physician Volume, and Patient Outcomes: Assessing the Evidence.* Chicago: Health Administration Press (1990)
27. *Statistical Abstract of the U.S.,* Washington, DC: U.S. Bureau of the Census, nos. 2 and 189 (1993)
28. L. K. Rolfe and P. Wehner, *Making the Physician Network Work: Leadership, Design, Incentives.* Chicago: American Hospital Publishing (1995)
29. Association of American Medical Colleges, *AAMC Databook: Statistical Information Related to Medical Education, January 1998.* Washington, DC: Association of American Medical Colleges, Table G7 (1998)
30. L. K. Rolfe and P. Werner, *Making the Physician Network Work: Leadership, Design, Incentives.* Chicago: American Hospital Publishing (1995)
31. S. M. Shortell, *Effective Hospital-Physician Relationships.* Chicago: Health Administration Press (1991)
32. L. R. Burns and L. R. Beach, "The Quality Improvement Strategy." *Health Care Management Review* 19(2), pp. 21–31 (1984)
33. S. M. Shortell, *Effective Hospital-Physician Relationships,* Chicago: Health Administration Press, Chapter 6, pp. 79–93 (1991)
34. J. Balint and W. Shelton, "Regaining the Initiative. Forging a New Model of the Patient-Physician Relationship." *Journal of the American Medical Association* 275(11), pp. 887–91 (March 20, 1996)
35. J. R. Griffith, *Moral Challenges of Health Care Management.* Chicago: Health Administration Press (1993)
36. BDC Advisors, *Physician Hospital Integration Models.* San Francisco: BDC (1993)
37. L. R. Burns and D. P. Thorpe, "Trends and Models in Physician-Hospital Organization." *Health Care Management Review* 18(4), pp. 7–20 (1993)
38. H. S. Luft and M. R. Greenlick, "The Contribution of Group- and Staff-Model HMOs to American Medicine." *Milbank Quarterly* 74(4): 445–67, (1996)
39. D. G. Cave, "Vertical Integration Models to Prepare Health Systems for Capitation." *Health Care Management Review* 20(1), pp. 26–39 (Winter, 1995)
40. F. McCall-Perez, "Physician Equity Groups and Other Emerging Equity." New York: McGraw-Hill, pp.183–200 (1997)
41. L. R. Burns and D. P. Thorpe, "Trends and Models in Physician-Hospital Organization." *Health Care Management Review* 18(4), pp. 17–18 (1993)
42. A. Herman, "IRS Memorandum Limits Joint Ventures." *Healthcare Financial Management* 49(8), pp. 51–2 (1992)

43. C. MacKelvie, "Fraud Abuse and Inurement." *Topics in Health Care Financing* 16(3), pp. 49–57 (1990)
44. Joint Commission on Accreditation of Healthcare Organizations, *Comprehensive Accreditation Manual For Hospitals.* Oakbrook Terrace, IL: The Joint Commission (1997)
45. J. R. Griffith, *Designing 21st Century Healthcare.* Chicago: Health Administration Press (1998)
46. L. R. Burns and D. P. Thorpe, "Physician-Hospital Organizations: Strategy, Structure, and Conflict." In *Integrating the Practice of Medicine, A Decision-Maker's Guide to Organizing and Managing Physician Services*, R. B. Connors, ed. Chicago: American Hospital Publishing, p. 352 (1997)
47. Ernst and Young, *Physician Hospital Organizations: Profile 1995.* Washington, DC: Ernst and Young (1995)
48. J. C. Robinson and L. P. Casalino, "Vertical Integration and Organizational Networks in Health Care." *Health Affairs* 15(1), pp. 7–22 (Spring, 1996)
49. Ernst & Young, *Physician Hospital Organizations: Profile 1995.* Washington, DC: Ernst & Young (1995)
50. L. R. Burns and D. P. Thorpe, "Physician-Hospital Organizations: Strategy, Structure, and Conflict." In *Integrating the Practice of Medicine: A Decision-Maker's Guide to Organizing and Managing Physician Services*, R. B. Connors, ed. Chicago: American Hospital Publishing, p. 352 (1997)
51. L. R. Burns and D. P. Thorpe, "Trends and Models in Physician-Hospital Organization." *Health Care Management Review* 18(4), pp. 15–17 (1993)
52. J. R. Griffith, V. K. Sahney, and R. A. Mohr, *Reengineering Health Care: Building on CQI.* Chicago: Health Administration Press, pp. 253–287 (1995)
53. G. D. Brown, "Independent Practice Associations." In *Integrating the Practice of Medicine: A Decision-Maker's Guide to Organizing and Managing Physician Services*, R. B. Connors, ed. Chicago: American Hospital Publishing, pp. 289–306 (1997)
54. M. Komaromy, K. Grumbach, M. Drake, K. Vranizan, N. Lurie, D. Keane, and A. B. Bindman, "The Role of Black and Hispanic Physicians in Providing Health Care for Underserved Populations." *New England Journal of Medicine* 334(20), pp. 1305–10 (May 16, 1996)

CHAPTER

9

CLINICAL SUPPORT SERVICES

Modern healthcare is a team activity employing several dozen specialized professionals other than attending physicians in clinical support services (CSSs). CSSs produce the intermediate products of care. They include activities such as laboratory tests, surgical operations, and physical therapy. They also include behavioral and psychological services such as social service, pastoral care, and health education to patients. Most, but not all, CSSs are ordered by an attending physician. They support prevention, diagnosis, treatment, rehabilitation, and daily living and are available to patients at several sites, including outpatient offices, the acute hospital, long-term care facilities, and home. Healthcare organizations must provide CSSs correctly, promptly, cheaply, and attractively. They must also seek the optimal number and kind of CSSs for each patient. Too many or too few, the wrong CSS, or poor quality CSS will reduce overall quality and increase total cost of care. Optimization of care is often a matter of providing exactly the combination and timing of CSSs required, but each unit of CSS must be provided at excellent quality and minimum cost.

Each CSS is supervised by a professional, often a specialist physician. Each has it own technology and procedures discussed extensively in its professional literature. Clinical support services also have a number of common characteristics. This chapter discusses management of CSSs in light of those common characteristics. It is organized around the following topics:

- definition and purpose
- functions
- management and organization
- measures and information systems

Definition and Purpose

A clinical support service is a set of patient care activities organized around one or more medical specialties or clinical professions providing individual patient care on order of an attending physician or physician extender. Large numbers of CSSs are used as part of the plan for seriously ill patients; almost every patient uses at least one.

Under this definition, nursing is a support service. It is so large and complex, however, that it merits discussion on its own, provided in Chapter 10. Many observations about support services apply to nursing as well.

The purpose of CSS is to extend the capability of the total healthcare system by improving quality or reducing cost of each specific service. CSSs are specializations that arose when one person with unique training, skills, and equipment could handle one part of the care for many patients better than several people with general skills. Simply put, a CSS comes into existence or continues to exist because it does something better or cheaper than alternatives.

This purpose is intuitively clear, but it contains a hidden complexity. Many of the less elaborate support services can be provided by several professions, and it is often both cheaper and more convenient for the patient to receive them from generalist caregivers. At the same time, many CSSs require heavy fixed costs in professional salaries and specialized equipment. They become quite costly if they are not widely used. Quality of care also often depends on volume; the more practice the CSS team gets, the better its skills.[1,2] The healthcare organization must balance the availability of expensive CSSs as it does medical referral specialists (Chapter 8), weighing community desires for convenience against quality and cost. Thus, the purpose implies that the profile of services offered must be consistent with the strategic plan. It also implies that the domain of each CSS must be defined by the organization as a whole, trading off the advantages of specialization for those of generalist care.

While a consequence of the purpose is that smaller healthcare organizations will have fewer CSSs than large ones, most will have several dozen, including critical services such as clinical laboratories, radiology services, pharmacies, electrocardiography services, and operating rooms. It is not necessary that the healthcare organization employ personnel or own the equipment for CSSs; it may obtain them through service contracts or alliances. A useful classification of the non-nursing CSSs categorizes them broadly into diagnostic, therapeutic, and general community activities. Figure 9.1 shows the types of CSSs all large healthcare organizations would be likely to have. About 30 separate CSSs are identified.

Functions of Clinical Support Services

A serious illness may require several hundred separate services from CSSs listed in Figure 9.1. It is obvious that these activities have very different characteristics. Yet at one level of abstraction above these differences, similarities emerge. Despite the difference in their products, the managers of social service and megavoltage therapy, for example, share eight common functions identified in Figure 9.2. Despite the length and complexity of the list, these are functions each CSS must perform to maintain effectiveness. The distinction between clinical and managerial functions should not be overdrawn. Clinical functions draw more heavily on the CSS's specific professional area, but both are essential.

FIGURE 9.1 Non-Nursing Clinical Support Services in a Large Healthcare Organization

Diagnostic Services	Therapeutic Services
Cardiopulmonary laboratory	Anesthesia
Electrocardiology	Birthing suite
Pulmonary function	Blood bank
Heart catheterization	Emergency service
Clinical laboratory	Operating suite
Chemistry	Surgery
Hematology	Recovery
Histopathology	Pharmacy
Bacteriology and virology	Dispensing
Autopsy and morgue	Intravenous admixture service
Diagnostic imaging	Radiation therapy
Radiography	Megavoltage radiation
Tomography	Therapy
Radio-isotope studies	Radio-isotope therapy
Magnetic resonance imaging	Rehabilitation services
Ultrasound	Physical therapy
Other	Respiratory therapy
Electroencephalography	Speech pathology
Electromyography	Occupational therapy
Audiology	Social and counseling services
	Social service
	Pastoral care
	Psychological counseling

Technical Quality: Effective and Reliable Completion of Orders

One can construct four important aspects of CSS quality:[3] technical quality, appropriateness, satisfaction, and continuity or integration of care. Although they are interrelated, each is approached by separate means, and each deserves a separate function. Technical quality, a concept essentially analogous to product consistency and service reliability, is the proper starting point; the other three depend on it. Technical quality is a matter of doing the correct thing for the patient consistently over a wide variety of situations. Technical quality is measured by a variety of process and outcomes indicators, as discussed below. It is achieved by sound procedures, correct equipment and supplies, training, and practice.

Many CSS professionals have extensive formal education and certification. Their knowledge and skill are a major part of technical quality assurance. The education includes mastery of relevant theory and supervised practice so that the student learns the processes, patient indications and contraindications for them, expected outcomes, and the rules governing process design. To reduce costs, many of the actual CSS procedures are performed by aides and technicians who do not have professional training. The staffing of most CSS units consists of one or two levels of professional training and one or more levels of nonprofessional personnel, allowing each professional to serve a larger

FIGURE 9.2 Functions of Clinical Support Services

Function	Description	Examples
Clinical Functions		
Quality	Provision of technically correct clinical interventions	Outpatient pharmacy: Correct drug, dosage, count, and patient instruction Operating room: Correct patient preparation, trained staff, equipment
Appropriateness	Provision of the most appropriate service for each patient	Outpatient pharmacy: Formulary, drug use education and consultation, generic drug substitution Operating room: Correct surgical implants and supplies; capability to do laparascopic and laser substitutes for more invasive procedures
Managerial Functions		
Facility, equipment, and staff planning	Projection of future equipment and facility needs, review of acceptable volumes of demand	Outpatient pharmacy: Number and location of sites, hours of operation, staffing required, costs Operating room: Number of suites, staffing, inpatient and outpatient demand
Amenities and marketing	Additional services for patients and doctors	Outpatient pharmacy: Comfortable waiting area, drug usage literature, consultation to patients; telephone and electronic order systems for doctors, advertising services to doctors and patients Operating room: Doctors' lounges, family waiting rooms, advertising services to doctors
Patient scheduling	Timely service, integrated with other CSSs	Outpatient pharmacy: Limit on patient service delays Operating room: No delay after patient admission; complete lab, x-ray, and anesthesia work-up; on-time start
Continuous improvement	Monitoring performance measures, benchmarking, and devising process changes to improve	Outpatient pharmacy: Evaluation of new drugs, inventory, packaging, and dispensing methods Operating room: Evaluation of new surgical supplies, techniques, and staffing roles
Budgeting	Developing expectations for each dimension of performance	Outpatient pharmacy: Implementing new hours of service or staffing Operating room: Implementing new preparation procedures or employee cross training
Human resources management	Recruiting, retaining, and motivating an effective work group	Outpatient pharmacy: Pharmacist recruitment, technician training, work group empowerment, worker scheduling Operating room: Nurse recruitment, technician training, work group empowerment, worker scheduling

volume of patients. Three issues of quality assurance beyond formal education emerge:

1. maintenance of skill for qualified professionals;
2. resolution of differences between professionals; and
3. training and supervision of nonprofessional personnel.

Intermediate product protocols are used to address these issues. As shown in Chapter 7, Figure 7.5, these are step-by-step procedure statements developed by continuous improvement teams. The protocols have several advantages. Developing the protocols is an educational exercise for the group. Review of recommended practice helps keep all participants current. Exploration of variation in performance clarifies the causes and builds consensus. Protocols are excellent classroom aids; they follow accepted training principles of breaking the learning into small parts and making each action explicit. Protocols simplify the logistics: they specify the exact demand for supplies and equipment, making it possible to identify the least cost alternatives and to prepare uniform set-ups in advance. When written copies or computer screens are used directly, protocols provide recognition rather than recall. Time requirements and error rates are reduced by recognition.

Monitoring performance reveals uniformity, compliance with protocols, and opportunities for improvement. There are several approaches to measuring technical quality of CSSs:

- *Performance measures built into protocols*, such as radiation monitors, temperature records, and reagent tests
- *Process inspections*, preferably following explicit methods and carried out by trained, unbiased observers
- *Record inspections*, including patient medical records and departmental records, to reveal delayed or unfilled orders, adverse results, or complications
- *Counts of repeat tests and unsatisfactory results*
- *Tests of output for compliance with expectations*, such as accuracy of values on known, or control, lab specimens or accuracy of prescription drugs delivered

These measures can be developed from either samples or universes, as appropriate, and subjected to statistical analysis (described in Chapter 7). A well-run CSS identifies a variety of measures of technical quality and uses the least expensive ones on a daily or hourly basis to ensure consistent performance, even though the validity of these measures is imperfect. It bolsters this short-term effort with periodic studies introducing greater scope and validity. The frequency and extent of these depends on the cost of unsatisfactory performance as well as the cost of the studies.

For most applications, the goal of technical quality should be to attain as high a quality as is consistent with the patient benefit. For example, although one wishes to get as many satisfactory x-ray films on the first try as possible, retake has a finite price, the variable cost of another film plus some allowances for patient discomfort and delay. Unsatisfactory exposures can result from improper dose estimation, improper machine calibration, variation in the power supply, or movement by the patient. One would not invest more in improving the protocol than the cost of eliminated retakes. Similarly, one would not make the examination unnecessarily unpleasant by frightening patients into absolute immobility. Satisfactory performance will be something greater than 0.0 percent retakes. The best reported performance, or benchmark, is often used as a guide, but even it must be tested against the cost to achieve it.

Zero-defect goals are appropriate only when failures are life-threatening or cause very high cost consequences. For example, the blood level of a certain enzyme is used to confirm a heart attack. The test is inexpensive, but expensive treatment is started immediately if the enzyme level is elevated. Delays increase fatality rates.[4] Zero defect is an appropriate goal for both accuracy and timeliness. Understated enzyme values and delay may increase fatalities; overstated values will trigger unnecessary expensive treatment.

Appropriateness

Any CSS indicated but not ordered can reduce quality or add to cost of care. Any CSS ordered unnecessarily adds to the cost and can potentially decrease quality because there is at least a small risk of negative result attached to each procedure. Final product protocols or individual patients' care plans address the correct selection and timing of CSSs. CSS professionals must be expert on the contribution of their services to total patient care.[5]

CSS performance contributes to appropriateness of care in four areas, as shown in Figure 9.3. Low technical quality is a barrier. The errors that result are costly. Low quality destroys physician confidence, leading to avoidance of services that would be used if they were felt to be reliable. In the case of diagnostic services, unreliable tests are repeated, raising costs. High unit costs are a barrier to appropriate use. High patient satisfaction is a facilitator. Satisfied patients are more likely to follow orders[6,7] and more likely to remain in the market share of both the CSS and the referring physicians.

Finally, the well-run service participates actively in clinical discussions, provides routine consultation to physicians, and advertises its services and their appropriate use. Most physicians have several choices for CSS as well as substitutions among CSSs. The well-managed CSS deliberately advertises its capability and offers helpful advice about the use of its services. CSSs participate routinely in final product protocol development, advising on the most economical way to gain the benefits available from their service. Similarly, they are available to consult with physicians on individual care plans.

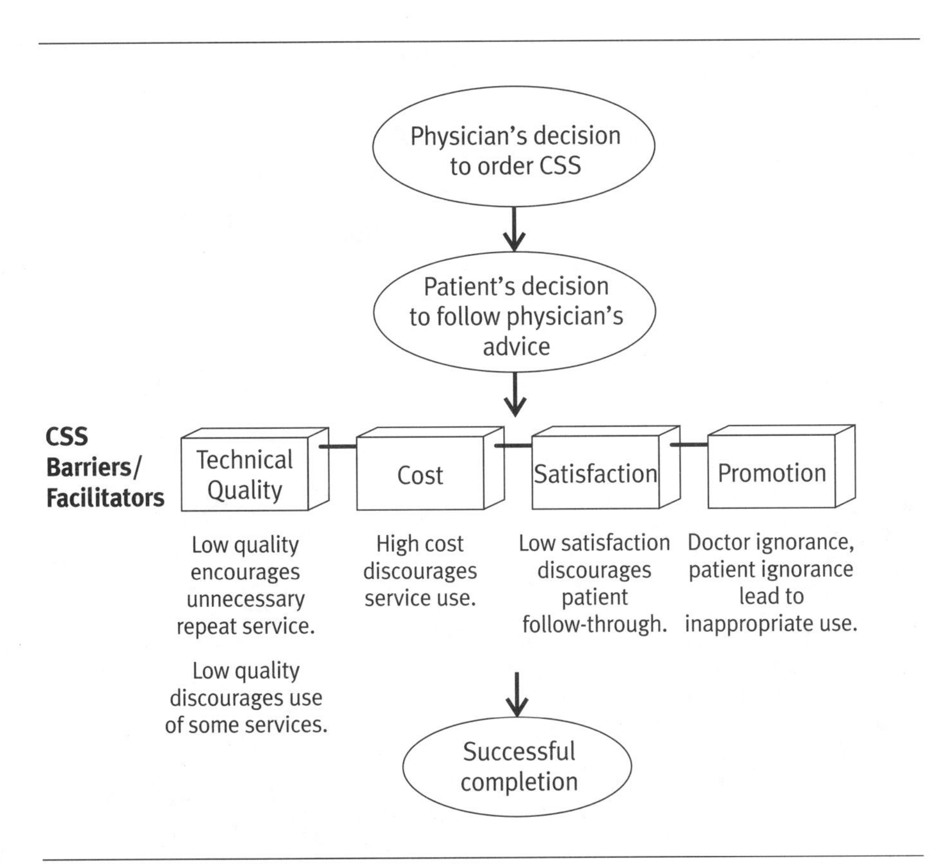

FIGURE 9.3 CSS Contributions to Appropriate Care

Examples of CSS assistance to physicians are now widespread. Pharmacists develop formularies, indications, and guidelines for selecting among drugs, and offer counseling about individual patients.[8,9] Rehabilitation services offer recommended protocols for specific conditions, evaluations of individual patients, and progress reviews.[10,11,12] Diagnostic services provide indications and counter-indications for various tests and consultation about complex cases.[13]

Facilities, Equipment, and Staff Planning

Planning matches the size and scope of each CSS to anticipated demand. It must strive to provide all the services the market can support, but only that level. Given the great importance of fixed costs in efficiency, the planning function is crucial. Services that are missing or too small cause loss of market share to competitors. Those that are too large draw insufficient demand to meet quality and cost standards.

Involving CSS personnel directly in the planning process helps them understand the problems which must be faced and improves the accuracy of the forecasts. CSS personnel are the most likely to know of technological changes that may affect the demand and the opportunities for improvement. Participating in the forecast preparation helps them understand the realism of the issue and convinces them of the need to improve. Because of the need to provide an optimal organization as a whole, the final decision on the existence or size of a CSS is always reserved to the parent organization.

Sizing clinical support services

CSS planning is based on the epidemiologic planning approach described in Chapter 6. The equation used to size each CSS is:

$$\left\{\begin{matrix}\text{Demand}\\\text{for a}\\\text{service}\end{matrix}\right\} = \left\{\begin{matrix}\text{Population}\\\text{at risk}\end{matrix}\right\} * \left\{\begin{matrix}\text{Incidence}\\\text{rate}\end{matrix}\right\} * \left\{\begin{matrix}\text{Average}\\\text{use per}\\\text{incidence}\end{matrix}\right\} * \left\{\begin{matrix}\text{Market}\\\text{share}\end{matrix}\right\}$$

For CSSs drawing directly from the community, populations are age-specific community censuses, the incidence rate is the occurrence of disease in the general population, and the market share is the institution's anticipated share of the particular market. For example:

$$\left\{\begin{matrix}\text{Outpatient}\\\text{pharmacy}\\\text{demand}\end{matrix}\right\} = \left\{\begin{matrix}\text{General}\\\text{community}\\\text{population}\end{matrix}\right\} * \left\{\begin{matrix}\text{Outpatient}\\\text{prescriptions/}\\\text{person-year}\end{matrix}\right\} * \left\{\begin{matrix}\text{Organization's}\\\text{market share}\end{matrix}\right\}$$

$$\left\{\begin{matrix}\text{Demand}\\\text{for specific}\\\text{surgical}\\\text{procedure}\end{matrix}\right\} = \left\{\begin{matrix}\text{Age/gender}\\\text{specific}\\\text{population}\end{matrix}\right\} * \left\{\begin{matrix}\text{Specific}\\\text{incidence}\\\text{rate}\end{matrix}\right\} * \left\{\begin{matrix}\text{Organization's}\\\text{market share}\end{matrix}\right\}$$

The inpatient and outpatient fractions of the surgical procedure can be determined from history, and the sums of all procedures will be the demand for the facilities.

For CSS demand arising from inpatients, the model is modified. The population becomes the anticipated number of admissions potentially needing the service (usually counts of specific diseases and conditions), and the incidence rate is the percentage of patients in the category likely to order the service. The market share is 1.0 within the inpatient population:

$$\left\{\begin{matrix}\text{Inpatient}\\\text{pharmacy}\\\text{demand}\end{matrix}\right\} = \left\{\begin{matrix}\text{Inpatient}\\\text{admissions}\end{matrix}\right\} * \left\{\begin{matrix}\text{Number of}\\\text{prescriptions/}\\\text{admission}\end{matrix}\right\}$$

The numbers on the right hand side of the equation must be forecast several years into the future. They are usually supplied from the institution's information base, using historical and comparative sources. The demand forecast is translated into a business plan for the CSS which provides forecasts of staff requirements by skill level, supply requirements, and facility requirements. These are translated into expected costs and unit costs. The unit costs can be compared to benchmarks and competitive data. Annual volumes can be compared to quality minimums. The final decision should be negative whenever quality is threatened and positive when both cost and quality comparisons are favorable.

With the radical changes that are occurring in healthcare today, many CSSs face falling demand trends. It will be necessary to close some services in many healthcare organizations. The planning process identifies the necessary downsizing, allowing an orderly reduction of resources. Executive managers must assist CSS in meeting the changes. There is a large gray area in which the continuation of the service depends on achieving minimum costs and attractive service. The competitive position of the institution as a whole is involved. Outsourcing and collaborative arrangements become realistic possibilities and must be evaluated. The final decision must be made at a governance level. The issue is discussed in Chapter 12.

Managing Amenities and Marketing CSSs

CSSs are in constant contact with both physicians and patients. Their success depends on maintaining the largest possible volume, and volume in turn depends on the ability to provide prompt, reliable, appropriate, and comfortable service.

Patient and physician amenities

All the eight functions can be viewed as marketing efforts to encourage doctors to select the service over competing alternatives. High quality, counseling on appropriateness, good scheduling, effective planning and budgeting are all aimed at making each CSS optimally attractive to patients and physicians. These will not succeed unless patients leave feeling well treated, willing to recommend the service to their friends, and willing to seek it out if they need it again.

Most CSSs have three types of competitors: units of other healthcare organizations, freestanding services, and doctors' offices. Patient amenities include scheduling, discussed separately below, and conveniences of access, such as parking, and attractive, comfortable surroundings. These factors are usually assessed by routine patient surveys. High percentages of satisfaction are anticipated and achieved. For laboratories, convenience usually means routine collection of specimens from doctors' offices, so that the patient has no travel requirement. Most other CSSs must limit waits, provide convenient sites and hours, and maintain comfortable surroundings. The attitude of CSS workers at all levels is often more important than the physical environment. Many patients are under stress because of their disease or problem. They are grateful for kindness and reassurance and are loyal to organizations that provide them. This means that all CSS personnel need training in sensitivity to patient reactions.

Physician amenities include advice and prompt reporting. They also include collaboration to improve patient satisfaction. Direct electronic communication with physicians' offices is becoming more common. It can be used to verify insurance coverage, ensure that the physician's order is complete, communicate special needs, and report promptly and efficiently on results.

Paper orders and reports are slow and costly, and telephone is inefficient and generates no permanent record. Both paper and telephone are subject to loss and misinterpretation. The goal is a system in which the doctor can order a test or treatment by a single keystroke, transmit all the necessary supporting information, be reminded of all procedural requirements, and get a scheduled date that can be confirmed immediately by the patient. He or she would then receive the results electronically as soon as the procedure is complete. Voice and face-to-face communication would be reserved for specific patient problems and discussions of improvements.

Collaboration with physicians on CSS availability

Competition between CSSs and physicians deserves special consideration. Many elementary CSSs can be performed in the physician's office.[14,15] Doing them there is often cheaper and almost always the most convenient to the patient. The objection is that quality standards are not met and errors add to the cost of care. These can often be overcome by specifying methods and training personnel. The site remains the cheapest, quickest, and most convenient for both patient and doctor. Healthcare organizations must negotiate the profile of their CSSs with their physicians in an effort to create an attractive joint offering for patients. The CSSs will emphasize the rarer and more expensive services. The doctor's office will provide any service that meets quality standards and is not cheaper to do at the CSS. Unfortunately, the concept is simpler than the application.[16] An important part of protocol development includes agreement on the site for minor CSSs and a deliberate effort to eliminate duplication, unreliable results, and unnecessary costs.

Promotion and sales of CSSs

A few CSSs where the customer has a choice of provider once the physician has made the order can benefit from direct patient advertising. Pharmacy and durable medical equipment suppliers are the most common examples. It is considered unethical for physicians to direct patients to a particular supplier unless they have an explicit contractual relationship to do so, such as being employed by the same organization or being in the same HMO. (The ethical issues are one of possible hidden gain or conflict of interest between the patient's needs and the success of a particular supplier, and one of restraint of trade. A physician should not advise patients on cost or convenience tradeoffs they are capable of making themselves.) Well-managed organizations respect the ethical problem and avoid placing their physicians in difficult situations. Advertising uses public media, capitalizes on the organization's relationship to the patient, but does not exploit the physician's relationship.

Promotion of CSSs to physicians and physicians' office staff is important. It tends to emphasize ways of maintaining efficient, high-quality relationships. Newsletters, personal contacts, and service assistants are used. There are ethical constraints; any activity that offers a reward to physicians or their personnel in return for CSS referrals is unethical, unless it is part of a savings-oriented managed care plan.

CSSs are increasingly sold as part of integrated contracts with HMOs, PPOs, and self-insured groups. Most healthcare organizations must solicit these sales to maintain a cost-effective total volume. Evidence of quality and satisfaction is important to these group buyers, but price is often the determining factor. For those selecting a fee-for-service payment mechanism, most healthcare organizations offer a variety of discounts in addition to their publicly posted price. The price is an important issue in determining costs. Managers of clinical service departments now understand the issues of price setting as described in Chapter 12 as a guide to cost constraints.

Patient Scheduling

Timing of the clinical support services is often critical and rarely irrelevant. Although delay is rarely fatal, it always reduces quality. The patient seeks prompt attention and rapid recovery. An extra day of illness is a loss of economic productivity. An extra hour in an operating room or intensive care unit, or an extra week in the nursing home adds substantially to cost and to the risk of adverse events. Coordination of CSSs is also important. Much of medical care is given in sequence—diagnosis precedes treatment, anesthesia precedes surgery, treatment precedes rehabilitation, et cetera. Interactions between the services abound: certain tests interfere with others, drugs interact, treatments impair organ systems not damaged by the disease itself. The more intense care becomes, the more critical sequencing and timing are. A long list of CSS orders must be completed prior to surgery. Delays in intensive care can be as life threatening as inaccurate reports.

Other timing issues are cyclic. Many activities, such as doctors' rounds, occur daily at regular times. Results of routine inpatient diagnostic tests are most useful if they are reported in time for rounds, usually about 24 hours after they were ordered. There is little benefit to 12-hour reporting cycles, and reports after 25 hours are no better than reports after 48 hours. Well-run support services determine when and in what order services are needed, measure actual response time, and make an effort to minimize delays that affect the attending doctor and the patient.

Two devices improve the ability of CSSs to meet timing and sequencing needs. Final product protocols and care plans are one. These often help CSSs understand their work load in advance. As soon as a myocardial infarction is diagnosed, a protocol like Figure 7.7 can be invoked. The patient's likely needs can be communicated to the CSS who will meet them, even several days hence. Eventually most complex patient care episodes will follow automated schedules from the point at which the protocol is selected or the care plan devised. The CSS involved will have substantial advance warning of demand.

Scheduling systems are the other necessary element. Scheduling systems improve CSSs' ability to meet both routine predictable needs and emergencies arising unexpectedly. As they grow in capability, they also improve in ability to coordinate between CSSs.

Healthcare demand can be classified by its urgency and predictability. Services that are both **urgent** and unpredictable by definition cannot be scheduled; they must be met when they occur. As discussed in Chapter 6, efficiency is lower in stochastic and life-threatening situations because resources must be on standby for an unpredictable surge of demand.

Despite the popular stereotype, most demands for healthcare are not stochastic and nondeferrable. Some are quite predictable, such as elective surgical procedures and preventive care generally. Others can safely and comfortably be deferred for several hours or days. If they are scheduled in advance, much greater efficiency can be obtained. Scheduled care is less prone to error than stochastic care, and it can be managed to the greater convenience of attending doctor and patient. Finally, scheduling permits prospective review of appropriateness. Any question about the desirability of the CSS can be settled during the period before the test occurs.

Scheduling systems work as shown in Figure 9.4. Demand is categorized by priority and is then met with appropriate timeliness. Emergency demand is met when it arises. Deferrable demand is scheduled for a time mutually convenient to the patient and the server. In very sophisticated systems, patients whose treatment could be improved by providing the service ahead of schedule are called in when emergency demand permits. This allows the service to use its resources almost fully. The reduction of variation in work load that results from scheduling is converted to lower operating costs.

FIGURE 9.4
Model of Sophisticated Scheduling Process

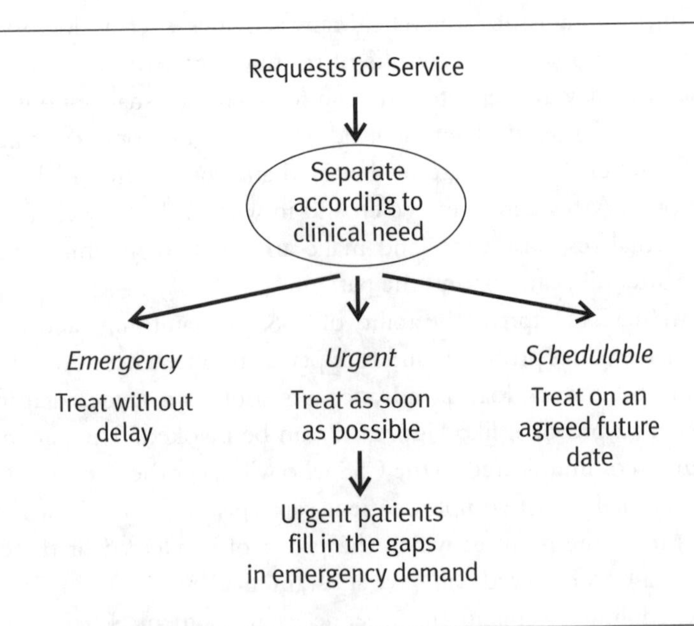

Scheduling requires an understanding of three areas: the nature of patient demand, the availability of scheduling resources, and the contribution of stabilized demand to quality and cost.

Analyzing and predicting patient demand

Scheduling models must be based on resources to be used, usually rooms, equipment, or specialized personnel. It is often necessary to consider several separate demands, scheduling the critical resource for each. A scale of priorities can be developed ranging from "immediate need" to "indefinitely deferrable." Three ordinal categories, called "emergency," urgent," and "schedulable," are often used. The scheduling objective for each category is as follows:

1. *Emergency*—to be treated without delay, despite the loss of efficiency that results. The term "emergency" can be applied to any situation for which first priority service is desirable; it need not be life threatening. The amount of standby protection will be adjusted downward for less serious priorities. As it is reduced, efficiency will rise. If the emergency category is life threatening, standby resources are available, or plans are made to divert resources from less critical activities. All the demand is met, but at substantial inefficiency.
2. *Urgent*—to be treated as soon as possible *without* serious impairment of either efficiency or the convenience of others. The category is appropriate where modest, controlled delay does not impair satisfaction or quality. It thus gets treated as soon as there is no emergency demand. Urgent becomes emergency if demand has not been met within a preestablished time period or if the patient's condition deteriorates.
3. *Schedulable*—to be treated at a mutually agreed future time. Once agreement is reached, care is delivered as scheduled in virtually every case. It is thus quite predictable for patient, doctor, and service. A subcategory of scheduled patients who are willing to accept an earlier date on short notice can be added. This subcategory actually improves efficiency in some situations, and it is attractive to some patients and doctors.

Uniformity of patient classification can be enhanced by published category definitions, examples, education, audits, and, if necessary, sanctions.

The support services differ in their priority profiles. Physical therapy, for example, is the opposite of the birthing suite. It has no emergencies and few urgent demands. The largest support service, the clinical laboratory, faces demand in a different sense because it works on specimens rather than patients and often provides several tests on each specimen. Its emergencies are called *stat* requests (from the Latin *statim*, immediately). It is difficult to define an urgent category. Schedulable is often defined in hours, but it permits substantial efficiencies from batching similar tests.

In addition to the priority categories, it is important to note that demand can vary by time of day, day of week, and season of year. The forecasts for cycles and trends are built into the scheduling system and, in turn, used to establish the required resources and the budget.

Elementary scheduling systems establish an allowance for combined urgent and emergency demand and schedule deferrable demand into the remaining capacity at mutually acceptable dates. They work well in situations in which a large fraction of the demand is schedulable. Sophisticated scheduling systems call in patients from the urgent list to fill in gaps in emergency demand, as shown in Figure 9.4.[17] For example, the office scheduling hospital admissions, seeing that fewer emergencies occurred during the night than expected, can summon urgent patients for admission. By doing this, a sophisticated admission scheduling system permits efficiencies of up to 95 percent of bed capacity, while still meeting both emergencies and prior scheduled commitments.[18]

The more sophisticated the scheduling system, the more it costs to operate. Data and processing requirements expand, personnel must be specially trained, and the costs of errors mount. However, well-designed systems are capable of 20 to 30 percent improvements in efficiency of use of fixed resources. 19 They also reduce variation, so labor needs are more stable and more easily predicted. This allows more predictable work schedules for employees and simplifies employee scheduling. Stable work flow reduces errors that result in repeat services. Predictable reporting reduces unnecessary emergencies or stat requests. Finally, they allow both doctors and patients to plan their activities. Except in cases in which danger or discomfort is high, a timely, reliable date is preferable to an unpredictable delay.[20]

Sophisticated automated scheduling systems are available for major support services and for admission and occupancy management. These programs keep records, print notices, and provide real-time prompts to scheduling personnel. They automatically monitor cancellations, overloads, work levels, and efficiency. They are integrated with ordering and reporting systems, so that the entire process of obtaining a CSS is automatic from the point of the doctor's decision to order it. Most scheduling systems can also be operated in a simulation mode to analyze the costs and benefits of alternative strategies. Simulation outputs are useful in both short-term and long-term planning to evaluate potential improvements in demand categorization, resource availability, and scheduling rules.

Continuous Improvement

CSSs participate actively in cross-functional teams to generate final product protocols and other general improvements in the organization.[21] They must also seek internal improvement opportunities, analyze them, and develop the best for implementation.[22] A key role of the CSS leader or manager is to stimulate specific initiatives that will change processes and generate improvements.[23,24] The initiatives are ongoing but ideally are coordinated with the budget process so that each year's efforts will culminate in measurable improvements in the budget parameters. The improvement opportunities stem from five major sources, as shown in Figure 9.5.[25] Monitoring the six dimensions of performance can reveal areas for improvement. External data from competitors or benchmarking may reveal an opportunity. New clinical technology can mean that an entire new process is required. Similarly, changes in the patient management guidelines usually require changes in the CSS. New equipment or the opportunity to replace old equipment often requires evaluation and detailed planning to get the best results from the new installation.

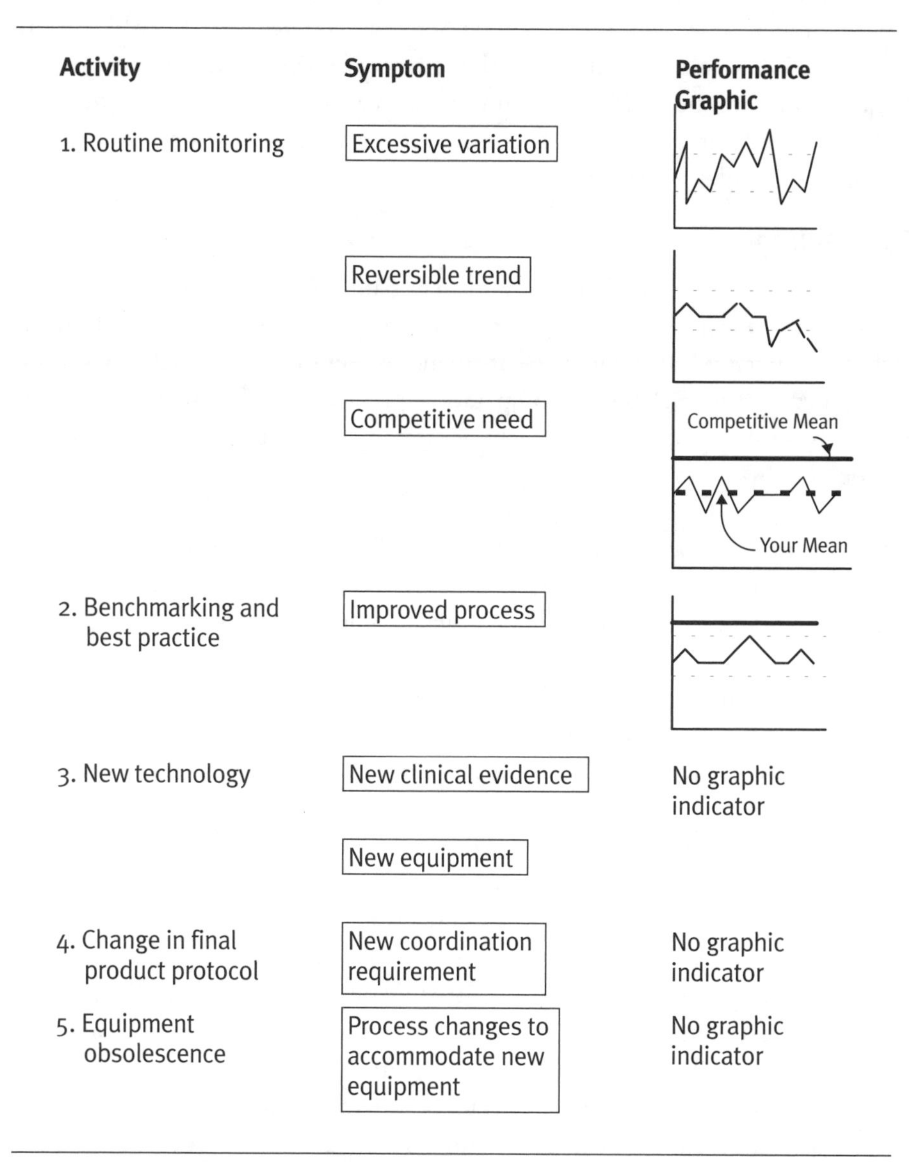

FIGURE 9.5 Sources of CSS Improvement Proposals

The internal initiatives themselves center on the intermediate product protocols. Revisions can improve quality, cost, patient satisfaction, physician satisfaction, or worker satisfaction. In some cases, they can promote an expanded market. The annual budget process and the reliance on six dimensions of measurement keep initiatives realistic. Any new process must not only improve an important measure of performance, but it must also satisfy all other performance constraints imposed by the market.

The best managed CSSs seek continuous improvement by using members of the unit as project teams. The group as a whole or designated subgroups study improvement opportunities constantly throughout the year. Consultation is available from planning, marketing, finance, and information services to help the groups develop new processes. Successes can be put on line immediately, but their real impact is to permit new expectations for the next budget cycle. The improvement activity becomes a part of the culture of the CSS. No one expects to do the same thing forever; rather, they expect that change will be continuous, and that they will participate in it. The sense of change and improvement becomes one of the rewards for working in a well-managed organization.

Budgeting

CSSs must establish their needs and negotiate a budget that allows the institution to meet guidelines approved by the governing board. CSS budgets should explicitly address all six performance dimensions. External and internal constraints, a formal budget preparation process, continuous improvement initiatives, and a method of reaching agreement are part of the budgeting process.

Constraints Constraints on productivity, quality, and satisfaction are essential; they are used as a basis for setting future expectations. External benchmark and competitor data should be used wherever possible. Comparative databases that show the CSS performance of similar healthcare organizations,[26] competitor data if available, and performance of freestanding CSSs are important. Internal constraints are often necessary to achieve organization-wide goals as healthcare organizations strive to meet global and capitation standards. These are justifiable when they do not exceed benchmarks, but they are more contentious. The CSSs will argue for advantage over each other. Exceeding a benchmark is dangerous, unless previous study has revealed a substantial improvement in processes that make the breakthrough realistic.

Constraints, history, and continuous improvement are all considered in setting the specific expectations for the coming year, as shown in Figure 9.6. The resulting expectations usually differ from the constraints. Reaching benchmark can be spread over several years, for example. A different pattern of cost/quality/satisfaction tradeoffs may be more appropriate to the local situation. Changes caused by patient management protocols may create temporary high-cost situations. Some CSSs may be continued indefinitely as high-cost, low-volume operations because the service is felt to be essential to the institution as a whole. Each of these compromises carries business risks of its own, however. The nature and extent of the risks should be clear to the CSS itself; in the long run, CSSs that thrive must find ways to meet the constraints.

Success begins with the strategic plan. Properly sized units can meet external comparisons. Continuous improvement projects reveal the opportunities and develop them in advance of the budget cycle. A unit that has been diligent in the preceding year will be able to formulate next year's budget quickly, drawing in large part on work that has already been done in continuous improvement. A few CSSs will need to ask for exceptions. These will be temporary, and unforeseen gains in others will be available to fund justified requests.

Roles of participants

Well-run organizations have clearly defined budget process roles for the CSS, the budget manager (a technical support person or office attached to finance), and the line supervisor.

The CSS manager and team are expected to:[27]

- Identify changes in the scope of services and the operating budget arising from the patient management protocol development, continuous improvement, and capital budgeting processes. Minor changes are incorporated in the operating budget. Major ones are addressed in the capital and new programs budget, discussed below.
- Review progress in quality, satisfaction, and appropriateness, setting improved expectations for the coming year.
- Review the demand forecasts prepared by the budget manager, extending them to the specific levels required in the department and suggesting modifications based on their knowledge of the local situation.

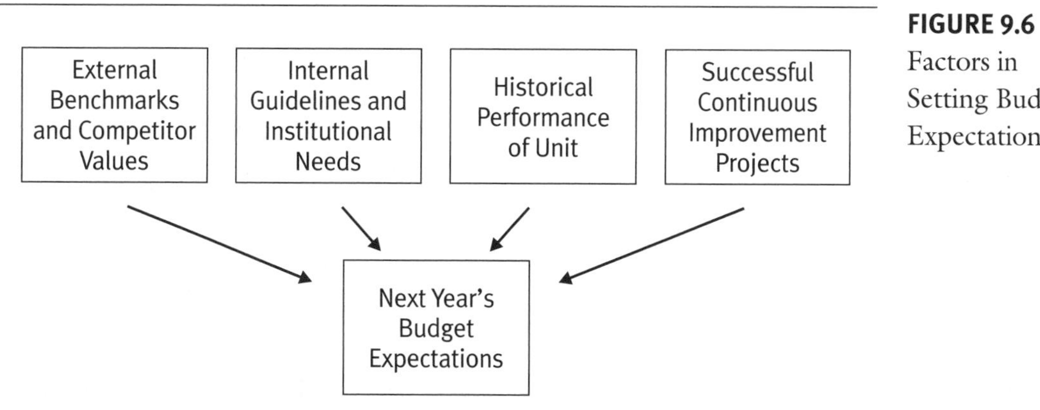

FIGURE 9.6 Factors in Setting Budget Expectations

- Propose expectations for staffing, labor productivity, and supplies consistent with demand forecasts and constraints.
- Identify initiatives that should be developed during the coming year.

The budget manager is expected to:

- Assemble historical data on achievement of last year's budget.
- Prepare hospital-wide forecasts of major CSS demand measures.
- Prepare benchmark and competitor data.
- Promulgate the budget guidelines for changes in total expenditures, profit, and capital investment approved by the finance committee of the board (Chapter 14).
- Circulate wage increase guidelines from human resources and supplies price guidelines from materials management.
- Assist in calculations and prepare trial budgets until a satisfactory proposal for the board has been reached.

The line superiors of the CSS are expected to:

- Ensure that budget proposals do not endanger quality or satisfaction.
- Assist the CSS and encourage steady but realistic improvement.
- Coordinate interdepartmental issues that arise from the budgeting process.
- Resolve conflicting needs between CSSs.
- Evaluate the progress of CSS to assist in the distribution of incentives.
- Identify interdepartmental opportunities for development during the coming year.

Using continuous improvement initiatives to meet constraints

The budget for a given CSS should reflect both continuous improvement and external events related to the service itself. For example, costs of pharmaceuticals have been rising rapidly. A pharmacy might have to pursue a number of initiatives to keep departmental cost increases at a minimum, and even so it might require an exception to internal constraints. Figure 9.7A shows some of the initiatives a pharmacy might support to minimize the impact of drug price increases. The strategy for pharmacy addresses four areas: price and inventory, formulary, final product protocols, and prescribing habits. Initiatives in each area might continue for several years. Figure 9.7B shows a set of initiatives for diagnostic radiology. Although all the initiatives are aimed at cost reduction, they take a number of different forms, both within and between these two important CSSs. Several in each department require cooperation with physicians and other CSSs.

Reaching agreement on expectations

Although the well-managed CSS invests heavily in improvement initiatives, it may still have difficulty meeting budget guidelines. In fact, the nature of the shifts occurring in the 1990s implies that some CSSs will grow in

FIGURE 9.7
Improvement Initiatives in Two CSSs

Issue	Initiative	Measures
A. Pharmacy		
Price and inventory management	Purchasing agreement Inventory management system Generic drug program	Unit cost versus wholesale Inventory turns/year Ratio of generic to proprietary
Formulary management	Identify and evaluate alternative therapies Control procedures for very expensive drugs	Average drug costs per dose
Final product protocols	Use lower cost drugs Avoid unnecessary drug use	Drug cost per specific treatment groups
Prescribing habits	Physician education, counseling, rules for prescribing	Drug costs per capita Drug cost per specific treatment groups
B. Diagnostic Radiology		
Improve patient scheduling and results reporting delays	Evaluate and install departmental information system	Patient delays for service hours from exam to report
Reduce retakes	Improve personnel training, intermediate product protocols	Count of retakes
Inappropriate exams	Final product protocols Physician education	Disease-specific exams per patient

size while others shrink. Many will face major revisions as the site of care moves from inpatient to outpatient. Thus, an arbitrary assignment of internal constraints across the many CSSs is not an effective strategy. Each CSS must maximize its own opportunities and defend its own needs, particularly in ensuring quality and satisfaction. If acceptable levels of quality and satisfaction require costs beyond the constraint, quality and satisfaction should get priority. The process of developing the budgets for CSSs must ensure that priority. This inevitably means a complex negotiation of conflicting interests between CSSs and usually results in compromises. The negotiation process has several important characteristics:

- Its goal is the optimization of patient needs as a whole as reflected in competitive needs and external benchmarks.

- It includes physicians and CSS personnel who can integrate both intermediate product and final product needs.
- It follows the functional accountability hierarchy, beginning with closely related departments and moving to very different ones.
- It assures responsible CSSs of a fair hearing.
- It offers at least intangible rewards for CSS managers and personnel who contribute to an effective solution.

If the negotiation is arbitrary, unilateral, or punitive, the CSSs will not be empowered to raise and address initiatives. If it fails to address genuine market needs reflected in the external measures, performance will fall short of competitive standards. A strong strategic plan is essential. If the strategic plan and the facilities, information, and recruitment plans derived from it are inadequate, it becomes impossible for the CSSs to reach competitive levels on all six dimensions. Thus, if a CSS falls short of its constraints, the first questions address the effectiveness of CSS operation; the second questions address the size and scope of the CSS itself, including issues of outsourcing or eliminating the service. Finally, attention turns to the strategy of the organization as a whole. Repeated and widespread failures in meeting CSS constraints are evidence of an organization or facility that is undersized or underfinanced for market needs. Affiliation with another organization or closure must be considered.

Preparing new program and capital budget requests

Managers of clinical support services are responsible for identifying opportunities and developing programmatic capital proposals. Technological improvements, aging of existing equipment, and revisions in the scope of service can require capital equipment or major shifts in the expectations. In well-managed organizations, these are developed in advance of the annual budget review and must compete with other investment opportunities. The following discussion assumes that the planning process resembles the one described in Chapter 12. It discusses ways in which good CSS managers identify, justify, and defend their proposals.

CSS personnel are in the best position to identify service opportunities and to develop proposals for those worthy of detailed consideration. They do this as part of their continuous improvement activities. They must monitor technological developments to identify innovations and obsolescence and respond to shifts in demand for individual services. They must also monitor physician and patient satisfaction, deliberately marketing the CSS and identifying ways in which service can be enhanced by changes in services, hours, and sites. They must also be prepared to reduce or close their service if demand is no longer sufficient to meet cost and quality standards. Expansion was encouraged under the payment systems before competition. As a result, many CSSs are oversized, and deliberate reductions are in order. These reductions may require capital or new programs to facilitate the change. For example, an imaging department may encounter declining demand for inpatient x-ray, increasing demand for convenient ambulatory x-ray and ultrasound, and increasing demand for magnetic and emission tomography. Substantial capital would be required to remove x-ray equipment no longer needed, purchase new equipment, and recruit and train staff for the expanded operations. It would prepare detailed business plans for these changes, documenting both the capital and operating cost changes, and also changes in other performance measures, such as process quality and patient and primary physician satisfaction.

Proposals are reviewed by the organization in several iterative steps of increasing rigor and complexity. While the CSS can undertake a preliminary evaluation on its own, consultation should be available from the planning-marketing group. Technical assistance will be necessary to prepare most competitive programmatic requests. The technical issues of preparing the business plan are discussed in Chapter 12. The forecasts must be translated into convincing benefits to win approval and support of the other parts of the organization. Most benefits are justified as quality improvements, cost reductions, or competitive improvements. Completely quantitative estimates of benefits are rare. Rather, the justification quantifies as much as is practical and describes the rest as compellingly as honesty permits. The proposal must then be ranked by review panels, starting within the CSS and moving to progressively broader participation, as shown in Figure 9.8. Only a small fraction of the possible investments get developed as business plans and only a fraction of those are funded. A broad search for ideas must be balanced by an efficient process for selecting winning ones. Attention to best practices and external data are important. As the proposal progresses upwards, its fit to potential changes in final product protocols is also considered.

Quality-related benefits

Although many technological advances are described as improvements in outcomes quality, or contribution to patients' health and well-being, the reality is that most proposals involve only convenience and competitive advantage. Benefits must be compared to the treatment alternative with the next lowest cost.[28] A service that supplements another one that is available ten minutes away has a quality value equal to ten minutes' travel, even if the service is lifesaving. (It may have a much higher competitive value.)

If in fact the proposal changes the number of people in the community who will achieve a more favorable outcome, its contribution can be quantified if disease prevalence rates, population reached, and probabilities of success are known:

$$\text{Contribution} = \left\{ \begin{array}{c} \text{Demand} \\ \text{for a} \\ \text{service} \end{array} \right\} \times \left\{ \begin{array}{c} \text{Probability that} \\ \text{service will} \\ \text{improve outcome} \end{array} \right\} \times \left\{ \begin{array}{c} \text{Value of} \\ \text{improvement} \end{array} \right\}$$

For example, if a new diagnostic process with a demand of 1,000 tests per year will reduce length of stay by one day for one-third of those on whom

FIGURE 9.8
Flow Chart of Programmatic Proposal Review

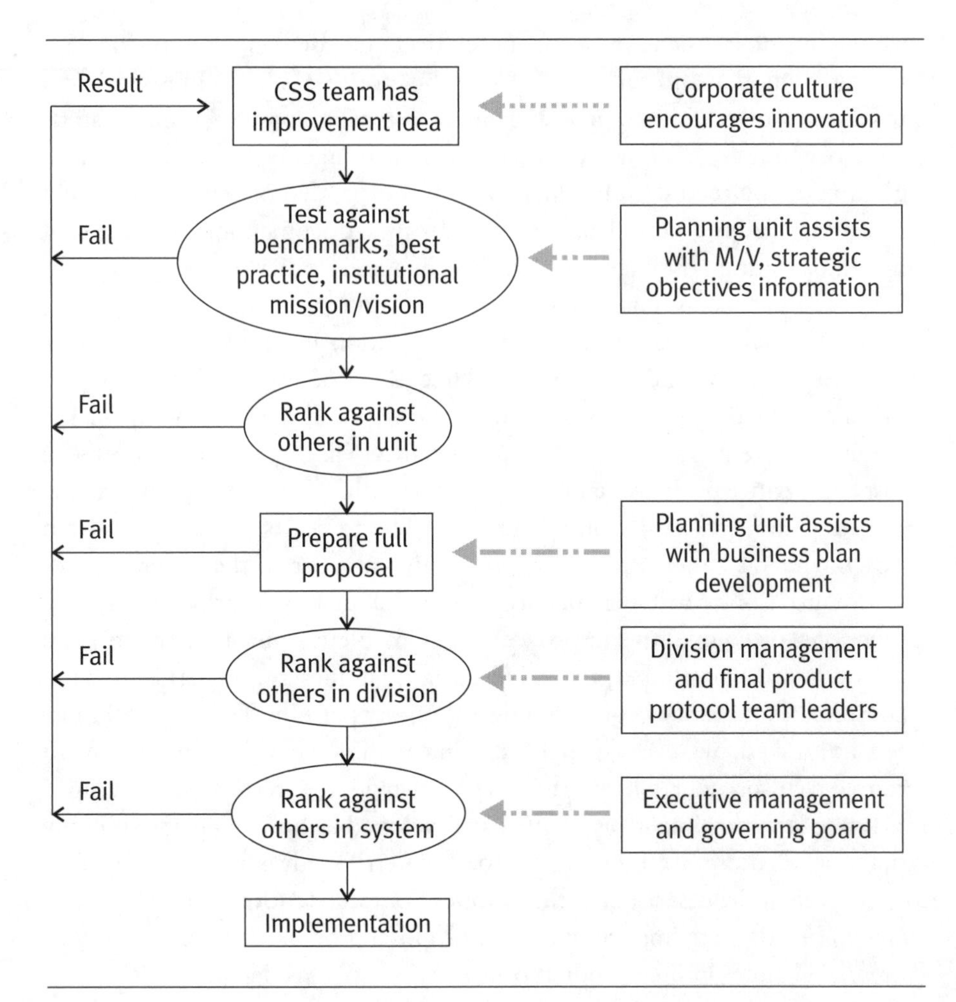

it is used, and a day of stay is worth a marginal cost of $200, the contribution of the process is $67,000 per year:

$$\text{Contribution} = 1{,}000 \times .333 \times \$200 = \$67{,}000$$

If the demand is forecast from the epidemiologic planning equation, only the probability of success and the value of the benefit require new information. Precise estimates of value and probability are often impossible, but at least subjective comparisons can be made between competing alternatives. Then the number of people to be helped and as accurate a description of the gain as possible constitute the justification. Descriptions of the benefit and the probabilities of success should be available in the scientific literature. (Clinical proposals not supported in the scientific literature are suspect, except in explicit research situations. Among other problems, managed care plans may deny coverage to questionable services.)

Quality benefits can theoretically be scaled by a variety of techniques, including forced choice surveys and Delphi analysis. Years of healthy life restored can also be used to scale benefits, but most new services improve the quality of life rather than extend life itself. Income loss avoided helps evaluate benefits, but it is problematic for retired persons. Because of the difficulties, precise measurement of gain is usually not worth the effort; the proposal must compete on the basis of the verbal description.

Cost-related benefits

Because of fixed costs and marketing implications, cost and demand are interrelated. First, CSS costs after adoption of the proposal must be competitive with other sources of the same services. If they are not, the proposal is inadequate to insure long-run survival. The CSS must find a way to deliver services competitively. If they are, a benefit is return on investment, the savings a proposal generates expressed as a return on its capital investment over the years of the life of the project or the capital equipment.[30] (Return on investment calculations are included in most spreadsheet routines.) Care must be taken to estimate all costs and demands accurately, including hidden ones, and to be sure the claims for savings can truly be met. The proposal will be incorporated as an operating budget reduction when it is implemented. The best justification of a cost savings is a prototype for the revised operating budget.

Some cost improvements occur outside the CSS that must support the service. For example, an improved diagnostic test may reduce drug costs or length of stay. In this case, the cost savings must be traced to the responsibility center where they will occur, and that unit must agree to actual budget changes.

Competitive improvements

Competitive improvements are those that improve market share or forestall a loss of market share. Replacing equipment that is critical to continued operations is an obvious, high-priority example. If a modern laboratory must have an automated, multichannel blood chemistry analyzer, and the existing one is no longer reliable, the proposal to replace it will not generate much debate.

A claim that a specific capability will attract or protect market share is a justification for capital investment if it can be shown that the advantage will actually shift market share. The value depends on the magnitude of the shift and the fixed cost involved. The justification is based on the return on investment, calculated from a forecast of the change in cash flow over the project life. Under global and capitation payments, change in cash flow must be calculated at the level of the final products involved or the actual capitation membership. Because only dramatic differences in CSSs are likely to sway people signing up for HMO coverage, most projects must be sold to physician panels who stand to lose or gain income for the total operation of plan. The panel must be convinced subjectively that the improvement is worth the cost.

Other examples are also complicated. The proposal may be a service that has become generally accepted as part of the protocol for a specific disease or procedure. The justification must be based on service for the final product, rather than the operation of the CSS. The budget for the final product protocol becomes the critical document, rather than that of the CSS. If it reflects competitive cost and quality, the proposal is worth further consideration. For example, a special laboratory for in vitro fertilization is a CSS. It can be justified only as a complete service, including evidence of epidemiologic need, evidence of sufficient actual demand, medical staff recruitment, all costs for couples seeking the service, payments allowed by various insurers, and evidence of competitive rates of successful fertilization. The studies to justify the proposal go well beyond the single CSS. As a result, these kinds of proposals are usually considered as strategic, and ad hoc teams are established to evaluate them.

Defending capital proposals

The support service manager and the planning-marketing representative are proper advocates of the proposal in the evaluation process. It is their job to prepare the analysis and the justification in the most favorable light. As advocates, they should be prepared to answer questions and make modifications as the proposal progresses. They also must be prepared to accept rejection. By the same token, it is management's obligation to see that their role as advocate is accepted by others, that they do not overstep the bounds of honesty, and that all projects get a fair and judicious hearing.

The procedures supporting annual review of capital and new program opportunities are described in detail in Chapter 12. Well-run organizations emphasize these elements:

- The CSS is clearly responsible for identifying opportunities.
- Planning-marketing assistance is readily available to develop proposals.
- The organization's mission statement:
  - is used routinely as the guide to rank new opportunities,
  - makes the preferred direction of growth clear to the CSS, and
  - is kept up-to-date in changing markets.
- There is medical review and ranking of clinical projects, and final product teams are fairly represented on the review panel.
- Clinical and nonclinical proposals are judged competitively with one another, in a common review process that includes medical and CSS representation.

Consistency of both process and judgment is the hallmark of success. In most organizations, there is always somebody claiming an urgent need to make exceptions to the review process. A wealthy donor, an unexpected breakdown, a unique technological breakthrough are frequent rationalizations for exceptions. Organizations that yield often to these pleas discover that there are soon enough exceptions to engulf the process. At that point, political influence and persuasive rhetoric become the criteria guiding investments.

One major benefit of consistency is that the dialogue helps the CSS to shape its service to complement others. This contributes, in turn, to an overall market appeal. The feedback to the CSS comes in two ways: through evaluation of its proposals and through participation in the evaluation of others' proposals. Over time, the CSSs learn to identify winning proposals earlier, making the process less onerous.

Human Resources Management

CSSs must recruit, train, and motivate both professional and nonprofessional personnel. The skills of the manager have much to do with success in attracting and retaining workers.[31] The role of the group leader is critical in the unit's atmosphere or culture.[32] Maintaining an effective work force also depends on several more tangible characteristics, such as training, rewards, scheduling, and job security.

Recruitment, orientation, and initial training

Although centralized human resources departments can assist with initial recruitment and selection, each CSS must handle the final selection and attract well-qualified workers. Deliberate orientation programs assist in establishing new workers. CSS members should be trained in guest relations and elementary continuous improvement concepts. Nonprofessionals must be trained in specific tasks they perform.

Much of the recruitment and retention success depends on actual performance. Success builds on itself. A unit that meets quality and satisfaction standards and has high levels of appropriate demand is more likely to attract and keep good workers than one that is struggling. Success also requires strong support from the central organization. These armies run not on their stomachs, but on their databases and information systems.

Cross training of personnel

Many of the CSS professions have licensure or certification requirements. They need continuing education; it is usually purchased from outside professional organizations as an employment benefit. Licenses assure customers of trained personnel and provide economic protection for the profession. In other services, prevailing standards of practice have the same effect. The system of professionalization tends to create inflexible job assignments and tasks, not only among the professions themselves but also among their nonprofessional assistants. Highly specialized personnel can sit idle because they are not trained to provide the specific service that is needed.[33]

Cross-training of personnel provides an important opportunity for cost reduction. Nonprofessional workers can be taught specific tasks originating from several CSSs. They may legally provide care limited to licensed professionals if they are appropriately supervised. For example, a technician can be trained to perform electrocardiographs, draw blood for laboratory analysis, and take simple x-ray films. Such a cross-trained person would be useful in a moderate sized ambulatory clinic or emergency department. Doctors' offices have long supported generally trained personnel. Larger healthcare organizations are expanding cross-training. Patient-focused units train workers to master all the needs of a disease group, rather than all the skills of one CSS.

With proper training, protocols, and adequate supervision, the cross-trained individual will have results comparable to the professionals.

Rewards and formal incentives

Extra effort on the part of individuals and groups should always be encouraged, but the methods of doing so are less clear than one might expect. The most powerful compensations are non-monetary. Recognition, praise, and non-monetary reward are compelling motivators, particularly in a unit where the culture itself supports change and improvement. The sense of a job well done and of belonging to a winning organization are important. CSS leaders and managers play a critical role in recognizing effort and encouraging team members. Many CSSs face grueling emotional and moral pressures related to their work; good leaders often assist with advice, reassurance, and respite opportunities.

Monetary compensation is widely used, but it has recognized drawbacks. Measurement is difficult, gaming (maximizing the compensation system rather than the real performance) is a constant danger, and the incentive tends to become expected rather than an opportunity. The incentive can easily create competition between workers or between CSSs that impairs overall mission achievement (Chapter 16). Well-managed CSSs use monetary incentive compensation, but the contributions to the whole organization are emphasized, and the program supplements strong non-monetary incentives.

Personnel scheduling

Personnel scheduling systems are important in meeting worker needs as well as maintaining efficient operations.[34] CSS workers are frequently women with child-rearing commitments; flexible hours and part-time assignments are popular and increase recruiting ability. Many CSSs must operate around the clock. Automated personnel scheduling systems improve capacity to handle these needs. They increase ability to cover for absences and provide reasonable advance notice of work assignments. The systems require human management of initial work requests and staffing needs, and final review of schedules. They are often interactive; the manager can revise schedules and choose between computer-generated options.[35]

Job security

Job security is an important foundation for retaining qualified workers. It stems from effective organization-wide and departmental planning. Competition will require prompt adjustment of the work force as changes in care occur. The better the planning, the longer the lead time for these changes and the easier the task of recruiting or elimination of jobs. There are six ways to adjust a work force to changes in patient demand:

1. Gain greater output per hour from improved procedures and productivity.
2. Change the number of part-time or temporary employees.
3. Adjust the effective number of full-time employees by using voluntary or involuntary furloughs or increasing overtime.

4. Transfer personnel from assignments with declining volume to those with increasing volume, with appropriate retraining.
5. Terminate workers or undertake new hiring.
6. Use contract, or agency, personnel.

It will be important for most CSSs to systematically use all six. Although the cost of a specific approach depends on the situation, the higher numbered responses are generally more expensive for short-term applications. The costs may appear in training, turnover, quality, or other indirect considerations. The use of agency personnel should be a last resort because of the costs, which frequently include losses of quality as well as premium hourly labor costs.

The strategy of the well-managed clinical support service should be to:

- Develop long-term forecasts of employment needs and limit permanent employment to the lowest reasonable forecast. These steps will avoid forced terminations and improve morale among permanent workers.
- Develop a cadre of trained part-time or temporary workers. These workers may require a premium over the hourly rate for standby, training time, or similar services, but they will be less costly than agency personnel and more familiar with the hospital's needs and standards of quality.
- Provide systems support and incentives for increased output, particularly when it is necessary to meet short-term fluctuations in demand.
- Use overtime to accommodate short-term increases in demand.
- Cross-train employees in several operations so that jobs can be reassigned without loss of quality.

These strategies will require substantial support from the human resources system, as discussed in Chapter 16. For the larger services, they will also require both personnel and patient scheduling systems to manage the complex logistics.

Management and Organization

The larger CSSs are significant organizations in themselves, providing a substantial management challenge. CSS leaders must combine management and professional skills. The history of CSSs has created a tangle of compensation approaches. The complex technology and the spread to multiple sites convenient for patients, and the need to coordinate between CSSs raise challenging organizational questions.

Requirements of CSS Managers

The manager of each support service is usually an experienced leader in the healthcare profession associated with it. Many CSSs—clinical laboratories, radiology and imaging, radiation therapy, anesthesiology, rehabilitation, and cardiopulmonary laboratories—have nonphysician managers subordinate to physician managers. Some services—operating rooms, delivery rooms, emergency services, and intensive care units—have used specially trained nurses as their professionals. They now collaborate closely with their physician counterparts. Pulmonologists, cardiologists, and neonatologists have assumed leadership roles in intensive care. Pharmacists, respiratory therapists, and medical social workers have less direct medical involvement, probably because they serve a broad array of specialties.

These people are accountable for the eight management functions. The range of skills and knowledge reflected in the functions is impressive, from arcane technology to delicate human relations. Not surprisingly, CSS management is a recognized career for both physicians and other professionals, challenging, professionally rewarding, and comfortably compensated.

Beyond their professional training, CSS managers need supervisory skills, including personnel selection, management of committees, continuous improvement concepts, data analysis, and participative management styles. Managers of the larger CSSs often have master's degrees in healthcare management or their specialty. Learning effective management styles requires more than coursework. Well-managed organizations reinforce good practice through line superiors and consultants from management support services, helping CSS managers to grow more effective over time.

Organizing Clinical Support Services

Figure 9.9 illustrates the common alternative structures for the larger CSSs. In CSSs with both physician and nonphysician managers (Figure 9.9A), both managers must collaborate on all eight functions. Priorities tend to be assigned by function, with the nonphysician manager responsible for amenities and marketing, patient scheduling, and human resources management. Physicians manage physicians, both within the CSS and as customers, and deal with the clinical issues of both final product and intermediate protocols. Quality, appropriateness, planning, continuous improvement, and budgeting must be shared. In CSSs with nonphysician managers, there is usually a specific medical committee, such as the pharmacy and therapeutics committee or an operating room committtee, to resolve questions affecting both customers and caregivers (Figure 9.9B). Larger CSS groups can assemble both models under a line superior, as shown in Figure 9.9C.

Integrating Clinical Support Services

Clinical support services vary widely in size and activity. Most CSSs, large and small, provide care in both outpatient and inpatient settings. The larger ones, like the clinical laboratory, imaging, and emergency services, can have more than 100 members working in several sites and at several subspecialties. The smallest have only one or two professionals. Large services are usually

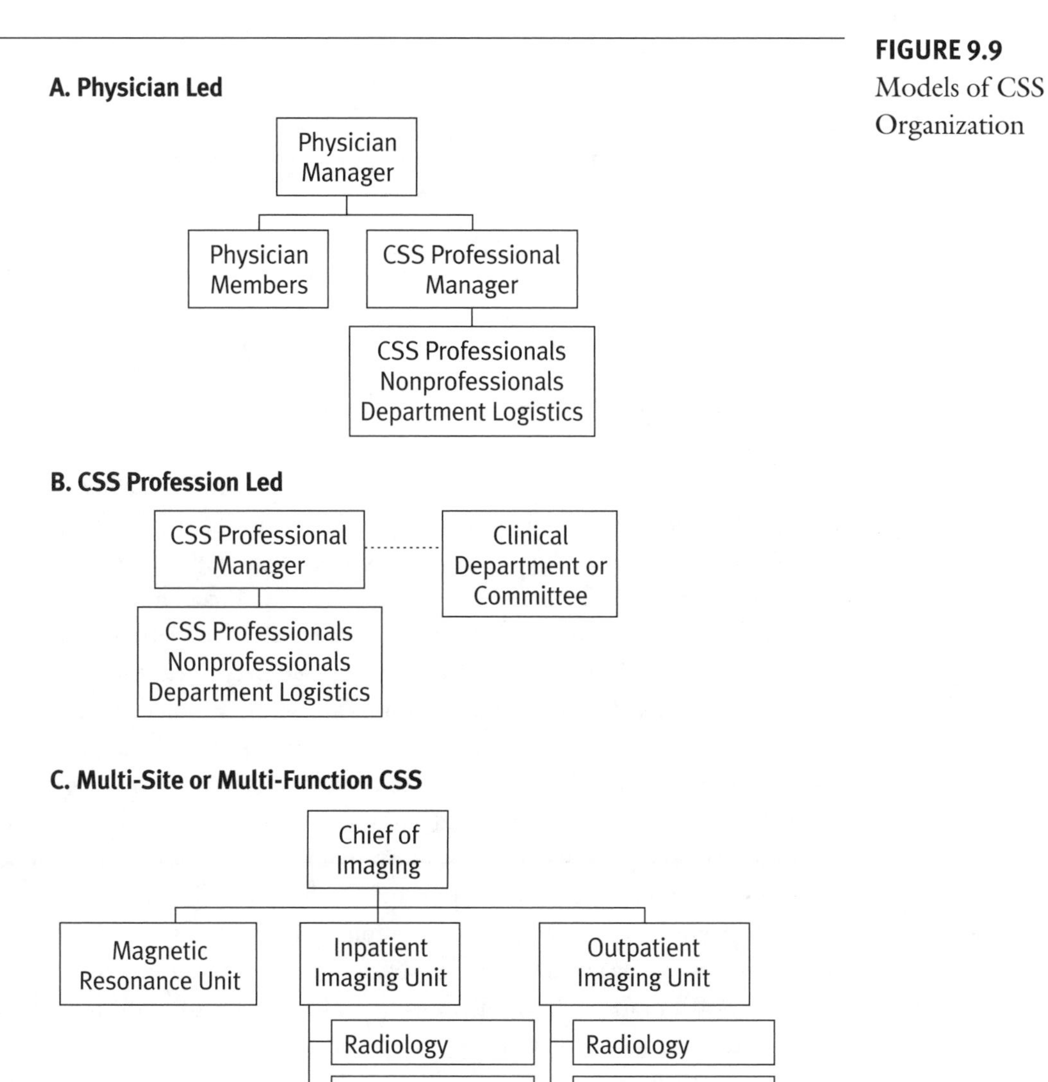

FIGURE 9.9 Models of CSS Organization

organized on the basis of their techniques, tools, or modalities. The less common techniques are centralized in one location; the more common may be distributed to serve patients and referring physicians better. There is an increasing tendency toward cross-training and team structure. Team collaboration allows greater efficiency and is preferred unless a clear and cost-effective quality improvement from specialization can be demonstrated.

Each CSS is relatively self-contained. It should have a complete set of performance measures and perform its own services autonomously, but it should participate actively and democratically in cross-functional teams. Guidance from the central organization might be necessary in several areas:

- relating the CSS goals to the organization's mission and vision, and implementing service plans, budget guidelines, and capital budget priorities;
- ensuring adequate technical (planning, marketing, and finance) and logistic (human resources and plant) support;
- recruiting or promoting a leader of the CSS itself;
- resolving conflicts arising from decisions of cross-functional teams or other CSSs; and
- correcting repeated failure to meet performance goals.

Except in the last item, the contribution of the central organization is supportive, rather than authoritative.

A traditional functional hierarchy such as Figure 9.10 associates CSSs that, for the most part, address related problems and serve the same physician and patient clientele into groups. It places seven group managers below a vice president who would report to the chief operating officer (not shown). It has three steps between the levels of CSS teams and chief operating officer.

The design in Figure 9.10 has largely been replaced by a much more fluid approach encouraging collaboration with service units and cross-functional teams, as shown in Figure 9.11. The new approach emphasizes the autonomy of individual CSS and relies on negotiated performance expectations. Several CSSs, such as birthing and the cardiopulmonary lab, are directly attached to service units. Others must maintain complex cross-functional relationships. Only the more important of these are shown by the dashed lines. Although Figure 9.11 looks complicated, it represents the reality of healthcare more clearly than the traditional model because it identifies the need for collaboration. It eliminates one or two levels of management. The vice president might remain in very large organizations to assist in resolving difficulties arising between the CSS and the service units. Group manager positions are generally replaced by service unit managers. This form requires exceptionally clear objectives, multidimensional measures of performance, and skill on the part of CSS managers.

FIGURE 9.10 Traditional Organization of Clinical Support Services

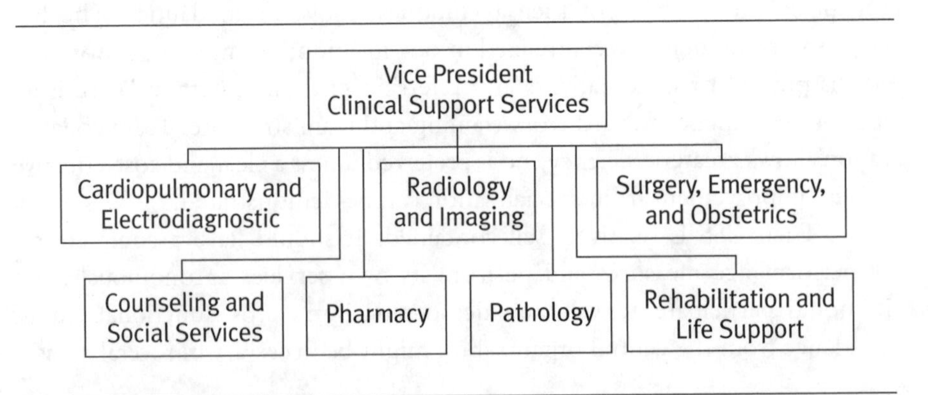

FIGURE 9.11 Emerging Organization of Clinical Support Services

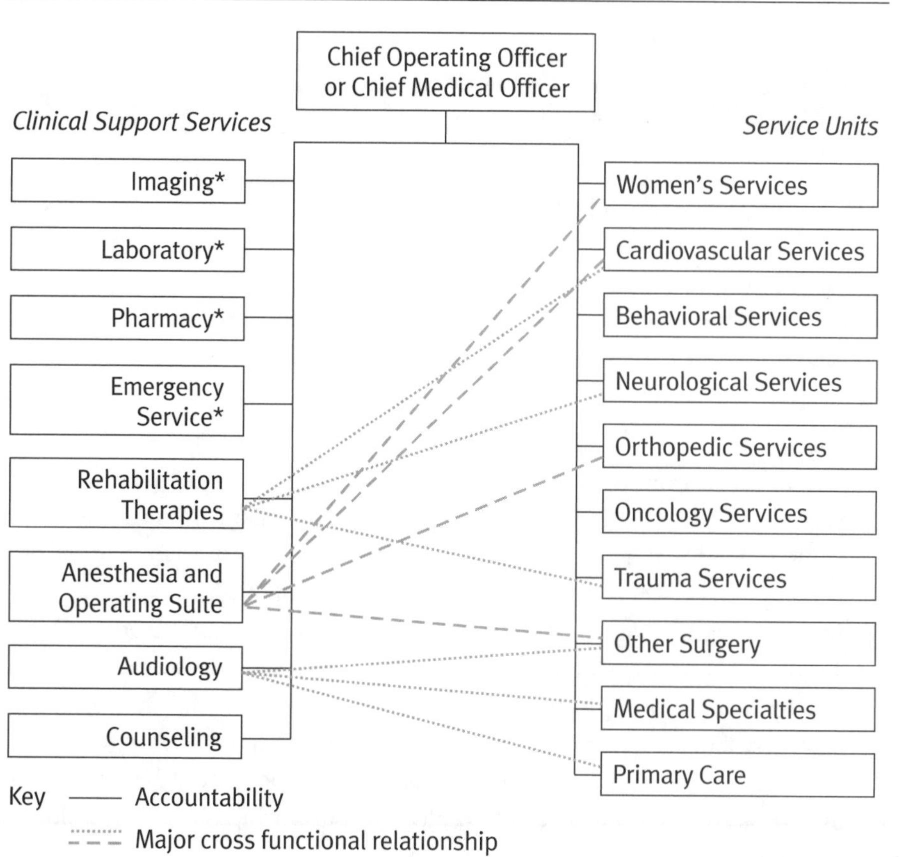

*Imaging, Lab, Pharmacy, and Emergency Service serve all service units.

Compensation of Support Service Personnel

CSS professionals often command high compensation and a wide variety of compensation mechanisms have developed over several decades. Method and amount of compensation of hospital-based physician specialists are recurring topics in the management of support services. Although it gets less attention, the subject of compensation for nonmedical professionals leading these services is also important.

Compensation for managers in an effective organization should meet two general criteria, and hospital-based physician specialists and CSS managers are no exception:

1. Compensation should equal long-run economic opportunities for similar positions elsewhere. That is, the test of compensation is the market. Compensation consistently below market rates will create difficulty in recruiting and retaining professionals. Compensation consistently above market rates will impair the competitive position of the organization.

2. Compensation should encourage professional growth and fulfillment consistent with organizational needs. Incentives to improve performance in directions consistent with exchange needs are part of a good compensation program.

Compensation for physician managers

The historical distinction in compensation contracts for hospital-based specialists was between employment and independent contractor status. Employment compensation from the organization for managing or participating in CSSs now prevails.[36] A third category, the joint venture, arose in the 1980s but is now limited in its applicability to CSS.[37] Each of the major forms is quite flexible, with a number of common variants.

1. *Employment.* Employment contracts include regular payment of salary or wages and participation in benefits. Healthcare organizations are often liable for the malpractice of their employees and insure them as part of their general coverage. Employee status is not established simply by the wording of the contract; it depends on the locus of specific responsibilities. Employees cannot bill patients or third parties for services covered under employment, although the organization may bill intermediaries for their direct patient services. It is possible for a specialist to be both an employee and a contractor, for different responsibilities. Doctors can be established as a separate class or classes of employees, permitting almost unlimited variation in designing the employment contract.
   a. *Status.* Doctors may be full time or part time. The employment contract may permit or restrict other employment or private practice.
   b. *Compensation.* Employment compensation can be by either wage or salary.
   c. *Benefits.* Doctors as employees can be included in group retirement, health, accident, and life insurance. Almost any other benefit or perquisite can be specified, sometimes with important tax consequences.
   d. *Incentives.* Compensation can be increased through year-end bonuses for achieving specific or general goals.
   e. *Limitations.* Compensation in the form of equity tends to be more difficult under employment contracts. It is impossible under not-for-profit corporations. This can be a tax disadvantage for the doctor.
2. *Independent contractor.* The contractor arrangement allows the doctor to operate as a business for tax purposes, changing the rules for deductible expenses. The aproach is very flexible and can offer strong performance incentives to the physician. Variants include arrangements that involve hospital payment to the physician, physician payment to the hospital, and those where there is no monetary transaction between the two.

a. *Fee-for-service.* The specialist and the hospital separately or jointly arrange for payment directly with the patient or the third-party carrier. Such arrangements are not uncommon where the analogy to surgery is strong, such as cardiopulmonary services and radiation therapy. The hospital may compensate for supervisory and teaching services by employment or other contract.
b. *Franchise and lease.* The specialist pays a fee to the hospital, either as rent for the facilities and equipment used or as a franchise for privileges. Franchise and lease arrangements are relatively rare. Barriers to covering the department's operating costs under the physicians' part of Medicare place the parties at a competitive disadvantage.
c. *Shared revenue.* Historically, CSS physicians and hospitals developed contracts involving joint billing for services and division of the proceeds. Two versions developed:
   1. *Percent of gross*, which divides the revenue before deducting the costs of operating the service department
   2. *Percent of net*, which divides revenue after deducting departmental expenses

Compensation of nonphysician managers

The compensation of nonmedical managers is not different conceptually from that of physician managers, except employment is by far the usual arrangement. Although many of the nonmedical specialty groups have indicated interest in fee-for-service compensation, the combination of their weaker bargaining power and increasing public concern over the cost of healthcare has prevented significant growth of any payment method other than salary. Viewed from the perspective of corporate enterprise generally, the use of a nonsalary mechanism is desirable when salaries fail to produce the desired behavior, usually when powerful, specific incentives can be devised. Thus, one might contemplate piece rates or productivity bonuses in repetitive, management-defined tasks like pharmacy order fulfillment or laboratory tests. The useful incentives can be achieved through employment contracts rather than fee-for-service arrangements. Fees are becoming less relevant, even within the practice of medicine, as a result of the growth of capitation insurance.

Measures and Information Systems

Measures for demand, cost, human resources, productivity, quality, and satisfaction exist for each CSS. Many are the same or similar across all CSSs. Others, particularly demand and process quality, are unique to the service. Figure 9.12 summarizes information available to CSSs. Well-managed organizations are tracking more and more of these measures. Under the continuous improvement concept, realistic and convincing expectations are established for the entire set in the budget process. The intent, as discussed in Chapter 6, is to set achievable goals consistent with long-run market needs.

FIGURE 9.12 Measures Available to CSS

Dimension	Measures Routinely Reported	Available in Database
Demand	Trends of major services Schedule status, delays, and rework	Referral and payment sources Detail for study of causes
Market Share	Share of ambulatory markets	Competitor and services, if available
Competitor Information	Services offered by competitors	Detail as available
Costs and Productivity	Total, unit, and final product physical and dollar costs by fixed/variable, direct/indirect	Time, shift specific Unit costs by individual service
Human Resources	Trends in retention, absenteeism, satisfaction Recruitment records	Worker groups, cross training, individual records
Outcomes Quality	Specific outcomes by case group	Patient, referral source, demographic and disease sub categories
Incidents and Hazards	Adverse event counts for patients and employees, safety surveys	Demographic and disease categories
Process Quality	Trends by services, sites, process	Item, worker, time, patient categories
Patient Satisfaction	Trends in overall satisfaction and specifics of service	Time, referral, and patient categories
Physician Satisfaction	Trends in overall satisfaction and specifics of service	Physician, patient categories

Demand and Market Measures

It is important to maintain detailed measures of demand to support scheduling processes, to identify competitors and measure market share, and also to evaluate appropriateness of service. A radar plot of typical measures is shown in Figure 9.13.

Measures for demand logistics

Measures of demand should be maintained in two areas:

1. *Level of demand.* Counts of orders or requests for service arise from automated scheduling or order entry sources. They should be reported monthly or weekly, by type of service, referring source, patient category, and pay sources. Statistical histories of demand trends for specific data groups should be accessible when needed.
2. *Rates of delay and demand failure.* Times to service routine and stat requests, cancellations by source, delays, and services repeated because of failure or unreliable results. Automated clinical service systems collect

all these measures. Statistically valid comparisons against history or expectations are needed in the larger units. These may require additional software and analysis.

Measures of market share

Both market share and competitor profiles are important demand information, but an annual cycle of reporting and thorough analysis would be appropriate. Monthly reports might focus on growth areas or special concerns. The share of ambulatory markets for each CSS must be estimated. (Inpatient markets are determined by the site of hospitalization.) It is a difficult task, most accurately and most expensively accomplished by household survey. Surveys of referring physicians frequently provide useful estimates and can identify market advantages of competitors, such as location, hours, or parking.

The mix and scope of CSSs are frequently important in marketing the healthcare organization as a whole as well as maintaining demand for each service. Thus, it is useful to survey as formally as possible the services offered by other providers serving the same market. Competitor services, prices, and locations are all important for detailed study when indicated.

FIGURE 9.13 Typical CSS Measures and Performance Reporting

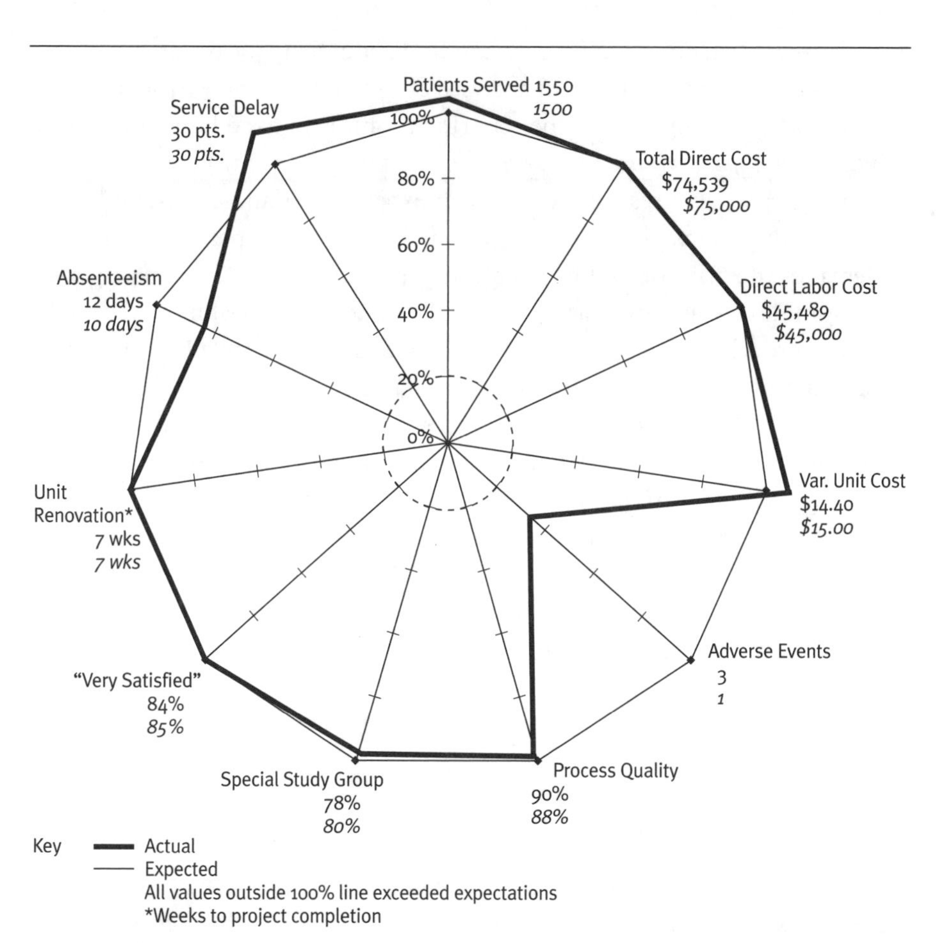

Cost and Productivity Measures

The measures for cost and productivity are collected by the accounting system, but the support service manager participates in determining how detailed the data should be. Issues involving the support service include application of accounting definitions and selection of productivity standards (see also Chapter 14).

- *Account center definition.* Stable groups within a CSS should have their own cost centers with detail on various physical resources and their dollar cost. Revenue by source of payment is useful for some purposes but is not available under global and capitation contracts. The use of multiple cost centers provides accurate detail for planning and for contracting with intermediaries. It also allows small groups to develop their own budgets and accept accountability.
- *Physical and financial direct cost measures.* The cost of labor, supplies, equipment, and contracts is reported to each cost center in detail and used to analyze unexpected results as well as in continuous improvement and preparing new budgets.
- *Cost productivity and facility utilization.* Productivity measures are necessary for comparative and analysis. Selected variable costs, such as supplies or overtime, might be reported monthly in fixed buget systems.
- *Flexible budget variance measures.* Flexible budget systems emphasize productivity measures (unit costs) over expenditures and are useful for CSSs with predictable volume variation. They report variances for the demand, the price or unit cost, and the physical quantity. The manager must minimize all three variances. Flexible budget applicability is limited. The approach is effective only when the CSS can accurately forecast output and has the ability to control resource scheduling to affect unit costs. This usually means the ability to schedule personnel. Few CSSs have either the forecasting accuracy or the scheduling flexibility required.
- *Indirect costs or overhead.* Overhead expectations were traditionally reported as fixed costs, but this provides no incentive for economy to either the overhead department or the CSS. Well-run organizations are moving to "sell" as much overhead service as possible to the support services on a transfer price basis, making the supplying department responsible for the price and the CSS responsible for the quantity used. The remaining overhead is of little concern in managing the CSS (Chapter 14).

Human Resources Measures

Measures of recruitment, retention, absenteeism, employee cross-training, and employee satisfaction are important. They are generally obtained by central human resources staff on an annual cycle. Comparisons for nonprofessional personnel can often be made across CSSs; there is no inherent reason why the reported values for each should be different for different CSSs. Monthly reporting might focus on a particularly sensitive area or an issue under study.

Quality Measures

Clinical outcomes

Leading CSSs are now using disease-specific and procedure-specific patient outcomes to validate process evaluation of technical quality. Outcomes measures for stroke patients receiving rehabilitation therapies include tests of ambulation, activities of daily living, and speech. The specific tests are unique to the patient; a patient with no ambulatory limitation at admission cannot be counted an ambulation success on discharge. Each test is of the form, "Percentage of patients not meeting the goal on admission who met it on discharge," for example, "Percentage of patients entering with speech impairment who were discharged without impairment." While failure on the measure can have a number of causes, the CSSs must collaborate with the cross-functional team to approach benchmark performance.

Outcomes give an absolute standard, but are subject to reporting delays, bias from changing patient populations, and the need for a cross-functional response. The role of one CSS in a given outcome may be unclear, and time lags to measure outcomes are often longer than a month. Therefore, process scores are generally more appropriate for monthly reporting if their relationship to outcomes is understood.

There are many areas in which no outcome statistic exists. Diagnostic services, for example, do not directly change outcome. It is hard to specify and measure outcomes in many diseases. These difficulties mean that outcomes measures should be used whenever possible as a guide toward absolute performance, but they must be extensively supplemented by process quality and satisfaction measures.

Incidents and hazards

Counts of unexpected adverse events are outcomes that sometimes relate directly to a CSS. These are accidents of all kinds, including clinical misadventures. They occur to patients, visitors, physicians, and employees. Support services account for significant fractions of the hospital's malpractice, workers' compensation, and general liability. Data on hazards and unexpected events can be compiled monthly, with a "zero tolerance" expectation. Annual review is necessary to identify trends and possible improvements. Case-by-case review may suggest avenues for improvement more often than statistical analysis. Comparative data are not reliable unless definitions and accounting procedures have been carefully standardized.

Safety surveys can reveal processes prone to adverse events. These are conducted by government agencies, including the federal Occupational Safety and Health Administration and state workers' compensation programs. Insurance companies often offer surveys and private consultants can be engaged.

The surveys can be scored, but they are done infrequently and do not lend themselves to routine reporting.

Process quality

Process measures of technical quality are generally compliance statistics, that is, attributes counts of acceptance against CSS specific criteria. Interim product protocols generate many such measures. Often a criterion is established by the profession and is a subjective consensus, for example, "Is the exposure correct on this radiograph?" Occasionally absolute tests are available, as with laboratory blind tests. The measures often cover a diverse array of considerations. If several dozen are evaluated for a single patient, worker, or setting, a score can be constructed and treated as a continuous or variables measure.

Well-run CSSs are implementing the following steps to obtain relatively frequent assessments of process quality:

1. The aspects of the service most clearly contributing to outcomes and satisfaction are included in interim product protocols. Although models for these are usually published in the literature of the profession, collective review and local consensus on the items selected are important.
2. A survey instrument establishing compliance with the interim protocol from automated information, written records, or direct observation is devised, and surveyors are trained to administer it in an unbiased manner.
3. A sampling strategy is formulated. The strategy identifies how frequently results are needed and at what levels of detail. It specifies a random selection of patients designed to meet the reporting needs at minimum cost. (Consultation with a qualified statistician is usually required.)
4. The strategy is implemented, frequently through automated ordering or scheduling systems, which also support recording, analyzing, and reporting results.
5. Global process quality scores are reported on the shortest horizon consistent with the sample. Data are aggregated over longer periods to reveal information about specific personnel, activity, or patient groups.

Customer Satisfaction Measures

Patient satisfaction

Customer response to a CSS can be obtained through reliable surveys and should be reported at least annually. The cheapest method is a general, organization-wide survey, with specific questions addressing at least the largest support services.[38] Both inpatients and outpatients can be contacted after an episode of care. The questions should be sufficiently detailed to identify correctable characteristics. Convenience, timeliness, and attitudes of personnel appear to be the most important concerns. Questions should be constructed from previously published sources and modified only as necessary for the specific situation.[39] Alternatively, a household survey (drawing a sample of all households in the community, and thus deliberately including patients who use competing sources) can provide information both on satisfaction and on competitor use and weaknesses.

The larger CSSs are used by almost all patients and therefore can be included in general surveys. These are done by mail or phone, with deliberate efforts to ensure high response rates and representative samples. Responses can often be tallied by site, referral source, and other categories of interest.

Smaller CSSs can use questionnaires directed specifically to their patients at or shortly after service. A universal rather than a random sample may be appropriate. A sample with careful attention to the response rate may be more effective than a universal survey. Response rates to universal surveys such as opinion cards tend to be low, and patients with extreme views may be more likely to respond than those who were simply served according to their expectations. Some CSSs encounter problems resulting from their patient population. Operating room and intensive care patients are often unconscious. Social service clients are often chronically ill, and hospice patients are dying. Special efforts need to be made in these cases to assess satisfaction. Often close relatives are surveyed, rather than or in addition to the patients.

Focus groups can complement or, if necessary, replace sample surveys. These involve direct meetings with much smaller numbers of CSS users, usually between 10 and 20. The approach trades statistical rigor for more depth of understanding and is more commonly an annual than a monthly activity. The loss of rigor means that comparisons with earlier data or benchmarks is suspect; the smaller sample and different approach will not yield the same percentage of satisfied patients. The gain is often that ideas for improvement come to light.

Physician satisfaction

A formal survey of referring physicians' views on support services is desirable annually in larger organizations. The topics are usually reliability and timeliness of response, acceptability to patients, and quality of professional advice and guidance. Well-designed surveys pursue negative responses with follow-up questions and comment opportunities to identify correctable matters. Comparison with results from prior years is useful, and survey questions can address the hospital's standing relative to its competition. ("Rank the five clinical laboratories listed below according to your preference.")

The survey should include all possible users rather than just the group referring routinely. A question indicating frequency of referral can be used to compare results by high and low users. Supplementary information from the viewpoint of the doctor who is already a high user can be obtained from focus groups or direct interviews. Anecdotal and idiosyncratic evidence on physician satisfaction should not be ignored. Those services that provide adequate professional advice and guidance tend to hear of problems and opportunities through that process. The formal mechanisms in such cases simply protect against failure of the informal contact.

Sources of Constraints

Cost constraints

If CSSs sell directly to patients and compete for market share, revenue and profits are a measure of success. Such competition is rare; most patients are covered by insurance, referred as part of a general plan of care, and financed through global payment mechanisms. The charge or price for the service is not reliable under those conditions. Even in fee-for-service environments, years of distortion under health insurance reimbursement schemes mean that charges, and even prices paid, are anything but market determined. Thus, revenues are not a reliable constraint.

Most CSSs must rely on cost constraints developed from multiple sources. These should be realistic and convincing, but they should be tailored to each CSS. Sources of information for establishing the guideline include:

1. *Unit cost history.* Cost per unit of service is available from the accounting system. Analysis of fixed and variable cost trends may reveal opportunities and new targets.
2. *Comparative costs.* Comparative cost data are difficult to find and use. Consultants and alliances with noncompeting institutions open opportunities to compare costs, but care must be taken to ensure comparability. Data on physical resource consumption, such as labor hours, are the most immediately useful. Publicly available Medicare cost reports permit study of the relative contribution of the CSS to the total for similar hospitals.
3. *Cost per episode.* The measure can be trended over time to indicate the CSS's contribution to improved final product efficiency. Consultants and alliances can provide case-specific comparisons.
4. *Price per episode or per member per month.* Payments like the Medicare DRG are close to market determined prices, although they apply to an episode of care rather than a CSS service. Similarly, capitation payments are market prices, but they apply to even larger aggregates. Trends and forecasts assist in understanding future operational limits.

The cost constraint or target for a given CSS budget must be established subjectively, reviewing all of these sources.

Quality constraints

Information on outcomes quality is increasingly available from consultants and associations and is being made available to the public.[40] It is the focus of accreditation efforts, and as a result is more standardized. The target for outcomes quality should be at or near benchmark. Although the market implications for continued below-benchmark quality are still unknown, it seems likely that poor performance will rapidly erode market share.[41] The implication for the individual CSS is to continue to collaborate on cross-functional teams toward the benchmark performance.

Process targets must be set subjectively, with an understanding of their contribution to outcomes and satisfaction. When outcomes data are satisfactory, continued effort to improve process measures may or may not be appropriate. Targets should be carefully evaluated in terms of their cost and the real contribution to the patient. Consultants and alliances may be able to offer comparative data on process quality scores.

Satisfaction constraints

Using independent surveyors for patient satisfaction not only makes the results more acceptable to discerning buyers, it also provides comparative data. Most vendors provide careful analysis and comparison. Patient satisfaction should be kept as high as possible. The number of patients "very satisfied," "willing to return to this service," or "willing to refer to others" is critical. Patients simply "satisfied" are easily lured to another vendor.

Physician satisfaction is often subjectively assessed, and valid quantitative estimates are difficult to obtain. Given the importance of physicians as referring sources, a "zero defect," or perfect satisfaction goal, is appropriate.

Information Systems

The information needs of many support services are now clear, and the technology is available to deliver them. All the larger CSSs have departmental decision support systems that not only collect the performance measures but also handle appropriate patient scheduling, personnel requirements and scheduling, sampling for quality and satisfaction, cost analysis, and trial budget development. The list of major components of the information system is relatively long, but several components interact, either with each other or with other services. Departmental systems handle all components on an integrated basis, taking advantage of data quality and efficiency.

- *Patient scheduling.* The level of sophistication is tailored to the individual CSS demand. In the future, the scheduling function will be integrated with other CSSs for both inpatients and outpatients so that a patient with several needs can have them met in an orderly and prompt manner. The scheduling component records historical data on demand by several important characteristics. A forecasting algorithm indicates personnel needs and schedules. The system also reports repeat examinations, cancellations, and delays.
- *Personnel scheduling.* Software recording the personnel available to the department, with data on skills, cost, employment history, and scheduling preferences, accepts short-term demand forecasts and calculates a reasonable schedule of personnel to meet them. Many systems accept individual requests. The schedule is presented to the CSS manager for review and correction and printed in convenient form for each worker. The software is capable of listing overtime, special request and shift assignments for each employee, allowing equitable distribution of these elements.

- *Order processing.* Descriptive data on patients obtained from the scheduling software will be attached to each order for service. When the service is performed, these data will be used to post the patient's account, capture patient characteristics, and build historical files for protocol development.
- *Results reporting.* Results can be electronically reported to the referring physician. In the diagnostic services, prior tests can be summarized, permitting analysis of trends. Historic results files will also be accessible, leading to improvement of intermediate product protocols.
- *Patient medical accounting.* Summaries of support service activity for episodes of illness will be incorporated in a master clinical abstract file. This file, augmented automatically with billing information, will form the historical resource for patient group protocols.
- *Clinical performance assessment.* An algorithm identifies sample patients for outcomes measures of quality and satisfaction, generates the survey instrument and accepts responses to it efficiently. It prepares summary reports and analysis of trends, calculates statistical significance, and provides early warning of departures from important quality measures.

Suggested Readings

A Guide to Performance Improvement for Pharmacies: Hospital Pharmacies, Home Care Pharmacies, Long Term Care Pharmacies. (1997). Oakbrook Terrace, IL: Joint Commission on Accreditation of Healthcare Organizations.

Pharmacy Information Systems: Justifying, Evaluating, and Implementing a System. (1993). Bethesda, MD: American Society of Hospital Pharmacists.

Adams, H. G., and S. Arora. 1994. *Total Quality in Radiology: A Guide to Implementation.* Delray Beach, FL: St. Lucie Press and American Healthcare Radiology Administrators Education Foundation.

Bozzo, P. 1998. *Cost Efffective Laboratory Management.* Philadelphia: Lippincott-Raven.

Kitchell, P., N. D. Landrum, and A. M. Schmidt, Jr. (eds.). 1995. *Outcome-Oriented Rehabilitation: Principles, Strategies, and Tools for Effective Program Management.* Gaithersburg, MD: Aspen.

Snyder, J. R., and D. S. Wilkinson. 1998. *Management in Laboratory Medicine,* 3rd ed. Philadelphia: Lippincott-Raven.

Tonges, M. (ed.). 1998. *Clinical Integration: Strategies and Practices for Organized Delivery Systems.* San Francisco: Jossey-Bass.

Notes

1. A. B. Flood, W. R. Scott, and W. Ewy, "Does Practice Make Perfect? Part I: The Relation Between Hospital Volume and Outcomes for Selected Diagnostic Categories." *Medical Care* 22(2), pp. 98–114 (1984)

2. H. S. Luft, D. W. Garnick, D. H. Mark, and S. J. McPhee, *Hospital Volume, Physician Volume, and Patient Outcomes: Assessing the Evidence.* Chicago: Health Administration Press, pp. 102–4 (1990)
3. A. Donabedian, *The Definition of Quality and Approaches to Its Assessment.* Chicago: Health Administration Press (1980)
4. ———. *Staffing and Equipping Emergency Medical Services Systems: Rapid Identification and Treatment of Myocardial Infarction: National Heart Attack Alert Program.* Bethesda, MD: U.S. Department of Health and Human Services; National Institutes of Heath, National Heart, Lung, and Blood Institute. (1993)
5. K. H. Vydareny, "New Tools from the ACR (American College of Radiology): Appropriateness Criteria and Utilization Analysis." *Radiology Management* 19(2), p. 40–5 (1997)
6. W. M. Macharia, G. Leon, B. H. Rowe, B. J. Stephenson, and R. B. Haynes, "An Overview of Interventions to Improve Compliance with Appointment Keeping for Medical Services." *Journal of the American Medical Association* 267(13), pp. 1813–7 (April 1, 1992)
7. X. M. Huang, "Patient Attitude Towards Waiting in an Outpatient Clinic and Its Applications." *Health Services Management Research* 7(1), pp. 2–8 (February, 1994)
8. S. Y. Crawford and C. E. Myers, "ASHP National Survey of Hospital-Based Pharmaceutical Services—1992." *American Journal of Hospital Pharmacy* 50(7), pp. 1371–404 (July, 1993)
9. T. L. Skaer, "Pharmacoeconomic Series, Part 3: Applying Pharmacoeconomic and Quality-of-life Measures to the Formulary Management Process." *Hospital Formulary* 28(6), pp. 577–84 (June, 1993)
10. K. A. Stern and P. Kramer, "Outcomes Assessment and Program Evaluation: Partners in Intervention Planning for the Educational Environment." *American Journal of Occupational Therapy* 46(7), pp. 620–4 (July, 1992)
11. M. G. Stineman, J. J. Escarce, J. E. Goin, B. B. Hamilton, C. V. Granger, and S. V. Williams, "A Case-Mix Classification System for Medical Rehabilitation." *Medical Care* 32(4), pp. 366–79 (April, 1994)
12. N. Harada, S. Sofaer, and G. Kominski, "Functional Status Outcomes in Rehabilitation. Implications for Prospective Payment." *Medical Care* 31(4), pp. 345–57 (April, 1993)
13. B. Portugal, "Benchmarking Hospital Laboratory Financial and Operational Performance." *Hospital Technology Series* 12(17), pp.1–21 (December, 1993)
14. T. M. Bailey, T. M. Topham, S. Wantz, M. Grant et al, "Laboratory Process Improvement Through Point-of-Care Testing." *Joint Commission Journal on Quality Improvement* 23(7), pp. 362–80 (July, 1997)
15. S. Rosen, "Point-of-Care Testing: Managing People and Technology, A Win-Win Approach to Successful Point-of-Care Test Management." *Clinical Laboratory Management Review* 11(4), p. 225–31 (July–August, 1997)
16. S. Rosen, "Point-of-Care Testing: Managing People and Technology, A Win-Win Approach to Successful Point-of-Care Test Management." *Clinical Laboratory Management Review* 11(4), pp. 225–31 (July–August, 1997)
17. R. H. Edwards, J. E. Clague, J. Barlow, M. Clarke, P. G. Reed, and R. Rada, "Operations Research Survey and Computer Simulation of Waiting Times in

Two Medical Outpatient Clinic Structures." *Health Care Analysis* 2(2), pp. 164–9 (May, 1994)

18. W. M. Hancock and P. F. Walter, *The "ASCS" Impatient Admission Scheduling and Control System.* Chicago: Health Administration Press (1983)
19. W. M. Hancock and M. W. Isken, "Patient-Scheduling Methodologies." *Journal of the Society for Health Systems* 3(4), pp. 83–94 (1992)
20. A. V. Lewis, J. White, and B. Davis, "Appointment Access: Planning to Benchmark a Complex Issue." *Joint Commission Journal on Quality Improvement* 20(5), pp. 285–93 (May, 1994)
21. L. H. Bernstein and F. I. Scott, Jr., "Strategic Considerations in Clinical Laboratory Management: A Laboratory Leadership Role in Clinical Pathways: Establishing the Laboratory's Direct Contribution to the Institution's Performance. *Clinical Laboratory Management Review* 11(2), p. 116–24 (1997)
22. P. B. Batalden, E. C. Nelson, and J. S. Roberts, "Linking Outcomes Measurement to Continual Improvement: The Serial 'V' Way of Thinking About Improving Clinical Care." *Joint Commission Journal on Quality Improvement* 20(4), pp. 167–80 (April, 1994)
23. T. P. Gibson, "Continuous Quality Improvement at Work in Radiology." *Radiology Management* 14(4), pp. 48–51 (Fall, 1992)
24. R. T. Preston, "Patient-Centered Care Through Consolidation of Outpatient Services." *Radiology Management* 16(1), pp. 20–22 (Winter, 1994)
25. D. L. Kelly et al, "Reengineering a Surgical Service Line: Focusing on Core Process Improvement." *American Journal of Medical Quality* 12(2), pp. 120–29 (1997)
26. ———. "When Data Were Scarce, ED Managers Formed Group." *Healthcare Benchmarks* 4(2), pp. 21–24 (February, 1997)
27. E. M. Travers and D. S. Wilkinson, "Developing a Budget for the Laboratory," *Clinical Laboratory Management Review* 11(1), pp. 56–66 (1997)
28. K. Castaneda-Mendez and L. Bernstein, "Linking Costs and Quality Improvement to Clinical Outcomes Through Added Valued." *Journal for Healthcare Quality* 19(2): pp. 11–6 (1997)
29. D. L. Patrick, *Health Status and Health Policy: Quality of Life in Health Care Evaluation and Resource Allocation.* New York: Oxford University Press (1993)
30. F. A. Butros, "The Manager's Financial Handbook: Cost Concepts and Breakeven Analysis." *Clinical Laboratory Management Review* 11(4), pp. 243–9 (July-August, 1997)
31. M. M. Shanahan, "A Comparative Analysis of Recruitment and Retention of Health Care Professionals." *Health Care Management Review* 18(3), pp. 41–51 (Summer, 1993)
32. C. McDaniel and G. A. Wolf, "Transformational Leadership in Nursing Service: A Test of Theory." *Journal Of Nursing Administration* 22(2), pp. 60–5 (February, 1992)
33. E. Ginzberg, "Health Personnel: The Challenges Ahead." *Frontiers of Health Services Management* 7(2), pp. 3–20, discussion pp. 21–2, 38 (Winter, 1990)
34. J. Chen and T. W. Yeung, "Hybrid Expert-System Appraoch to Nurse Scheduling . . . NURSE-HELP." *Computers In Nursing* 11(4), pp. 183–90 (July, 1993)

35. J. J. Gray, D. McIntire, and H. J. Doller, "Preferences for Specific Work Schedules: Foundation for an Expert-System Scheduling Program." *Computers in Nursing* 11(3), pp. 115–21 (May, 1993)
36. G. Roback, L. Randolph, and B. Seidman, *Physician Characteristics and Distribution in the U.S.—1981.* Chicago: Division of Survey and Data Resources, American Medical Association (1982)
37. D. B. Higgins and M. L. Hayes, "Practical Applications of Stark II to Hospital Operations." *Healthcare Financial Management* 47(12), pp. 76–8, 81, 83–5 (December, 1993); J. E. Steiner, Jr., "Update on Hospital-Physician Relationships Under Stark II." *Healthcare Financial Management* 47(12), pp. 66-8, 70–2, 74–5 (December, 1993)
38. M. Zviran, "Evaluating User Satisfaction in a Hospital Environment: An Exploratory Study." *Health Care Management Review* 17(3), pp. 51–62 (Summer, 1992)
39. S. Strasser and R. M. Davis, *Measuring Patient Satisfaction for Improved Patient Services.* Chicago: Health Administration Press (1991)
40. National Commission on Quality Assurance, Internet home page: www.ncqa.org, (accessed July 28, 1998)
41. D. R. Longo, G. Land, W. Schramm, J. Fraas, B. Hoskins, and V. Howell, "Consumer Reports in Health Care. Do They Make a Difference in Patient Care?" *Journal of the American Medical Association* 278(19), pp. 1579–84 (November 19, 1997)

CHAPTER

10

NURSING SERVICES

Definition, Purpose, and Scope of Nursing Service

In the healthcare field, nurses are as ubiquitous as doctors, and about four times more numerous. There is virtually no place that they have not made a contribution. Nursing is almost always critical to inpatient care, usually relevant to outpatient care, central to hospice, home, and long-term institutional care, and important to prevention. Nurses make major contributions to case management, patient care guidelines, and health promotion. Organizationally, nursing is by far the largest professional employee group. Their contribution is clearly recognized by patients. Most people, when asked to evaluate their inpatient care, speak first not of the doctor, but of the nurse. Furthermore, if they think well of their nursing care, they tend to rate the whole experience, even the bill, more favorably. While the patient's emphasis is in some ways naive, it is not entirely misplaced.

The competitive environment has produced a more varied and more influential role for nursing, defined by patient needs and professional skills rather than the site of care or traditional restrictions. The mature profession of nursing has a broad purpose of helping individuals deal most effectively with the risks and consequences of illness. It will pursue that purpose in teaching, counseling, curing, and supporting in venues ranging from well baby clinics to hospices.

Definition

Defining what nursing service is has proved troublesome to both nurses and non-nurses. In part this may be a result of the extraordinary breadth of nursing's contribution. Nursing can be defined by its willingness to undertake almost anything necessary to help the patient return to or sustain independence. The patient need not be sick; nursing services include prevention. The patient need not survive; nursing service is important for the dying. Florence Nightingale saw the nursing role as stretching from emotional support to control of hazards in the environment. She articulated the objective of assisting the patient to homeostasis, a state of equilibrium with one's environment, saying in 1859 that nursing is those activities that "put the patient in the best condition for nature to act upon him."[1] This concept prevails in most of the more modern definitions, which add the goal of independence.[2]

> Nursing is the provision of physical, emotional, and cognitive services that support or improve the patient's equilibrium with his or her environment and that help the patient gain independence as rapidly as possible.

The definition is limited only by the patient's needs and the services provided by others. As the support services grew to technical and professional maturity over this century, nursing relinquished responsibility for many of them. More remains than has been given away.

Purpose

It is obviously better to prevent loss of equilibrium than to try to regain it. Prevention of illness and promotion of health has always been important in nursing. Nurses' work with individuals and families includes immunization, education, environmental safety, and disease screening. For the sick patient, the route to homeostasis includes a nursing assessment or diagnosis, the development of an individualized care plan, and the implementation of the plan by specific nursing care or activities requested of other services. Even for the sick patient, preventing the spread of disability is superior to correcting losses. Nurses instruct patients in adapting to disease and disability, speeding their own recovery, and minimizing the risk of further impairment.

The nursing process of diagnosis and response resembles the medical one conceptually, but the details of a nursing care plan seek to complement rather than duplicate a medical protocol. Medicine's focus on technology has stimulated nursing's emphasis on access, mental and emotional considerations, education, motivation, acceptability, and satisfaction. As medicine has become high-tech, nursing has become high-touch.

The purposes of nursing are as follows:

- to promote health, including emotional and social well-being;
- to prevent disease and disability;
- to provide environmental, physical, cognitive, and emotional support in illness;
- to minimize the consequences of disease; and
- to encourage rehabilitation.

Scope

Nursing can be classified into two categories: personal nursing services, or what nurses do for patients as individuals such as bedside care, and general nursing services, or what nurses do for people in groups such as educational and public health activities. The first is far larger and historically the center of hospital nursing activities, but the second is important in its own right and is receiving increased attention from healthcare organizations seeking to maintain community health.

Personal nursing service

Personal nursing service employs about two-thirds of this nation's 2.6 million working nurses.[3] Personal nurses specialize both by activity and by patient characteristics, as shown in Figure 10.1. Some specializations, like operating rooms and intensive care units, emphasize technical skills. Others, like extended care of the chronically ill, emphasize human relations skills and empathy, but most blend both. All facets of personal nursing require an understanding of physiology, pharmacology, and disease processes. Nonprofessional personnel, licensed practical nurses, aides, and technicians, support almost all specializations. The aides and technicians now are likely to have training specialized for the site.

Historically, most nursing employment has been in acute intensive and intermediate medical and surgical care, the upper sections of Figure 10.1. At present, intermediate care is declining and intensive care is relatively stable. Growth is in the balance of the sites. A leading healthcare organization is likely to have almost all the sites indicated. Many of them will be specialized

FIGURE 10.1 Categories of Personal Nursing Service

Site	Nature of Activity	Common Sub-Specialization*
Acute Hospital		
Operating Rooms	Assist surgical team	Pediatric, surgical specialty
Birthing Suite	Pre- and post-partum care, assist delivery	None
Intensive Care and Recovery	Demanding, technically complex bedside care	Surgical, cardiovascular, and neonatal
Intermediate Care	Less demanding bedside care, patient instruction, emotional support	Medical, surgical, and pediatric
Emergency Services	Wide variation	None
Ambulatory Unit	Direct care, patient instruction, emotional support	Surgery, oncology, and cardiology
Primary Care Office	Screening, case management, patient instruction, limited direct care	By primary care specialty
Rehabilitation Unit	Direct care, patient instruction, emotional support	Cardiovascular, stroke, and trauma
Long-Term Care Facility	Bedside care, emotional support	Skilled and extended care
Home Care	Bedside care, emotional and family support	None
Hospice Care	Bedside care, emotional and family support	Inpatient and home

* Other specializations, such as pediatric sub-specialization, also occur.

by patient group creating about 30 different nursing work assignments. The individuals filling these posts use specialized skills and draw on unique as well as general nursing experience, so organizations would seek related experience when recruiting or promoting them.

General nursing services

General nursing services emphasize prevention and health promotion for the well population. Contacts are often in groups and outside the healthcare framework, although the personal and general approaches merge at individual counseling and preventive care. Efforts are made to reach populations at particular risk, and financing often includes elements outside the usual health insurance structures. The scope of general nursing services is shown in Figure 10.2. Nonprofessional assistants are used less often. Nursing is only one of several professions who can supply the activities in Figure 10.2. Its advantages lie in the respect for nurses among the target populations and in the nurses' ability to relate the specific topics to a broader context of health and disease.

Well-run healthcare organizations have moved decisively toward preventive services, not only as a contribution to their public health goals, but also as a way of reducing total cost of care.

Extended nurse roles

The nurse providing personal or general service in patient care and community settings fills a familiar role. Three more independent professional nursing roles have emerged. One group of extended roles involves more clinical responsibility. **Clinical nurse practitioners** receive extra training for medical diagnosis or treatment. Nurse practitioners conduct patient examinations, counsel patients, manage prevention and minor illnesses, and supervise routine chronic care. **Nurse midwives** handle uncomplicated obstetrics. Both have demonstrated competence equal or superior to that of physicians within these domains. **Nurse anesthetists** are trained to work under general medical supervision.

The second extended role is that of **case manager**. The case manager is a coordinator and overseer who assists other healthcare professionals in finding the least costly solution at any particular juncture in a lengthy and complex treatment. Patients with permanent or long-term illness or disability develop complex medical and social needs. They often require services from several medical specialties, and social services are necessary to allow them to function at the highest possible level. Nurses, particularly those with postbaccalaureate education and considerable clinical experience, are well positioned to become case managers. Case management is emerging as routine for severe workers' compensation and auto injuries, for AIDS and other chronic diseases, and for many aged persons with multiple diseases and impairments.

The third extended role is in healthcare organization management. Nurses comprise a significant group of middle management. Some are **nurse clinicians**, specialists in the problems of certain patient groups. Others are general line managers, supervising large staffs and accountable for a broad

FIGURE 10.2 Categories of General Nursing Service

Activity	Common Subjects	Benefit
General Education		
Prenatal and neonatal education	Preparation for pregnancy, delivery, breast feeding	Reduced complications and infant distress
Parenting and child health	Infant care, home safety, immunizations	Reduced disease, injury, and abuse
Child and adolescent development	Nutrition, learning, sexuality	Improved child health and learning performance
Lifestyle and adult health	Menopause, aging parents	Reduced anxiety, fewer office visits
Sexual expression and contraception	Family planning, sexually transmitted diseases	Reduced pregnancy complications, STD incidence
Exercise and fitness	Diet, weight control	Reduced cardiovascular and bone and joint disability
Self-examination and self-care	Breast examination, home medication	Improved survival, fewer office visits
Chemical dependency and substance abuse	Smoking cessation, alcohol use	Reduced serious illness
Screening	Hypertension, diabetes	Improved management and reduced complications
Social and Home Services	Community centers, home meals, transportation	Reduced institutional care needs
School Nurse Services	Care, counseling, and education for schoolchildren	Communicable disease control, improved health, improved learning
Occupational Nurse Services	Care, counseling, and education for workers	Reduced accidents and disabilities, reduced substance abuse, improved health

range of expectations. It is wise to remember that an acute care nursing floor will involve 50 or more employees, have an annual budget in excess of $2 million, and relate routinely with many physicians and most clinical support services as well as finance, human resources, and plant services. The nursing department constitutes half the work force in most hospitals and is accountable for at least half the expenses.

Plan of the Chapter

This chapter describes the functions nursing must perform in a well-managed healthcare organization, the personnel and organization of nursing departments, the measures of nursing performance, and the information systems it requires.

Nursing Functions

Nursing and the Eight Functions of CSSs

As shown in Figure 10.3, nursing must perform all of the eight CSS functions. Nursing's emphasis on homeostasis, its commitment to control of the environment, and its central role in the care process have given it a unique profile in six of the eight functions. Coordination, both of its own extensive services and between medicine and other CSSs, is an important element of nursing activity. In quality management, appropriateness management, patient scheduling, and continuous improvement, nursing contributes not only to its own services but also to medicine and other CSSs. In budgeting and planning, its heavy dependence on human effort as opposed to equipment and supplies requires an elaborate scheduling and work force management capability. In human resources management and amenities and marketing management, nursing differs from other CSSs mainly in scale, but because nursing is the most visible service to the patient and employs nearly half of the typical healthcare organization work force, the scale is impressive.

General nursing, although growing rapidly, is much smaller than personal nursing. Its eight functions tend to resemble those of other CSSs. Marketing is stressed. The intent of general nursing is to maximize health behavior, making the number of persons reached per dollar of effort a critical measure.[4]

Direct Patient Services: The Nursing Quality Function

The services nursing provides include:

- an independent diagnosis and plan;
- personal nursing care;
- communication with doctors and support services;
- assistance to the patient's family;
- control of the care environment;
- preventive education; and
- case management.

Nursing diagnosis and plan

All CSSs are expected to make an assessment of patient needs. Nursing's assessment is particularly encompassing, including many personal and social elements not often emphasized in medicine. These dimensions are important in prevention, management of chronic disease, and building patient satisfaction. The activities comprising the nursing assessment are discussed below, as part of protocols and care plans.

Personal nursing care

Nursing's strength lies in the breadth of its services to patients. Figure 10.4 shows the extraordinary scope of nursing care to patients as individuals. Much

FIGURE 10.3 Nursing and the Eight CSS Functions

Function	Nursing Implications	Personal Nursing Examples	General Nursing Examples
Clinical Functions			
Quality	Identify and provide personal nursing service and care ordered by physician; support and coordinate care by other CSSs	Develop and implement care plan or protocol; administer drugs and treatments; maintain safe care environment; transport CSS orders, specimens, patients, and reports	Provide accurate, effective teaching and counseling; provide safe, effective screening; identify most critical needs and develop attractive programs for them
Appropriateness	Provide timely and complete service; identify and eliminate obstacles to compliance	Meet protocols; instruct patient on care plan	Identify higher risk, more receptive groups; encourage appropriate use of healthcare services; identify and address patient's unmet needs
Managerial Functions			
Facility, equipment, and staff planning	Projection of future personnel and facility needs; review of acceptable volumes of demand	Plan service size, facility, and personnel needs; monitor employee skill levels and case experience	Plan number, locations, and timing of programs
Amenities and marketing	Additional services for patients and doctors	Family and visitor support; monitor or participate in food service	Maximize attendance by attention to location, time, cost, and promotion
Patient scheduling	Timely service, integrated with other CSSs	Maintain protocols and schedules for each patient; coordinate with other CSSs	Does not apply
Continuous improvement	Monitoring performance measures, benchmarking, and devising process changes	Improve final and intermediate protocols; meet budget guidelines Provide data for medicine, other CSSs	Monitor changing public needs and tastes, revise programs as indicated
Budgeting	Developing expectations for each dimension of performance	Maintain efficient staffing and use of expensive supplies	Maintain revenues or meet unit cost goals
Human resources management	Recruiting, retaining, and motivating an effective work group	Maintain a recruitment plan, training program, incentive program, effective supervision for workers	Recruit and retain effective teachers

FIGURE 10.4
Scope of Personal Nursing Care

Organ System	Example
Physical Care of Afflicted Organ Systems	
Respiration	Postoperative breathing, coughing exercises
Circulation	Ambulation, passive exercise
Digestion and elimination	Dietary consultation, catheterization
Feeding and nutrition	Meal planning, parenteral nutrition
Skin care	Turning, positioning, massage
Bones, joints, and muscles	Ambulation, passive exercise
Sensation	Pain management
Sex and reproduction	Prenatal and newborn care
Emotional Care and Support	
Counseling Activity	**Example**
Reassurance and motivation	Presurgical
Illness related disability and disfigurement	Cancer, AIDS
Grieving and death	Treatment alternatives, bereavement
Supporting general mental health	Stress management
Detection of mental illness and substance abuse	Family support, encouragement of treatment
Psychiatric nursing	Anxiety, depression management
Treatments Ordered by Attending Physician	
Treatment	**Example**
Explicit drug orders	Intra-muscular antibiotic
Judgmental (PRN) drug orders	Pain medication
Other treatments	Wound dressing
Care Related Teaching	
Activity	**Example**
Self-care	Diabetic insulin, nutrition management
Rehabilitation	Poststroke, posttrauma recovery
Infant care	Breast feeding, safety
Sex and reproduction	Contraception alternatives, avoidance of sexually transmitted disease
Home care	Nursing family members
Environmental Control	
Activity	**Example**
Infection control	Isolation procedures
Medical hazard control	Security and sterility of supplies Proper disposal of hazardous waste
Narcotics control	Control of narcotics inventory
Patient, staff, visitor safety	Lighting, floor condition, equipment maintenance Surveillance of home hazards

of this care is managed independently by the nurse, coordinating as necessary with the attending physician and other CSSs. All of it is important. Emotional, educational, and personal care elements contribute to improved outcomes and patient satisfaction.

Family assistance

Nursing shares with medicine responsibility for communicating with the family or other significant persons in the patient's life. Nursing success in this communication is a critical element of overall patient satisfaction. The more stressful the illness, the more nursing attention the patient's family is likely to need. Terminal illness provides a unique and extreme case, and well-run hospitals are moving systematically to minimize the emotional trauma, guilt, and anxiety associated with the death of relatives. When death is almost certain, this effort frequently centers on the hospice, home, or nursing home care designed to make death as emotionally bearable as possible. In less predictable situations, the patient is in the hospital or nursing home. Nursing support for the family is as important as for the patient, for it is the surviving family whose health can be improved.

Generally, the assistance falls into two categories, cognitive and emotional. The family needs a variety of specific facts, ranging from the name of the responsible nurse to care needs after discharge. Well-run nursing units, including outpatient units, anticipate most of these factual needs and provide educational materials, both verbal and written. The broad outline of the care plan is given to the family, including the anticipated dates of key events such as surgery and discharge. This serves a dual function, relieving anxiety and permitting the family to prepare. Nursing shares with the plant system responsibility for treating visitors hospitably.

The key to provision of emotional support to the family is thoughtfully developed protocols that anticipate common problems and provide the staff with solutions. Well-run hospitals are developing protocols for family support in terminal illness and other high-stress events and are incorporating them into in-service education.[5] Such programs include:

- Identifying significant personal relationships:
  - Evaluating the family structure
  - Recognizing important non-familial relationships
- Identifying family stress:
  - Stress-producing medical events
  - Symptoms of stress in family members
- Role of cognitive information in relieving stress
- Specific cognitive requirements for common events
- Professional affect and behavior allaying stress
- Techniques for assisting individuals in stressful situations
- Policies on stress-producing situations, for example:
  - Post surgical notification
  - Terminal care
  - Emergency resuscitation
  - Orders not to resuscitate
  - Assistance available to family members

- Assistance available to staff
- Dealing with professional guilt and grief.

Prevention and health education

Nursing has extensive and important educational responsibilities relating to the consequences of specific diseases and events. It teaches diabetics how to adjust and administer their insulin; heart attack survivors how to regain full activity; hypertensives the importance of their medication; new mothers how to care for and enjoy their babies, how to maintain their own health, and how to avoid unwanted pregnancies; and many other useful programs. If these activities are well done, future disease is reduced. Under managed care, healthcare organizations receive direct financial benefits from their successes in this area. Under any insurance, patient, professional, and community satisfaction is improved. Thus, expectations for patient education are an essential part of care plans. With much shorter hospital stays, the site for education has moved to the primary care office.

Well-run organizations go beyond the disease-specific teaching in the care plan. They educate the patient about the risk defined by existing disease, sex, age, occupation, and other demographic characteristics. Patient-specific education providing individual patients with information they need at a time when they are most receptive to it is an important supplement. General education, offered to the public at large and usually done in group settings, is one vehicle. Support groups for stressful events other than disease (divorce, childbirth, job) have become popular following the disease-oriented model (postcolostomy, Alcoholics Anonymous, hemophilia). Nurses provide educational programs and counseling and organize and assist support groups.

Environmental control

Although Florence Nightingale and her followers scrubbed the floors themselves, maintaining a safe and effective institutional or ambulatory environment is now the responsibility of the plant system. Nursing, however, is properly held accountable for reporting any failure in patient care areas. The inpatient or outpatient head nurse is responsible to patients, visitors, and staff for general safety, effectiveness, and expected amenities in the floor environment.

In addition to general environmental control, nursing is responsible for clinical aspects of the environment. Certain sites—for example, surgery, premature nursery, and coronary care—have become highly complex. Electronic, mechanical, and chemical environments are created for intensive patient care. They are frequently the responsibility of specially trained and experienced nurse managers. Control of microbial, radiation, and chemical hazards on nursing units is a nursing responsibility. Special techniques for avoiding contamination are part of the clinical procedures of nursing. They often involve other professions and usually require coordinated development. Nursing must enforce these procedures.

Certain addictive drugs called *controlled substances* or, less formally, *narcotics* are regulated by the federal government. Nursing shares with medicine and pharmacy the reporting and control obligations. Well-run hospitals, recognizing that doctors and nurses have a high risk of addiction, provide preventive and rehabilitative programs.

Protocols and Care Plans: The Nursing Appropriateness Function

Nursing emphasizes the development of an individual care plan based on independent patient assessment, but the plan is increasingly built around disease-specific protocols such as the one shown in Figure 7.6. The nursing care plan documents the needs of each patient and establishes the expectations for nursing procedures and outcomes.[6] The care plan incorporates a discharge plan. In more complicated cases, the discharge plan is segregated to help coordinate the several professions who must complete their work before the patient can leave. It establishes realistic treatment goals and timetables to meet them, ending if possible with the termination of nursing support. The care plan is developed early in the disease episode and is revised as needed. It is more formal in inpatient and long-term outpatient care and is often left unwritten in brief, uncomplicated outpatient encounters. A good care plan strives to do the following:

- incorporate all care that is cost-effective;
- exclude any care or service that is less than cost-effective;
- anticipate individual variations and prevent complications;
- organize the major events in the hospitalization or disease episode to minimize overall duration; and
- identify potential barriers to prompt discharge and plan to investigate and remove them.

Nursing diagnosis

Each nursing care plan begins with a thorough nursing diagnosis, that is, the identification of actual or potential departures from homeostasis. The nurse evaluates the patient using a paradigm that reflects the scope of personal nursing services (Figure 10.4) and takes into consideration the patient's total set of diseases and disabilities, general physical and emotional condition, and family and social history. Sources of information include observation of the patient, physical examination, patient and family interviews, and the physician's history, physical examination, provisional diagnosis, and diagnostic test and treatment orders. Family views are important, and a description of the patient's home environment is frequently required.

The plan as part of the patient management protocol

The nursing care plan has obvious parallels to the patient management protocol or medical care plan. Nursing will participate actively in most management protocol design. Nursing care plans must be closely coordinated with the protocols, and nursing will monitor protocol achievement. The nursing plan emphasizes physical, emotional, and environmental aspects of treatment as well as disease. The nursing plan tends to be less specifically related to the disease at hand and more broadly directed to the full needs of the patient and may be tailored more often to changes in the patient's condition, because nursing must deal with side effects and potential complications of treatment. If the emotional impact of the disease on patient and family will be severe, the diagnosis should recognize this as an element of comprehensive care and a potential barrier to prompt discharge. Similarly, the plan addresses family and general environmental needs. If the spouse is ill or the apartment has narrow doors, return home may be more difficult.

Even more than the doctor's protocol, the nursing plan can be significantly aided by computer programs. Models for specific diseases, analogous to the patient management protocols discussed in Chapter 8, can be available on computer as a pattern. Components of the care plan can be assembled from standard nursing intermediate care protocols. Nurses can develop a plan more quickly and with less risk of oversight by modifying a disease model to individual needs. They can control the specific content of several thousand activities by relying on intermediate protocols.

Nursing's contribution to economic care

The nurse's professional skill and judgment contribute substantially to economic care. Although the doctor's approval may be required for a specific response, a significant amount of care can be given or withheld at the nurse's discretion. If the nursing diagnosis is well made, patient observation is thorough, and the responses are prompt, necessary care can be given and unnecessary care avoided.

As an illustration, an otherwise well 60-year-old woman with hip joint deterioration will receive a replacement. If all goes well, she will walk that evening and be ready to go home in a few days. Nursing will avoid the following hazards: circulatory complications from inactivity, respiratory complications from anesthesia, infections at the wound site, imbalances in body chemistry, insecurity and anxiety related to postoperative condition, postdischarge complications from poor dietary habits, and drug dependency. Should any of these occur, an expanded course of treatment will be required. The new treatment will introduce new hazards, starting the cycle over. Stay and cost will escalate, and patient satisfaction will deteriorate. Should the patient be older, her systems will be more fragile, and the range of tolerance to nursing error diminishes. If she has an intercurrent disease or complication, nursing needs mount exponentially. Two new groups of hazards must be avoided, one relating to the other disease, the second to interactions between the two. The patient's hip problems create one list; a complication such as diabetes creates a second. Having both creates a third because surgery profoundly endangers the homeostasis of diabetes.

Coordinating with the final product protocol

The nursing care plan is an extension of the final product protocol. Automation will assist in these steps. An automated protocol, an automated nursing care plan, and automated monitoring will steer most patients on uneventful, minimum cost courses to recovery.

Case management

Case management is the comprehensive oversight of an individual patient's care from the perspective of long-term cost-effectiveness. It is emerging as an effective device for very complicated patients. It is used primarily with patients at high risk for very expensive care, especially AIDS and trauma patients. Case management begins with a sophisticated care plan, often developed by a multidisciplinary team of caregivers. The plan identifies specific goals, CSS and medical services to meet them, measures of improvement, and timetables. Nurses often manage the cases once the plan has been agreed upon, working to see that the various servers are effectively coordinated.

Case management is also attractive as a way of providing comprehensive but economical long-term care to the aged. The term first arose in experimental HMOs for the aged called social health maintenance organizations (SHMOs). Effective care of the aged must dedicate itself to lengthening and improving biological and emotional life while minimizing lifetime healthcare expenditures. Although evidence is far from complete, it appears that the best solution is one that guides the patient continuously from late middle age. The case manager maintains a long-term relationship with the patient, one that emphasizes prevention and fitness to the greatest possible extent, treats the deteriorating organ systems thoroughly but economically, provides increasing support as several organ systems begin to fail simultaneously, and arranges the last months of life in response to the patient's own wishes.

Patient and Family Support: The Nursing Amenities and Marketing Function

Nursing's constant contact with patients and their visitors gives it a prime role in amenities and marketing. Nursing's dominance of the satisfaction survey stems from the fact that patients and families see more of nursing than any other CSS and from the supportive design of the nursing role. People expect nursing to be sympathetic and sensitive to human needs. They are vocally grateful when it is and disappointed when it is not.

Patient care logistics are an important part of both care and amenities. The delivery of drugs, medical supplies, and food usually involves nursing. Drugs for pain relief are frequently prescribed *PRN*, when necessary, at the nurse's discretion. Parenteral fluids present a particularly critical challenge, both to cost and outcome quality. The consequences of error can be life threatening. Food is important symbolically and emotionally as well as nutritionally. The patient's ability to maintain maximal nutritional status is often important in health education and disease prevention. Nurses do nutritional education more often than dietitians.

Nursing has a direct concern with environmental safety for patients and visitors in the institution and in the home. Cleanliness, lighting, state of repair, odors, heating, and cooling are part of nursing's concern. Personal safety and security are also part of nursing's general monitoring function. It generally relies on plant services or other CSSs to carry these concerns out in the institutional setting, but it retains responsibility for monitoring both safety and comfort. Nurses are responsible for stopping any unsafe or threatening activity, whether it be caused by an outside agent or an employee or physician.

The amenity and marketing functions are almost automatic in well-managed organizations. They are supported by effective work in plant services and other CSSs, by training for nursing personnel in guest relations, and by executive managers who support the goals of patient and family satisfaction with specific assistance when problems arise and go uncorrected.

Coordinated Care: The Nursing Patient Scheduling Function

Nursing generally coordinates the episode of care, whether it is in an inpatient, outpatient, or home setting. Regardless of the setting, the goal is to organize all elements of care, including nursing care, in the least costly and most patient-satisfactory elapsed time. Patient-related logistics and communications can be grouped into three major functions: communication with CSSs, CSS scheduling, and transportation.

Patient-related communication

During the patient's episode of inpatient or outpatient care, it is necessary to maintain a comprehensive, current medical record for the many services participating in diagnosis and treatment. Generally the information must include symptoms and complaints, concurrent disease or complication, working diagnosis, medical orders and nursing plan, diagnostic orders and results, treatment to date, and the patient's response. The record is increasingly automated. In automated form, it is accessible to all caregivers and is constantly up to date.

The medical records department (Chapter 17) is responsible for the design of the automated medical record as a document, securing the confidentiality of its contents and arranging access among the clinical services. It also manages permanent storage and certain summarizing functions. The attending and house physicians, nursing, and the individual support services are responsible for their own entries into the record, although nurses and clerical personnel under nursing supervision may make entries for physicians.

Nursing transmits orders to services and receives responses back. The cost and time involved in nursing's responsibility is often overlooked. In fact, prior to the advent of computer assistance, communication of all kinds required about half the time of inpatient nurses. Similar problems affect scheduling of ambulatory patients. There are fewer transactions, but more independent schedules to be coordinated.

Patient scheduling

Most inpatient and outpatient support service scheduling is still done by clerks on telephones. The information they get usually comes through nursing, and in inpatient settings the clerks are part of the nursing team. The scheduling must accommodate limitations in the patient's physical condition and competing demands. Most of the services require direct contact with the patient, and many of the services have requirements affecting others, such as being performed before meals or before certain other services.

The support service departments are rapidly developing their own computerized scheduling systems. Coordination of these into a master schedule for each patient is technically possible and can be expected to emerge piecemeal over the next several years. As it does, nursing's responsibility can shift to active monitoring of the automated process and to more effective preparation for each patient. Substantial reductions in clerical personnel appear feasible. Quality will be enhanced as oversights and conflicts are eliminated. The advance schedule permits prospective review of compliance with the patient group protocol, even though it may be only a few hours before the events are to take place. A reduction in duplicated and spoiled tests and orders can be expected. Prompt fulfillment of scheduled orders also reduces stat requests.

Patient transportation

Nursing is also responsible for the safe transportation of inpatients. Although many outpatients can follow guidance from plant services to reach the various clinical support services, inpatients are frequently impaired by their illness and must be moved by hospital personnel. The task is time consuming but important to patient satisfaction. Employees who do it are usually unskilled and may be supplied by a unit of plant services (Chapter 15). They should be trained both in guest relations and in handling the medical emergencies that may arise while the patient is in transit.

Staffing: The Nursing Planning and Budgeting Functions

Nursing units like other responsibility centers should prepare annual budgets covering all six dimensions of effective performance and longer range plans for major resource requirements. Because up to 90 percent of nursing costs are labor costs, staffing decisions and personnel scheduling become a critical function in cost control. They are also critical to quality; too few nurses cause the care processes to break down and outcomes to deteriorate. Finally, staffing and scheduling are important in human resources management; nursing personnel appreciate predictable work schedules, choice of time off, and flexible working arrangements that require automated scheduling systems. A three-step staffing, scheduling, and assignment process moves toward progressively shorter time horizons:

1. *Staffing* decisions establish the number of professional, technical, and clerical nursing employees required for each nursing floor or unit. The results of staffing decisions establish scheduling and daily assignment requirements and set the nursing expense budget. Combined with forecasts of patient demand they generate long-range personnel plans.
2. *Scheduling* decisions develop plans for daily availability of personnel and establish the work schedules of individuals over horizons of a few weeks.
3. *Assignment* decisions adjust shift-by-shift variation in personnel requirements of each floor.

Staff modeling, planning, and budgeting

Conceptually, a well-designed staffing plan is based on expectations of what activities nursing will perform, how frequently these will occur, what indications support them, and what outcomes in quality, efficiency, and economy are anticipated. Decisions about the nurses needed for outpatient care are easy to comprehend and can serve as a model for the vastly more complicated inpatient staffing decisions. For example, a small clinic decides to staff day shifts Monday through Friday with two classes of personnel, licensed practical nurse (LPN) and clerk, a level historically sufficient to provide satisfactory service. This decision sets the budget—two FTEs—and establishes the scheduling that must occur. If the staffing were upgraded to one registered nurse (RN) and a clerk, one would expect greater nursing responsibilities and more procedures, such as an increase in patient education. Further, one would expect the clinic to attract more patients, or to care for them with less hospitalization, or to be more satisfactory to patients and doctors, or in some way to show a measurable improvement for the increased cost.

Similarly, an inpatient unit might have a staff of 25 or 30 nursing FTEs with various skills. Adding staff or increasing skill levels would be undertaken to shorten length of stay, improve outcomes, or improve patient or physician satisfaction. Staff would be reduced to save costs, if it could be done without impairing those measures.

The personnel budget is derived directly from staffing policies. Fixed personnel budgets establish expectations for monthly consumption of nursing in total hours and total costs. They are used in many settings where demand does not vary, such as outpatient clinics and long-term care, and where demand cannot be predicted, such as obstetrics and intensive cardiac care inpatient units. Flexible labor budgets set the expectation in a productivity ratio, like hours/patient day. They assume that short-term variation in patient demand will be met by changes in schedule and assignment. The best real nursing budgets have a fixed component and a flexible component. All supplies and some labor costs vary with patient census and acuity (individual patient need) and are in the flexible component.

Inpatient nurse staffing decisions are made for each floor and shift. They establish the number and mix of personnel (baccalaureate, registered, and practical nurses, nurse aides, and clerks) required for the expected range of acuity and census. Patient requirements are radically different in long-term care, intensive care, the emergency room, and the recovery room. In many of these areas, requirements differ by day of week and by random variation in patient arrivals and acuity. Team approaches are aimed at reducing costs by substituting less skilled personnel under the supervision of professional nurses.[7] The desired staff for a nursing unit and shift is usually expressed in a table, such as Figure 10.5.

The solution in the figure treats staffing as an integer problem, making no changes smaller than eight hours, or one full shift. The table keeps staffing between 3.9 and 4.0 hours per patient, and between 40 and 45 percent RN level or better. Staffing for odd numbered censuses is the same as preceding even numbers; hours per patient day drops to about 3.9. Shading shows the changes as census varies. At extreme lows, few and not very sick patients, only 20 FTEs will be needed; when the floor is full and patients are very sick, 30 FTEs will be needed. Given weekends, holidays, and random fluctuation, a typical inpatient unit can be expected to vary over at least this large a range over a year. (The acuity weighting is discussed below.)

The same computer aids that develop the work assignments generate the forecasts of census and acuity necessary for budgeting. Most software programs have simulation features, which allow evaluation of alternative strategies. The labor expense budget is determined almost automatically once the staffing pattern and the forecasts of demand are selected.

Evaluating individual patient need

The demand for nursing care is a function of two elements: the **census**, or number of patients, and how sick they are. Sicker patients require more nursing care. There are two approaches to weighting. Acuity weighting is based on an assessment of the patient's condition. Care planning draws on the time required for individual elements of the care plan. Under either approach, patient needs are expressed as a percentage of a standard patient. A patient with twice average needs would count as two standard patients in a weighted census.

Acuity approaches use binary or simple ordinal scales indicating departure from normal function in several physiological and psychological factors known to influence nursing time.[8] Items include therapeutic and diagnostic needs as well as those involving eating, dressing, and elimination; the emotional state; and the amount of observation ordered by the doctor. Values for each patient are assessed subjectively and reported by the head nurse. A patient with a high score requires increased nursing care. Representative acuity

FIGURE 10.5 Example of Nurse Staffing Model for Inpatient Floor*

Weighted Patient Census	Head Nurse	BSN Team Leader	RN	LPN	Aide	Clerk	Total Hours	Hours/ Weighted Census	Percent RN
40	8	32	32	16	56	16	160	4.00	45%
42	8	32	32	16	64	16	168	4.00	43
44	8	32	32	24	64	16	176	4.00	41
46	8	32	40	24	64	16	184	4.00	43
48	8	32	40	24	64	24	192	4.00	42
50	8	40	40	24	64	24	200	4.00	44
52	8	40	40	24	72	24	208	4.00	42
54	8	40	40	32	72	24	216	4.00	41
56	8	40	48	32	72	24	224	4.00	43
58	8	40	48	40	72	24	232	4.00	42
60	8	40	48	40	80	24	240	4.00	40

*Day shift. Assumes 8-hour increments. Shading highlights changes in numbers of personnel by category.

variations for obstetrical labor and delivery care are shown in Figure 10.6. The computer software forecasts both census and acuity and develops specific work assignments a shift or two in advance.

Care planning approaches use standard times required to complete care plan elements. As the nurse prepares the patient's care plan in an automated system, the time required for each element is added to the total for the patient. Allowances are made for general care not specified in the plan, and the result is an estimate of the actual time nursing personnel will spend with each patient. It is possible to adjust the calculation to skill level as well.[9] The sum of these hours for the floor can be used directly to generate staffing requirements. A file of historic census variation is used to generate the budget and the expected range of staffing by personnel class, similar to Figure 10.5.

The subjective nature of the patient evaluation is an important limitation of weighting schemes. Although acuity assessment is relatively inexpensive, requiring only a few minutes of time per patient, it depends on human memory, which is fallible and can be distorted by bias. Similarly, the nursing care plan is by definition a subjective evaluation. The nurse can add elements, and each element is likely to produce some gain for the patient. The question of how much the patient and the payment system can afford is far removed

FIGURE 10.6 Patient Acuity Variations

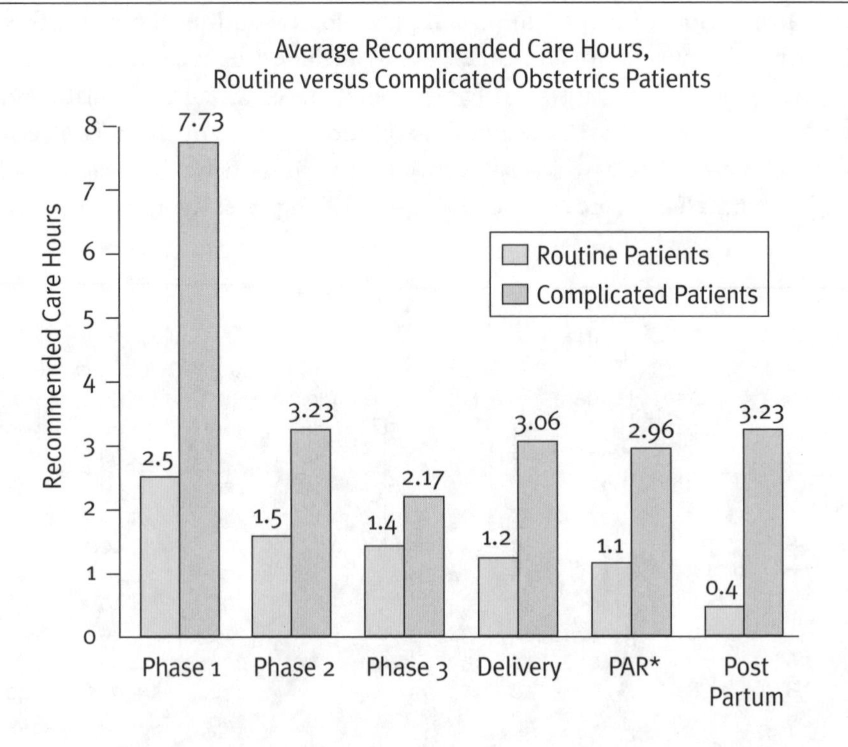

* Post Anesthesia Recovery

SOURCE: © Copyright, *LADPAQ™. National Comparative Data Book, Fifth Edition. Medicus Systems Corporation, 1995.*

from the point of decision. Scores tend to creep upward in an unmonitored system, inflating the nursing staff requirement. Identification and correction of creep is possible, but at added system cost. Well-designed computer systems routinely test the means and variances of weighting scores for statistical trend. In addition, protocols represent consensus on appropriateness, providing a guideline and a point of reference.

Scheduling

The staffing plan must be translated to work schedules for specific employees. This step requires a short-range (usually four to eight weeks) forecast of weighted census. For purely stochastic units like obstetrics and coronary care, each shift must be scheduled for the average conditions. On other floors scheduling is adjusted to day of week and shift. The scheduling system develops work schedules for specific employees for several weeks in advance. Predictable absenteeism, holidays, and non-patient care assignments must be accommodated in the schedule. Part-time personnel, and 12-hour or 8-hour shifts are also accommodated.[10]

Nurses desire predictable schedules, but they also want to request special days off. Scheduling systems that help them do this are an important recruitment and retention device.[11] A well-designed staffing and scheduling program has the following characteristics, listed in approximate order of importance[12]:

- Staffing matches the forecast requirement; overstaffing and understaffing are minimized.
- Personnel are scheduled consistent with their designated specialization, professional competence, and agreed-upon work commitment (that is, full-time or part-time).
- Schedules for individuals are maintained four or more weeks in advance.
- Schedules minimize unnecessary transfers between units and shifts.
- Weekends, late shifts, and other less desirable assignments are equitably distributed. ("Equitably" is usually not "equally"; one nurse's preferences are not the same as another's.)
- Personal requests for specific days off are accommodated equally, so long as they are submitted in advance, can be met within cost and quality constraints, and do not exploit other workers.

Assignment

Assignment makes the final adjustment of staff on each floor and shift to the best available estimate of immediate need by changing the number of personnel on a given floor or unit, or, in some cases, by changing the number of patients on a floor or unit. Thus, if the floor shown in Figure 10.5 had absenteeism or an unpredicted increase in census or acuity, extra personnel would be moved there to help meet the load.

It is important to note that problems of variability of staff and reliability of measurement are greatly reduced by aggregating individual values by unit. Although individual patients vary three- or four-fold, aggregates of 30 patients vary only 20 percent as much, and aggregates of 60 patients only 12 percent as much. If patient need averages four hours per shift and ranges from one to 12 hours, a 30-patient aggregate will range only between 2.5 and 3.5 hours per patient. It will be staffed with 15 people, and the range will be plus or minus three people. A similar 60-patient aggregate will have 30 people and range fewer than four people. Staff absenteeism will add to this requirement, in both cases. Thus, larger units significantly reduce the need for assignment changes. They have a lower overall variation and more personnel to reassign internally to meet emergencies.

It is also true that some variation can be handled by the ability of the nursing staff on the floor to work harder. It is clearly understood that workers can sustain peak outputs up to 40 percent higher than the average demand.[13] The 25 people assigned to the Figure 8.5 floor for the average of 50 patient equivalents can treat 60 patient equivalents acceptably for a day or two; they cannot sustain that level without quality, patient satisfaction, and personnel satisfaction problems.

Using the law of large numbers and the flexibility of workers further reduces the need to assign staff. The remaining staffing flexibility is usually obtained by:

- developing float pools of nurses trained to work at several different locations. Float pool nurses are often given extra compensation recognizing their flexibility;
- using call-in and agency personnel when needed;
- assigning overtime to available workers; and
- transferring workers between floors.

Census adjustment is more complex. It combines the patient-scheduling system and the nursing-staffing system to reduce variation in weighted census. Although its greatest application is in outpatient unit management, it offers several possibilities. The patient scheduling system can stabilize both the number and individual needs of the incoming patients. Outpatient visits are usually scheduled as separate events. Inpatient units typically turn over about one-third of their census each day.

- The counts and needs of incoming patients can be coordinated to the staffing level, so that variation in demand is reduced.
- Units can be designated for specific ranges of need. For example, the scheduling system assigns the sickest arriving inpatients to intensive care units. This reduces variation on routine care floors, although ICUs themselves are subject to widely fluctuating need for staff.
- In organizations with several similar treatment units, incoming patients can be placed when they arrive to units with surplus staff.

In general the fewer changes at the assignment level, the more efficient the system and the higher the quality is likely to be. The more effective the staffing, personnel scheduling, and patient scheduling, the narrower the range of differences and the less adjustment by assignment.

The use of float pools, call-ins, and transfers is necessary, but it should be minimized. Float pools are difficult to sustain and generally increase costs. Call-ins from outside pools of temporary employees or agency personnel brought in on contract are even more expensive. At best, the training of agency personnel is outside the hospital's control, and the individuals are less efficient because they are not familiar with their work environment. Transfer of personnel from one location to another within the hospital presents similar difficulties. Most nurses do not like to be transferred, and the problems of cross-training and unfamiliar workstations remain. Quality deteriorates as a result.

Well-run healthcare organizations now have computer support for staffing, scheduling, census weighting, and assignment. Commercial software offers assignment, acuity, and quality assessment; simulation for budgeting; and basic personnel records in a single package.[14] The same software frequently supports quality assessment as well. Combining the software with well-developed nursing procedures, formal nursing care plans and protocols, flexible personnel budgeting, and patient scheduling, they are in a position to specify improvements in cost and quality measures that might result from changes in staffing.[15,16]

Observation: The Nursing Continuous Improvement Function

Nursing's frequent contact with the patient places it in a unique informational situation. It has the opportunity to make a comprehensive assessment of patient needs that is often broader based than the doctors'. It is in the best position to identify oversights, omissions, and failures in the care process. It can use this information to monitor not only its own performance, but also that of the team as a whole, and to identify improvement opportunities for other units as well as its own. In effect, nursing contributes a focal point for improving its own processes and those of others.[17] A significant part of nursing resources goes to supporting continuous improvement in its own activities and those of other CSSs.

Auditing the medical care process

The inpatient nurse is responsible for the following kinds of information activities:

- reporting clinical observations to the physician;
- understanding and reporting family-related factors of clinical importance;
- recording drug administration and nursing treatments;
- receiving, coordinating, and transmitting orders for clinical support services;

- preparing patients or specimens for support services;
- knowing patients' locations and receiving them back from support services;
- receiving and transmitting results of reports from support services;
- preparing and forwarding incident reports for any untoward events;
- maintaining the paper medical record;
- recording and storing patients' possessions; and
- assisting visitors to the floor.

Nurses working in outpatient, home, and long-term care settings have similar lists. Only details of scheduling, transportation, and reporting, and some elements of family contact differ because of the site of care. Completing this list of information generates nursing's unique perspective on the patient.

Nurses use the information to identify omitted, inconsistent, and incorrect actions, and actions that had unexpected results. They actively monitor the course of care. Although this puts them in a position of criticizing other professionals, they have learned to do this diplomatically and effectively.[18] Nurses catch omitted, wrong, lost, conflicting, and delayed reports and orders on a daily basis. They are the first to see unexpected results and unsatisfactory treatments. They remind, persuade, cajole, and convince others to correct these problems quickly so that they do not escalate. Only rarely do they draw anger or resistance to their efforts.

From a management perspective, two things are important about this ongoing audit. The first is that it is essential to any high-quality system of care, and therefore must be actively supported by management. When nursing cannot get a constructive response from another service, management must investigate and correct. The problem may lie with nursing, with the other service, or both, and the change may involve anything from a revised ordering system to new equipment and processes to a more diplomatic alert. In any case, the cause of any serious failure in this mechanism needs to be identified and fixed. If this system breaks down, quality, cost, and satisfaction will deteriorate rapidly. If it has broken down, the culture of the institution is in a dysfunctional state, and immediate, extensive efforts are required to fix it.

The second issue important to management is that much of this communication represents "rework," the unproductive repetition of something that could and should have gone right the first time. The higher the volume of audit alerts from nursing, the more things have gone wrong and the more resources from nursing or another service will be consumed fixing them. The ideal is that nursing rarely or never detects a failure or omission. Things are so well done the first time that the monitor does not generate alerts, or generates them only rarely, with very complex and unusual cases. The key to the ideal, of course, is well-designed processes.

Improving intermediate product protocols

Nursing is responsible for the continuous improvement of its own care plans and protocols. It is so central to most complex care that it is a major contributor to final product protocols. Its central position gets it involved with many CSS intermediate protocols.

Nursing has a large number of internal processes and procedures, intermediate care protocols of its own. Leading institutions are computerizing these, allowing nurses the opportunity to recover the procedures quickly and follow written instructions rather than memory. The list of desired procedures can constitute the nursing plan for the patient and, as noted above, can be used to develop staffing needs. A historic data file generated under this system identifies both the frequency and cost associated with each procedure. Improvement priorities will be directed to the most numerous and expensive procedures. The improvement question is, "Can this procedure be eliminated, improved or replaced?" In many cases, the answer will be yes.

Contributing to final product and other protocols

It is probably impossible to write a final product protocol without active participation by nursing. Nurse specialists have a particular role here because their specialization makes them expert on particular diseases and conditions.[19] As Figure 10.7 shows, nursing can suggest existing problems (Plan), ways to solve them (Do), and experiments to check new protocols and their comments (Check). Nursing will inevitably implement much of the plan, and monitor implementation of the rest (Act).[20]

Similarly, nursing often has a role in the intermediate products of other CSSs. It should be readily available to consult on new protocol design.

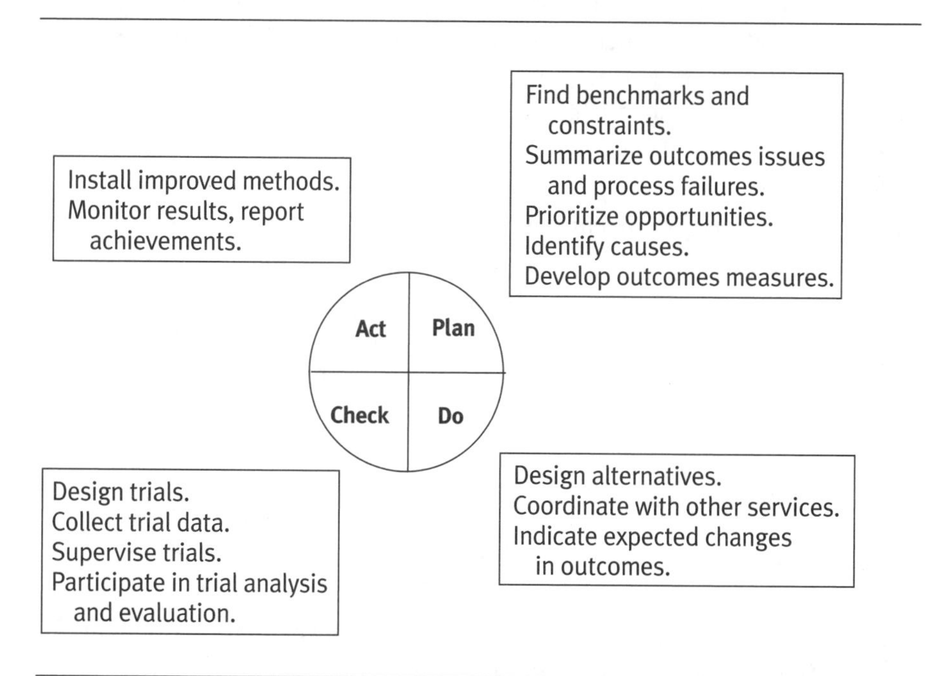

FIGURE 10.7 Nursing Roles in the PDCA Cycle for Final Product Protocols

Management must see that appropriate consultation occurs and is constructive. Because the interface often involves transfers of responsibility from one unit to another, mediation and consensus building are important.

Recruiting and Retaining: The Nursing Human Resources Function

Human contact is the central element of all nursing, and the recruitment, retention, training, and motivation of nursing personnel are critical functions. Nursing human resources management is not different from other CSSs or from other workers; the activities outlined in Chapters 10 and 16 apply. There is periodic national concern about shortages of professional nurses; the key to avoiding local shortages is ongoing effective relationships.

A healthcare organization needs to recruit and retain nurses, particularly the staff RNs who provide most acute inpatient care. A medium-sized organization will employ 400 or more individual nurses. Most of them will be inpatient nurses, a job that is both physically and emotionally demanding. Compensation is now comparable with similar professional opportunities, such as teaching and pharmacy, although neither of those jobs combines the hours, physical demands, and critical responsibilities of a staff nurse. It is not surprising that staff nurse turnover is high, sometimes exceeding 50 percent per year. Well-managed organizations keep turnover in the 10 to 20 percent range,[21] but they still must hire substantial numbers of new nurses.

Well-managed organizations do not have difficulty recruiting sufficient nursing personnel.[22] They attract new people and retain old ones because they are desirable places to work. An effective nursing culture attracts and keeps qualified personnel, but there appear to be several elements in the culture.[23,24,25,26] Management style is important; nurse managers like others must learn to support and respond to their subordinates.[27] Empowerment is an important attraction.[28] Efforts to maintain a sufficient cadre of qualified nurses begin with a deliberate effort to reduce turnover and increase work satisfaction.[29,30] Retention is generally cheaper than recruitment. More important, the satisfaction of current staff is quickly sensed by potential recruits, and a reputation as a good place to work is a powerful asset. Most important, there is evidence that nurse satisfaction is related to outcomes measures of patient care quality.[31] Well-run organizations strive for a recruitment and retention advantage over their competition by repeated attention to the following concepts:

Planning

- Human resources planning identifies recruitment needs well in advance.
- Special efforts are made for undesirable shifts and assignments.
- Job security is used to increase loyalty. Turnover, voluntary retirement, and retraining are used to reduce the work force when necessary.

- Promotions ladders provide opportunity for advancement. Subsidies are often offered for formal education, and inservice education is available to cross-train personnel.

Operations

- Clarity of roles, procedures, and expectations is used to reduce job stress.
- Effective supervision provides prompt, reasonable response to job-related questions and maintains motivation.[32,33,34]
- Comprehensive, effective nursing care plans and protocols increase the staff nurse's contribution to patient care and make the contribution more visible.
- Scheduling systems make the work assignments attractive.

Compensation

- Base wages and salaries are kept competitive.[35]
- Intangible rewards, chiefly praise and public recognition, reinforce self-respect and collegial recognition of professional achievement.
- Tangible rewards can be used to encourage improved job performance and to undertake less desirable assignments.

The underlying philosophy of this list is that good nursing is its own reward and that the job of nursing management is to provide opportunities to do good nursing. The functions described in the preceding sections, and the systems that implement them efficiently and effectively, are the tools for the job.

Personnel and Organization

Nursing as a profession and as a unit of healthcare organizations is almost as diverse as medicine. As Figures 10.1 and 10.2 show, the profession contains within it careers reaching from high-tech in the operating room and ICU to high-touch in the home, and include general and public health services that do not involve individual patient care. In addition, there are significant numbers of managerial jobs. The patterns of training and the modes of nursing organization reflect this diversity.

Educational Levels of Nursing Personnel

Formal educational opportunities in nursing, as in most other professions in the United States, have increased since World War II. Unique among the professions, nursing has retained all of its original levels, rather than simply adding years to the training requirement. There are now three professional and four nonprofessional educational levels (Figure 10.8).

FIGURE 10.8
Educational Levels of Nursing Personnel

Name	Degree or Certificate	Education Required
		Nonprofessional Levels
Nursing aide	None	Only hospital in-service training is required
Licensed practical nursing	LPN	One year junior college program Also called "Licensed Vocational Nurse"
Diploma in nursing	RN	Hospital-based program of three years post–high school, qualifying for RN but not the baccalaureate degree
Associate in nursing	RN, AAN	Junior college–based program of two years qualifying for RN and associate degree; the degree is accepted as partial fulfillment of the baccalaureate
		Professional Levels
Baccalaureate nursing degree	BSN	Four years beyond high school in an accredited college or university are required
Nurse anesthetist	BSN, CNA	One year after the baccalaureate degree is required
Nurse practitioner	BSN, CNP	At least one year after the baccalaureate degree is required
Nurse midwife	BSN, CNM	Less that one year post-baccalaureate
Clinical specialist	MSN	One or two years post-baccalaureate study Fields parallel the major specialties of medicine
Public health nurse	MPH	Two years post-baccalaureate study
Nurse manager	MSN	Two years post-baccalaureate study
Doctor of nursing	PhD	Four or more years post-baccalaureate study

Several attempts to rationalize this structure have led to a career ladder that accommodates repeated return to formal education, via LPN, associate, bachelor's, master's, and doctoral degrees.[36] The growth of junior colleges has made this career ladder more accessible. Almost all hospitals have abandoned diploma programs in favor of participation in associate and baccalaureate programs. Certification has not kept pace with these developments. Registration, the traditional recognition of professional nursing qualification, is available with as little as two years' study after high school. Well-run healthcare organizations are specifying BSN degrees for many assignments such as intensive care, team leaders, supervision, and primary nursing. Practical experience as a substitute for formal requirements can be judged on an individual basis.

Nursing Organization

Nursing tends to follow a consistent accountability hierarchy in its many sites and specialties. A team led by a staff nurse (sometimes called a primary nurse) constitutes an informal work unit below the responsibility center. The team varies in size and skill levels depending on patient needs. Several geographically adjacent teams comprise a floor or clinic, the usual designation for a responsibility center. The responsibility center manager is usually called head nurse. The hierarchy beyond the responsibility center usually follows clinical specialty lines. Figure 10.9 shows the functional organization of a medium-sized hospital or a large multispecialty clinic.

Functional hierarchies can be modified to fit home care, hospices, rehabilitation, and extended care facilities. Specific policies, procedures, and skills differentiate the various services. Clearly, the procedures for operating rooms are very different from those for outpatient psychiatry, but the structure of teams and accountability hierarchy is the same. The staff nurse for chronic care is usually an LPN; for acute units, an RN or BSN; and for intensive care, a BSN or MSN. The skill required for outpatient care depends on the role and can be LPN, RN, or BSN.

Nurses from all levels are drawn to cross-functional teams to develop final product protocols, work on nursing intermediate protocols, and consult with other CSSs. Matrix structures emerge from close alliance between the nursing and medical organizations. These identify dual accountabilities and use the matrix and cross-functional teams to gain continuous improvement. Matrices can evolve to product line groups including a line management person responsible for marketing and logistics.[37] An example tracing just one line of accountability from birthing services to women's services to the executive management team is shown in Figure 10.10.

Measures and Information Systems

The growth of automated support for patient scheduling, medical records, care plans and protocols, nurse scheduling, quality assessment, and detailed

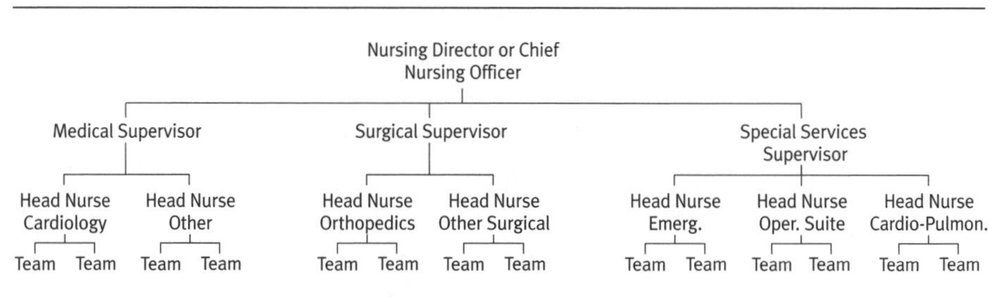

FIGURE 10.9 Nursing Functional Accountability Hierarchies*

*With minor changes in specialization, the hierarchy describes larger ambulatory facilities as well as medium-sized to smaller inpatient units.

FIGURE 10.10
Nursing in the Matrix/ Product-Line Organization

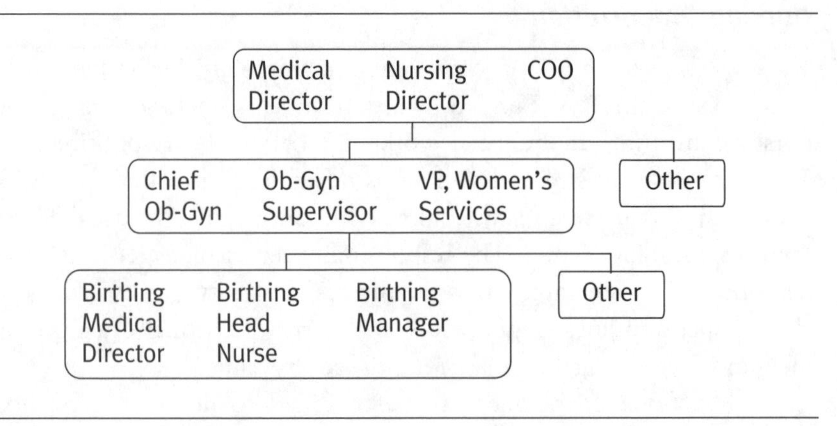

cost accounting has provided a platform for major advances in quality and cost-effectiveness for nursing.[38] It is possible to measure much of what was only conceptual a few years ago, and to use the measures in the routine solution of nursing problems. Both measurement advances and processing advantages have contributed to this development. The discussion that follows summarizes the measures by the usual six dimensions: demand, cost, human resources, output and productivity, quality, and customer satisfaction. Nursing's major data processing systems are described in terms of their applications.

Measures

The typical responsibility center can measure, set expectations, and achieve improvements on all six dimensions. A "nursing management minimum data set" includes standardized definitions for many of the necessary measures.[39] Examples are shown in Figure 10.11.

- Demand measures such as the average and the variation in demand, delays for scheduled and urgent service, and counts of cancellations or disruptions in the scheduling process. Expectations are set through, and achieved by, patient-scheduling systems.
- Costs by functional account (that is, labor, supplies, and facilities) for both the total dollars per accounting period and, under flexible budgeting, the costs per unit of nursing output. Well-managed nursing units, supported by the full array of computer aids, now find the achievement of cost expectations routine. Summary levels of performance are monitored, and modern payroll, materials management, accounts receivable, and general ledger systems permit the exploration of any level of detail necessary.
- Human resources are routinely monitored through absenteeism and turnover data and satisfaction surveys. Staffing, scheduling, and assignment systems monitor overtime, understaffed situations, and shift assignments.

- Nursing output is measured in terms of patients treated. Automated systems allow classification by disease or condition and weighting for patient need in both inpatient and outpatient settings. Nursing activities are recorded by automated patient care plans, protocols, and order entry systems and can be aggregated reliably at the patient group level.
- Productivity is measured in costs or hours per case, per visit, or per day of care. Final product costs are aggregated from unit costs. While precise unit costing remains difficult (Chapter 14), cost estimates for nursing interim products and components of final products are increasingly reliable.
- Outcomes quality is assessed by condition-specific achievement rates such as recovery of mobility and activities of daily living and failure rates, such as infections, or bedsores.
- General failure rates, such as incidence reports and nosocomial infections are routinely measured in most settings. The data are used by organization-wide risk management programs and infections control committees.[40,41]
- Process quality is routinely assessed through inspection of both patients and nursing records. Reliability has been improved by using specific questions to guide the inspection and by developing numerous questions to cover the range of patient needs. Cost and time requirements have been reduced by automation of question selection, sampling procedures, tallying, and analysis.
- Structural measures of quality such as hours per weighted output and percentage of hours by professional personnel are available from staffing and scheduling systems. Occurrences of values below preset minimums are the most sensitive indicators. The JCAHO lists a number of other structural standards designed to encourage good nursing practice.[42]
- Patient satisfaction is assessed by survey. Continuous surveying permits monitoring by small nursing units. Questions can address components of satisfaction, such as personal care, reassurance, and patient education.
- Physician satisfaction with nursing is assessed as part of formal surveys of the attending and house staffs. Informal and subjective evaluation of performance is also useful. It should occur at all levels of the accountability hierarchy. Evaluations of nursing supervisors include review of relations with physicians.

Constraints for nursing continue to require review of benchmarks, competition, and history, integrated into a negotiated agreement. Leading organizations are using both functional cost histories and final product cost limits imposed by the marketplace.[43] Benchmarking remains difficult in many nursing units, but is feasible in others.[44]

The rich measurement set depends heavily on information systems. As the systems are installed, obvious avenues of improvement appear and are explored. These are initially at the level of a single process. Integrated

FIGURE 10.11 Nursing Performance Measures

Dimension	Inpatient Examples	Outpatient Examples (Home Care Program)	General Nursing Examples
Demand	Number and acuity of patients, pct. emergencies	Scheduled home visits, delay for visit	Enrollment in programs, pct. eligibles attracted
Costs	Labor hours, by pers. class medical supplies	Payroll costs, home supplies, travel costs	Faculty cost, facility cost, promotional cost
Human Resources	Satisfaction, turnover vacancies	Satisfaction, turnover vacancies	Satisfaction, turnover vacancies
Output/ Productivity	Discharges, cost/discharge, cost/member month	Visits, visits/patient, patients/visiting nurse, costs/patient month	Number of presentations, attendance, cost/member
Outcomes Quality	Return to work, recovery of function, infections	Daily living scores, hospitalizations, transfers to long-term care	Pct. members smoking, pct. seeking prenatal care, child trauma
Process Quality	Pct. complete care plans, medication errors, pct. presurgery pt. education	Pct. visits late or missed, errors in equipment, supplies	Member awareness, curriculum evaluation, facility evaluation
Patient Satisfaction	Pct. "very satisfied," number of complaints	Pct. "very satisfied," family satisfaction	Audience evaluation, member satisfaction
Physician Satisfaction	Pct. of referring physicians and attending physicians "very satisfied," complaints	Pct. of referring physicians "very satisfied," complaints	Phys. awareness, satisfaction, complaints

and final product opportunities appear later. The process of identifying and addressing these opportunities appears to take several years in most organizations. The best organizations are only now reaching the conclusion of this phase. A third, more rewarding, and more challenging phase is now beginning, where medicine, nursing, and other CSSs collaborate toward a goal of cost-effective care.

Information Systems

Nursing now requires a set of automated systems interlocking with those required elsewhere in the hospital, as discussed in Chapter 17. A summary list may be helpful here.

Patient information systems

- Patient registration (also called admission, discharge, and transfer) records basic registration information, assigns identification number, identifies hospital location of patient, communicates arrival and initial orders, and initiates both patient ledger and patient order file.

- Medical information (also called order entry and results reporting) records physician's and nurse's orders and care plans, transmits orders to support services, receives reports back from support services, supports the patient ledger and prompts recurring nursing activities. More advanced systems permit tailoring of individual care plans from a patient group protocol and will record nursing progress notes.
- Patient scheduling records classification of demand (usually emergency, urgent, or scheduled) and scheduled future date, if any. Support service scheduling records future support services, resolves conflicts in preparation and transportation needs, and shows availability of service. Advanced systems establish current and future availability of admission opportunities and prompt call in from the urgent list. (Chapter 9)

Managerial support systems

- General accounting and budgeting supports flexible budgeting and cost reporting by physical and dollar units.
- Final product analysis groups clinically similar patient data for cost, quality, and satisfaction according to any of several dimensions such as responsibility center, physician, payment category.
- General patient satisfaction surveys include specific questions on kinds of nursing service and are maintained at a frequency that allows analysis at the unit level.
- Physician satisfaction surveys include questions that allow evaluation at the unit level.
- Personnel satisfaction surveys provide evidence of nursing employee morale at the unit level, by job classification for larger classes.

Nursing management systems

- Staffing and scheduling algorithms support long-range nursing needs, budgets, work schedules, and assignment. They generate structural measures of staffing. Advanced models accept employee preferences and special requests.
- Nursing personnel records include special training and assignment capabilities, work preferences, evaluations, and other data on individual employees.[45]
- Nursing procedure descriptions are instantly accessible. They replace the paper procedural manual and can be used to weight census, construct care plans, and support staffing models. Continuous improvement teams review these and keep them current.
- Acuity assessment and assignment accepts tallies of patient acuity by floor and shift, and records time series data on acuity scores to provide statistical quality controls to detect significant change in recorded acuity.

- Process quality assessment identifies samples of patients and questions, prints survey questionnaires, accepts responses, and tallies quality scores following preset rules.

Well-managed healthcare organizations are moving rapidly on this list and have at least elementary systems in place for most of the list.

Suggested Readings

American Nurses Association. 1997. *Implementing Nursing's Report Card: A Study of RN Staffing, Length of Stay, and Patient Outcomes.* Washington, DC: American Nurses Pub.

Birdsall, C., and S. P. Sperry. 1997. *Clinical Paths in Medical-Surgical Practice.* St. Louis: Mosby.

Deloughery, G. (ed.). 1998. *Issues and Trends in Nursing,* 3rd ed. St. Louis: Mosby.

Grohar-Murray, M. H., and H. R. DiCroce. 1997. *Leadership and Management in Nursing,* 2nd ed. Stamford, CT: Appleton & Lange.

Katz, J. M., and E. Green. 1997. *Managing Quality: A Guide to System-Wide Performance Management in Health Care,* 2nd ed. St. Louis: Mosby.

Price, S. A., M. W. Koch, and S. Bassett (eds.). 1998. *Health Care Resource Management: Present and Future Challenges.* St. Louis: Mosby.

Stamps, P. 1997. *Nurses and Work Satisfaction: An Index for Measurement, Second Edition.* Chicago: Health Administration Press.

Swansburg, R. C. 1997. *Budgeting and Financial Management for Nurse Managers.* Sudbury, MA: Jones and Bartlett.

Toni, G., H. A. Cesta, L. Tahan, and F. Fink. 1998. *The Case Manager's Survival Guide: Winning Strategies for Clinical Practice.* St. Louis: Mosby.

Notes

1. Florence Nightingale, quoted in V. Henderson, *The Nature of Nursing.* New York: MacMillan. p. 1 (1966)
2. V. Henderson and G. Nite, *Principles and Practice of Nursing,* 6th ed. New York: MacMillan, pp. 1–25 (1978)
3. U. S. Department of Health and Human Services, Health Resources and Services Administration, *The Registered Nurse Population.* Hyattsville. MD: U.S. Dept. of Health & Human Services, Public Health Service, Health Resources and Services Administration, Bureau of Health Professions, Office of Data Analysis (March, 1996)
4. V. J. Numinen, D. L. Haas, L. Yaroch, and P. Fralick, "Building Community-Based Service Systems for Children with Special Needs: The Michigan Locally Based Services Program." *Issues in Comprehensive Pediatric Nursing* 15(1), pp. 17–37 (January–March, 1992)
5. M. M. Seltzer, L. C. Litchfield, L. R. Kapust, and J. B. Mayer, "Professional and Family Collaboration in Case Management: A Hospital-Based Replication of a Community-Based Study." *Social Work in Health Care* 17(1), pp. 1–22 (1992)

6. P. Hanisch, S. Honan, and R. Torkelson, "Quality Improvement Approach to Nursing Care Planning: Implementing Practical Computerized Standards." *Journal for Healthcare Quality* 15(5), pp. 6–13 (September-October, 1993)
7. F. C. Munson, J. S. Beckman, J. Clinton, C. Kever, and L. Simms, *Nursing Assignment Patterns, User's Manual.* Chicago: Health Administration Press (1980)
8. C. Y. Phillips, A. Castorr, P. A. Prescott, and K. Soeken, "Nursing Intensity: Going Beyond Patient Classification." *Journal of Nursing Administration* 22(4), pp. 46–52 (April, 1992)
9. P. Hanisch, S. Honan, and R. Torkelson, "Quality Improvement Approach to Nursing Care Planning: Implementing Practical Computerized Standards." *Journal of Health Care Quality* 15(5), pp. 6–13 (September-October, 1993)
10. J. Chen and T. W. Yeung, "Hybrid Expert-System Approach to Nurse Scheduling . . . NURSE-HELP." *Computers in Nursing* 11(4), pp. 183–90 (June, 1993)
11. J. J. Gray, D. McIntire, and H. J. Doller, "Preferences for Specific Work Schedules: Foundation for an Expert-System Scheduling Program." *Computers in Nursing* 11(3), pp. 115–21 (May-June, 1993)
12. Medicus Systems Corporation promotional literature. Evanston, IL
13. M. W. Isken and W. M. Hancock. "A Heuristic Approach to Nurse Scheduling in Hospital Units with Non-Stationary, Urgent Demand, and a Fixed Staff Size." *Journal of the Society for Health Systems* 2(2), pp. 24–41 (1991)
14. NPAQ: A Product of Medicus Systems Corporation. Evanston, IL
15. K. G. Behner, L. F. Fogg, L. C. Fournier, J. T. Frankenbach, and S. B. Robertson, "Nursing Resource Management: Analyzing the Relationship Between Costs and Quality in Staffing Decisions." *Health Care Management Review* 15(4), pp. 63–71 (Fall, 1990)
16. S. F. Hollander, M. Smith, and J. Barron, "Cost Reductions, Part I: An Operations Improvement Process." *Nursing Economics* 10(5), pp. 325–30, 364 (September, 1992); "Part 2: An Organizational Culture Perspective." 10(6), pp. 401–5 (November-December, 1992)
17. S. H. Taft, E. L. Minch, and P. K. Jones, "Strengthening Hospital Nursing: The Planning Process." *Journal of Nursing Administration,* Part 1 22(5), pp. 51–63 (May, 1992); Part 2 22(6), pp. 36–46 (June, 1992); Part 3 22(7/8), pp. 41–50 (July, 1992)
18. E. M. McMahan, K. Hoffman, and G. W. McGee, "Physician-Nurse Relationships in Clinical Settings: A Review and Critique of the Literature, 1966–1992." *Medical Care Review* 51(1), pp. 83–112 (Spring, 1994)
19. E. A. McFadden and M. A. Miller, "Clinical Nurse Specialist Practice: Facilitators and Barriers." *Clinical Nurse Specialist* 8(1), pp. 27–33 (January, 1994)
20. G. L. Ingersoll, M. T. Bazar, and J. B. Zentner, "Monitoring Unit-Based Innovations: A Process Evaluation Approach." *Nursing Economics* 11(3), pp. 137–43 (May, 1993)
21. J. R. Griffith, *Designing 21st Century Healthcare.* Chicago: Health Administration Press, pp. 32–36 (1998)
22. M. L. McClure, M. A. Poulin, M. D. Sovie, and M. A. Wandelt, *Task Force on*

Nursing Practice in Hospitals, Magnet Hospitals: Attraction and Retention of Professional Nurses. Kansas City, MO: American Nurses Association (1982)

23. H. Van Ess Coeling and L. M. Simms, "Facilitating Innovation at the Nursing Unit Level Through Cultural Assessment," *Journal of Nursing Administration:* 23(4), pp. 46–53 (April, 1993); "Part 2: Adapting Management Ideas to the Unit Workgroup" 23(5), pp. 13–20 (May, 1993)
24. C. T. Kovner, G. Hendrickson, J. R. Knickman, and S. A. Finkler, "Changing the Delivery of Nursing Care: Implementation Issues and Qualitative Findings." *Journal of Nursing Administration* 23(11), pp. 24–34 (November, 1993)
25. J. E. Johnson, L. L. Costa, S. B. Marshall, M. J. Moran, and C. S. Henderson, "Succession Management: A Model for Developing Nursing Leaders." *Nursing Management* 25(6), pp. 50–5 (June, 1994)
26. M. A. Blegen, C. J. Goode, M. Johnson, M. L. Maas, J. C. McCloskey, and S. A. Moorhead, "Recognizing Staff Nurse Job Performance and Achievements." *Research in Nursing and Health* 15(1), pp. 57–66 (February, 1992)
27. M. K. Kohles, "Redefining Management through Redesign of Patient Care Delivery Systems." *Seminars for Nurse Managers* 5(1), pp. 39–48 (March, 1997)
28. R. S. Morrison, L. Jones, and B. Fuller, "The Relation Between Leadership Style and Empowerment on Job Satisfaction of Nurses." *Journal of Nursing Administration* 27(5), pp. 27–34 (May, 1997)
29. J. A. Alexander, "The Effects of Patient Care Unit Organization on Nursing Turnover." *Health Care Management Review* 13(2), pp. 61–72 (Spring, 1988)
30. J. R. Bloom, J. A. Alexander, and S. Flatt, "Organization Turnover Among Registered Nurses: An Exploratory Model." *Health Services Management Research* 1(3), pp. 156–67 (November, 1988)
31. C. S. Weisman and C. A. Nathanson, "Professional Satisfaction and Client Outcomes." *Medical Care* 23, pp. 1179–2 (October, 1985); R. W. Revans, *Standards for Morale: Cause and Effect in Hospitals.* London: Oxford University Press for Nuffield Provincial Hospitals Trust (1964)
32. L. Chase, "Nurse Manager Competencies." *Journal of Nursing Administration* 24(4S), pp. 56–64 (April, 1994)
33. C. McDaniel and G. A. Wolf, "Transformational Leadership in Nursing Service: A Test of Theory." *Journal of Nursing Administration* 22(2), pp. 60–65 (February, 1992)
34. J. C. McCloskey, M. Mass, D. G. Huber, A. Kasparek, J. Specht, et al, "Nursing Management Innovations: A Need for Systematic Evaluation." *Nursing Economics* 12(1), pp. 35–44 (January–February, 1994)
35. M. A. Blegen, C. J. Goode, M. Johnson, M. L. Maas, J. C. McCloskey, and S. A. Moorhead, "Recognizing Staff Nurse Job Performance and Achievements." *Research in Nursing and Health* 15(1), pp. 57–66 (February, 1992)
36. M. C. Kreider and M. Barry, "Clinical Ladder Development: Implementing Contract Learning." *Journal of Continuing Education in Nursing* 24(4), pp. 166–9 (July–August, 1993)
37. M. P. Charns, L. J. Smith, and Tewksbury, *Collaborative Management in Health Care: Implementing the Integrative Organization.* San Francisco: Jossey-Bass (1993)

38. K.H. Bowles, "The Barriers and Benefits of Nursing Information Systems." *Computers in Nursing* 15(4):191–6 (Jul–Aug, 1997)
39. D. G. Huber, C. Delaney, J. Crossley, M. Mehmert, and S. Ellerbe, "A Nursing Management Minimum Data Set: Significance and Development." *Journal of Nursing Administration* 22(7/8). pp. 35–40 (July, 1992); D. Huber, L. Schumacher, and C. Delaney, "Nursing Management Minimum Data Set (NMMDS)." *Journal of Nursing Administration* 27(4), pp. 42–8 (April, 1997)
40. J. M. Welton and S. Jarr, "Automating and Improving the Data Quality of a Nursing Department Quality Management Program at a University Hospital." *Joint Commission Journal on Quality Improvement* 23(12), pp. 623–35 (December, 1997)
41. S. E. Feldman and D. W. Roblin, "Medical Accidents in Hospital Care: Applications of Failure Analysis to Hospital Quality Appraisal." *Joint Commission Journal on Quality Improvement* 23(11), pp. 567–80 (November, 1997)
42. Joint Commission on Accreditation of Hospitals, *Accreditation Manual for Hospitals*. Chicago: Joint Commission on Accreditation on Hospitals (published annually)
43. D. G. Anderson, S. F. Hollander, and P. Bastar, "Customized Productivity Feedback Systems Improve Nursing Performance and Reduce Costs." *Nursing Economics* 9(5), pp. 367–70 (September–October, 1991)
44. J. C. Ziegle and N. K. VanEtten, "Implementation of a National Nursing Standards Program." *Journal of Nursing Administration* 22(11), pp. 40–6 (November, 1992)
45. H. A. De Groot, L. Forsey, and V. S. Cleland, "The Nursing Practice Personnel Data Set: Implications for Professional Practice Systems." *Journal of Nursing Administration* 22(3), pp. 23–8 (March, 1992)

CHAPTER

11

PREVENTION AND NON-ACUTE SERVICES

The vision of most healthcare organizations is to offer seamless, comprehensive care across the full spectrum of services. The ideal shown in Figure 11.1, adapted from Figure 2.4, would see each member of the community accessing what he or she needed from an integrated delivery system, financing it comfortably, and moving freely from one element to another as necessary to achieve the best possible outcome. The reality is that the provision and financing of services has been skewed by economics, politics, and technology so that certain needs and certain populations get preference and others are more or less severely disadvantaged. Figure 11.2, adapted from Figure 3.4, shows the reality, distinguishing the traditional "have" and "have not" services. The three shaded activities consume the lion's share of healthcare resources.

A great many analysts believe that an integrated strategy, with more emphasis on the neglected services, would pay off in better health, if not in lower costs. Scientific proof and popular acceptance of these beliefs are mixed

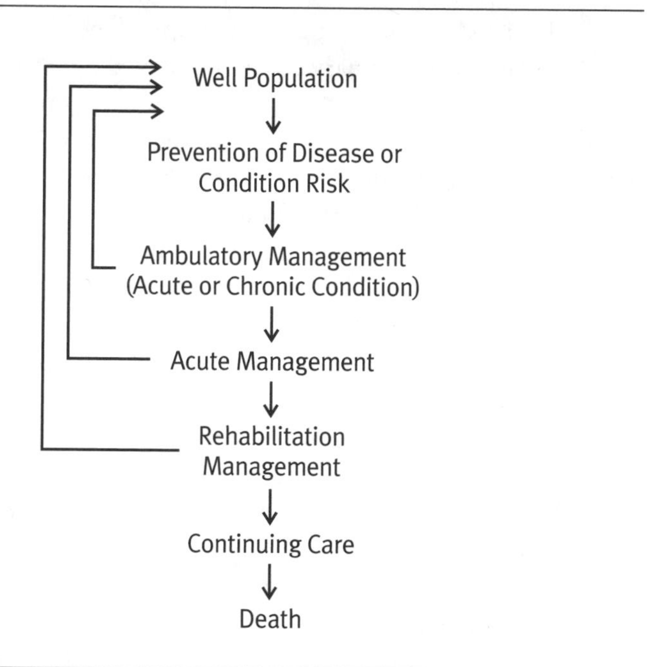

FIGURE 11.1 The Ideal of Seamless Service (Adapted from Figure 2.4)

FIGURE 11.2
The Reality of Distorted Emphasis (Adapted from Figure 3.4)

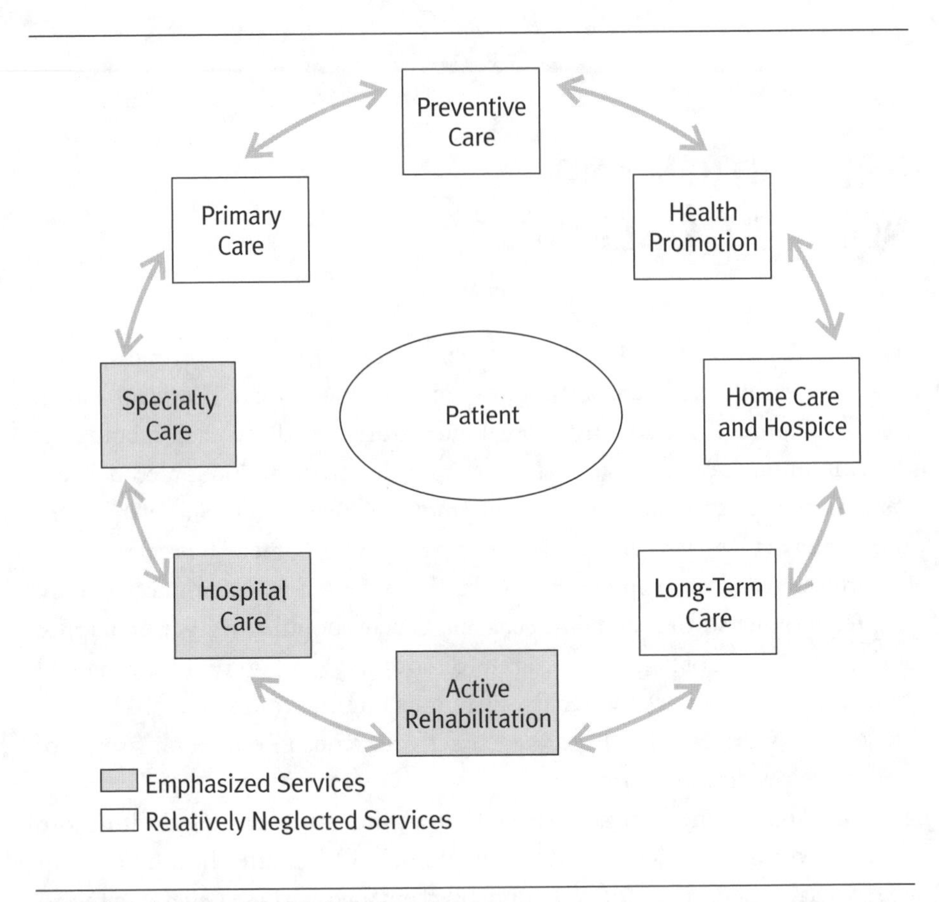

SOURCE: American Health Care Association.

at best. There is strong scientific evidence and emerging consensus on primary care. Well-supported primary care practitioners can achieve economy, quality, and patient satisfaction.[1] Leading organizations are implementing primary care models successfully, and Chapters 7 through 10 incorporate primary care. The public supports such efforts, although "gatekeeper" systems that rigidly limit access to specialists have only a limited market.

The case for prevention and health promotion is summarized in Chapter 7; specific prevention activities may be cost effective if they include both efficient delivery mechanisms and targeting to populations at high risk. Large-scale proof is lacking, but demonstrations are encouraging, both in evidence of results and popular acceptance.[2]

Despite many experiments, the case for integrated non-acute care—the home, hospice, and long-term care portions of Figure 11.2—is neither scientifically proven nor sold to the public. A comprehensive analysis of published studies on community-based long-term care concludes that "in almost all cases, community based long-term care does not increase survival and does not . . . slow the rate of deterioration in functional status," and "overall costs *rose* an average of 13 percent." (emphasis added)[3] Actual market demand, as reflected in the sale of insurance benefits and the actions of legislatures designing government programs, was historically biased toward acute services and continues that bias in many recent decisions.

On the other hand, the evidence of the opportunity is compelling. Large amounts of acute care are consumed on diseases and problems caused by substance abuse, poor nutrition, undesirable sexual behavior, and violence. Over one quarter of all Medicare funds are spent on the last year of life.[4] Aging of the population will increase in the number of persons needing long-term care more than half again by 2020. Unless more effective patterns are developed, economic limitations will reduce quality and satisfaction not only of non-acute care, but of all healthcare. At least one example, the Arizona Long-Term Care System, has shown that, "Home and community-based services appeared to save substantial amounts on costs of nursing home care. Estimates of savings were very robust and did not appear to be declining as the program matured."[5] But the savings were achieved in a rigorously controlled capitated environment for Medicaid patients. Eligibility was determined by the state, all clients needed at least three months of nursing home care, and caps were placed on both quantity and price of home and community services in addition to the global capitation limits.[6]

This chapter outlines the opportunities for a strategy to integrate prevention and non-acute care into community healthcare organizations, in light of the realities. It discusses the purposes of prevention and non-acute care, the special competencies of various kinds of agencies, the strategic possibilities open to healthcare organizations that expand from an acute base, and measures of performance in prevention and non-acute care.

Purposes of Non-Acute Care and Prevention

In prevention, health promotion, and long-term care the emphasis shifts from the cure of a specific disease or problem to the maintenance of functional status. Acute care efforts usually are directed toward cure—that is, return to full functionality—and are guided by a specific clinical diagnosis and treatment protocol. The purpose of non-acute services of all kinds is to maintain or improve function, preventing deterioration or restoring a limited and often declining capability. Non-acute care is guided in large measure by the individual's nonclinical risks and problems. Whether the individual can walk, shop, manage relationships with others, or escape addiction or destructive habits is more important than the diagnosis. Whether a person is a candidate for sex education, diabetes screening, asthma management, home care, hospice, or nursing home depends on the person's life style and functional limitations. People enter nursing homes because they have difficulty with activities like toileting, moving from bed, and eating. Others with similar disability but different support structures remain in community settings; their needs met by family, friends, and hired assistance.[7]

Although the shift may appear subtle, it profoundly affects the delivery of all non-acute services. Three questions emerge:

1. What replaces the disease/treatment model of medicine, which no longer fits individuals' needs? Clear endpoints are missing; solutions are idiosyncratic; professional skills of health caregivers are incomplete at best and irrelevant at worst. Functional needs suggest a social model, similar to education or welfare, but healthcare organizations are not familiar with social models and are not financed to explore them.
2. How much service is enough? In an open market, individuals buy as much as they want, but under health insurance there must be a consensus on the limits of benefits to pool risk. A large percentage of people most in need of non-acute services are poor.[8] Their needs must be supported by government. They have extensive needs for housing, education, safety, nutrition, and reasonable social opportunities. When both the open market and the medical model are abandoned, limits such as the quality of nursing home care or eligibility for hospice become issues of government, not healthcare.
3. Who will pay? The health insurance mechanism is designed to address medical, not social, problems. Social services in America are provided on a limited basis to people who are not capable of self-sufficiency. Their funding has a long history back to seventeenth century English Poor Laws. That history is of services that are deliberately minimal, and often delivered stingily and reluctantly in drab, mean surroundings. It does not fit well with customer satisfaction and competition for patients.

While these questions are rarely frontally addressed, they lie behind most of the issues and problems of **outreach programs**, that is, programs designed to integrate and extend services beyond the traditional focus. In both prevention and non-acute care, they are compounded by problems of class, the tendency to identify certain groups of people as socially desirable or undesirable. Healthcare organizations providing outreach care must thread their way between the limits of available funding, the prejudices of various constituencies, and the opportunity to improve health for some of the most needy.

Coordinating Outreach Services

The problem of outreach services is not trivial. About 10 percent of the cost of health care is involved in tobacco abuse alone.[9] Other preventable diseases contribute significant amounts. Similarly, about 10 percent of total cost is associated with non-acute care. (The estimates overlap and cannot be added.) Disability is strongly associated with age. About 20 percent of the total population over 65 need help with daily living, and about half those over

85. One in ten persons over 65 needs assistance approaching inpatient care levels. The aged population is increasing rapidly. There are 35 million over 65 now, and 50 million, a 40 percent increase, projected for 2020. The average age of the elderly population is expected to grow, further increasing demand.

The set of services that can be offered is extensive, as shown in Figure 11.3. The articulation is the result of tailoring to different functional needs, and additional articulation occurs by source of payment or income level. For example, some long-term care facilities target Medicaid markets, and others private pay, and congregate care comes at a range of price levels. Many agencies specializing in non-acute care offer several different services, but they usually focus within a major group or two. Only a few large integrated health systems make any effort to provide a wide range of the Figure 11.3 services; probably none provide all.

Most large American communities already have a high percentage of the services shown on Figure 11.3. The issues facing a healthcare organization are more likely to be those of coordination and extension of access than of supplying major unmet needs. In efforts to find each patient the least intensive care necessary to sustain function, the problems encountered will be those of locating the appropriate services, overcoming limitations or barriers to access, managing multiple sources effectively, and meeting financial constraints. The task is complicated by the limitations of the agencies. Most are small, and all operate under stringent financial constraints. Many have adopted niche survival strategies, focusing on specific needs for specific people. The patient at hand may or may not fit the focus of the service. Compounding this problem, the most needy people tend to be poor and often live in unattractive neighborhoods. Case managers and social services play a major role here, developing a plan for each patient with extensive needs.

Non-acute care presents a surprising mixture of Samaritan and profit motives. About two-thirds of nursing home beds and almost one-third of home care agencies are for-profit.[10] Many are owned by publicly listed national corporations. At the same time, a vibrant volunteer effort supports many prevention, health promotion, transportation and recreation activities. The vast majority—about three quarters—of care is provided informally by family, friends, and neighbors, without monetary compensation.[11] Organized services need to support this Samaritan network because it substantially reduces the portion of care that must be financed through insurance or governmental assistance.

Prevention and Health Promotion Programs

As indicated in Chapter 7, a wide variety of prevention and health promotion opportunities exist. By category, roughly in order of importance, they are:

- *Immunization.* A wide variety of serious diseases can be reduced or avoided by immunization. Most immunization is delivered to infants and

FIGURE 11.3
Components of Extended Services

Prevention and Health Promotion Programs

These programs target specific groups that generally must be functional in an open community environment. They are usually disease-specific and require clinical skills as well as educational and counseling skills.

- Immunization Programs—efforts to immunize children not reached through the usual infant and child care mechanisms.
- Screening—secondary prevention programs for chronic disease carried to non-clinical sites such as malls or workplaces.
- Smoking Cessation Programs—education and psychological support for tobacco-addicted individuals.
- Alcoholics Anonymous and methadone clinics—specialized facilities for alcohol and substance abuse care.
- Support Groups—educational, counseling, and mutual assistance groups for patients and families with chronic or fatal disease.
- Educational Programs—condition- or age-specific programs emphasizing prevention and management of risks related to specific conditions or ages, such as teen health, safe sex, prenatal, infant care, child care, menopause, and Alzheimer's.
- Parish Nursing—outreach to chronically ill or at-risk individuals by registered nurses through religious congregations.

Expanded Ambulatory Services

These programs target highly functional individuals and are often combined with clinical care opportunities. They have little or no clinical content and can be operated by volunteers or unskilled personnel.

- Day Care—support for impaired elderly who return to their homes at night.
- Senior Centers and Membership Programs—recreational and social facilities for well aged.
- Transportation Programs—assistance in shopping, medical care, etc.
- Resource Centers—information on available programs and assistance.
- Telephone Contact and Emergency Response—routine and emergency communication with at-risk individuals living at home.
- Senior Volunteers—support activities encouraging mutual support among senior citizens.

Home Care Programs

These programs target homebound persons and are designed to keep them out of institutional settings. They include some nonprofessional services but often require clinical skills and can involve extensive technology.

- Home visitors—volunteers who provide social opportunities and minimal assistance to the homebound.
- Meals on wheels—meals delivered to the homebound.
- Homemaker and personal care—non-professional services to the homebound.
- Respite care—temporary support in the home to relieve family caregivers.
- Home nursing—vocational or professional level nursing, rendered in the home.
- Durable medical equipment—sick room supplies leased for home use.
- High-technology home therapy—Advanced medical support provided in the home, usually drugs or total nutrition through intravenous infusion or naso-gastric intubation.

Hospice Programs

These are programs expressly designed to assist terminally ill patients and their families. They require professional clinical skill, and special skills in counseling for grief, depression, and bereavement.

- Home hospice—services delivered to the patient's home.
- Institutional hospice—inpatient support for terminal patients, usually because of an inadequate home situation.

continued

FIGURE 11.3 continued

Chronic inpatient care
These programs are targeted to two groups of people, those recovering and being rehabilitated from serious acute episodes and those who face long-term chronic disability. Both require clinical skill; long-term chronic care relies heavily on vocational and specially trained personnel.

Rehabilitation programs—services to achieve specified functional recovery goals from conditions such as heart surgery, orthopedic surgery, heart attack, and stroke. Services usually last a few weeks and are continued as long as progress is made against the disabilities. Sometimes provided through hospital "swing beds" or step-down units.

Skilled nursing programs—continuing service to recovering patients who usually return to home living after a few weeks. Sometimes provided through hospital "swing beds" or step down units.

Extended care—continuing service to patients with severe disabilities.
Stays are measured in months or years, and return to home living is unlikely.

Alzheimer's and mental deterioration programs—continuing service to patients with impaired and usually deteriorating mental capacity.

Housing
These are programs for the elderly that provide varying levels of assistance to individual apartments or home units. Although some housing organizations also provide chronic inpatient care, housing itself requires no clinical skill. Individuals in organized housing often participate in expanded ambulatory services, prevention and health promotion, home care, and hospice.

Independent senior housing—housing for seniors capable of independent living.

Congregate care facilities—housing for seniors needing or desiring support such as meals, transportation, social and recreational support.

children and is combined with review of development, preventive instruction for parents, and secondary prevention for problems such as home violence, developmental disorders, and chronic diseases.

- *Smoking and tobacco use cessation.* Tobacco-related diseases (heart and lung disease and several cancers) can be prevented or reduced through assistance for tobacco-addicted individuals and education to prevent adolescent smoking.
- *Adolescent health.* Guidance in substance abuse, nutrition, safe sex, contraception, and exercise is believed to be effective in helping young people develop into healthy and productive citizens. Counseling may be useful in detecting disease, assisting with emotional development, and preventing violence.[12]
- *Alcohol and other substance abuse.* Assistance to addicted persons appears to reduce the high social costs of addiction, which include crime, accidents, domestic violence, loss of income, and increased risk of other disease.
- *Improved nutrition and exercise.* Obesity is a contributing factor to heart disease, arthritis, diabetes, and some cancers. Exercise is recognized as contributing to long life. Poor nutrition and lack exercise are health risks that are not sufficiently recognized.[13]
- *Safety.* Death and disability from accidents can be reduced through

education and promotion of home, auto, workplace, and environment safety.
- *Prevention of impaired newborns.* Contraception, prenatal care, and prenatal education are believed to reduce the incidence of immature or deformed infants.
- *Domestic violence.* Education for young families and women may reduce domestic violence. While data on the topic are lacking, it is repeatedly referenced by citizen groups from disadvantaged areas.[14]
- *Disease-specific screening.* A variety of diseases can be detected for secondary prevention. Uterine, colon, prostate, and breast cancer; hypertension; asthma; and diabetes are among the most common outreach programs. Less frequently employed are genetically related diseases, such as sickle cell anemia or Tay-Sachs disease.

Obviously, most Americans do not need special programs for these matters. They already have their immunizations, have learned to manage their sexuality, understand the dangers of smoking and alcohol, and know to get screening specific to their risks. Successful programs must identify the population in need to be cost effective. The fact that every risk on the list is strongly associated with poverty reveals that preventive programs must be directed to the most disadvantaged members of society. Only slightly less obvious is the overlap between populations and risks. Teen health and impaired newborns are related; alcohol underlies several other risks; nutrition, exercise, and substance abuse are related.

The constellation of needs suggests a strategy of focused effort to improve health habits of the poor. (It also suggests the elimination of poverty as a national goal.) This strategy runs counter to the prevailing attitudes and politics of the country; we have traditionally aided the "deserving poor," a concept called "pauperization." The addict, the welfare teen, and the homeless person are stigmatized and marginalized in our society. Successful prevention and health promotion strategies must deal with this reality, one way or another.

Expanded Ambulatory Services

Many people with moderate disability can be supported in a home setting with modest assistance in activities like social and recreation events, shopping, home meal delivery, and transportation to medical care. Others with greater disability can live with family overnight, but need attention during the day when family members work. The expanded ambulatory services are intended to fill those needs. With the exception of day care, capital requirements are small and skill levels are within volunteer capabilities. The goal of the healthcare organization should be to support the range of needs apparent in the community. It fills that goal by promoting volunteer opportunities, training and supporting volunteers, and investing in equipment and insurance protection.

The demand for adult day care appears limited. Two models exist, one emphasizing a health/rehabilitation approach, and the other social support for mentally impaired. As of 1989, the most recent data available, 42,000 people used day care each weekday, about 20 persons per 100,000 population.[15] About 3,000 centers serve this population, with an average census of 14. Almost all are not-for-profit and have financial problems related to their low census.[16] Large programs appear possible only in urban areas with large aged populations. Costs vary by the level of service, but were estimated at $30 to $70 per day. Only a quarter of costs were covered by user fees. Day care is not a Medicare benefit, although Medicare HMOs may elect to cover it. Medicaid, federal funds available through the Older Americans Act, and other public funds provide almost two-thirds of costs. The balance is met by charity.[17] The possibility of expanded demand financed by health insurance apparently has not been explored; it is dimmed by the issues of transportation time, mingling of populations with different impairments and different classes, and erosion of previous family support.

Home Care Programs

A second group of persons with chronic disease and disability can be supported with specific services delivered to the home. If services are limited, it is cheaper to provide in the home than to institutionalize, and patients generally prefer it. The notion of home care as an inexpensive substitute for institutional care is widespread, although unsupported by evidence. The reality is that home care in fee-for-service environments adds to the total cost of care, probably because services are extended to needs that were previously unmet, or met by informal sources.[18] Managed care patients under home care have lower utilization and costs but inferior outcomes than similar patients under fee-for-service Medicare.[19]

Home care can be limited to non-health services, such as housekeeping, or nonprofessional services, such as personal care. Much home care currently goes beyond those levels, which are not supported by Medicare and rarely included in private insurance. Skilled nursing, counseling, and physical, occupational, and speech therapies are routinely provided in the home. "High tech" home care, which includes intravenous or intubated nutrition, ventilation or respirator, renal dialysis, and intensive drug management for antibiotics and chemotherapy, has become available in recent years.

Nearly two million Medicare beneficiaries, or about 545 per 10,000 persons over age 65, or about 5 percent, were on home care in 1991. Home care is also used by younger persons, but the incidence is substantially lower. They received almost 90 million visits, about 45 per person. Home care is well-supported by private insurance, Medicare, and Medicaid. Although the incidence of home care use appears to have stabilized, the number of visits has been mounting exponentially.

As might be expected with a subsidized service and three to four million potential patients, costs have been mounting rapidly, although expenditure increases have slowed in recent years. In 1980, a million recipients received an average of $1,000 of care per person. In 1992, the last published recipient counts indicated that two million recipients received $7 billion of care, or an average of $3,500 per person per year. By 1996, the total had grown to half again 1992 levels. Much of the growth has been in high-tech services, which grew fivefold in the decade ending 1996 and consumed almost one-third of the 1996 expenditures.[20]

A substantial portion of payments are questionable under insurance benefit definitions. The U.S. Office of the Inspector General (OIG) ranks home care payments as the second largest source of improper Medicare payments. The OIG estimate is that $2.5 billion was improperly paid in FY 1997; almost all because of "lack of medical necessity."[21] The amount would be about one-sixth of the Medicare payment. As a result of federal concern with rising costs and potential fraud, Medicare home health payments were reduced 4 percent from FY 1997 to FY 1998, and a prospective payment system is to be developed.[22]

Home care agencies must be certified to receive Medicare funds, and most states license agencies. There are about 8,700 certified agencies, with an average 1996 Medicare reimbursement of about $4 million per year.[23] Thirty percent of agencies are for-profit. Many are linked to major pharmaceutical or hospital supply companies, particularly for high-tech services. Almost as many, 28 percent, are hospital owned. (They, like the hospitals, are usually not-for-profit.) The remaining agencies are either not-for-profit or government owned. Visiting Nurse Associations, voluntary agencies that began home care around 1900, have fallen to 10 percent of the total.[24] There are an approximately equal number of agencies providing home care without Medicare certification.[25] These are likely to be much smaller, unsponsored agencies.

Home health represents a competitive area where healthcare organizations and other voluntary organizations have been successful, but where for-profit organizations have made substantial gains. Given the evidence of overcharging and the increasing concern with cost, the market share is likely to go to those agencies that can provide attractive service efficiently. Case management, well-trained personnel, honest billing, and reasonable profit margins all contribute to those goals.

Hospice Programs

Hospice care is provided to terminally ill patients and is a deliberate alternative to curative or life-extending treatment. Hospice care accepts the reality of death, provides physical, emotional, and spiritual support to the patients in their homes or home-like settings, emphasizes comfort and quality of life, and supports family members during the dying and bereavement process.[26]

Services include the less technical home care services, with augmented counseling and emotional support.

As of 1992, the most recent data available, hospice organizations served 250,000 persons, slightly less than 100 per 100,000 total population. Growth was at 12 percent per annum, but the total number of predictable deaths per year is only around 600,000, or 240 per 100,000 total population. Three-quarters of hospice patients were over age 65, and 80 percent had diagnoses of cancer. Hospice care is supported by Medicare and most private insurance, with a restriction that the patient will not simultaneously seek curative treatment and physician attestation of a life expectancy less than six months. Medicare hospice coverage has recently been extended to nursing home patients. Hospice care is relatively inexpensive and may save money. One systematic review of the published studies noted the limitations of the data, but concluded, " . . . [T]he existing data suggest that hospice and advance directives can save between 25% and 40% of health care costs during the last month of life, with savings decreasing to 10% to 17% over the last 6 months of life and decreasing further to 0% to 10% over the last 12 months of life."[27] That is, the sooner hospice is started, the less it saves, but the author noted that hospice care and advance directives "certainly do not cost more and they provide a means for patients to exercise their autonomy over end-of-life decisions."[28]

In 1992, about 2,000 hospices served about 125 persons each per year, with an average employed staff of 20, and approximate costs averaging less than $1 million per agency. Ninety percent were nonprofit. At least a few were affiliated with hospitals or home care agencies.[29] Hospices encourage volunteers and received an average of 25 hours of volunteer service per patient in 1990.[30]

Hospice is a small but critical part of healthcare in any community. For patients with predictable death—about one quarter of all deaths—it provides an attractive and less expensive alternative. It may also assist people in coming to terms with death, promoting the use of advanced directives and personal representatives to avoid futile and expensive terminal care. Given the unique requirements of hospice patients, programs need to operate with considerable autonomy, but healthcare organizations can and should assist them by facilitating referrals, encouraging appropriate use, and recognizing their contribution.

Chronic Inpatient Care

Long-term care is provided by several different kinds of facilities. The traditional nursing home is the most common, but nursing homes have expanded to assist Alzheimer and other mental disability victims, and to emphasize rehabilitation, particularly for stroke, heart attack, accident, and orthopedic repair patients. According to the principal trade association, the American Health Care Association,[31]

> In 1997, there were 17,176 Medicare and/or Medicaid certified nursing facilities with 1.8 million beds and 1.5 million residents. Based on the total population in 1996, there were roughly 57 nursing facility beds per 1,000 persons aged 65 to 84, and 454 nursing facility beds for persons aged 85 and over. 1995 survey results indicated that the two most frequently reported admission diagnoses for nursing facility residents were hypertension and cerebral vascular disease for both Medicare and Medicaid beneficiaries.

Functional disability is the cause of nursing home use. The Association reports that:

> In 1997, the average nursing facility resident required assistance with 3.67 activities of daily living (ADL)—a figure that has changed very little over the past five years. . . . Nearly 93 percent of all nursing facility residents in 1997 were either dependent or required some assistance from nursing staff to bathe. . . . Nearly 85 percent of residents also . . . require staff assistance to dress. . . . [A]nother 25 percent require some level of assistance with eating. . . . Since 1995 . . . the percentage of residents who were ambulatory has increased from 45 percent in 1995 to 55 percent in 1997. Forty-two percent of nursing facility residents suffer from some level of dementia and 25 percent have documented symptoms of depression. The percentage of residents receiving preventative skin care has risen noticeably since 1994, from 28 percent to 53 percent of the total resident population.

Ownership of nursing homes is shown in Figure 11.4. Government and small proprietary homes have declined as a percentage of the total, and hospital-owned homes have slowly increased, although recent changes have not been large. About 10 percent of the industry by revenue is in large publicly listed corporations. Four large companies—Beverly Enterprises, Manor Care, Health Care and Retirement Corporation, and Integrated Health Services—provide almost 10 percent of all care. In 1997, 77 percent of the 17,176 nursing facilities were dually certified for both Medicare and Medicaid. Nine percent were certified for Medicare only and 14 percent were certified for Medicaid only. The Association reports that 68 percent of the patients in nursing homes were supported by Medicaid in 1997. Nine percent were on Medicare, and the balance were principally private pay.

The Association notes that the average nursing facility had a daily census of 88 residents and average facility bed size of 107. The nation's nursing facilities have experienced a 3 percent decline in median facility occupancy since 1993. The occupancy decline is significant; profit margins are slim and a few points' difference in occupancy can mean financial collapse. The four largest for-profit chains managed to sustain their net profits, however. In part, this was the result of increased revenue from specialty services. The Association

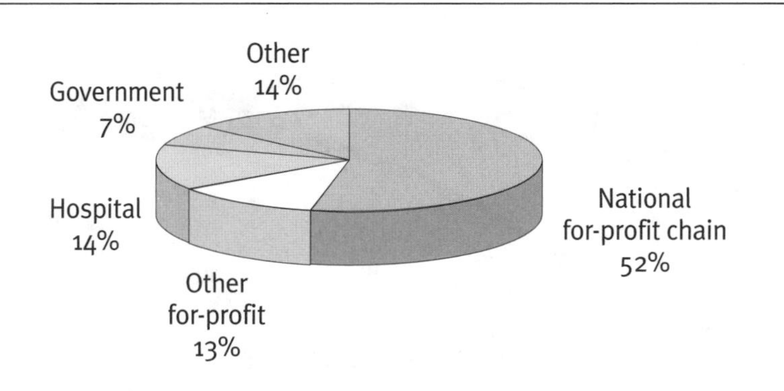

FIGURE 11.4 Ownership of Nursing Homes, 1997

reports that special care beds were about 6 percent of the total in 1997, and of these, two-thirds were in Alzheimer's special care units.

Quality of care in nursing homes is often criticized, and one leading chain, Beverly Enterprises, has been frequently cited by state licensing agencies and individual lawsuits.[32] The Association maintains records on citations against homes by state licensing agencies and claims that most citations for medical conditions, such as incontinence management, pressure sores, physical restraints, and unnecessary drugs, have declined since 1992. Reduced range of motion has declined substantially, from 7.5 percent in 1992 to one percent in 1997.[33] The decline is likely to be related to the increase in ambulation and the decrease in physically-restrained residents, but also to the shift to specialty care.

The Association reports that the average nursing facility employs 54 direct care staff personnel—which includes 36 nurse aides, 11 LPNs, and 7 RNs—for a staff-to-bed ratio of .50 to 1 and an average of 3.5 total direct care staff hours per resident day. Although this represents a lot of attention, the skill and motivation of aides is dependent on the management of the home. They are among the lowest paid workers, and they deal routinely with incontinence, disorientation, and physical burdens moving patients. Strong incentives, including excellent training and supportive supervision, are essential to help aides perform effectively.

The financing of nursing home services is shown in Figure 11.5. In 1996, total national health expenditures for nursing facility care were $78.5 billion dollars, or 7.8 percent of health and health services expenditures. Thirty-eight percent of payments were private, 48 percent Medicaid, and 11 percent Medicare. Five percent came from private health insurance. Medicaid payments for nursing facility care in 1996 equaled 25 percent of the nation's total Medicaid spending. The average per diem Medicare reimbursement for skilled nursing facilities was $253.84 in 1995. The routine portion of the per diem reimbursement, deducting the special services Medicare patients must receive to be eligible, averaged $126.42. Medicaid payment averaged $92 per day, based on the HCFA expenditures report and the Association's estimate of 409 million Medicaid patient days.

FIGURE 11.5
Trends in Nursing Home Finance

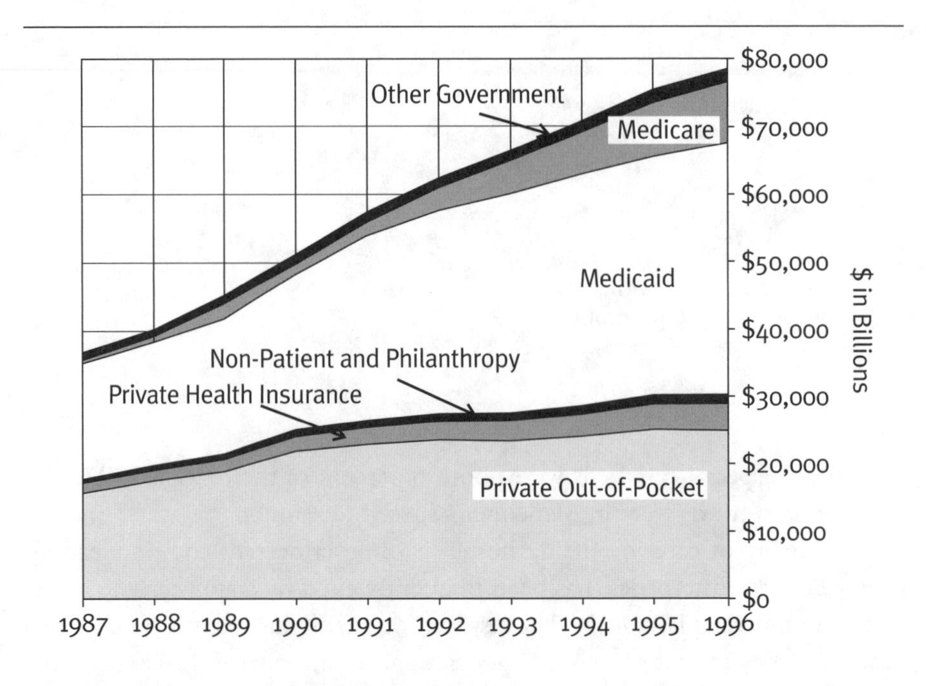

SOURCE: American Health Care Association.

The number of nursing home patients differs widely by state. Against a U.S. average of 53 beds per thousand elderly population, the range was from 24 (Nevada) to 86 (Nebraska). Twelve states had more than 75 beds per thousand elderly, and eight had less than 35. Similar variation occurs in Medicaid expenditures, which had a mean of $623 per recipient in 1992, but ranged from $302 (Florida) to $1,382 (Connecticut). The differences are driven by state Medicaid and certificate of need policies. States with generous Medicaid benefits tend to restrict construction of beds as a way of limiting the Medicaid burden on state taxes.[34] Nationwide, the share of Medicaid funds devoted to nursing homes has fallen steadily since 1980.[35]

These figures reveal the essential problem of financing chronic inpatient care. If one takes the routine cost of Medicare patients as an indicator, Medicaid reimburses less than three-quarters of long run average costs. Also, the amount available differs dramatically by state, and states with generous payment tend to use certificate of need programs to constrain access. The consequences of underfinancing are clear in the quality and access problems and the stringent limits for Medicaid eligibility. Individuals seeking Medicaid must expend virtually all of their assets to be eligible, although certain limited protections are available for the spouse. The long-run solution appears to be increased private and Medicare financing, coupled with strong case management of chronic disease aimed at reducing the need for nursing home care.

The role of the healthcare organization is to see that adequate nursing home care is available for their patients. That includes quality assurance and patient satisfaction for the rehabilitation-oriented services, and at a minimum avoidance of the worst quality situations for continuing care patients. The leading organizations are pursuing this role by operating some inpatient care themselves, and by careful affiliation and partnership with the better independent or national chain suppliers.

Housing

More than three-fourths of older persons own their own homes. The majority of the balance live in rented apartments. The clear preference of the aged is to retain these situations as long as possible. Estimates of housing arrangements with support services vary because of differing definitions. About three million housing units have supportive features, of which possibly two million offer board and continuing care. Only about half a million live in continuing care retirement communities, specially designed facilities with meal, recreational, transportation, and chronic inpatient services. About two million units of government assisted housing exist.[36] As their tenants age, federally assisted complexes have been adding services, but "the overall pattern was a patchwork of services that were relatively unplanned and uncoordinated."[37]

The issues in housing can be divided into three parts: helping homeowners and financially self-sufficient apartment dwellers retain their independent living, providing supportive facilities for those who desire them, and assisting those who cannot afford private solutions.

Almost 90 percent of the aged population of a typical community will own or rent private housing. They will be the backbone of the outreach services in ambulatory care, home care, hospice, and rehabilitative chronic inpatient care. Counseling and modest home modification programs are the only additional services to be considered. Many of these people have a substantial financial asset in their home that can be liquidated through reverse mortgages allowing them to remain in the homes. Financial counseling may assist in tapping this resource. Home modification programs include safety inspections and range from handbars to bathroom revisions and lifts for moving between floors. Much of the work can be done by volunteers from the building trades or with specific training. It can also be purchased from construction contractors. Purchased services may be covered under some Medicare HMO contracts.

A small fraction of people, apparently around 5 percent of the aged, are candidates for congregate living of some kind, short of chronic inpatient care. Apparently only one or 2 percent of the aged population desire and can afford continuing care retirement facilities. Their needs are frequently met by for-profit companies, although there are a number of successful not-for-profit models. Large cities and retirement areas like Florida and Arizona offer a variety of prices. While healthcare organizations can collaborate with these ventures, supplying many services and facilitating transfers when necessary, few will choose to invest capital in them directly.

Subsidized housing, while important in meeting the needs of poor aged, is not generally accepted as part of the healthcare organization mission. It is undertaken by the federal government through state and private collaborative programs and is also supported by some private charities. Again the healthcare organization role is collaborative, supplying services and facilitating transfers.

Strategy for Integrated Healthcare Organizations

The overview of the range of non-acute services reveals a clear strategy for healthcare organizations with a vision of high quality, low cost, comprehensive care. As one of the largest organizations in most communities, and the focal point of health-related activity, the healthcare organization should undertake all of the following:

1. Monitor all community health needs and non-acute services, comparing actual services against national averages and benchmarks, collecting evidence of needs met, client satisfaction, quality of service, and problems encountered.

The intent of this step is to allow the healthcare organization to use its market influence and relationship to the power structure in support of community goals. If nothing else, this step identifies what the issues are, allowing the board to establish priorities for their solution. The annual environmental surveillance should include statistics on availability and use of services, satisfaction, quality, and problems such as delays in arranging appropriate service or access problems for specific groups. Measures of preventive needs and activities should be included with those of non-acute care. As indicated below, a substantial data collection effort is required. Much of the data are available from public sources or by relatively simple surveys. Other important measures can be constructed from the organization's own database and performance assessment activities.

The overall needs of the community should be assessed periodically. The best instrument for this is the Behavioral Risk Factor Survey, developed by the Centers for Disease Control.[38] The survey is used to establish state-level data; a local sample is necessary to estimate needs at a community level. Public health departments often maintain community health assessments and will collaborate in expanding these.[39]

A collaborative effort with other interested agencies can be mounted to collect and share the necessary data. It may be appropriate to support a neutral agency such as local universities or United Way for the data collection. Such an effort is useful in building broader community consensus on priorities. Economic pressure, exercised through referrals and direct assistance, may be important in gaining support of the surveillance effort.

2. Work collaboratively with other agencies to ensure a full spectrum of services in appropriate quantities.

A wide variety of agencies and informal groups address non-acute care needs. The posture of the healthcare organization should be to stimulate these activities and to make them more effective by careful coordination and supplementation. Replacing them would reduce charitable contributions, decrease enthusiasm for meeting real community needs, and substantially increase the demands on the organization's capital. It might also reduce the flexibility and variety of services.

Substantial skill is required to support community-wide collaboration.[40] Many of the groups are focused on idiosyncratic goals that are highly valuable to small numbers of people. They tend to view the healthcare organization as a bureaucratic behemoth and to guard their objective zealously against potential competition. Others may see the healthcare organization as a convenient excuse for diverting their energies to other causes, actually reducing the total commitment. For-profit companies may feel profit margins are threatened by collaboration that strengthens competitors. The organization's own caregivers may feel non-acute care is an unjustified encroachment on acute needs. These responses must each be met with tact, diplomacy, evidence of benefit from collective effort, and extensive but candid discussion.

Subsidies and joint ventures may be important in supporting collaboration. Healthcare organization capital can be donated or invested to assist in meeting newly identified needs. Various devices can ensure the independence of groups fearful of being consumed or corrupted by affiliation. The healthcare organization can pass funds through a community foundation, fund central agencies focusing on collaboration, provide favorable contracts for referrals, supplies, or facilities, provide direct grants, encourage matching grants from others, and establish joint ventures or shared subsidiaries with explicit board representation. All of these devices offer stimuli, and each can be managed in ways that encourage rather than threaten the efforts of others. It may be wise for healthcare organizations to limit their investments, explicitly taking no action until collaborative opportunities have been thoroughly explored.

3. Provide aggressive case management of chronic patients with functional disabilities.

The patients who combine chronic illness and functional disability consume large amounts of healthcare. Because their care is so expensive, financial problems often complicate medical ones. Even modest co-payments mount to levels beyond the family's economic reach. The demand on private or government insurance is routinely in excess of $100,000 per patient. These patients are clearly worth identifying as individuals and adopting specific plans including family and all community resources to provide optimal support at minimal cost.

The largest fraction of the money, and the most critical elements of care, are provided through the acute sector, including primary care, making the integrated healthcare organization an appropriate site for case management. Non-acute care management goes beyond the usual clinical care, and patients involved in it often do not fit the usual protocols. Case management should begin when the seriousness of the patients' conditions are first identified, making it integral with management of acute care. Ideally the plan should be proactive, rather than recovering after the disability has occurred.

Individual programs of care should draw on existing agencies throughout the community, using carefully developed predictors of need to identify specific services.[41] Solutions utilizing standard products will work for many patients, integrating multiple protocols and resources to provide a comprehensive program of care. For others, extensive individualizing and collaboration between agencies will be necessary. The case management program automatically develops a database of the patients most at risk, facilitating surveys of performance.

4. Develop and support focused primary prevention activities.

Important primary prevention activities include immunization, tobacco use, alcohol use, illicit drug use, safe sex, and contraception. As noted, domestic violence is a concern raised by the people at risk. Target audiences are preschool children, teens, and new mothers, with secondary prevention for adults who have encountered problems. Persons most in need are often poor. Racial prejudice and moral or religious concerns complicate the issue. Still, success in these activities can result in major savings, not only in healthcare costs, but in other social costs. Every community should have the most effective possible programs in these areas. Healthcare organizations fulfill their missions by making sure that these programs exist.

Leading organizations have found success in collaborative activities that commit several agencies to the objective. The assistance of government, schools, churches, and community organizations is important in promoting acceptance and use of programs. Support from within the target community is inexpensive and highly effective; opposition is often fatal. Support is built by soliciting participation in the environamental assessment and gaining consensus around shared goals. The data may suggest these goals; they may come from national goals such as "Healthy People 2000" reviewed for local appropriateness; or they may arise from the perceptions of local leaders.[42]

Support often depends on packaging the programs in ways that allay concerns about moral issues. Participation of community representatives helps design attractive programs. Programs aimed at broader goals such as "Family and Child Health" or "Teen Health" appear to be more successful than narrower interventions, although programs that deal explicitly with moral concerns, such as the STARS program (Students Today Aren't Ready for Sex), have also been successful.[43]

5. Expand appropriate secondary prevention.

Most healthcare organizations now support cost-effective programs of secondary prevention. These include a battery of screening tests targeted to specific age and sex groups, and also various activities to support patients and families with chronic disease, including optimum medical care. Actual patient participation in these programs is often less than desirable. Active promotion is necessary to gain compliance with screening objectives, and the promotion must be carefully designed to reach the target audience without stimulating demand from persons for whom the activity is not cost effective. Systematic use of patient records to identify potential users and carefully designed person communication have been effective.

Support groups are often run by volunteers. Some, like Alcoholics Anonymous, deliberately avoid affiliation with the healthcare establishment. Others use medical endorsement to promote their cause. The role of the healthcare organization in both cases is to support the success of these groups. They are important in motivating both patients and family caregivers, and thereby reducing institutionalization. Where direct support, such as space and advertising, is acceptable, the organization can provide it. It can stimulate the formation of groups where need exists. Where less direct intervention is in order, the healthcare organization can rely on community agencies. It may support those agencies that in turn support groups like AA.

6. Support voluntary activities for outreach ambulatory services.

The voluntary activities in transportation, home meals, and social and recreational services can be assisted through community agencies. The healthcare organization should strongly support agencies like Urban Ministry and United Way. In many communities, governing board seats in these organizations are available to the healthcare organization or its members. These provide a vehicle for coordinating and stimulating the broader goals of health. Many specific programs can be supported through these agencies. Some institutions provide direct support through grants or a community foundation.

7. Ensure the provision of effective home care, hospice, and nursing home services.

These services are now provided in many communities, although sometimes in less than fully effective ways. They are essential to cost-effective healthcare because the provision of equivalent services in acute settings would be more costly, and because the financing of care now requires separation. Medicare, for example, pays additional funds for rehabilitation without reducing payments for acute care to the same patient. The issue of cost effectiveness must be addressed through case management. The underlying issue of the amount people are willing to spend for these services must be addressed through market and legislative decisions.

The role of the healthcare organization is to promote healthy competition to the extent possible. It is clear that in home care and nursing home care, the two largest components of outreach care, buyers will exert strong downward pressure on prices. The healthcare organization should ensure that price pressure leads to increased efficiency, rather than simply diminished service. To achieve that, the organization must monitor the existing array of services, identify shortcomings on all measured dimensions, and selectively employ its resources to overcome the weaknesses. A range of options is usually open. The healthcare organization may:

- Start and support a subsidiary for a specific set of services, either to fill a gap or to compete with an inadequate provider.
- Develop preferred partnerships with some existing providers, deliberately strengthening them in competition with others, or to meet evolving needs.
- Supply support in kind, such as facilities, purchasing services, or information services.
- Provide direct cash subsidies, or use its influence with community funding agencies to subsidize promising providers.
- Joint venture with existing providers to facilitate their expansion.

The goal of the healthcare organization is to make all necessary services available while maximizing the use of external capital and ensuring acceptable quality and satisfaction. The key to achieving the goal is the comprehensive measurement of community needs and existing services.

Implementing the goal will mean that the healthcare organization operates selected services in many communities. It has some important advantages, such as space available at reduced cost, control of referrals, low cost overhead services, and a reputation for quality as a direct provider. Operation of a service with a small market share can provide a benchmark for quality and satisfaction. There are also some important disadvantages. Acute care organizations have had difficulty adjusting to the cost limits of subacute care.[44] In states with particularly constrained Medicaid support, the acute care organization may be linked to an underfinanced subacute activity that is either a financial drain or a quality and satisfaction liability. Established providers are often difficult to dislodge, even when a superior service is offered. Entry into a saturated market may weaken all competitors, reducing rather than enhancing quality.

A sound strategy is one carefully articulated in light of local needs and opportunities. It generates improved results for the whole community, on all healthcare issues.

8. Support the provision of appropriate housing.

While housing is obviously important to health, it lies at the extreme of healthcare priorities, and it is more central to those of other social agencies. As a result, healthcare organizations should be alert to the health impacts of housing problems, be positioned to make these problems known to others, and be supportive of corrective efforts. The case for congregate living and continuous care retirement centers is simply not as compelling as those for hospice, rehab, and prevention, and the healthcare organization's commitment should be proportionate. Direct entry into housing is the establishment of new business, less relevant to healthcare than, say, the acquisition of optometry stores or dental practices. Any organization that enters the housing market should justify the entry as a sound business venture, a difficult task at best and impossible for most healthcare organizations. Various forms of collaboration may be useful to meet specific needs in particular communities.

Measuring Prevention and Non-Acute Care

The first step in an integrated care strategy, and the normal requirement of any program, is comprehensive measurement of outreach care needs and services. Figure 11.6 shows the kinds of data desirable and their sources.

Demand and Output

Many communities maintain a community survey of agencies as part of United Way or similar activities and produce a handbook with descriptive data for public use. The listings form an inventory of resources and a database for further work. Licensure and certification records help identify appropriate entries.

Epidemiological estimates of need can be based on data about the existence of specific needs, such as the number of persons with severe disability, obtained from household surveys or medical record surveys. They can also be inferred from national data. Disability measurement is now standardized. Activities of daily living (ADL) include bathing, dressing, eating, continence, getting in and out of bed or chair, and toileting. Instrumental activities of daily living (IADL) include walking, going outside meal preparation, shopping, money management, telephone use, and housekeeping.[45] Chronic disease and disability estimates are always based on age- and gender-specific populations, as are most prevention and health promotion estimates. As more institutions implement integrated care strategies, intercommunity comparative data and benchmarks will become available. They are currently difficult to obtain.

Acceptance delays—the number of days between request for service and actual delivery—are an important indicator of unmet need. They are superior to waiting lists, which are subject to inaccuracy and manipulation.[46] Data can be obtained from the referring agency, which is often the healthcare

FIGURE 11.6
Measures of Outreach Care

Dimension	Measures	Examples	Data Source
Demand	Inventory of available services	Handbook for patients, families, and counselors	Community survey
	Epidemiological estimates of need	Surveys of disability and disease incidence applied to local population	Population census and comparative use rates; survey of functional status
	Acceptance delays and waiting lists	Transfer delay from acute inpatient care	Referral sources
		Waiting list for hospice, home care	Agency operators
	Unmet need	Persons without immunization or appropriate secondary screening	Household survey Survey of medical records
Costs/ Resources	Supply of facilities	Beds, units	Agency survey, licensure reports
	Costs	Annual costs by type of resource	Agency reports
	Prices charged	Nursing home charge and Medicare reimbursement	Agency publications Medicare and Medicaid regulations
	Charitable funding	Annual donations received	Agency reports
	Profits/deficits	Annual profit and financial ratios	Agency reports
Human Resources	Volunteer hours	Number of volunteers and hours contributed	Agency reports
	Employment by skill level	Number of paid employees by class	Agency reports
	Worker satisfaction	Survey, turnover, vacancy statistics	Agency reports
Output/ Productivity	Number of persons served	Admissions	Agency reports
	Units of service delivered	Patient days, visits	Agency reports
	Cost/person or unit	Charges or cost/patient-year	Derived
	Cost/capita	Charges or cost/person insured	Derived
Quality	Case evaluation of patient progress	Change in functional disability status at quarterly or annual intervals Adverse events	Case management reports Agency reports, licensure and insurance reports
	Process quality scores	Patients ambulated, bedsores Scores on procedural audits	Agency survey
	Structural quality measures	Staffing hours/patient, by class Counts of license citations by type Licensure status	Agency reports State licensure data
Customer Satisfaction	Patient and family satisfaction	Satisfaction surveys	Agency reports, healthcare organization surveys
	Referral physician satisfaction	Physician satisfaction surveys, anecdotal reports	Physician survey or informal contact
	Community perception	Recognition and impression of non-users	Household surveys

organization itself, and documented from medical records. Delays in discharge from acute inpatient care and transfer to nursing home, sometimes called "administrative days," are particularly important and are routinely monitored in most institutions. Many communities measure unmet immunization at school enrollment, when the problem must often be corrected by law. Age five or six is too old for optimum results, however. Surveys and databases constructed from birth certificates allow earlier correction. They are difficult to construct for the populations most at risk, however.[47]

Data on the number of persons served, units of service, and acceptance delays must be compiled by the agency, and release must be negotiated. Some agencies may resist release. However, licensure, certification, and Medicare data are public, and the growing databases of healthcare organizations allow tracking of patients and insured members, so that agency resistance is limited. Integrating data collection with community funding such as United Way encourages participation. The statistics should be available by cause of use, geographic area of patient residence, patient age and sex, and source of payment. These categories permit construction of use and productivity statistics for specific populations of interest.

Costs and Productivity

Descriptions of the physical resources, including staffing, are sometimes available from licensure and certification records. The costs of outreach care are part of the global cost of healthcare, and conceptually should be monitored as closely as the cost of any other clinical service. Most cost data is internal to the agency, and release must be negotiated. A central agency can ensure confidentiality of detail, and charitable donations, such as United Way support, can be tied to the provision of data. Donations available through centralized sources are measured routinely, and most central sources insist on release of records of direct gifts. Gross prices must be public, but discounts and net prices are frequently concealed for competitive reasons, along with profitability. Net prices paid by Medicare are public, can be compared with other communities, and can be used as a rough guide to fairness of other charges. Prices paid by Medicaid are at best marginally adequate; their relative size and the number of Medicaid recipients are an indication of the financial adequacy of outreach care support.

Unit costs, including cost per capita, are derived from output and cost statistics. They are the basis for evaluating efficiency of outreach care. They can now be compared to national averages for specific groups; increased attention to data collection will allow intercommunity comparisons and benchmarking.

Quality

The most rigorous evaluation of outreach care is the progress of the patients, in absolute terms and against expectations. An individual care plan, a program, or a community can be said to be effective if the patient recovers functional capability, or recovers as much functional capability as expected. In practice, substantial progress has been made implementing the concept, but only among the least sick or disabled patients. It is now common to evaluate recovery of patients with trauma, orthopedic repair, stroke, heart attack, and heart surgery by assessing their functionality after 90 days. The assessment requires special planning but can be made in routine primary care follow-up. Similarly, more permanently disabled patients can be monitored for functionality in each of the various outreach settings: recreational, day care, home care, and nursing home. Medicare certification requires the routine use of a patient assessment instrument in nursing homes, and many states have extended it to all patients.[48] The concept does not apply to hospice. However, data collection on this scale is expensive. It draws from already severely limited funds, takes a long time to collect, and is difficult to interpret. As a result, outcomes evaluation of care beyond the rehab level is usually limited to research projects.

Adverse events, such as patient falls, skin deterioration, and infections, are easier to track. Litigation over the quality of care is relatively rare, but lawsuits or insurance settlements can be monitored. Licensure agencies monitor such records, and the American Health Care Association maintains reports from licensure agencies and its members. With customer satisfaction, these measures provide the basic assurance of quality in outreach care. Licensure and certification requirements also include structural measures, such as the availability of professional nurses and the safety of the facility. Their reports are public information.

Customer Satisfaction

Patient and family satisfaction can be surveyed either by outreach care agencies or by integrated healthcare organizations. Including questions on outreach care in the surveys of acute care is relatively inexpensive and allows a broader sampling base than most outreach care agencies can afford. Similarly, referring physicians are routinely surveyed, formally and informally, by the healthcare organization. Household surveys can address recognition of the availability of outreach care and of specific providers, as well as perceptions of overall adequacy. At present, formal surveys are rare, but informal data from families and physicians helps to detect unacceptable service.

Role of the Healthcare Organization

Community-oriented healthcare organizations are obligated to collect or support the collection of data on the dimensions of Figure 11.6, to monitor such data as are available, to identify problems in quality and satisfaction, and to use their influence as referring sources to get problems corrected. The routine review of outreach care performance is the first step of any sound strategy, as indicated above. It underpins priorities and supports the collaborative efforts essential to improvement. Under managed Medicare, it is likely that integrated healthcare organizations will take those obligations more seriously, because expensive episodes of acute care are often the result of outreach care failures.

Suggested Readings

Beaton, S. R., and S. A. Voge. 1998. *Measurements for Long-Term Care: A Guidebook for Nurses.* Thousand Oaks, CA: Sage Publications.

Binstock, R. H., L. E. Cluff, and O. von Mering (eds.). 1996. *The Future of Long-Term Care: Social and Policy Issues.* Baltimore: Johns Hopkins University Press.

Bogue, R., and C. H. Hall, Jr. (eds.). 1997. *Health Network Innovations: How 20 Communities Are Improving Their Systems Through Collaboration.* Chicago: American Hospital Publishing.

Curran, C., K. W. Kuhn, N. Miller, A. Skalla, R. O. Thurman. 1999. *Shaping an Integrated Delivery System: Home Care's Role in Improving Service Outcomes and Profitability.* Chicago: Health Administration Press.

DiGuiseppi, C., D. Atkins, and S. H. Woolf (eds.). 1998. *Guide to Clinical Preventive Services 1996: Report of the U.S. Preventive Services Task Force 2nd ed.* Available on the National Institutes of Health website: text.nlm.nih.gov/ftrs/pick?collect=cps&cc=1&ftrsK=53235&t=910194751 (Nov. 4, 1998).

Fox, D. M., and C. Raphael (eds.). 1997. *Home-Based Care for a New Century.* Malden, MA: Blackwell Publishers.

Institute of Medicine. Committee on Using Performance Monitoring to Improve Community Health. 1997. *Improving Health in the Community: A Role for Performance Monitoring.* Washington, D.C.: National Academy Press.

Jolt, H., and M. M. Leibovici (eds.). 1997. *Long-Term Care: Concept and Reality.* Health Care Management Series v. 3, no. 1. Philadelphia: Hanley & Belfus.

Lerman, D., and C. Tehan (eds.). 1995. *Hospital-Hospice Management Models Integration and Collaboration.* Chicago: American Hospital Publishing.

Mason, V. 1997. *Marketing the Continuum of Care: Strategies for Developing Community Services.* New York: HFMA/McGraw-Hill.

Mills, R. E. (ed.). 1996. *Long-Term Care Investment Strategies: A Guide to Start-Ups, Facility Conversions and Strategic Alliances.* Chicago: Irwin Professional Pub.

Minkler, M. (ed.). 1997. *Community Organizing and Community Building for Health.* New Brunswick, NJ: Rutgers University Press.

Notes

1. J. Kupersmith, M. Holmes-Rovner, A. Hogan, D. Rovner, and J. Gardiner, "Cost-Effectiveness Analysis in Heart Disease, Part II: Preventive Therapies." *Progress in Cardiovascular Diseases* 37(4): 243–71 Jan–Feb, 1995; P. W. Newacheck, J. J. Stoddard, D. C. Hughes, and M. Pearl. "Health Insurance and Access to Primary Care for Children." *New England Journal of Medicine* 338(8):513–9, (Feb 19, 1998); B. A. Bartman, C. M. Clancy, E. Moy, and P. Langenberg. "Cost Differences Among Women's Primary Care Physicians." *Health Affairs* 15(4):177–82, (Winter, 1996)

2. ———. "Assessing the Effectiveness of Disease and Injury Prevention Programs: Costs and Consequences." *MMWR-Morb-Mortal-Wkly-Rep.* 44(RR-10): 1–10 (Aug. 18, 1995)
3. W. G. Weissert, S. C. Hedrick, "Outcomes and Costs of Home and Community-Based Care: Implications for Research-Based Practice." In *New Ways to Care for Older People*, E. Calkins, ed. New York: Springer Publishing Co. (1999)
4. E. J. Emanuel. "Cost Savings at the End of Life. What Do the Data Show?" *JAMA* 275(24):1907–14 (Jun 26, 1996)
5. W. G. Weissert, T. Lesnick, M. Musliner, and K. A. Foley, "Cost Savings from Home and Community-Based Services: Arizona's Capitated Medicaid Long-Term Care Program." *Journal of Health Politics, Policy and Law* 22:6 1329–57, 1330 (Dec, 1997)
6. *Ibid*, p. 1330
7. C. J. Evashwick and L. G. Branch, "Clients of the Continuum." Ch. 2 of *The Continuum of Long-Term Care: An Integrated Systems Approach*, C. J. Evaswick ed. New York: Delmar Publishers, p. 17 (1996)
8. J. W. Lynch, G. A. Kaplan, and S. J. Shema, "Cumulative Impact of Sustained Economic Hardship on Physical, Cognitive, Psychological, and Social Functioning." *New England Journal of Medicine* 337(26):1889–95 (Dec 25, 1997)
9. W. G. Manning, E. B. Keeler, J. P. Newhouse, E. M. Sloss, and J. Wasserman, "The Taxes of Sin. Do Smokers and Drinkers Pay Their Way?" *JAMA* 261(11):1604–9 (Mar 17, 1989)
10. C. J. Evashwick, "Nursing Homes." Ch. 4 of *The Continuum of Long-Term Care: An Integrated Systems Approach*, C. J. Evaswick, ed. New York: Delmar Publishers, p. 45 (1996)
11. Survey of Income and Program Participation, quoted in P. Doty, R. Stone, M. E. Jackson, and M. Adler, "Informal Caregiving," ch. 4 of *The Continuum of Long-Term Care: An Integrated Systems Approach*, C. J. Evaswick, ed. New York: Delmar Publishers, p. 127 (1996)
12. M. D. Resnick, P. S. Bearman, R. W. Blum, K. E. Bauman, K. M. Harris, et al, "Protecting Adolescents from Harm. Findings from the National Longitudinal Study on Adolescent Health." *JAMA* 278(10): 823–32 (Sep 10, 1997)
13. J. O. Hill, and J. C. Peters, "Environmental Contributions to the Obesity Epidemic." *Science* 280(5368):1371–4 (May 29, 1998)
14. C. Warshaw, "Domestic Violence: Changing Theory, Changing Practice." *Journal of the American Medical Women's Association* 51(3):87–91, 100, 1996 (May–Jul)
15. National Institute on Adult Day Care (NIAD) of the National Council on Aging. Website: www.utmb.edu/aging/adacare.htm (undated as of 9/9/98)
16. W. G. Weissert et al, *Adult Day Care: Findings from a National Survey.* Baltimore: Johns Hopkins University Press, (1990)
17. J. Tedesco, "Adult Day Care." Ch. 6 of *The Continuum of Long-Term Care: An Integrated Systems Approach*, C. J. Evaswick, ed. New York: Delmar Publishers, pp. 84–96 (1996)
18. W. G. Weissert, E. A. Miller, and M. Chernew, "Managed Care for Elderly People: Extant Evidence and Its Implications for the Role of Government."

Paper presented at the Panel on Politics of Families and Family Care, American Political Science Association, Chicago (April, 1998)

19. R. E. Schlenker, P. W. Shaughnessy, and D. R. Hittle, "Patient-Level Cost of Home Health Care Under Capitated and Fee-for-Service Payment." *Inquiry* 32(3):252–70 (Fall, 1995)
20. S. Hughes "Home Health." Ch. 5 of *The Continuum of Long-Term Care: An Integrated Systems Approach*, C. J. Evaswick, ed. New York: Delmar Publishers, pp. 66–72 (1996)
21. Office of the Inspector General, "Report on the Financial Statement Audit of the Health Care Financing Administration." Washington, DC: OIG (preliminary report released July 28, 1998)
22. Balanced Budget Act of 1997 Medicare and Medicaid Provisions. Washington DC: Health Care Financing Administration (December 3, 1997)
23. Health Care Financing Administration, Annual Statistics (1996). Another unit of Health and Human Services suggests a total of 19,000 agencies, but non-Medicare agencies are likely to be much smaller. (U.S. Administration on Aging, Department of Health and Human Services Directory of websites on Aging: www.aoa.dhhs.gov/aoa/webres/in-home.htm, (9/10/98; last modified: March 6, 1998)
24. S. Hughes, "Home Health" p. 68
25. SMG Marketing Group, Inc., "Institutional Digest." Hoechst Marion Roussel Managed Care Digest Series (1997)
26. G. Miller, "Hospice." Ch. 7 of *The Continuum of Long-Term Care: An Integrated Systems Approach*, C. J. Evaswick, ed. New York: Delmar Publishers, p. 98 (1996)
27. E. J. Emanuel. "Cost Savings at the End of Life. What Do the Data Show?" *JAMA* 275(24):1907–14, p. 1907 (June 26, 1996)
28. *Ibid*, 1907
29. G. Miller, "Hospice," p. 102
30. G. Miller, "Hospice," pp. 99–101
31. American Health Care Association, *The Nursing Facility Sourcebook, 1998*, Executive Summary, www.ahca.org/research/nftoc.htm (9/10/98)
32. B. Feder, "What Ails a Nursing Home Empire?" *New York Times* Sec. 3, pp. 1, 8 (Feb. 11, 1988)
33. American Health Care Association, *The Nursing Facility Sourcebook (1998)*
34. B. Burwell, W. H. Crown, C. O'Shaugnessy, and R. Price, "Financing Long-Term Care." Ch. 13 of *The Continuum of Long-Term Care: An Integrated Systems Approach*, C. J. Evaswick, ed. New York: Delmar Publishers, pp. 198–207, 218–9 (1996)
35. *Ibid*, p. 207
36. J. Pynoos, "Housing and the Continuum of Care." Ch. 8 of *The Continuum of Long-Term Care: An Integrated Systems Approach*, C. J. Evaswick, ed. New York: Delmar Publishers, pp. 110–113 (1996)
37. *Ibid*, p. 113
38. J. S. Marks, G. C. Hogelin, E. M. Gentry, J. T. Jones, K. L. Gaines, M. R. Forman, and F. L. Trowbridge, "The Behavioral Risk Factor Surveys, I: State-Specific Prevalence Estimates of Behavioral Risk Factors." *American Journal of Preventive Medicine* 1(6):1–8, (Nov–Dec 1985); E. M. Gentry, W.

D. Kalsbeek, G. C. Hogelin, J. T. Jones, K. L. Gaines, M. R. Forman, J. S. Marks, and F. L. Trowbridge, "The Behavioral Risk Factor Surveys, II: Design, Methods, and Estimates from Combined State Data." *American Journal of Preventive Medicine* 1(6):9–14, (Nov–Dec 1985) Also see the Centers for Disease Control website: www.cdc.gov/publications.htm (October 29, 1998)

39. M. E. Cowen, M. Bannister, R. Shellenberger, and R. Tilden, "A Guide for Planning Community-Oriented Health Care: The Health Sector Resource Allocation Model." *Medical Care* 34(3):264–79 (Mar 1996); National Association of County Health Officials, *Assessment Protocols for Excellence in Public Health.* Washington, DC: National Association of County Health Officials (1991)
40. M. Minkler, ed., *Community Organizing and Community Building for Health.* New Brunswick, NJ: Rutgers University Press (1997)
41. W. G. Weissert and C. M. Cready, "Toward a Model for Improved Targeting of Aged at Risk of Institutionalization." *Health Services Research*, 24:4, 485–510
42. ———, *Developing Objectives for Healthy People 2010.* Washington, DC: US Dept. of Health and Human Services, Office of Disease Prevention and Health Promotion (1997). Electronic access: www.health.gov/healthypeople/Guide/TOC.htm (October 1998)
43. J. R. Griffith, *Designing 21st Century Healthcare: Leadership in Hospitals and Healthcare Systems*, Chicago: Health Administration Press, p. 147 (1988)
44. S. Milder, "Look Before You Leap." *Health Care* 24(2):20–1 (Mar 19, 1982)
45. D. Dawson, G. Hendershot, and J. Fulton," Aging in the Eighties: Functional Limitations of Individuals 65 and Over," *Advanced Data*, No. 133. Washington, DC: National Center for Health Statistics (June 10, 1987)
46. S. Frankel, "The Natural History of Waiting Lists—Some Wider Explanations for an Unnecessary Problem." *Health Trends* 21(2):56–8 (May, 1989)
47. J. R. Griffith, *Designing 21st Century Healthcare*, p. 148
48. J. E. Allen, *Long-Term Care Facility Resident Assessment Instrument: User's Manual for Use with Version 2.0 of HCFA Minimum Data Set Resident Assessment Protocols and Utilization Guidelines October 1995, Plus HCFA's 249 Questions and Answers, August 1996.* New York: Springer Pub. Co., (1997)

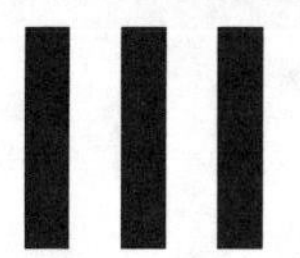

PART III

Learning: Meeting Information and Support Needs

An organization committed to open systems, community-focused strategic management, and continuous improvement is by definition a learning organization. As stakeholder needs change, the organization must change, and changing requires understanding the new needs, developing processes to meet them, and improving the processes over time. New facts and new skills must be learned to support the change.[1] The learning includes a sometimes painful readjustment of individual goals and values to the group objectives that allow the organization to continue.[2] Handling the change and learning is a core competency of any modern organization.[3] In the rapidly moving world of healthcare, it is the hallmark of success. Those organizations that handle change and learning continuously and smoothly are well managed. Those that procrastinate or are snarled in crisis and controversy are failing.

At least nine different functions underpin successful operations and crisis-free change. Figure III.1 shows them in terms of the tasks that must support a successful clinical service line or support service. As the figure shows, they can be grouped in three parts: those functions necessary to track and respond to external needs (on the left), those necessary to support the internal improvement (on the right), and those that provide the physical workspace and supplies. The physical environment is created, not learned, but it too must change to meet new needs.

These functions are largely creations of the last century and, in many cases, the last few decades. They depend heavily on computers, and will depend more on them. Although none of them provide healthcare and few of them interact directly with patients, they consume a substantial chunk—about 20 percent—of healthcare resources. The functions are arrayed and labeled differently in different organizations. In this text, they are grouped into planning, marketing, finance, information systems, human resources, and plant. The grouping reflects their historical origins, and probably the functional hierarchy in most institutions. The hierarchy and its labels are less important than the existence of the resources and the ability to integrate them smoothly.

There are skeptics in the world who feel that the learning functions are overblown or even in some cases unnecessary.[4] It is unquestionably possible to spend too much on them, and it is unfortunately possible to waste even what has been spent well by failures in governance or management. Leading

FIGURE III.1 Learning Support for Successful Clinical Operations

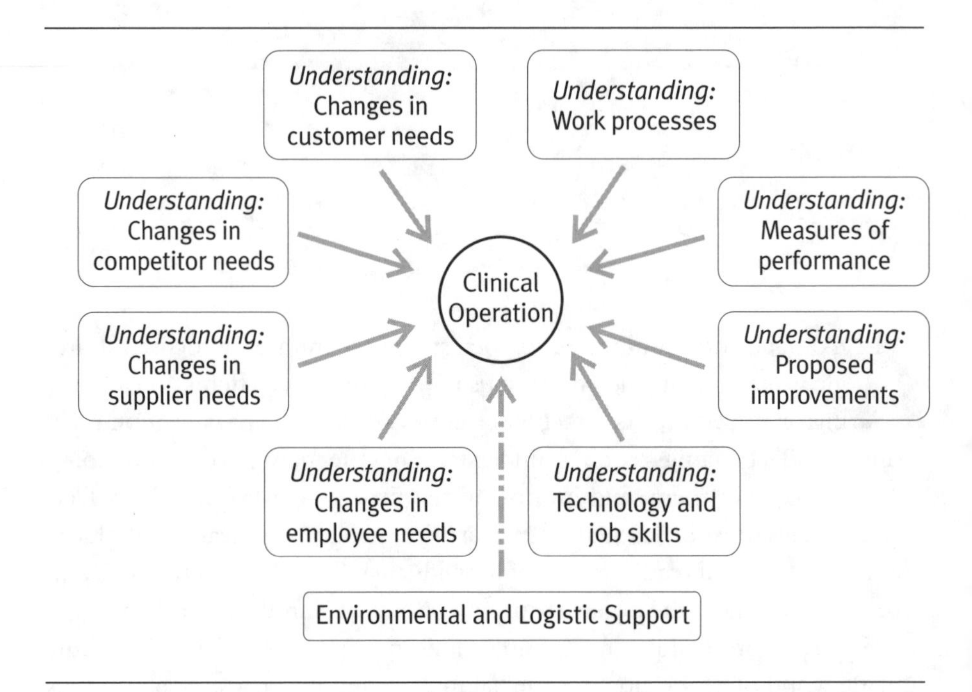

organizations demand as much justification from the technical support units as they do from clinical operations, insisting upon performance measures, expectations, and continuous improvement. But they have found the justification, invested heavily, and seen their market share and profit rise, not only in healthcare,[5] but in many industries.[6]

Notes

1. P. M. Senge, *The Fifth Discipline: The Art and Practice of the Learning Organization*. New York: Doubleday/Currency, (1990)
2. R. Pascale, M. Millemann, and L. Gioja, "Changing the Way We Change." *Harvard Business Review* 75(6):126–39 (Nov–Dec, 1997)
3. J. Barnsley, L. Lemieux-Charles, and M. M. McKinney, "Integrating Learning into Integrated Delivery Systems." *Health Care Management Review* 23(1):18–28 (Winter, 1998)
4. C. R. Miller, J. Epstein, and S. Woolhandler, "Costs at For-Profit and Not-For-Profit Hospitals." *The New England Journal of Medicine* 337 (24): 1779 (Dec 11, 1997; S. Woolhandler and D. U. Himmelstein, "Costs of Care and Administration at For-Profit and Other Hospitals in the United States." *The New England Journal of Medicine* 336: 769–74 (Mar 13, 1997)
5. J. R. Griffith, *Designing 21st Century Healthcare* Ch. 5, pp. 247–265 (1998)
6. J. Pfeffer, *Competitive Advantage Through People*. Boston, MA: Harvard Business School Press, pp. 27–65 (1994)

CHAPTER

12

PLANNING FUTURE DIRECTIONS

Planning and marketing define the healthcare organization's basic response to its environment. They are resource allocation decision processes that must meet the twin tests of realism (fit with the realities of the customer and provider markets) and conviction (convincing individual patients and workers that the decisions are in their personal best interests; this concept is discussed more fully in Chapter 5). Excellent planning and marketing must not only lead to rewarding exchanges between the organization and its community, but also encourage a timely, responsive, consistent, and even-handed process for resource allocations resolving many potentially conflicting interests. In the context of open systems theory, community-oriented strategic management, and continuous improvement (Chapter 2), they must be proactive, emphasizing foresight and placing the thinking of management in the future compared to the present. They are always market oriented; that is, they assess the real interests of the community and search for ways to meet them.

Planning and marketing are such extensive activities that it is difficult to develop uniform definitions. Different authors use different, sometimes conflicting, terminology. Planning often refers to the process of making resource allocation decisions about the future, particularly the process of involving organization members to select among alternative courses of action. The term **marketing** has an unfortunate sharp distinction between its technical and common usage. In common usage, as the term might be understood by doctors, nurses, and some trustees, marketing generally implies sales, promotional, or advertising activity. In contrast, as it appears in professional texts and journals,[1] marketing incorporates the entire set of activities and processes normally ascribed to planning plus those relating to sales and promotion.

Both of these concepts are important. Recognizing the importance of marketing in its broad sense of establishing fruitful relationships with patients, intermediaries, other stakeholders, and potential competitors, Chapter 13 is devoted to that subject. This chapter covers decision making about mission, vision, services, products, locations, and prices. These are the subjects often labeled "planning." The chapter covers purpose, functions, performance measures, and organization for planning.

Purpose

The purpose of both planning and marketing is to optimize the organization's future exchange relationships. Only the word "future" distinguishes this purpose from the purpose of the entire governance system. Planning includes analysis of future community needs and interests, response to external threats and opportunities, design and promotion of new programs, assembly and recruitment of necessary resources, and acquisition of required permits and certificates. Compounding planning's broad scope, the subtlety of the concepts that lie behind the word "optimize" makes planning one of the most fascinating activities in healthcare management.

The word "optimize" implies finding the best possible achievement of some good or benefit through decisions allocating scarce resources. One optimizes the benefits of a specific activity relative to its costs, but in the final analysis, both benefits and costs are in the eye of the beholder. Especially for the not-for-profit healthcare organization, a key part of the planning process consists of understanding and reaching consensus on the benefits to be achieved. This understanding is embodied in the mission, a statement of the preferred good or benefit couched in terms of community, service, and finance (see below, and Chapter 3). The mission provides a guide that is used routinely and consistently to make resource allocation decisions.

The concept of optimizing is to design each healthcare project to have the greatest possible benefit to cost ratio, and to rank order possible projects, identifying and implementing the ones that have the greatest ratio of benefits to costs, as shown in the center box of Figure 12.1. Conceptually, one finds a project, evaluates it in terms of the mission, and, if the benefits exceed the costs by more than any other project, adopts it. Practically, the process is almost never so simple. Selection is less critical than discovery; the best projects often require laborious and frustrating search. Neither the benefits nor the costs are easy to measure. They are even less easy to compare against one another and against other projects.

The simple concept leaves two formidable questions, shown in the upper and lower boxes of Figure 12.1: "How much is a healthcare benefit worth in terms of non-healthcare opportunities?" and "Given that the future is always uncertain, how do I deal with the risk that my forecasts are incorrect?" These questions are outside the control of the organization. The value of the benefit is set by market pricing mechanisms; it is worth what the customer is willing to pay for it. Risk is what cannot be foreseen. Whenever a given proposal is accepted, a decision is made that the risk is tolerable and that the objective can be reached within the customer's price limit. The ideal is to make these decisions in such a way that even with complete hindsight, none would be changed. Real organizations fall substantially short of the ideal, but well-managed organizations come closer than others. In other words, they thrive because they plan well, choosing and delivering healthcare that the customer is comfortable buying and they can comfortably deliver.

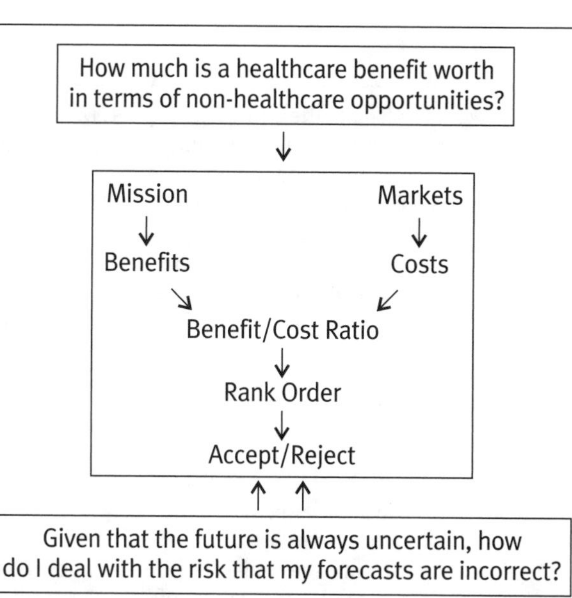

FIGURE 12.1 Optimization Concept

Functions

The functions of planning are shown in Figure 12.2. The six major functions can be summarized as surveillance, strategy, and four levels of responses, where the purpose of strategy is to give coherence to the individual actions. The functions are sequentially interrelated. Achieving optimal planning decisions is the result of a continuous cycle that begins with surveillance, continues through to regulatory compliance, and starts again. Many elements are on a formal annual schedule, but events may force a change in mid-cycle.

An oversight or failure at a low numbered function usually causes problems at higher numbered functions. For example, failure to recognize a competitor decision may lead to suboptimal decisions about the scope of clinical services, a missed partnership opportunity, and eventual difficulties with selecting and funding programmatic proposals. Efforts to enhance the effectiveness of planning usually begin by improving the surveillance function. The intent is to increase awareness among the decision makers, thereby enhancing the number of potential opportunities and creating demand for improvement in the other functions.

Surveillance

Surveillance is the sensory function of the healthcare organization. It is a continuous process that monitors the open systems relationship of the organization to its environment. It attempts to identify all changes in the environment that may require responses from the organization. It also identifies the perspectives of stakeholders and influentials in the community on

FIGURE 12.2
Planning Functions

Function	Description	Example
1. Surveillance	All activities to understand changing stakeholder needs	Monitoring plans of competitors
a. Environmental assessment	Formal annual review of changes and trends affecting future performance	Summary of insurance coverage and price trends
b. Community-based epidemiologic planning	Analysis and forecasting of community demographics and disease incidence	Trends in births
2. Strategic positioning	Crafting a response to stakeholder needs that will be effective in the long term	Limiting the scope of clinical services
a. Revising the mission and vision	Stating the underlying purpose and values of the organization	Adding primary care to a traditional hospital mission
b. Strategy selection	Agreeing on a set of price, quality, and service goals	Forming a strategic partnership
3. Implementing the strategy through long-range plans	Describing future plans for facilities, personnel, and information services	Description of expansion and renovation plans
4. Responding to external opportunities	Evaluation of events that change the strategic risks or benefits	Acquiring a faltering competitor
5. Developing and evaluating programmatic proposals	Systematic review of equipment replacement, program expansions, and new technology	Replacing x-ray equipment
6. Maintaining relations with government and accreditation agencies	Compliance with regulation and criteria, monitoring and reacting to proposed changes	Lobbying

these changes, with particular attention to those of other healthcare agencies, patients, doctors, and employees. All members of the strategic apex are responsible for surveillance. Trustees and directors bear a particular responsibility, because of their contacts in the community. Excellent CEOs and chief planners often devote substantial personal time to surveillance.

Surveillance should be both broad and timely. No risk is as great as the risk of the unnoticed idea. Thorough surveillance opens opportunities for revision and compromise that might otherwise be overlooked. The missed trend away from an old product or service, the overlooked interest in a new one, the too-narrow perception of capability underlie many wrong investments and the demise of entire industries. The earlier a change is identified, the longer the organization has to respond. As a result, good surveillance includes large amounts of vague, rapidly changing information. (It can include deliberately misleading information placed by competitors.) Evaluating the information to decide what to act upon, what to monitor, and what to ignore is part of the process. In addition to the dangers of omitting or dismissing important changes, there is a danger of too rapid response, of overreacting to a transient variation. Yet, perversely, this danger often arises from incomplete surveillance. The transient fad is more likely to be identified as such when one's knowledge is broad.

Environmental assessment

Environmental assessment is a formal surveillance review of the organization and its environment. It is undertaken annually by the planning unit, and supported by detailed factual and quantitative analysis. As much as possible should be quantified, but the appeal of numbers should not overshadow the importance of changes in unmeasurable topics, particularly attitudes, beliefs, and technology. Good environmental assessment takes into account the following:

- *Community demography, epidemiology, and economy.* See community based planning, below. A thorough description of the market being served, identification of all major trends in demographics and disease incidence, and forecasts to the future are essential to the environmental assessment. A quantitative database is maintained, analyzed, and used to support forecasts of the future.
- *Patient and health insurance buyer attitudes.* Trends in total purchases of healthcare, sites of care, and market share should be described and quantified as much as possible. Communities vary substantially, even within a single state. Particular attention should be paid to the attitudes of unions, employers, and governments, whose decisions affect large groups of individual consumers. While state and national trends are important, the view of local groups on key matters such as service, debt, price, and amenities is often the final determinant of planning and financial strategy. These major customer stakeholders are often on the governing board, but explicit efforts to solicit their opinion are useful.[2] Household surveys are a useful, although expensive, vehicle for assessing attitudes and behavior, and their popularity is growing rapidly. Focus groups can provide in-depth understanding of customer perspectives, although it is difficult to get complete representation.
- *Trends in insurance intermediary activity.* Insurer and intermediary arrangements such as the development of capitation, preferred provider contracts, and limits on government programs are important influences on

strategy. The rapid growth of managed care has resulted in radical revisions in strategies of many providers. Payment limits imposed by Medicare, Blue Cross, and Medicaid have important financial and managerial consequences. The trends in market share of the various insurance products and the payment policies of the larger intermediaries must be examined and forecast.

- *Trends in clinical practice.* Technology and the attitudes of practitioners and patients interact to create demands for new services and new modes of delivery. In the 1980s, for example, patients began to prefer outpatient over inpatient care. At the same time, technology supported rapid growth in complex procedures like cardiac catheterization, in vitro fertilization, and orthopedic replacements. While clinical trends are difficult to forecast quantitatively, describing them improves decision making.
- *Member attitudes and capabilities.* Trends in the skills and attitudes of current employees, physicians, and volunteers are important background to planning decisions. Formal surveys are frequently used, but additional insights can be gained through focus groups and informal discussion.
- *Trends in physician availability and organization.* The number of physicians in practice, by specialty and other characteristics, is a critical indicator of both cost and quality of care. A database is maintained to support physician organization planning functions described in Chapter 8.
- *Trends in other health worker availability.* Well-managed institutions forecast their need for professional workers of all kinds. The lead time allows them to adapt to shortages and surpluses, using advance warning to plan work force recruitment or reduction.
- *Role of other provider organizations.* Other provider organizations can complement the mission, be competitors, or allies. Any given organization must choose between avoidance, competition, or collaboration modes of interacting with all others serving its population. To make these decisions, it needs accurate descriptions. Mission, ownership, location, and services are usually public information. Population surveys and historic use data are the sources for market share information. Financial strength of competitors is frequently available from public sources. Because detailed data are often kept secret, quantitative forecasts are not always available and subjective observations become important in their absence. Strategic positioning, discussed below, identifies the mode of interacting with each other's provider.

The planning unit is accountable for a thorough and current database of all of these elements and a written annual review highlighting important trends and developments. It should also be accountable for reporting and, where possible, integrating insights or beliefs regarding future trends offered by other members of governance.

Community-Based Epidemiologic Planning

The planning department is the "source of truth" for demographic, disease incidence, and market share data. It maintains the databases that support epidemiological planning (Chapter 6, with applications in Chapters 8, 9, and 10). It generates forecasts for almost any service demand on request and routinely produces short-run and long-run forecasts for a number of important demand measures. These are used in strategic positioning, the development of facility and service plans, and the construction of expectations for the next budget year. The reliability of the forecasts, the advice available from the planning department, and the speed with which requests can be serviced are critical elements in long-term success of the organization. Planning staff offer alternative estimates of incidence rates, advice on segmentation of the population, and ranges of current practice on use that help operators understand the dynamics of demand and the uncertainty of forecasts. These services are frequently available from national consulting services, but an in-house source is usually cheaper and develops expertise in the local situation. Calculation and presentation software are also available to make construction of forecasts, sensitivity analysis, and exploration of alternative scenarios quickly and easily.

Strategic Positioning

The mission, vision, ownership, scope of services, location, and partners of the organization define its **strategic position**. Surveillance information and the environmental assessment are used to review the strategic position at least annually but also as opportunities arise. Many of the opportunities arise from the actions of others—changes of service, closures, offers to partner, changes in healthcare financing, partnering strategies of competitors—that are outside local control. Being able to respond to those opportunities requires a thorough knowledge of internal and environmental realities.

***Hoshin* perspective**

The continuous improvement approach to strategic planning has been called *hoshin* planning, an effort to link all levels of resource allocation closely to customer needs.[3] *Hoshin* means a core belief, an intellectual pole star or reference point. In continuous improvement, the *hoshin* is customer needs. The best examples of *hoshin* perspective go far beyond meeting immediate customer requests to anticipate and even implant ideas customers would never have thought of on their own. Examples abound in high-tech manufacturing, Sony's Walkman being one of the most dramatic. The *hoshin* perspective involves a sophisticated interplay of market analysis, technology analysis, creativity, and role-playing leading to breakthrough inventions and fundamental redesigns.

In *hoshin* planning, both existing and proposed activities are modeled in business plans against market and price trends.[4] Realism centers on the assumptions for the models. Benchmarking information on the performance of competitors and market leaders becomes essential to achieve realism. Quality measures establish minimums for acceptable performance, and the costs of meeting those minimums are tested against market price realities. The long-range financial plan provides the acid test for the enterprise as a whole. The achievable cost trend will be plotted against a stakeholder-determined price trend. The difference must generate the capital the organization needs for survival. That set of services or products that passes the acid test becomes the services plan.

Healthcare organizations have a long way to go to reach a true *hoshin* perspective.[5] They may be no different from organizations generally in that respect; Hamel and Prahalad point out that corporations that thrive in competitive markets have greater ambition and follow a rigorous program of focused, complementary innovation.[6] In healthcare, provider logic, rather than customer logic, has traditionally driven innovation. That is, new products and services are often driven from the perspective of a technological challenge, rather than one of what the customer might want given a full understanding of the options. (Caesarean sections, circumcisions, prostatectomies, and executive physicals are among the more glaring examples.) What is missing, so far, is creativity, roleplaying, and breakthrough innovation oriented around customer realities. There are methods and styles of delivering healthcare we have not dreamed of yet.

Flexibility in strategy

Effective strategy is a highly dynamic, responsive activity. Planning in itself does not define strategy, it merely identifies likely outcomes of varying possibilities. The fact that the databases are historic gives planning a strong bias toward the status quo. Numerous companies have become trapped in their own data, missing opportunities to change in ways that eventually proved fatal.[7] *Hoshin* ideas are intuitive; they do not arise from databases. At the same time, many advocates of intuitive innovation have failed, at least in their first attempts. Installing new ideas in complex existing systems is simply harder than it usually looks at the outset. Success lies in balancing the two risks, exploring the new, but retaining the old until the new is tested. The problem is how to do that. Simon suggests that every manager, and by implication, every organization:

> . . . needs to be able to analyze problems systematically (and with the aid of the modern arsenal of analytical tools provided by management science and operations research). Every manager needs also to be able to respond to situations rapidly. . . . The effective manager does not have the luxury of choosing between "analytic" and "intuitive" approaches to problems. Behaving like a manager means having command of the whole range of management skills and applying them as they become appropriate.[8]

The leading healthcare organizations follow Simon's advice. They use the analytic tools, but constantly search for intuitive ideas. Some of these they develop on their own. They probably steal a larger number from each other. Even if the first trial of an idea succeeds, it usually takes longer and is more expensive than the second. Alliances with other leaders provide a mechanism for sharing the risks of exploration.

Revising the mission and vision

The mission set by the governing board (Chapter 3) identifies the community to be served, the level of service, and the financial limits. A vision statement often adds the philosophic goals and style by which the mission will be achieved. Together, these statements represent the most central desire of the owners and stakeholders and, as such, become the cornerstone for all subsequent planning decisions. To fulfill that function, they should be as permanent as possible. But in a dynamic environment, even the most carefully set mission may lose its relevance. Acquisitions and divestitures may change the community. Changes in demography, technology, and the competitive environment make certain services essential and others redundant. Growth of effective community concern about cost forces revised perspectives on productivity.

Even though major change is infrequent in the mission and even rarer in the vision, well-run organizations review the need for change annually. They contemplate mission revision far more often than they actually revise, because it is wise to consider many scenarios that in the end do not materialize. The process helps keep key decision makers familiar with the mission, as well. Given the mission's central role of setting values and directing the optimization process, it is important to deal decisively with possible changes. Actual revisions of mission require formal board action. The governing board planning committee should discuss the mission consequences of each year's environmental assessment. The planning staff marshals the arguments for and against revision and suggests appropriate wording for any revision.

Strategy selection

Strategy selection begins with a review of the organization's strategic options and responses, using a framework such as the strengths, weaknesses, opportunities, and threats (SWOT) analysis.[9,10] The SWOT analysis makes judgments about the implications of the data using both the environmental assessment and the *hoshin* principle. Strengths and weaknesses describe internal characteristics, and threats and opportunities external ones. These are described briefly, but as realistically as possible. The judgments arise from comparison of performance against the prior year's expectations, the changes noted in the environmental assessment, and the progress against benchmarks and the vision. The SWOT is a profile of the extent to which the organization's reach (goals) exceeds its grasp (performance). It recognizes that weaknesses and threats are part of life, not a cause for criticism. Reach must exceed grasp for improvement to occur. When the SWOT analysis is translated to action goals and prioritized, it establishes the improvement agenda.

Figure 12.3 shows a recent SWOT analysis for a successful healthcare organization serving about half of a community of 750,000 persons. The community has not expressed strong interest in managed care and has been ambivalent in past efforts at cost control, but the organization, here called Excalibur Health System, expects that attitude to change. The mission and vision commit the organization to retaining local service, income, and control with a nearly comprehensive scope of services and the use of managed care insurance to stimulate high-quality, cost-effective care.

The resulting display is checked against the mission and vision and used to identify broad goals or strategic directions for the institution. A key part

FIGURE 12.3 SWOT Analysis for Excalibur Health System

Strengths	Merger of two facilities now completed Single governance and medical staff established for system Strong medical staff support Recent reduction of 400 personnel, 200 more in view $50 million available cash, plus $30 million to correct existing deficiencies Rapidly developing information system Owns small HMO Medical school affiliation, strong primary care program Loyal and satisfied personnel
Weaknesses	No COO or visible second-in-command Ineffective physician-hospital organization Dissatisfaction among primary care physicians Low volume, high costs at smaller facility Poor ambulatory patient amenities at larger facility Serious OR shortages/deficiencies at larger facility Despite cost reduction, Medicare patients are served at a small financial loss Some aggressive HMO/PPO contracts are served at a loss
Opportunities	Strong community support, 50 percent market share Community loyal to local care, doctors, and traditional healthcare finance Recent alliance with leading institutions in region Possible link with large regional HMO/PPO Generally favorable patient attitudes Several smaller hospitals in region are in marginal condition Primary care doctors seeking organization help
Threats	Major competitor in city gained market share during merger years Largest intermediary in region has linked with competitor Regional competitors in adjacent city to north threaten northern edge of primary market and several specialties State reform may require new low-income/Medicaid HMO Federal reform may cause severe Medicare losses Shortage of primary care physicians Probable oversupply of referral specialists and specialty residency training

SOURCE: Based on a real organization, 1993. Identity concealed.

of the exercise is the study of overall patterns, raising the questions shown in Figure 12.4. The answers to these questions will determine the strategic direction. Various ways to improve the SWOT, usually called **scenarios**, will be proposed and evaluated against the environmental assessment. Some will die quickly, as major flaws appear. Others will receive detailed and quantitative review, even constructing market and financial forecasts of their implications. The SWOT description and the environmental assessment are used to test the scenarios for realism—consistency, fit with the environment, fit with accessible resources—and conviction—acceptance and support of members and stakeholders.[11] Those with the best fit will carry forward, perhaps to reality. The process of review and discussion develops conviction about the organization's direction. People become convinced, and consensus builds as the scenarios are described and tested.

The strategic direction that emerges from a healthcare organization's decisions reflects an attitude or business philosophy. The philosophy should be consistent with the mission and vision. It is important to communicate the philosophy to organization members and potential members so that they know what the organization stands for and what kinds of proposals for change are likely to gain support. If EHS's strategy continues to emphasize local control, notions of sale or merger with healthcare organizations in other cities need not be considered. If it continues to encourage managed care, partnering with established HMOs who can market effectively must be weighed against expansion of the owned HMO. If developing primary care continues to be an important goal, proposing a new transplant surgery program is probably a

FIGURE 12.4 Questions Arising from the EHS SWOT

Service position	Affiliate with regional HMO/PPO? Sell or expand own HMO? Build a low income/Medicaid HMO? Attempt to recover link to largest intermediary? Provide primary care organization support? Defend traditional medicine and health care finance? Promote local specialty capability?
Geographic position	Close, or find new uses for smaller facility? Use as OR/ambulatory site? Develop alliances with smaller hospitals in area? Pursue regional alliance? Affiliate with strong competitor from adjacent city to north? Acquire or affiliate with leading local competitor?
Operating position	Continue aggressive personnel reduction? Develop program to change clinical behavior, break even in Medicare, HMO patients? Correct ambulatory care amenities at larger facility? Correct OR deficiencies at larger facility? Expand primary care physician supply? Refocus medical training program to primary care? Continue information system development?

waste of time. Proposing a service corporation to support owned and affiliated primary care practices will be much better received.

A matrix allowing consideration of two dimensions of desirability is sometimes desirable to array scenarios. There are several alternatives for defining the axes. The versions of the Boston Consulting Group[12] or General Electric[13] are popular. Both lead to a display such as that illustrated in Figure 12.5, where the axes are market attractiveness (opportunities for growth or profit) versus organizational advantage (internal resources, sometimes called "competencies"). Such displays are useful in selecting the optimum portfolio of services. For example, a small rural hospital, noting both that there was a high demand for home care and respite care in its community and that it had the skills for such services (Situation A), would include them in its plans. Obstetrics, important to the customers but expensive for the hospital (Situation B), would be retained. A high-tech service only infrequently needed and requiring specialists who would be difficult to recruit (Situation C) would be avoided. But a service already in place, with specialists attracting market share from elsewhere (Situation D) would be retained or expanded. The resource barrier that exists in C has been met in D, and the investment gives the hospital an advantage.

The strategic direction of an institution can always be described by the specific proposals selected to improve its SWOT. It is also possible to describe strategy according to one of several available paradigms. Miles and Snow have characterized strategies according to risk and aggressiveness, describing four archetypes, "prospector, analyzer, reactor, and defender."[14] Eastaugh has modified the archetypes based on actual characteristics of hospitals.[15] The differences between the archetypes are two-dimensional, as shown in Figure 12.6. One dimension is externally focused and intuitive, the willingness to seek innovation outside the traditional parameters. The other is internal and analytic, the concentration on meeting quality and cost standards in the core business.

Shortell, Morrison, and Friedman note that the effectiveness of the Miles and Snow types depends on the environment, and that among healthcare systems prospectors and analyzers have the advantage in a turbulent healthcare environment.[16] Eastaugh notes that single hospital prospectors have not fared as well as analyzers, and defenders have done better than either.[17] Reactors fare badly in both studies.

One could consider adopting a Miles and Snow style as a strategy, "We want to be an analyzer healthcare organization." This is dangerous because it substitutes labels and generalities for a set of specific actions that are realistic and convincing in the specific setting. As the study by Shortell and others suggests, the critical issues in strategic direction are realistic appraisal and response to external forces, consistency in application, and congruence with internal resources. Saying "We are analyzers" is less important than doing the analysis and selecting some actions. The lesson from the research is that

FIGURE 12.5 Matrix of Market Attractiveness and Advantage

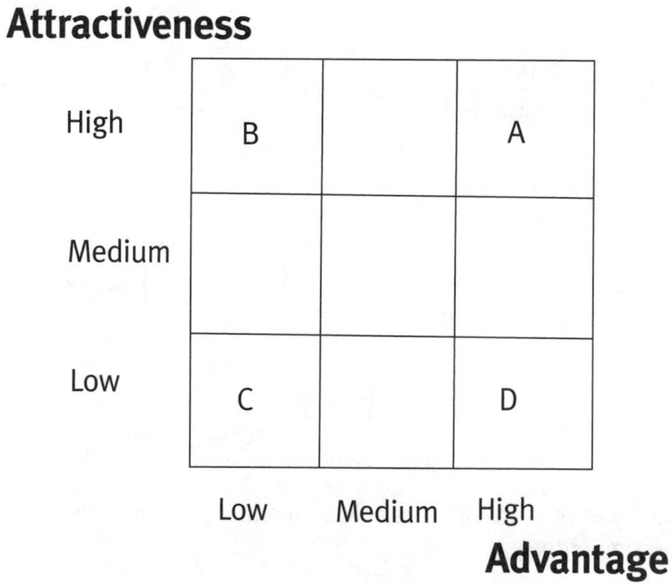

Attractiveness

High	B		A
Medium			
Low	C		D
	Low	Medium	High

Advantage

Service A, where the market is attractive and the hospital has a strong advantage, would be selected for further investment.

Service B, where the market is attractive but the hospital faces a large or difficult investment, would be judged on its importance to overall market share.

Service C, where both market and advantage are low, would be phased out or avoided.

Service D, where the attractiveness is low but the hospital has an advantage, would be supported but expanded only to the extend market support could be foreseen.

a willingness to change is essential when the environment around you is changing.

The Miles and Snow taxonomy is probably the most useful for integrated healthcare organizations. Other strategic philosophies include Porter's "cost leadership versus [quality] differentiation"[18] and Miller and Friesen's "adaptive, dominant, giant, conglomerate, and niche innovator."[19] Quality differentiation may be elusive in healthcare. It is difficult to document and even harder for the average patient to perceive. Differences based on satisfaction and prestige, being the carriage trade provider, are feasible for some institutions in larger cities. Many institutions dominate their market as local monopolies, and even some that don't have explicit strategies to keep out competition.[20] Dominating by deliberate emphasis on customer needs is legitimate, and when combined with control of price leads to exceptional healthcare systems.[21] Dominating by directly excluding or hampering competitors is potentially a criminal violation of the Sherman Antitrust Act. Very large corporations

FIGURE 12.6
Miles and Snow's Typology of Strategic Types

External Focus	Low	Medium	High
High diversification (Beyond industry)	Prospectors		
Moderate diversification (Selective targets)		Analyzers	
Rare diversification (Stick to knitting)	Reactors*		Defenders

Focus on cost, productivity, quality
Internal Focus

*Reactors do not have a strong strategy in either direction. They respond passively to actions of competitors.

frequently spin off niche innovators to develop risky ideas. The new company escapes the rigidity of the larger one, and the parent limits its risk against failures.

The strategic direction of most successful organizations is now toward integrated acute care services for a broad spectrum of health insurance including several varieties of managed care. The change occurred during the 1990s for most of the nation. The leading organizations became convinced that comprehensive control of acute care is essential to meet customer demands for economy and quality. The success of examples such as Henry Ford Health System and Intermountain Health Care has reinforced that belief.

The shift represents major revisions in physician organization and compensation, collaborative management of patient care, assignment of caregiver tasks, and the use of quantitative performance measurement. It is the most profound shift since the emergence of the hospital as the provider of clinical support services several decades ago. Shortell, Gillies, et al., have identified eight barriers limiting the success of the strategy.[22] The list, shown in Figure 12.7, is a useful catalogue of the problems faced by all strategic change, with suggestions about how to deal with them. Generally, the barriers and responses can be understood in three groups. Failures to win internal conviction about the new strategy are addressed with education and consensus-building techniques, plus efforts to stimulate a more articulate customer market. Failures to progress with the implementation are addressed by specific actions to strengthen critical resources. Finally, internal resistance or prolonged inability to meet critical new goals is met with the deliberate use of power. Rules and procedures are changed, and obstructing personnel are replaced. Implementation is a thread that runs conspicuously through the facilitators; clearly selecting the strategy is only the beginning.

The alternative to the integrated service strategy is a niche strategy, deliberately seeking highly specialized services that can be delivered to a receptive market. Specialty hospitals serving children, mentally ill, cancer patients, and the like are following niche strategies.[23] Small rural healthcare organizations offering primary care and limited hospitalization are also niche strategists. So are independent home care and hospice organizations. Although both the label and reality suggest that niche strategies are associated with smaller organizations, some niche strategies can be quite large. For-profit chains pursue niches in several markets simultaneously. Columbia HCA had acute care hospital facilities in several dozen different cities.[24] National Medical Enterprises attempted a niche strategy with a for-profit chain of mental health facilities.[25] Both encountered ethical, legal, and managerial difficulties. Several for-profit chains pursue similar niches in chronic care. The leader, Beverly Enterprises, has also encountered severe difficulties,[26] suggesting that niche strategies have inherent limits.

The strength of niche strategies is the ability to respond quickly and excellently within the limited service. Niches tend to emerge around new services and to sustain themselves when unique factors in the service are difficult for competitors to copy. The problem with niche strategies is the risk that the comparative advantage will disappear. The technology may change, making it possible for every integrated health system to achieve results as good as the niche specialists. (The service line strategy of integrated systems is an attempt to gain advantages of niching while retaining those of the larger organization.) The financing may change, leaving the niche company with insufficient funds to finance expansion. Customer judgments may change, so that people who were willing to travel for a specialized service decide not to or, in the case of rural institutions, decide the trip to the big city is worth the effort. The result is that niche strategy institutions are a relatively small part of the total; integrated comprehensive strategies prevail.

Validating the strategic position

The strategic position must meet the twin tests of realism and conviction. A realistic strategy must represent a broadly accepted consensus about what should be done, incorporating not just the customer *hoshin*, but also the needs of providers and organization members. The strategy need not please all, but no group can be sufficiently disaffected that it will withhold critical support.

Strategic realism is tested repeatedly, using the long-range financial plan. Realistic strategies increase the organization's financial resources, either by reducing costs or by increasing demand and revenues. The impact of a strategy on the institution's financial plan should be tested as soon as the changes it requires in expenditures and revenue are clear. The process is iterative. The first check is almost intuitive, "Do we have, or can we get, the resources to do this, and will we be paid the cost?" The final check

FIGURE 12.7
Barriers and Facilitators of Organized Delivery Systems*

Barrier	Facilitator
Understanding and Acceptance	
Failure to understand primary care and wellness as the new core business	Invest in educational programs and consultants emphasizing new core.
	Deliberately involve "naysayers" in strategic discussions.
	Change the incentive of key managers.
	Seek new appointments experienced in new core.
Inability to overcome the hospital paradigm	Revise mission and vision.
	Limit capital expenditure toward old uses, expand it toward ambulatory care.
	Increase influence of primary care physicians.
	Stimulate growth of managed care insurance.
Implementation	
Lack of strategic alignment	Expand performance measures
	Centralize planning effort and planning staff.
	Develop realistic and convincing strategies for each subsidiary.
	Close or divest subsidiaries not fitting new core business.
Ambiguous roles and responsibilities	Expand and clarify roles.
	Strengthen incentive system and relate to performance measures.
	Eliminate redundant managers
Inability to manage managed care	Expand/revise quality improvement activities.
	Improve cost data.
	Hire experienced manager.
	Partner with experienced, effective HMO.
Inability to Execute the Strategy	
	Replace/reassign middle management.
	Revise the strategic position.
	Replace the CEO.
Resistance	Select committees, committee chairs.
Resistance by system board members	Deliberately confront and resolve board ambivalence.
	Replace board members.
	Restructure board.
Resistance by subsidiary units	Centralize capital budget, budget authority.
	Replace local board members.
	Expand subsidiary CEO responsibilities.
	Remove uncooperative executives.

* S. M. Shortell, R. R. Gillies, D. A. Anderson, and K. L. Morgan, "Creating Organized Delivery Systems: The Barriers and Facilitators." *Hospital & Health Services Administration* 38 (4): 459.

incorporates the details of specific plans into the financial plan, and shows the capital required and the impact on measures of financial strength, as described in Chapter 14. The "Reality Check" shown in Figure 3.6 should be a major element in the governing board's decision.

Conviction about strategy is expressed through stakeholder commitment. People learn the strategic direction by participating in the annual environmental assessment and some of the strategic discussions that arise then and during the year. Iteration of the mission and vision and the environmental assessment over several years helps both members and customers understand the strategy. The best organizations share their strategic exercise broadly. The review helps a large number of members and customers understand the organization's profile of needs and achievements and the possible improvements. The result is that the strategic position is not secret. In the words of the Intermountain planner, Greg Poulsen, "It's in our competitors' portfolio tomorrow morning."[27] The Intermountain approach is to win not on secrecy but on sound implementation.

Documenting strategy

Many organizations have no formal statement of strategy. Consensus about the strategic direction is documented by the actions taken. Yet a large number of people know the organization's direction in considerable detail. If they do not, the strategy fails the test of conviction and is difficult or impossible to implement. The decisions that result from the planning process are incorporated in a set of documents that are sometimes called the long-range or **strategic plan**. The documentation includes the following parts:

- *Mission and vision*—broadly distributed, brief statements to provide consistent direction
- *Environmental description and forecasts*—a database for the planning activities of all units derived from the environmental assessment, covering about five years, and identifying potential directions of change for a second five years
- *Services plans*—specifying the clinical services and other major activities in which the institution will engage.
- *Long-range financial plan*—summarizing the expected financial impact on income statements, cash flow, long-term debt, and balance sheets (Chapter 14)
- *Information services plan*—describing the future capability and hardware array of information service, including plans for collection, standardization, communication, and archiving of data (Chapter 15)
- *Human resources plan*—showing the expected personnel needs, terminations, and recruitment requirements (Chapter 16)
- *Medical staff plan*—a part of the human resources plan focusing on physician replacement and recruitment (Chapter 8)

- *Facilities plan*—detailing the construction and renovation activities (Chapter 17)

Although the plans may be separate documents, the processes generating the decisions must be integrated. In general, mission and vision drive services and finances, and these, in turn, drive facilities, human resources, and information needs. Thus, the plans can be portrayed in a hierarchical relationship as shown in Figure 12.8.

The planning unit is responsible for coordinating the long-range plans as a set and preparing the annual environmental assessment with its required forecasts. The other technical and logistic support services are responsible for their components.

Responding to Strategic Opportunities

Strategic opportunities arise from the strategy process, from improvement activities and from external events. Many must be evaluated on a timetable outside the organization's control. They often involve sums of money several times the normal operating and capital budget decisions. They usually involve more than one functional unit and imply disruption of the lives of many members of the organization. They also may require secrecy because premature public knowledge would substantially change the nature of the transaction. Finally, they are often irreversible. The opportunity, once passed, will not soon return.

External strategic opportunities generally require high-risk decisions that test the governance structure and the skills of its leaders as no other activity does. The uniqueness of each opportunity makes rules impractical, but some characteristics are common to successful responses:

- Criteria for all opportunities are the mission and vision. In some cases (mergers, for example) it is necessary to go beyond the mission and vision to the customer *hoshin*.

FIGURE 12.8
Hierarchical Relationship of Long-Range Plans

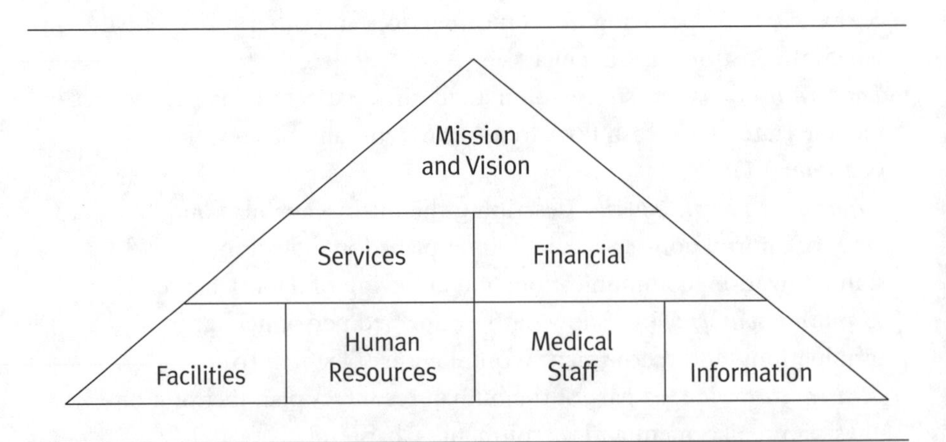

- Surveillance of market and political trends gives advance warning. Many opportunities can be predicted some years in advance. Surveillance of competitors' activity can alert the organization to many partnership opportunities. Who is growing, failing, buying, selling, or approaching a critical organizational juncture can usually be detected in advance.
- The general opportunities can be debated in advance and broad positions established as part of the strategic position. A well-written mission statement, long-range plan, and fiscal plan, plus the history of discussion surrounding them, provide the criteria for evaluating most specific strategic opportunities.
- Well-run organizations can assemble a knowledgeable response team for each specific opportunity. The team membership emphasizes maturity in business decisions. The CEO is usually team leader, although a senior board officer occasionally assumes this role. Trusted senior physicians should be included. Senior line officers often contribute. Planning, marketing, and finance staff make up the work force. Outside consultants are frequently useful, particularly in situations without parallels in the organization's history. The need for conviction and the complexity of most opportunities has led to larger teams, often organized into task forces.
- Response teams may be limited in size if necessary and be accountable only to senior governance officers until the project has undergone initial review. This arrangement preserves confidentiality where that is necessary. The usual result of the confidential review is a larger scale, more public review.

In short, preparation allows the well-managed institution to make prudent evaluations of opportunities within externally imposed time frames.

Developing and Evaluating Programmatic Proposals

Programmatic proposals are detailed specifications of resources and processes for projects usually involving only a single functional unit and coming from that unit. Much of the strategic position is implemented by selecting those proposals that best fit. Programmatic proposals arise as strategies are implemented and as a result of continuous improvement projects, technological advances, and simply aging equipment and facilities. They have to be justified, compared against alternative uses of funds, approved, and implemented. Large ventures like new facilities or products are often made up of many smaller projects. While these would follow a different approval process, the same sort of analysis and justification are in order. Figure 12.9 gives examples.

Well-managed organizations encourage programmatic proposals because they reflect an alert, flexible work attitude and because they provide an opportunity for continuous improvement. An abundant supply of programmatic proposals minimizes the danger that the best solution will be overlooked. Hundreds of programmatic proposals originate each year in large healthcare organizations. Dozens survive initial review and are formally documented.

FIGURE 12.9 Examples of Programmatic Proposals

Proposal	Description	Approximate Cost	Possible Justification
Renovate ORs	Enlarge operating suite into adjacent inpatient unit, modernize	$10,000,000	Increase attractiveness to ambulatory surgery patients
Replace flat-work ironer	Replace old ironer with faster machine less likely to break down	$50,000	Essential to laundry operation; more reliable service; lower unit cost
Laser surgery equipment	Specially designed laser for gynecological surgery	$50,000	Match competitor's investment
Expand parking lot	Add 50 spaces for visitors	$1,000,000	Relieve crowding for ambulatory patient visits

As the organization becomes familiar with the process, the fraction of documented proposals rises to well over half, but it should never be 100 percent.

Developing programmatic proposals

Programmatic proposals are developed by operating units, as described in Chapter 9. The role of planning is to encourage a broad search for promising ideas, assist proposal development teams in preparing cases for competitive review, support, ensure accuracy in forecasts and claims, and support fair review.

Encouraging promising ideas

Many ideas should be considered; only the most promising should be formally developed. The following procedures encourage managers to seek intuitive ideas and evaluate them:

- The general management environment encourages line supervisors to seek imaginative ideas. Ideas are respected even when they are unusual.
- Planning staff are readily available to discuss concepts informally.
- The planning unit systematically communicates the mission and vision, the environmental assessment and evidence of the strategic direction. Planning staff are a source of knowledge about the plans in existence and the discussion that surrounded the decisions.
- Planning staff assists managers to articulate benefits in terms of the mission, to specify the market, and to forecast performance measures.

Assisting proposal development

For those projects deemed worth the effort, planning provides extensive assistance, guiding line management with concepts, facts, and methods. Marketing textbooks note that introducing a new product or service successfully requires a comprehensive approach to its design summarized by the four Ps[28]:

- *Place*—the segment of the market to be served and issues of style, location, and amenities that make the service maximally attractive to the customer.
- *Product*—the exact definition and design of service to be offered.
- *Price*—the total cost the customer is willing to pay for given services, including transaction costs such as travel time, and in healthcare including an analysis of the insured and out-of-pocket portions of costs.
- *Promotion*—the advertising, public relations, and communications that make customers aware of the service and its desirability.

Planning's role is to remind line management that while this approach may seem grandiose, it is quite valuable. A replacement flatwork ironer in the hospital laundry looks simple, but it should prompt a thorough review of the laundry's future demand, the price of competitive laundry services, the desirability of closing the laundry and purchasing the service elsewhere, and the possibility of actually expanding laundry volume by selling the service to others. For a proposal like a new primary care clinic, omitting a step suggested by the mnemonic is likely to be a fatal error.

As the mnemonic is pursued, a long list of technical questions develops. Figure 12.10 shows a standard list of review questions. Planning staff help line managers answer these questions. They are expert in the data available to analyze specific issues or opportunities, analytic techniques to use the data effectively, and persuasive methods of presenting the information. Their job is to see that all formally developed proposals are presented in their best light.

Ensuring accuracy and fairness

Given the competitive review, the temptation to overstate benefits and underestimate costs is always present. Planning staff provide the "source of truth" for demand and market numbers. They coordinate cost estimates with accounting, human resources, and purchasing. They ensure that plant personnel have checked facility and equipment proposals for safety and feasibility needs.

Supporting review teams

The proposals that survive initial, informal review are usually evaluated by a planning team that begins as a simple consultation between an operating leader and a planner. In complex projects, the team can grow to a formal planning structure bringing in experts from other operational and technical support areas and outside consultants as needed. Major projects can be assembled from several smaller teams, making it possible to move programmatic proposals to strategic opportunities as necessary. Planning staff support all teams, assisting with records, responding to questions, and reminding the team of schedule requirements. They protect the process of review itself, discouraging attempts to subvert or avoid it and making the process as efficient and fair as possible.

It is important to note that the planning staff never judges the proposals themselves. They do provide facts and concepts to line managers and let them decide. They do the same, on a larger scale, to development teams and review

FIGURE 12.10
Issues in Evaluating a Programmatic Proposal

The assistance provided by the planning department to line supervisors considering programmatic proposals begins with a thorough checklist of the likely issues to be involved. There is no perfect list, but a schema such as the one below tends to reveal the important questions in an order which identifies those most likely to be disabling early, when the idea can easily be modified, deferred, or abandoned.

Mission, Vision, and Plan

What is the relationship of this proposal to the mission and vision?

Is this proposal essential to implement a strategic goal in the long-range plan?

If the proposal arises outside the current strategic goals, can it be designed to enhance or improve the current plan?

Benefit

In the most specific terms possible, what does this project contribute to healthcare? If possible, state:

- the nature of the contribution, the probability of success, and the associated risk for each individual benefiting; and
- the kinds and numbers of persons benefiting.

If the organization were unable to adopt the proposal, what would be the implication?
Are there alternative sources of care? What costs are associated with using these sources?
If the proposal contributes to some additional or secondary objectives, what are these contributions and what is their value?

Market and Demand

What size and segment of the community will this proposal serve? What fraction of this group is likely to seek care at this organization?

What is the trend in the size of this group and its tendency to seek care here? How will the proposal affect this trend?

To what extent is the demand dependent on insurance or finance incentives? What is the likely trend for these provisions? What are the consequences of this proposal for competing hospitals or healthcare organizations?

What effect will the proposal have on the organization's general market share or on other specific services?

What implications does the project have for the recruitment of physicians and other key healthcare personnel?

What are the promotional requirements of the proposal?

Costs and Resources

What are the marginal operating and capital costs of the proposal, including startup costs and possible revenue losses from other services?

Are there cost implications for other services or overhead activities?

Are there special or critical resource requirements?

Are there identifiable opportunity costs associated with the proposal, or other proposals or opportunities that are facilitated by this proposal?

Are there other intangible elements (positive or negative) associated with this proposal?

Finance

What are the capital requirements, project life, and finance costs associated with the proposal?

What is the competitive price and anticipated net revenue?

What is the demand elasticity and profit sensitivity?

What are the insurance or finance sources of revenue, and what implications do these sources raise?

What is the net cash flow associated with the proposal over its life, and the discounted value of that flow?

continued

FIGURE 12.10 continued

What are the opportunities to enhance this proposal or others by combination?
Are there customers or stakeholders with an unusual commitment for or against the proposal?
Are there any specific risks or benefits associated with the proposal not elsewhere identified?
Does the proposal suggest a strategic opportunity, such as a joint venture or the purchase or sale of a major service?

Timing, Implementation, and Evaluation
What are the critical path components of the installation process, and how long will they take?
What are the problems or advantages associated with deferring or speeding the implementation?
What are the anticipated changes in the operating budget of the units accountable for the proposal? What changes are required in supporting units?

committees, but they strive not to influence the decisions beyond the provision of reliable facts and methodologies.

Maintaining Relations with Other Health Agencies and Government

Healthcare organizations have ongoing relationships even though they may be competing directly. They also are obligated to gain certain planning approvals and to comply with other laws affecting the planning process.

Assist in negotiations with competing or collaborating organizations

As noted above, strategic positioning should be based on thorough, ongoing surveillance of institutions with related or potentially related missions. This surveillance frequently includes considerable direct communication, and this in turn leads to collaborative relationships of various kinds (Chapter 13).

There is a long-standing tradition that community hospitals should collaborate with one another, principally because they share a common obligation to the same community and because such collaboration appears to be more economical. However, in the era of unlimited financial support and significant subsidization for growth, the tradition was exceptionally difficult to implement. In the newer, more restrictive and more competitive environment, collaboration appears, ironically, to be more successful, even as competition is more common.

Even bitterly competing healthcare organizations tend to communicate frequently. Any collaborative activity that is not a violation of the antitrust laws is a fair topic of conversation. Ad hoc allegiances to market specific products such as health insurance plans, or to meet specific needs such as clinical training programs, or serve specific populations such as programs for the disadvantaged are common. Within a framework of competition, communication and collaboration are used constantly.

The antitrust implications of dialogue between competitors are difficult to describe. The law on per se violations is clear: conversations between competitors cannot include collusion to set prices, divide or establish markets, or exclude other competitors. Such actions are criminal, and individuals have been prosecuted for them. On the other hand, exploration of merger or shared service possibilities is neither a criminal nor a civil violation of the acts if it can be defended as being in the public interest. A practical suggestion is that dialogue is necessary, but that the per se topics should be avoided in action, implication, and intent. Legal counsel is frequently necessary; many actions depend on details of presentation and content.

Activities other than the per se violations that tend to increase the services available for patients are generally defensible under antitrust, and are also important between healthcare organizations not directly competing, such as hospitals and nursing homes. Competitors can often improve specific services by mergers and affiliations. Legal counsel is indicated to keep the discussion consistent with the law. The actual negotiation of mergers and affiliations is usually reserved to the CEO and selected members of the governing board, but the planning executive is a member of the strategic response teams, and planning data are the appropriate bases for many of the decisions. As a result, the planning executive is frequently a participant.

Obtaining regulatory approvals

National laws enacted in 1966 and 1974, but repealed in 1988, encouraged the states to develop regulation of hospital investments. As a result, many states required certificates of need (CONs) for new services and construction or renovation. CONs are a form of franchise, a government-issued permission to proceed with capital investment. These laws are enforced with varying degrees of vigor, and their importance is diminishing. In those states where they remain, success depends on timing, well-designed and attractive services, technically well-prepared proposals, and the support of influential persons in the community. Strategies for dealing with HSAs and CONs vary. The influence of these laws is arguable.[29] Most well-run organizations have developed strategies and tactics for gaining the approval of all or nearly all their important options and proposals.

In some communities there are voluntary or other regulatory bodies, and in most cities, hospital construction requires zoning board approval, or construction permits, or both. These negotiations are clearly the responsibility of planning units.

Organization for Planning

Personnel Requirements

Even a large healthcare organization will employ only a few people in its planning activity. Other members of the governance system, particularly the CEO and CFO, will have important planning functions, and outside consultants are often used. Very small hospitals must assign planning and marketing responsibilities directly to the chief executive or one deputy. A small professional staff with an identified chief (usually called vice president for planning) is common even in smaller organizations and can often be justified by reduced expenditures for outside consultants.

Professional skills of planning executives

Effective institutional planning requires an ability to build consensus by negotiation, together with mastery of a growing body of professional knowledge and skill. Professional requirements include techniques for analysis, knowledge of healthcare administration, and understanding of community and individual opinion formation. Analytic techniques should include practical skills in epidemiologic analysis, cost accounting, present value analysis, statistics, forecasting, and business plan modeling. The complexity of healthcare also requires detailed knowledge: current status and trends in health insurance, government financial programs, health personnel availability, healthcare technology, sources of capital funds, the role of regulatory bodies, and prevention of disease. Finally, the planning executive must understand community power structures and decision processes, methods of information dissemination, and the uses of advertising and public relations.

Most of the professional subject matter is covered in an accredited master's degree program in healthcare administration. A graduate degree in business also covers many of the topics, although with important omissions in the specifics of the healthcare field. Competent individuals with a degree in either of these fields can improve their skill through continuing education and reading. The combination of both business and health administration degrees is increasingly relevant and becoming more popular.

Negotiating skills are learned by practice. Certainly the mature planning executive should be able to conduct fruitful meetings, identify and assist in the resolution of disputes, and present information clearly and convincingly, both orally and in writing. Beginners must learn those skills by observation and supervised experience, although community and extramural collegiate activities are useful.

Planning personnel are recruited in national markets. Deputies and beginners are often selected from among recent graduates. Planning executives are promoted from within, attracted from consulting firms, or hired from other organizations. Although experience and maturity are important, it is not uncommon to rely on the experience of the CEO to overcome immaturity in the planning unit. The centrality, breadth of scope, and requirements for planning suggest it as an excellent background for CEOs and COOs.

Outside consultants

The variety and extent of skills required in planning make it a fruitful area for the use of consultants. Many activities of planning can be assigned to outside firms. These include:

- *Surveillance*, demographic and economic forecasts, trends in technology and personnel availability, evaluation of future plant and equipment needs,

consumer demand and market surveys, and surveys of competitor's behavior;
- *Strategic positioning*, investigation of competitor's interests and positions, evaluation of partnership and acquisition options, advice on entering new markets or offering new services, and experience in strategic procedures and negotiations;
- *Proposal development and evaluation*, suggestions for new products and services, feasibility and cost-benefit analyses, and design of response evaluation protocol; and
- *Communication and consensus building*, assistance starting and maintaining a planning-oriented dialogue among organization influentials.

Consultants can specialize in understanding demographic, economic, and underlying attitudinal trends; act as extra hands; impart technical skills for specialized responses; bring knowledge of what others facing the same problem are doing; and mediate entrenched conflicts over the nature of the mission, the objectives, or a specific response. The possible uses of outside consultants are so extensive that specifying what they *cannot* do may be the easiest way to identify their contribution. Consultants cannot replace the judgment of either operating personnel or governing board members, and, of course, they cannot and do not accept accountability for the mission, vision, long-range plan objectives, or selection of specific programs. Thus, any consultant's recommendation must be carefully and fully evaluated by those responsible for the institution. Consultants cannot provide the continuity of an ongoing executive presence.

The keys to successful use of consultants are as follows:

1. The assignment should be clearly specified in terms of process, timing, and result. As a general rule, the clearer the assignment and the more details of the work specified in advance, the better the chances for success. It is occasionally wise to use consultants to gain fresh insights into vague, ill-defined problems, but such use should be limited to very short-term assignments.
2. To be cost-effective, topics assigned to consultants should require skills or quantities of effort not available locally. Using consultants as neutral third parties is essentially correcting a failure of the local process, and this should not occur often.
3. Consultant firms should be selected on the basis of relevant prior experience. In the absence of direct experience with a consultant, opinions of other clients should be solicited before any major assignment is made.
4. Consultant activities should be carefully monitored against the specifications throughout the project. This job is often assigned to the planning executive.

Organization

Most planning units in healthcare organizations are small enough that the internal organization is simply a single team with a few specializations or general assignments. In larger units, deputy planner-marketers can be held accountable for specifics along functional lines of surveillance, mission, and strategic options, and programmatic proposal development and implementation. Planning activities are sometimes merged with marketing, and two units covering planning and marketing under one vice president is not uncommon. A service line view designates individuals responsible for maintaining relations between planning and major clinical units. This suggests that a practical organization of a planning unit follows matrix organization principles, with each deputy of the planning executive accountable for a functional area and relations with specific line units.

The supervision of consultants should also be explicitly assigned to individuals, with accountability running through the planning executive. Failure to identify a point of contact slows the consultants, adds to their costs, and defeats the possibility of continuous monitoring during the contract period.

Well-run organizations keep planning activities very close to the CEO and the governing board. Split reporting of planning functions, some to the CEO and some to the COO, may cause some aspects to get less attention than they should. Assignment of planning to the COO risks an undesirably short-term focus and may result in insufficient attention to strategic options and community needs. Assignment of planning to the CFO increases the dominance of the financial aspect of decisions; in the long run, responsiveness to community need should determine the decisions more than financial implications.

Very large healthcare systems frequently centralize some aspects of planning to improve the technical skills of personnel, to provide economies of scale, and to ensure consistency when appropriate. Databases and methodological skills are easily centralized to form an internal consulting service. On the other hand, healthcare remains a locally generated and locally delivered product. Many chains operating in several communities retain local planning staffs in each.

Measures of Planning Effectiveness

The planning activity, like every other part of the well-run organization, should have established performance measures, short-term expectations, and regular reporting of achievement against these. For planning, this means that service quality, cost, customer satisfaction, and human resources should be measured as quantitatively and objectively as possible, and specific expectations should be set. A set of measures for a planning unit is shown in Figure 12.11.

FIGURE 12.11 Performance Measures for Planning Services

Dimension Measured	Measure
Demand for planning services	
	User satisfaction with response time
	Activity log
	Delays to respond to service requests
Cost measures	
	Total direct costs
	Labor costs
	Consultant costs
	Data and information acquisition costs
Human resources satisfaction	
	Satisfaction scores of planning personnel
	Vacancy, turnover, and recruitment effectiveness
Outcomes quality	
Demand and market share forecasts	Variations from annual forecasts of major measures of market share and demand for service
	Comparisons of rates of growth of demand and revenue for new services implemented with forecasts from programmatic proposals
Programmatic project forecasts	Actual project implementation costs against forecast
	Actual project operating costs and profit against forecast
	Project implementation timetables against forecast
Customer satisfaction	
User satisfaction	Attitudes toward overall planning service
	Attitudes toward timely recognition of opportunities and potential problems
	Attitudes toward timely completion of projects relative to community and market needs and opportunities
Patient and buyer influence	Attitudes of patients and buyers toward institutional mission and specific programs, with particular attention to attitudes of influentials

Demand, Output, and Productivity Measures

It is almost impossible to make objective measures of demand or output, and without those there is no measure of productivity. Milestones on major projects and time delays on programmatic requests are partial substitutes. A log of requests and responses must be kept, and the milestones established in advance. Goals for those dimensions, and others such as the unit's contribution to specific projects and to overall success, can be set by discussion and agreement. Evaluation of achievement remains subjective. One request is different from another, and a failed milestone can have a dozen causes outside planning's control.

Resource Measures for Planning

The planning activity should have an explicit cost budget, like any other unit in the organization. The budget must be fixed rather than flexible and established subjectively, based on the scope and quality of service desired. The principle costs are labor costs, and consultant services are often separately accounted. Costs of data and information are also important. Some information must now be purchased from outside sources and computer hardware and software is essential to effective service.

Satisfaction of planning personnel is a valid human resources measure for this unit, as it is for all others. Evidence of respect by peers, such as publications or presentations, is sometimes used.

Quality Measures

Quality of planning includes outcomes measures on how accurate, timely, and effective the planning contribution was and process measures on the methods and approaches used. A well-run planning unit will have expectations and routine measurement involving at least the topics listed in Figure 12.11. They call for accuracy in technical assistance and timeliness in project completion. Unfortunately, forecasts are rarely perfect, projects take years to complete, and both are subject to events outside planning's control. (Even a small programmatic proposal will be completed in a different year than proposed because of the capital budget review cycle.) The difficulties of measuring and isolating the planning contribution suggest strongly that these measures must also be considered subjectively. Often, evaluation must be limited to the events that are complete and self-contained enough to yield lessons for the future. These anecdotes are still enough for beneficial review and evaluation.

It is possible to evaluate planning units according to the technical proficiency of their work, such as the completeness of data, availability of analytic software, and the use of correct analytic techniques. Periodic evaluation by outside consultants and review against JCAHO criteria are useful.

Customer Satisfaction

The customers of planning are the users from other units, the executive office, and the governing board. They should have ample opportunity to provide confidential evaluation of planning. Written surveys, records of complaints, and review of performance on larger projects are appropriate. Again, these do not reduce well to objective data. They must be subjectively judged, but they provide important information both for evaluation and for identifying improvement opportunities.

Constraints

Despite the measurement difficulties, the planning unit should establish specific goals and demonstrate improvement. Timelines, databases, forecast accuracy, and customer satisfaction are appropriate targets. Cost reduction may also be important. Comparative data should be obtained from noncompeting organizations via alliances and participation in national meetings. Consultant's evaluations can be used to set goals. It is sometimes possible to specify a strategic objective—for example, that the unit must identify and develop several appropriate new sources of market share. Such an objective is probably more appropriate to a five-year horizon than to an annual one, but it could be included in the long-range plan and used to support more specific annual expectations.

The ultimate judgment of planning, that the organization is or is not positioned where it should be in the community, is based on the environmental surveillance itself. The evaluation of planning is inevitably bound up with that of the chief executive and the governing board. The overall success of the planning function may have less to do with the planning unit performance than with the value issues in planning, discussed below.

Value Issues in Planning

Success in planning occurs when the organization is led into fruitful endeavors. Failure comes in two ways: when weaker ventures are selected and when better ones are overlooked. From that perspective, a formal planning activity must justify its existence by being prompt and thorough: it must uncover the obscure and have new detail about the obvious. From one viewpoint, planning is an intelligence activity, uncovering hidden risks and overlooked opportunities. From another, it is a service to expedite a decision-making process. The model for success emphasizes surveillance, mission setting, and community-focused criteria. Experience with this model has revealed two groups of issues in which organizations differ. Extreme positions on these values have caused organizations to fail. The first group deals with the technical foundations and assumptions of the unit. The second relates to the premises or biases of the decision makers, particularly the governing board of community not-for-profit organizations.

Technical Foundations

Successful planning units seem to excel in four areas of planning activity: (1) they take extra pains to guard against oversights, (2) they use the most objective forecasts they can obtain, (3) they are rigorous in their evaluation of costs and benefits, and (4) they follow procedures that deliberately use comparison and competition to debate the best course of action.

Guarding against oversight

The first step in avoiding overlooking the best ideas is in recognizing the danger of doing so. Most planning and forecasting is done by extrapolating from past history, often assuming *ceteris paribus* (other things being equal). No other approach is practical or prudent as a mainstay of a planning unit, or of a governance activity generally. Truly radical departures requiring innovative solutions are rare; the past is usually prologue to the present. There are several ways to check for those few cases where innovation is the key to success:

- Radical change often occurs at different times in different places. A check of conditions elsewhere may show trends not yet evident in the local community.
- Radical change often arises from individuals with different views from the rest of the group, sometimes to the point of being outcasts. Careful study of the opinions of critics of the status quo can suggest practical improvements.
- The *hoshin* concept leads to a search for the ideal way to meet customer needs, perhaps using technology the customer could never think of on his own. At least a few hours each year should be devoted to *hoshin* thinking.
- Imagination can be prompted by deliberately trying to think the unthinkable. The most successful planners deliberately insert a step in major forecasting or planning exercises that asks two questions:

1. What could occur that would make this forecast totally wrong?
2. Is there any other scenario, however improbable, that would be significantly more attractive than this one, and what might make such a scenario more probable?

Successful institutions promote an environment in which ideas can be openly expressed. They open their plans to widespread debate and discussion, with the intention of finding conflicting views and evaluating them, and making sure that those who express unusual views are protected from personal insult or injury, such as losing promotions or salary increases.

Using objective forecasts

Subjective forecasts, those prepared intuitively by people working in the area under study, can be very accurate for periods of a year or less, if they are carefully prepared. Their accuracy deteriorates rapidly over longer terms and in unfamiliar applications. Successful organizations take pains to find independent sources of forecasts, to use several different sources, and to use rigorously unbiased methods to describe the future and to evaluate a range of possible scenarios. Such cold-blooded realism improves planning in two ways: it reveals projects based on fantasy soon enough to avoid them, and it develops a climate of credibility in which the surviving proposals can be effectively evaluated.

Factors influencing demand must be forecast as accurately as possible. These include community population by age and sex, birth rate and disease incidence, income, insurance coverage, and the need for goods and services other than healthcare. Most of these are forecast by several independent sources, and well-run organizations use these forecasts rather than their own. They discard predictions by groups with vested interests (such as the local power companies and the Chamber of Commerce) and use the remaining ones to project both an expectation and a range of possibilities. They then explore costs and benefits of proposed responses across the range of values, showing the sensitivity of the conclusion to forecasting assumptions. Graphic displays are important in helping people understand alternatives and their consequences. It requires sophisticated, well thought out data management to carry this out. Databases and forecasting models must be readily available, easy to use, and easy to understand. An important contribution of planning personnel is in knowing and using these tools and bringing them to bear in ways the line originators of the proposal can appreciate.

Using cost-benefit measures effectively

The costs and benefits of many different proposals must be assessed quickly and inexpensively. The iterative evaluation described above is one step toward this goal. Some others that well-run organizations adopt include:

- Adhering to a formal protocol such as Figure 12.10 that prompts recognition of obscure costs and hidden risks. The protocol should strongly encourage investigation of several areas known to be overlooked in less rigorous approaches:
  - Costs of borrowing or leasing
  - Costs of obsolescence, or unduly optimistic estimates of project life
  - Opportunity costs in committing irreplaceable resources
  - Overhead costs or burdens on other units
  - Promotional costs and the implications of competition for limited demand
  - Intangible costs, including possible political repercussions, member dissatisfaction, and malpractice liability
- Searching for combinations of projects that increase the attractiveness of all of the individual projects. Often a project that is too costly to be undertaken on its own is valuable when it is included in a package with others. Renovations, for example, create conditions in which many previously impractical revisions become cost-effective. They also represent windows in time. When the renovation is complete, overlooked projects may be forever lost. The well-run organization sees more possible combinations because it looks for them.
- Encouraging complete identification and description of benefits that cannot be assigned precise dollar valuation. Benefits that are difficult to evaluate in dollar terms can be identified and described, and the number of people likely to receive them can be forecast. These estimates are much less expensive than imprecise dollar estimates and probably as useful.
- Using staff experts, individuals from other healthcare systems, and outside consultants to enhance the accuracy of cost and benefit estimates. Physicians, industrial engineers, purchasing agents, finance department staff, and plant department staff can improve the reliability and the

credibility of estimates. Outside consultants bring objectivity and broader experience to bear.

- Using examples from other healthcare organizations. The most convincing evidence of accurate cost-benefit estimates is the existence of a smoothly operating example elsewhere. Many poorly run organizations are trapped by the "not invented here" syndrome, delusions of their own uniqueness or leadership.

Maintaining objectivity in the evaluation process

Objectivity and realism must extend to the entire process of response evaluation and selection. There are natural human tendencies not only to overstate the ratio of benefits to costs, but also to favor one's friends. The well-run organization must minimize both these risks. The following are specific steps:

1. Use line-staff teams to develop projects because their dual contribution tends to reduce bias.
2. Start comparative review as far down the accountability hierarchy as possible, preferably involving every responsibility center.
3. Provide formal review against broadening competition at higher levels of the accountability hierarchy.
4. Keep a broadly representative membership on the highest level committees. The committee that makes the final recommendation to the board frequently must weigh several expensive, strongly advocated projects, each of which has considerable merit. The credibility of this committee is essential to continued generation of proposals.
5. Encourage candid discussion of proposals by minimizing the negative consequences of honesty. Influential people must visibly respect the opinions of individuals who are less powerful. Power should not be rewarded in the planning process. Helpful techniques for encouraging candor include:
   - adhering to the established protocol for all proposals;
   - selecting planning committee members so that powerful people are balanced against one another rather than against groups of less powerful people;
   - chairing meetings competently, so that all can be heard;
   - using outside consultants to counterbalance local experts; and
   - instructing or sanctioning individuals who endanger the process of development and evaluation.

Values of Community Healthcare Organizations

It sometimes happens that very similar opportunities are attractive to one organization but not another. Examples are often in areas like prevention, facility location, human resources and physician relations, and some less visible aspects of quality of care. Assuming that both organizations are well run, considerations other than the opportunity itself must lead to this result.

There are four premises about planning decisions that are independent of the individual proposal or opportunity and related to the values or beliefs of the decision makers:

1. Community mission and values
2. Time horizon used for decision making
3. Willingness to accept risk
4. Willingness to assume debt

Well-managed healthcare organizations have consensus positions on these elements. Each position involves a set of tradeoffs in which certain proposals will face diminished chances of acceptance, while others will face enhanced chances. The tradeoffs are by definition intangible (that is, impractical to measure in dollar terms in most situations), and they are implicitly decided by any action taken, even an action to defer or delay. An institution's profile on the premises, reflected in its actual decisions, constitutes part of its style or corporate culture.

Community mission and values

The motivations for operating community healthcare organizations—classified in Chapter 2 as Samaritanism, personal health, public health, community economic gain, and healthcare economy—differ in the extent to which they benefit individual patients employees, and physicians.[30] Samaritanism, public health, and economy are goals that make communities attractive as a whole. For-profit organizations are justified in ignoring any benefits that do not contribute directly to profit; they can be penalized for diverting funds away from their owners. Not-for-profit organizations are explicitly rewarded by their tax exemptions to address the community benefits. The justification for tax exemptions is criticized by people who say that the true owners are the doctors and employees, who take the value of the exemption in enhanced salaries.[31] Leaders of not-for-profit healthcare have responded by increased emphasis on community values.[32,33]

It is possible to measure the community contribution indirectly by accounting data such as bad debts, uncompensated care, and investment in health education. It is also assessed by the existence or commitment to certain programs such as the willingness to meet needs of the disadvantaged. Scales for measuring community commitment have been developed by the Catholic Health Association and others. Evidence from California hospitals by Clement, Smith, and Wheeler suggests that the amount of community contribution declined during the 1980s, but in 1987 it remained more valuable than the tax exemption itself, or alternative investments.[34] Leading institutions are developing explicit community goals, analogous to dividend goals of for-profit companies, and committing a portion of their earnings.[35]

Closely related to the concept of community mission, a not-for-profit organization may protect certain assets, or resources, which will never have a precise accounting definition. The organization's religious commitment, or achievement of a certain mission, such as reduction of racial tension or deliberate assignment of jobs or economic opportunity to disadvantaged groups, are assets to the community that never appear on any balance sheet. Locating or keeping employment in inner city areas, supporting educational programs for unskilled workers, and assisting with housing or environmental needs are examples.[36] These decisions are unrelated to health; they deal solely with perceived community benefit.

There are many more philosophical issues than one would at first think. For example, what is the value of affiliation with a medical school or a religious organization? What is the importance of remaining in a certain location, such as a downtown site near the homes of poor patients and unskilled workers? Is it appropriate to recognize loyalty and partially protect employees and physicians against economic vicissitudes? How much is appropriate to spend on aesthetics, such as a statue or a traditional building? (The Johns Hopkins Hospital has kept its nineteenth-century entrance with the large marble statue of Christ and the famous dome over it at very high cost. How can one decide whether the cost is worthwhile? One cannot, except by voting yes or no on the specific proposal. Those who vote to save the entrance consider tradition, viable expression of a Samaritan commitment, and aesthetics to be more important than the benefits that might have accrued from alternative use of the space and funds.)

It is generally believed that not-for-profit organizations should place higher values on intangible assets. That is, one of the social functions of hospitals, Blue Cross Plans, universities, and private foundations is to uphold the values that may be overlooked in purely commercial transactions. There is by definition no evidence that this policy is correct, but it is widely accepted. The converse can be more convincingly stated: if healthcare organizations do not protect intangibles, they lose an important characteristic distinguishing them from for-profit organizations. Sooner or later, people will ask why they should continue to exist.

Time horizon used for decision making

Different benefits have different time horizons. Samaritanism, public health, economical healthcare and non-health benefits have the longest horizons, in the sense that only a small fraction of the total benefit is recovered in the short term. High-tech care and care of the dying tend to produce much shorter range benefits. Thus, a short-term style will emphasize proposals whose benefits lie in high-tech personal healthcare and direct economic benefits such as employment.

The correct time horizon depends on time and place, but well-run community healthcare organizations emphasize the long term. Actions that only yield immediate benefits are considered expedient and are usually avoided. Organizations that are in trouble tend to shorter horizons, but a sign of their recovery is a movement to longer perspectives.

Risk All proposals and strategies involve risks, but the amount and kind of risk can differ. In an oversimplified example, two projects are proposed. One may help thousands of people if it works, but it is difficult to estimate the chances that it will work. The other is virtually certain to help 200 people. If both cost exactly the same, and only one can be adopted, which should the organization choose? There is an underlying bias toward prudence, expressed in the law and tradition of not-for-profit organizations, which favor risk avoidance. Yet prudence itself must be defined. Time and place determine what is acceptable risk. In the example, a research hospital might accept much higher levels of risk than a community hospital, and hospitals in a wealthy community would take more risk than those in a poor one.

In real healthcare organizations, the odds are never clear, costs are never exactly the same, and benefits are rarely directly comparable. Each year the institution makes a series of specific decisions that reflect what the governance structure feels to be acceptable levels of risk. The accepted role of not-for-profit organizations emphasizes prudence; very high risks must be placed in organizations specially designed to deal with them, and to limit losses of community funds. Higher risks should be matched by higher potential gains. Consistency is important. The institution should not be unwilling to accept risk on one decision yet accepting a similar risk on another. And in the final analysis, it must invest its earnings. They cannot be given away, and a growing pile of cash is an asset frozen from any benefit.

Liquidity The issue of liquidity and borrowing is inseparably related to risk. Resources in their liquid form are usually invested in readily salable instruments earning a tangible return. When strategic and programmatic proposals are funded, funds transferred from liquid to illiquid assets are no longer available for spending. A decision to wait, or to remain liquid, is a decision that the benefits of the project will not overcome the loss of flexibility. It implies that a better, as yet unforeseen, opportunity will arise. A decision to spend is the opposite, and a decision to borrow, which itself carries a tangible cost, is a decision that the value of the project exceeds the cost of borrowing. The tangible costs and benefits of borrowing are handled by competent technical analysis. What complicates the decision is that borrowing has intangible costs that apply to all projects rather than to any specific opportunity. Borrowing reduces the future ability of the organization to borrow and, as a result, its ability to respond to unforeseen trouble. That is to say, the opportunity cost of borrowing is increased risk.

It is also important to understand the relationship of liquidity to expansion and to economical healthcare. Borrowing permits rapid expansion, which for healthcare organizations means increased costs to the community. A strong motivation for economy discourages borrowing. The cost of borrowing, and to a certain extent the risk, is set by the interest rate. The organization may add to the interest rate the intangible cost of borrowing, or preference for liquidity, sometimes called the **hurdle rate**. Organizations that prefer liquidity generally set a high hurdle rate: they expect any successful proposal to repay not only the interest, but also the hurdle. The result is that fewer projects are accepted; those that are tend to have higher benefits and lower risks.

Well-managed not-for-profit healthcare organizations tend toward higher liquidity. They use hurdle rates either explicitly or implicitly to avoid projects of limited return.

Importance of community representation in decisions

As major alternatives are debated at the governing board level, positions on these premises are identified by specific resource allocation decisions. The profile that emerges will ultimately reflect the relative weight placed on representation of different perspectives within the community. A representative profile of well-managed not-for-profit healthcare organizations is shown in Figure 12.12. Individual organizations and communities will differ but, in general, the not-for-profit vision is one of community support, community values, longer terms, prudence, and liquidity.

Many classifications of the community can be used. The consumer-provider dichotomy is an important but simplistic one. Whether decision makers are poor or rich, influential or not, religious or secular, male or female, or white or black also influences the final values placed on the premises. The ability to accommodate the views of others, however, appears more important than actual affiliation. Wise decision makers not only transcend their own self-interest and background, but they also recognize the need for compromise and the importance of understanding specifics to compromise effectively. One characteristic of well-run healthcare organizations is that they recognize when special interests are important and accommodate them in specific, rather than general, terms.

The subtleties of the question begin to emerge if one considers the issue of customer versus provider orientation. Customers and providers may have legitimately conflicting interests. Optimization will call for finding the balance that maximizes the totality of interests met. If too much is conceded to the providers, some community goals may not be achieved. In particular, costs will mount and some members of the community will drop their health insurance. If too much is conceded to the community, skilled providers will leave for more attractive situations. If too much conflict develops, the organization may fail to achieve either member or community goals. Through its planning decisions, a healthcare organization inevitably places itself on the community versus member continuum. That is, it implicitly trades off the values of the decision makers on questions such as the importance of hospital employment and the attractiveness of the community to other commerce.

The consistency, wisdom, and effectiveness that decisions such as these reflect distinguish the well-run healthcare organization. The predisposition of the governing board toward short-term or long-term, high-risk or low-risk,

FIGURE 12.12 Profile of Not-for-Profit Values

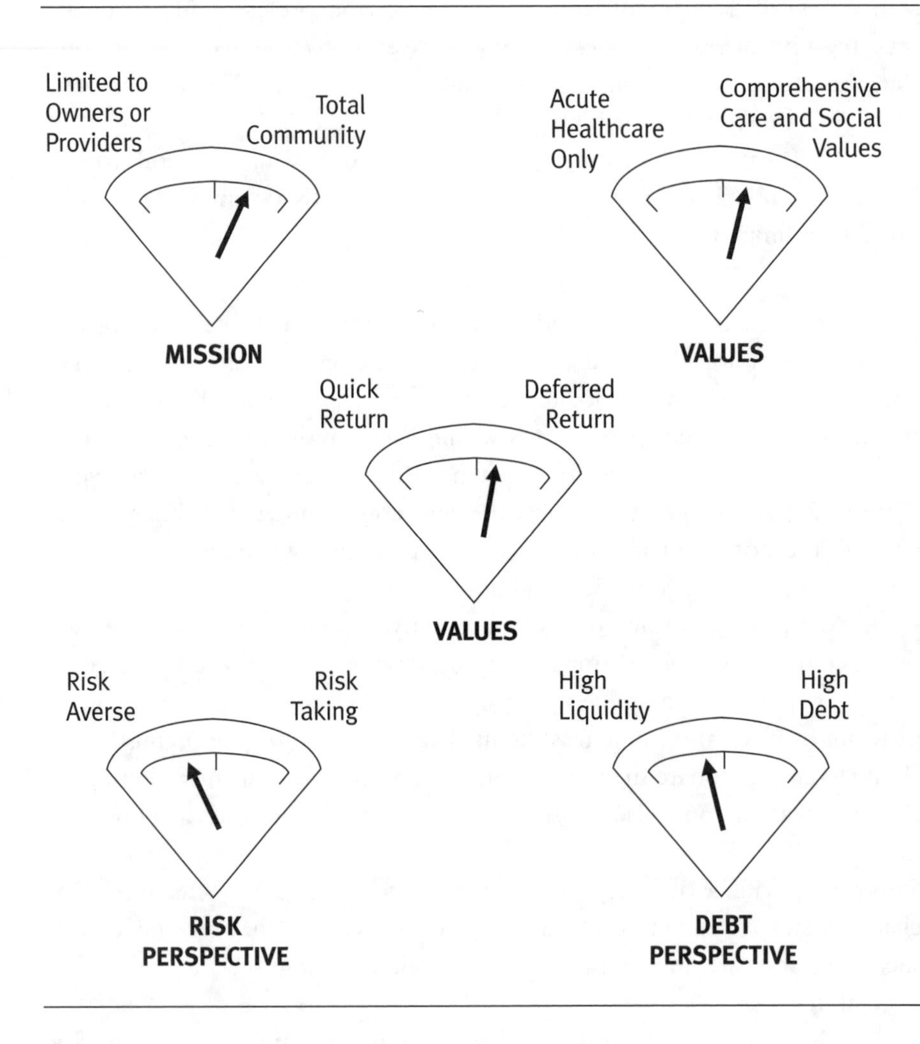

greater or less liquidity, and for or against certain missions and values, will determine the eventual shape of the organization.

Suggested Readings

Kotler, P. 1991. *Strategic Marketing for Non-Profit Organizations.* 4th ed. Englewood Cliffs: Prentice-Hall.

Kotler, P., and R. Clark. 1987. *Marketing for Healthcare Organizations.* Englewood Cliffs: Prentice-Hall.

Mintzberg, H. 1994. *The Rise and Fall of Strategic Planning: Reconceiving Roles for Planning, Plans, Planners.* New York: Free Press.

Pfeffer, J. 1994. *Competitive Advantage Through People: Unleashing the Power of the Workforce.* Boston: Harvard Business School Press.

Porter, M. E. 1998. *Competitive Advantage: Creating and Sustaining Superior Performance.* New York: Free Press.

Senge, P. M. 1990. *The Fifth Discipline: The Art and Practice of the Learning Organization*. New York: Doubleday/Currency.

Spiegel, A. D., and H. H. Hyman. 1991. *Strategic Health Planning: Methods and Techniques Applied to Marketing and Management*. Norwood: Aplex Pub. Corp.

Notes

1. P. Kotler, *Strategic Marketing for Non-Profit Organizations*, 4th ed. Englewood Cliffs: Prentice-Hall (1991)
2. J. R. Griffith, *Designing 21st Century Healthcare*. Chicago: Health Administration Press, 240–242 (1998)
3. See *Quality Management in Health Care* 1(4) (Summer, 1993). The issue is devoted to strategic quality planning and includes articles based on five different healthcare systems.
4. D. M. Demers, "Implementing Hoshin Planning at the Vermont Medical Center" *Quality Management in Health Care* 1(4): 64–72 (Summer, 1993). See especially p. 69.
5. See *Quality Management in Health Care*, 1(4) (Summer, 1993)
6. G. Hamel and C. K. Prahalad, "Strategy as Stretch and Leverage." *Harvard Business Review* 71(2): 75–84 (Mar/Apr, 1993).
7. H. Mintzberg, *The Rise and Fall of Strategic Planning: Reconceiving Roles for Planning, Plans, Planners*. New York: The Free Press Division of Macmillan, Inc, pp. 323–397 (1994)
8. H. A. Simon, G. B. Danzig, R. Hogarth, C. R. Plott, H. Raiffa, et al, "Decision Making and Problem Solving." *Interfaces* 17(5): 57–67, p. 63 (1997)
9. T. Proctor and P. Ruocco, "Generating Marketing Strategies: A Structured Creative Decision Support Method (Matching Organizational Strengths and Weaknesses with Opportunities and Threats)," *Management Decision* 30(5): 50–3 (1992)
10. J. Peters, "On Audits." *Management Decision* 31(6): 26–7 (1993)
11. M. E. Porter, *Competitive Strategy: Techniques for Analyzing Industries and Competitors*. New York: The Free Press, pp. xvi—xx (1980)
12. D. F. Abell and J. S. Hammond, *Strategic Market Planning: Problems and Analytic Approaches*. Englewood Cliffs, NJ: Prentice Hall, (1979)
13. H. Thomas and D. Gardner, *Strategic Marketing and Management*. New York: Wiley (1985)
14. R. E. Miles and C. C. Snow, *Organizational Strategy, Structure and Process*. New York: McGraw-Hill (1978)
15. S. R. Eastaugh, "Hospital Strategy and Financial Performance." *Health Care Management Review* 17(3): 19–31 (1992)
16. S. M. Shortell, E. M. Morrison, and B. Friedman, *Strategic Choices for America's Hospitals*. San Francisco: Jossey-Bass (1990)
17. S. R. Eastaugh, "Hospital Strategy and Financial Performance." Health Care Management Review 17(3): 27 (1992)
18. M. E. Porter, *Competitive Strategy*. New York: The Free Press (1980)

19. D. Miller, and P. H. Friesen, *Organizations: A Quantum View*. Englewood Cliffs, NJ: Prentice Hall (1984)
20. J. R. Griffith, *Designing 21st Century Healthcare*. Chicago: Health Administration Press, pp. 20–1, 80, 165, 237–8 (1998)
21. W. E. Welton, "The Impact of Organizational Factors on Community-Wide Medicare Costs." unpublished doctoral dissertation. Ann Arbor, MI: The University of Michigan, pp. 170–177 (1999)
22. S. M. Shortell, R. R. Gillies, D. A. Anderson, J. B. Mitchell, and K. L. Morgan, "Creating Organized Delivery Systems: The Barriers and Facilitators." *Hospital & Health Services Administration* 38(4): 447–66 (Winter, 1993)
23. R. Herzlinger, *America's Largest Service Industry*. Reading, MA: Addison-Wesley Pub. (1997)
24. B. C. Vladeck," Market Realities Meet Balanced Government: Another Look at Columbia/HCA." *Health Affairs (Millwood)* 17(2): 7–26 (Mar–April, 1998)
25. S. Lutz, "NME's New Day Dawns." *Modern Healthcare* 25(10): 68, 70, 72–4 (Mar 6, 1995)
26. B. Meier, "Big Nursing Home Company Is Accused of Mistreatment." *New York Times* (late New York edition), p. B7 (Jan 13 1995) G.L. Miles, "This Nursing Home Giant May Need Intensive Care." *Business Week* pp. 124 (Nov 7, 1988)
27. J. R. Griffith, V. Sahney, and R. Mohr, *Reengineering Healthcare*. Chicago: Health Administration Press, Chapter 4 (1995)
28. P. Kotler, *Marketing for Non-Profit Organizations*, 2d ed. Englewood Cliffs, NJ: Prentice-Hall (1982)
29. US General Accounting Office, Health Systems Plans: A Poor Framework for Promoting Health Care Improvements: *Report to the Congress by the Controller General of the United States*. Washington, DC: GAO (June 22, 1981)
30. H. Long, "Valuation as a Criterion in Not-for-Profit Decision-Making." *Health Care Management Review* 1:34–52 (Summer, 1976)
31. B. Arrington and C. C. Haddock, "Who Really Profits from Non-Profits." *Health Services Research* 25: 291–304 (June, 1990)
32. J. D. Seay, and B. N. C. Vladeck, eds., *In Sickness and In Health: The Mission of Voluntary Health Institutions*. NY: McGraw-Hill (1988)
33. A. D. Kovner, "The Hospital Community Benefits Standards Program and Health Reform." *Hospital & Health Services Administration* 39(2):143–57 (Summer, 1994)
34. J. P. Clement, D. G. Smith, and J. R. C. Wheeler, "What Do We Want and What Do We Get from Not-for-Profit Hospitals?" *Hospital & Health Services Administration* 39(2): 159–78 (Summer, 1994)
35. J. R. Griffith, *Designing 21st Century Healthcare*. Chicago: Health Administration Press, pp. 57, 133, 163 (1998)
36. J. R. Griffith *Designing 21st Century Healthcare*. Chicago: Health Administration Press, pp. 231–6 (1998)

CHAPTER

13

MARKETING THE HEALTHCARE ORGANIZATION

As noted in Chapter 12, the broad definition of marketing emphasizes a cohesive, integrated activity. Here is one favored by Philip Kotler, a noted professor of marketing, that includes not only planning but also implementation and control:

> . . . the analysis, planning, implementation, and control of carefully formulated programs designed to bring about voluntary exchanges of values with target markets for the purpose of achieving organizational objectives.[1]

Beyond the important concept of integrating planning and action, the unique contribution of marketing is the deliberate effort to establish fruitful relationships with exchange partners. It applies not just to customers, but to all exchanges, including competitors, employees, and other community agencies.

Market share is critical to price and profitability, and cost-effective processes require more complex exchanges at several levels. Healthcare organizations today work steadily on attracting patients to their doctors, linking doctors to the organization, winning profitable contracts with intermediaries, and persuading employers and insured groups of their advantages. They are collaborating with competitors and other agencies to expand service and meet price constraints. Well-run institutions market themselves to physicians and employees as well; it gives them the opportunity to select the best and to attract professionals in short supply. Seventy percent of hospitals were reported to have moderate to high marketing orientations in 1991. Larger hospitals reported an average of about 15 people in marketing, public relations, and planning activity, with seven devoted to marketing, five to public relations, and only three to planning.[2] In a different survey, about one-third of marketing expenditures were for advertising, and only one in four marketing people reported responsibility for planning. Most of the funds went for consumer marketing. Physician marketing received 20 percent of the funds, and employer marketing about 10 percent.[3]

This chapter emphasizes marketing's unique contribution, identifying the purpose, functions, and organization of marketing services and providing measures of marketing performance. The perspective is what marketing must do for the organization as a whole to succeed.

Purpose

The purpose of marketing, as Kotler suggests, is to build exchange relationships that forward the organization's mission and strategic position. It is all activities that encourage or improve the initial contact between exchange partners.

Several difficulties complicate this purpose, and overcoming them is an intrinsic part of healthcare marketing. Marketing healthcare must deal with:

- an intimate, life-shaping service about which people have strong and sometimes irrational feelings;
- differences of opinion among patients, buyers, providers, and society at large about what is appropriate care. Optimum treatment is only imprecisely known, and there may be serious disagreements about what is necessary;
- expenses that are often unpredictable and that fall disproportionately on a few people. These must be financed by insurance, bringing a third party into the transaction. The insurance mechanism raises the need for agreement about what is necessary;
- expenses that are financed largely through payroll deductions and employer contributions, bringing a fourth party into the transaction;
- delivery mechanisms that are highly capital intensive and as a result have high fixed costs. This requires careful adjustment of supply and demand, and opens the possibility of differential pricing;
- providers who are divided into a large number of competing professions, and who often compete within their specialty; and
- interests of other organizations and their members that may be in direct conflict with those of the organization represented.

Functions

In such a complex environment it would be disastrous to think of marketing as a simple or limited activity. It has five major functions, as shown in Figure 13.1.

Identifying Markets of Healthcare Organizations

As Kotler implies, targets are the key to marketing. The organization must identify specific groups of people or organizations seeking to make exchanges of value, and convince them to participate. Healthcare marketing pursues three distinct sets of exchanges, and each set is differentiated into particular subgroups based on the groups' exchange need, as shown in Figure 13.2. The process of identifying subgroups, called segmentation, is a critical function that underlies all the others.

Marketing deals with complexity by **segmentation**, the deliberate effort to separate target audiences by the message to which they will respond. The first marketing function is to identify, describe, and understand the exchange

FIGURE 13.1 Marketing Functions

Function	Description
1. Identifying markets	Marketing must begin with a solid understanding of the market structure with emphasis on recognizing target markets, groups of participants with similar goals.
2. Promoting the organization	Marketing must make the organization as a whole attractive to the entire community by finding and emphasizing the goals broadly shared and by identifying and meeting those unique but critical to particular groups.
3. Convincing patients to select the organization	Marketing must make potential patients aware of the service and persuade them to select the organization over its competitors.
4. Attracting capable workers	Marketing must ensure a steady stream of personnel seeking to join the organization. The successful organization will market itself so that it has a choice of qualified applicants, even in areas of personnel shortages.
5. Managing external relationships	Marketing must establish constructive relationships with other organizations, such as insurance intermediaries, employers, and providers of competing or noncompeting services.

partners of the community being served. Following the outline in Chapter 2, the general categories are patients, buyers, and caregivers, and each of these expands into several specific segments.

Purposes of segmentation

Each group of individual exchange partners must be understood in terms of its wants and needs, but also in terms of how it can be reached with information and how its opinions can be influenced. Exchange groups like patients or buyers are not homogeneous within themselves; they must be segmented further to understand them fully. The first goal of segmentation is to identify all segments of a market in terms of their interests, emphasizing the homogeneity of each segment, and identifying how it differs from others. The second goal is to understand how each target group will respond to specific healthcare alternatives. Understanding supports quantitative estimates of the four parameters of the planning equation in Chapter 6 for each of the dozens of unique services a healthcare organization offers:

$$\left\{\begin{matrix}\text{Demand for}\\ \text{a service}\end{matrix}\right\} = \left\{\begin{matrix}\text{Population}\\ \text{at risk}\end{matrix}\right\} \times \left\{\begin{matrix}\text{Incidence}\\ \text{rate}\end{matrix}\right\} \times \left\{\begin{matrix}\text{Average}\\ \text{use per}\\ \text{incidence}\end{matrix}\right\} \times \left\{\begin{matrix}\text{Market}\\ \text{share}\end{matrix}\right\}$$

The third goal of segmentation is to understand for each segment how changes in product, place, price, and promotion will affect the demand. That is, to predict the effect of changes on the four parameters, and from them the effect on demand for the service.

These purposes require a database that can be organized by market segment. The content and detail of that database tend to expand over time

FIGURE 13.2
Major Marketing Directions

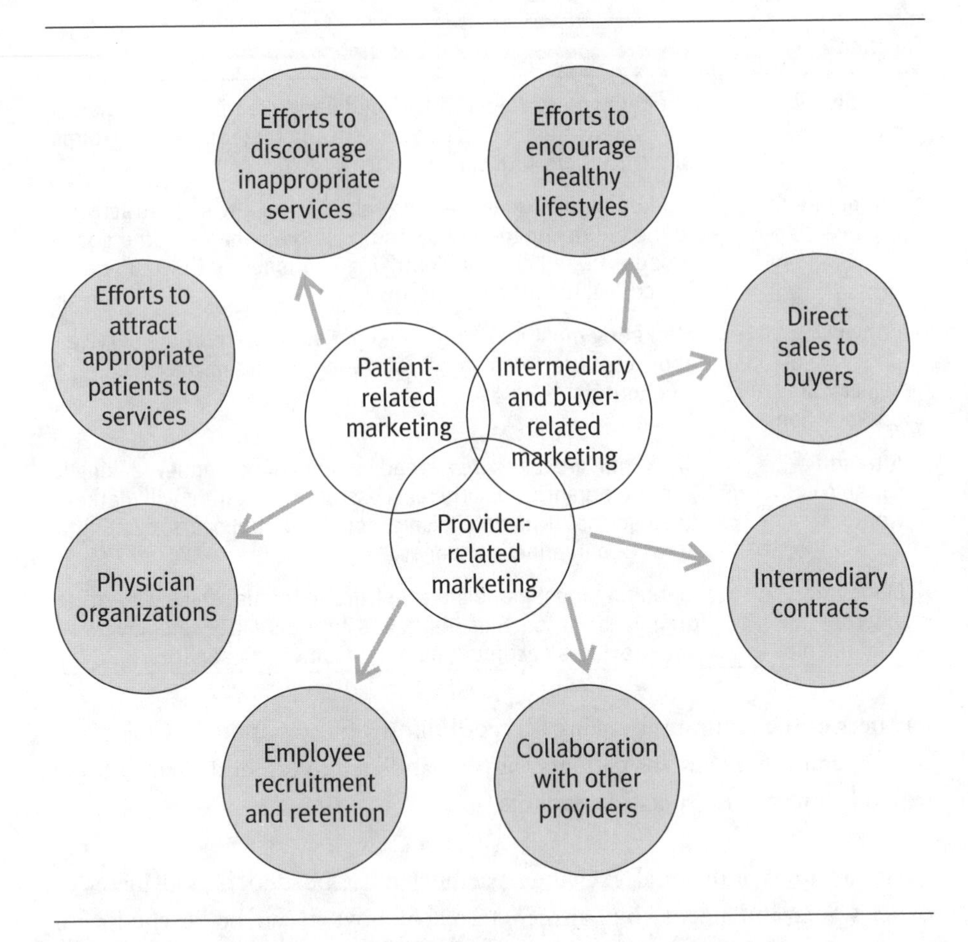

in the number of segments and combinations that can be examined and the amount of knowledge in each. It becomes a rich resource for fact-finding, analysis, promotion, and negotiation. It supports both the strategic planning and the marketing activities, making it possible to identify specific groups of people and organizations in the community with specific needs, interests, talents, and affiliations.

An example of segmentation

The epidemiologic models determine the customer demand and the required provider supply Many answers involve groups other than the patients or potential patients involved. Taking a relatively simple service, well-baby care, it is possible to reach an initial estimate of the demand relatively quickly. Using the parameters suggested in Figure 13.3 an initial forecast of well-baby visits can be constructed:

$$\left\{\begin{matrix}\text{Well-baby}\\\text{visits}\end{matrix}\right\} = \left\{\begin{matrix}\text{Number of}\\\text{births/year}\end{matrix}\right\} \times \left\{\begin{matrix}\text{Number of}\\\text{visits/baby}\end{matrix}\right\} \times \left\{\begin{matrix}\text{Pct. of}\\\text{all well-}\\\text{baby visits}\end{matrix}\right\}$$

The initial estimate treats the well-baby market as homogeneous; that is, it assumes all babies and mothers are alike. This is a doubtful assumption;

it is possible to identify a series of questions based on differences in the baby and mother market:

- What fraction of babies now receive care from some provider? Would they move from their present provider to a new service? What would make them move? More comprehensive service? Better hours or amenities? Lower price? Advertising or other promotion?
- What fraction of babies now do not receive care? Why? What would bring these mothers to a new service?
- Is there any condition that might discourage mothers from using well-baby care? How can it be avoided?
- Is there any condition that might strongly encourage mothers to use this service? How can it be incorporated into the well-baby program?
- How will well-baby care be financed? What price is practical for the patient? What are the chances of insurance coverage? Will employers and unions support well-baby care as an employment benefit? What is the price sensitivity for insurance or employment coverage?
- What agencies and individuals now provide well-baby care? What are the opportunities to collaborate with them? What collaboration mechanisms are likely to be rewarding? What will the terms of competition be? What will be the cost of meeting those terms?

The answers to these questions will lead to multiple market segments as shown in Figure 13.3. Some of the segments will be unique to the problem at hand, but all will be related to the identification of useful subgroups of exchanges. Out of the repeated segmentation of the market comes differentiated programs reflecting the needs of the segments. These have their own solutions of price, placement, and promotion even though the product, well-baby care, is the same.

As answers to the questions are developed the well-baby care proposal may change shape several times depending on the specific circumstances of the community. The fraction of babies not now receiving care (the right-hand group of Figure 13.3) will be much higher in certain rural and inner-city locations, for example. An extensive program of clinics to reach babies now missed may have substantial value to Medicaid and local government public health activities. To keep costs low, the clinics may emphasize nurse practitioner care. To reach an audience not already sold on the product, special outreach activities may be useful. Joint finance or collaborative relationships may emerge. Even direct competitors may wish to collaborate on a program if it reduces their costs and does not impair their market share. Schools, day care centers, and churches may be willing to advocate use of the well-baby service. A low cost promotional campaign may be designed among these groups. "New Program 1" of Figure 13.3 would meet this combination of needs.

FIGURE 13.3
Segmenting the Well-Baby Care Market

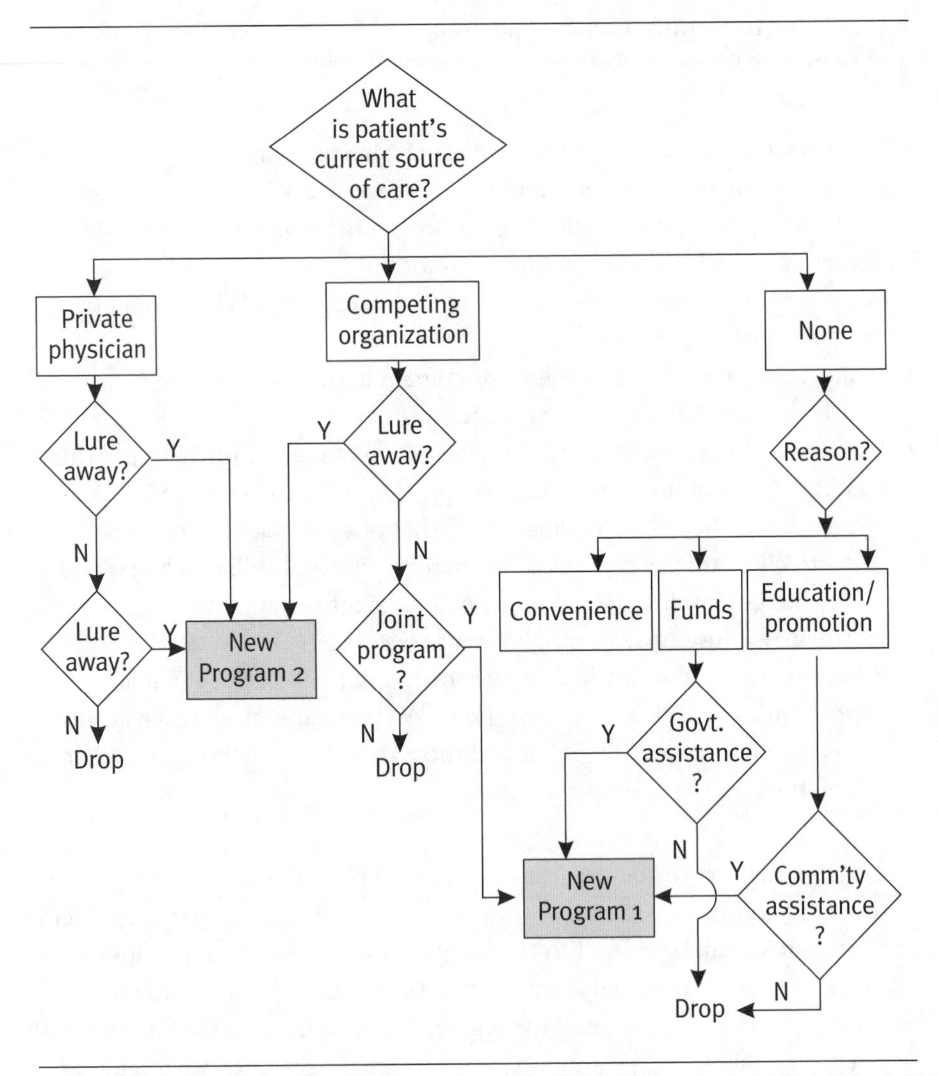

Other babies (the left of Figure 13.3) will have their need met by family practitioners and pediatricians in independent practice or by existing programs operated by competitors. Aggressively luring mothers away from their current physicians may be very costly, because these are primary care doctors who may be critical to the organization in other ways. A proposal to collaborate with current providers to support their current activities and fill the remaining unmet need by attracting it to existing sources may emerge. This pattern of market interest leads to "New Program 2" of Figure 13.3. Organizations normally peripheral to healthcare, such as schools and churches, may still have an important interest and position of influence. Financial and promotional support may be available for Program 2, if the partners are convinced the program will achieve important goals.

The Figure 13.3 analysis leads to two new programs. One addresses the needs of mothers not now being reached with broad community collaboration and innovative promotion. The other addresses the needs of mothers and providers in a market already being served and strengthens the ties to the organization and its doctors. Reflecting reality, the new programs fail to reach some mothers and babies who are not reached in either target market. The competitor still has some market share, and those babies outside the contacts through community organizations are still without care. If well-baby care is an important part of the mission, the next step is to study the unserved group further. New market segments will be developed, and Program 3 or 4 will be built to capture these groups.

Common segmentation taxonomies

Much market segmentation follows established taxonomies, or ways of subdividing patients and buyers. Figure 13.4 shows common patient taxonomies. These begin with demographics, but quickly expand to categories of health insurance or finance. Disease or condition is often the final stage of segmentation. Risk factors, such as smoking or drug use, are also used to identify groups that must be reached by promotion and attracted with services, placement, and price that meet their needs.

Service lines are a form of market segmentation; the services have been organized to meet a specific population, such as women, children, or cancer patients. MacStravic has suggested that a limited set of segments, such as young adults, older adults, seniors, physicians, and businesses, be identified as core businesses. A strategy for developing familiarity, attractiveness, and market share within the segment is developed, implemented, and assessed. Data

FIGURE 13.4 Patient-Oriented Taxonomies

Category	Classifications
Demographic	Age Sex Race Education
Economic	Income Employment Social class
Geographic	Zip code of residence Census tract Political subdivision
Healthcare finance	Managed versus traditional insurance Private versus government insurance
Diagnosis	Disease classification Procedure Diagnosis-related group (DRG) Ambulatory visit group
Risk	Health behavior attribute Preexisting condition Chronic or high-cost disease

monitoring performance and profitability are developed, and accountability is assigned. He notes that segment administration is time consuming and difficult, and has a heavy front-end investment compared to product line management. However, it builds broader support than most product-oriented strategies and is more focused than a general stance toward the market.[4]

It is often necessary to classify insurance intermediaries, employers, and community agencies. A variety of approaches can be used, but purpose, size, type, or industry are common, as shown in Figure 13.5. Often the classification of these exchange partners is a function of the proposal. HMOs, traditional private insurance, Medicare, and Medicaid are likely to offer different prices for a given service, have different criteria for necessity, and have different rules to enforce those criteria.

Providers and members as markets

Market segmentation techniques can be applied to relationships with physicians, employees, volunteers, and charitable donors. In open systems theory, these too are voluntary exchanges contributing to organizational objectives. Figure 13.6 shows common taxonomies for these groups. Because most successful proposals must fit both customer and provider needs, negotiation and promotion are likely to be necessary with these groups. Many healthcare organizations invest in promotional material to attract donors, recruit clinical specialists in short supply, and encourage volunteers. These markets are segmented by profession or type of work, and in the case of donors, by type and dollar level of giving.

The marketing role of physicians is unique and is discussed in Chapter 12. Segmentation is still important. It is possible to segment physicians by specialty, age, location, and organizational affiliation. The last is not necessarily permanent; proposals may involve winning physicians over to your organization to capture the demand they represent. Particularly primary care physicians exercising their gatekeeper role have an important influence on demand, as the well-baby example suggests.

FIGURE 13.5
Insurance Intermediary and Employer Taxonomies

Category	Classifications
Employers	Size Geographic location Industry Income level Union organization Health insurance benefit Health insurance type
Intermediary	Health insurance type Ownership or corporate structure Size Number of health insurance subscribers Employer groups covered

FIGURE 13.6 Healthcare Provider Taxonomies

Category	Classifications
Individual providers	Training, certification, or licensure Organizational affiliation Location Age
Donors	Interest Level of contribution
Organized providers	Scope of service Geographic location Ownership Size Market share Financial strength Competitive position

The segmentation concept applies to competitors and potential partner organizations as well. The twenty-first century healthcare organization is likely to include a much larger array of formal affiliations than the traditional hospital or freestanding medical clinic. Partnerships, joint ventures, and parent/subsidiary relationships will be common. Techniques of market segmentation apply here as well. Competitors and complementary organizations will fulfill a continuum of relationships ranging from collaborative to adversarial. As shown in Figure 13.6, they are classed by type of service, size, market served, financial strength, and type of relationship, where the last is understood to be flexible and subject to change.

Promoting the Organization

One function of marketing is to maintain the overall reputation or **image** of the organization so that it remains attractive to most members of the community at large. Recent decades have seen a major expansion of the public's right to know. The well-run healthcare organization must respond affirmatively to this trend, using the obligations to inform the public as an opportunity to promote broader support. Image building usually begins as a community-wide effort reflecting the mission. The activities include public and community relations, image advertising and promotion, and media relations. As groups in the community articulate special needs or are identified as important market segments, image building may be tailored to those groups. The message to those groups emphasizes both the general contribution of the organization and its ability to meet particular needs.

Public and community relations

A deliberate program of public and community relations includes descriptive information such as annual reports, web sites, and personal appearances by management and caregivers. It also includes deliberate contacts with influentials and opinion leaders, and direct assistance to community groups. It relates indirectly to lobbying (Chapter 4) because grass roots support depends on a favorable response by individuals in the community.

Public information is one of several sources from which people derive a positive image of the organization. Public information should be coordinated with advertising and media relations, and all three can be deliberately coordinated to promote use of specific services. Obviously, success begins with having a good story to tell. Although the information is slanted to emphasize the positive aspects, ability to be candid about weaknesses is recognized and respected.

Most members of strategic management are involved in public and community relations activity. Speeches, personal contacts, and participation in community affairs are important. The CEO has a uniquely important role. Specific accountability for coordinating public information and promotion should be assigned, and marketing has strong claims to the assignment. Coordination of themes, logos, and printing styles are important. The organization often issues material such as newsletters, annual reports, and regular mailings that describe the organization in general terms and highlight specific events.

The goal of image-building activity is to increase two dimensions of recognition of the institution: familiarity and attractiveness. The process is sometimes called "branding." Well-established scales and survey techniques allow the organization to monitor how familiar members of the community are with the organization, usually measured by ability to recall the name without prompting and ability to recognize the name in a list. Similarly, well-designed questionnaires allow profiling of what people think of the organization, how they compare it to competitors, and which attributes they like most or least.[5]

"Branding" is much more difficult than most people expect. Dozens or hundreds of exposures to the image are necessary to establish favorable independent recognition, the level that is felt to be necessary to attract and retain market share. A successful branding program identifies both goals and audiences. Segmentation is effective. Specific strategies to communicate concepts about the organization strengthen the familiarity built by general releases. Outreach activity such as healthcare screening vans, helicopter services, and open houses are used to reach specific audiences. Special community relations efforts may be directed to certain groups such as people living in the local neighborhood, people with special interests, or people who are influential with the organization's target markets.[6] Community relations relates to media relations; the activities are often chosen with an eye to attracting coverage in local media.

Image advertising and promotion

Image advertising and promotion has also become commonplace in recent years. It includes purchased media exposure that is not related to a specific sales objective, or that combines a specific and a general goal. It also includes association of the institution with various activities such as athletic events or public services, and distribution of products bearing the name and logo of the organization. Most well-managed organizations try to establish their name, mission, and an image of warmth and supportiveness. Some also emphasize their technological proficiency or convenience. Often the image message is combined with a specific promotion. Advertising techniques easily support dual concepts like, "Bring your baby for care while he's well to keep him well," and "Excalibur Health System cares about you and your family."

Image promotion is far from a panacea. It takes a large number of exposures even to increase name recognition, and changing attractiveness is harder. Kotler and Clarke note:

> Healthcare organizations seeking to change their images must have great patience, because images tend to last long after the reality of an organization has changed. . . . Image persistence is explained by the fact that once people have a certain image of an object, they tend to be selective perceivers of further data; their perceptions are oriented toward seeing what they expect to see.[7]

The implication is that an established reputation, being among the first two or three names people independently recall for healthcare, is a valuable asset, hard to replace and well worth protecting.

Media relations

Most organizations are acutely aware of what is said about them in the media, but the evidence suggests that the public at large is quite resistive to media statements. Nonetheless, the **media** can portray the organization favorably or unfavorably, and the result often depends on the quality of information supplied by the organization. There are two types of media communication. One is the planned release of information, where the organization wishes to have its story told by print or electronic media. Attractive, thorough releases, identification of visual elements for photos and television, access to knowledgeable, articulate spokespersons and identification of newsworthy elements all assist in improving the coverage. A deliberate program of regular information releases and efforts to draw media attention to favorable events promotes a positive image. The more information released, the greater the familiarity and attractiveness of the community is likely to be.

The second type of communication is response to media initiatives. These are often related to major news events such as healthcare to prominent personages or general disasters. In the worst case, they come as a result of unfavorable events such as lowered bond ratings, civil lawsuits, or criminal behavior. They can be quite hostile when journalists sense or assume something is wrong. Investigative journalism is an aggressive effort to dig out all the public might want to know, with emphasis on what the organization might want to hide. Effective handling of media initiatives is largely preventive. The organization should prevent or minimize events that will draw investigation. It should maintain a strong program of releasing newsworthy, positive information about itself. It should attempt to deal fully and candidly with issues, anticipating reporters' questions and preparing detailed responses. It should establish its spokespersons and equip them to give thorough, convincing replies to questions. Training and experience are necessary to handle the functions of media relations well.[8]

Marketing the Organization to Patients

Healthcare organizations have made deliberate efforts to attract patients for decades, but these were uneven, underfunded, and generally limited to promoting technological advances. Overt promotion was considered unethical by physicians and inappropriate by not-for-profit hospitals until 1978 when a ruling of the U.S. Supreme Court held the proscription to be in violation of antitrust laws.[9] Some ethical reluctance toward promotion remains, however, because indiscriminate promotion of healthcare risks generating unnecessary demand for services. While providing unnecessary services is highly profitable for providers under traditional insurance mechanisms, it is certainly unethical because it is dangerous for the patient. It is also self-defeating under managed care insurance because it increases cost without adding to revenue. These complexities limited direct marketing to patients until about 1990.[10] The field is still immature. Healthcare promotion has reached neither the level of funding nor the sophistication of approach of other consumer purchases.

The growth of competition and cost control made direct patient marketing an area of increasing importance, and one that will grow in skill and sophistication. Deliberate efforts to make patients aware of choices and to influence their behavior will be critical to success. They will take three principal forms. First, promotional activities will be used to convince patients to select insurance intermediaries, provider panels, and services affiliated with the organization. Second, they will be used to encourage wellness and disease prevention. Third, they will be used to adjust patient expectations about care.

Influencing patient selection of providers and insurers

As healthcare moves from atomistic markets of individual providers to oligopolistic markets with large integrated providers, the maintenance of customer allegiance becomes essential. Major thrusts toward winning and keeping allegiance must work through the purchasing and finance structure of healthcare.

Influence points in patient loyalty

A chain of market decision makers is shown in Figure 13.7. Integrated health systems manipulate all parts of the chain to attract the spouse or employee as patient. Employers are moving toward offering alternative insurance plans, with initial screening of price and quality, and often with price incentives toward lower cost plans.[11] The healthcare organization can market directly to employers, can own its own insurance plan, or can market itself through insurers. The objective will be to have the physicians and the institution prominently placed on the employee's selection list, either as a direct purchase option or through the intermediaries. The employee and spouse select between plans based on out-of-pocket premium share or copayment costs, panel image, and convenience issues. Women influence more of the decisions than men.[12] Consumers value loyalty to their historic providers, convenience, certain amenities such as waiting time and parking, alternatives in primary care, and reputation or credentials of specialists.[13] There is a strong tendency for the insurance plans to offer a broad array of panels. The larger the panel, the fewer patients will have to be lured from their historic relationship. Similarly, the successful healthcare organization strives for a large panel of popular physicians, convenient primary and secondary services, and a competitive price.

An attractive primary care panel is crucial. Patients want easy and prompt access for care and minimal waiting time. They also want choice of gender, age, and ethnic background, confidence in provider judgment, and prompt referral to specialists when required. Emergency coverage and off-hours access are important. Although many patients prefer physicians, there are growing roles for nurse practitioners and midwives. At the same time, the panel must be willing to accept risk for cost and quality of care. Only competent and well-supported physicians will be able to operate effectively under risk contracts. One job of the integrated healthcare organization becomes building and maintaining this panel. Its skills in meeting cost, quality, and patient satisfaction are a major factor in success.

Specialists are typically selected by primary care physicians under managed care, but are often selected directly by patients under traditional insurance. Patients judge specialists on credentials and placement amenities.[14] Employers judge them on cost and measurable quality outcomes. Primary care physicians judge specialists on cost, a broader range of outcomes and process quality, and patient satisfaction. Much care requires at least periodic consultation by a specialist, even if the primary care provider keeps control. Integrated healthcare organizations must balance the number of specialists to need, avoiding either shortages or surpluses, and provide the necessary support in equipment and staff. The inpatient hospital and large ambulatory services are increasingly the domain of the specialist. Effective management of the specialist and hospital services is a major support function appreciated by primary care physicians.

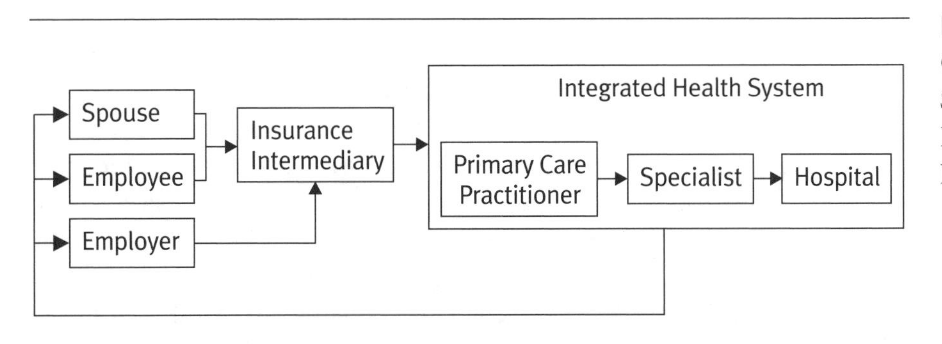

FIGURE 13.7 Chain of Buyer Selections and Provider Feedback

Larger healthcare organizations have substantial advantages. Larger primary panels can meet wider ranges of patient needs. They support in turn a fuller array of specialists and institutional services, with higher, more stable referral volumes. Finally, the larger organization can invest more in programs to control quality and cost.

Pricing strategies

Most prices between buyers and providers are now negotiated in contracts renewed annually. The buyer may attempt to divide providers to drive down price and to keep financial control (and profit) of the care management systems. The integrated system, including all provider groups, responds with customer attractiveness, reduced contract management costs to the buyer, and competitive price. The system may attempt to eliminate the intermediary, going directly to the employer. Strategies for specialists and hospitals encourage maintaining as broad a range of contracts as possible, and discounting some prices when necessary. High fixed costs make significant discounts possible, but only in the short run and only to the extent that variable costs are covered. Long-run success depends on customer attractiveness, clinical efficiency, and operational efficiency. There is strong pressure on the organization to remove physicians who cannot meet cost or quality standards and to lure physicians or services that are broadly attractive.[15]

Promotion issues

Primary promotion becomes a matter of making the advantages clear to the employee and spouse, beginning with convenient and attractive primary care. Specific promotion builds on branding, but can identify the sites and practitioners near each family's home. General media, like billboards, radio, and television, can be used; specific media reaching each company are likely to be less expensive. Referral specialists and tertiary services must be promoted both to patients and to primary practitioners. Promoting use of the panel to patients becomes important. There is growing emphasis on promotion to specific segments with material directly related to their medical need.[16] Promotion can be oriented around social class[17] and health attitudes,[18,19] and as noted in the well-baby example, collaboration can reduce or spread the cost of promotion. It is possible to share promotional expenses with suppliers when the service generates a demand for a specific product.[20] "Service recovery" approaches can reduce dissatisfaction with service and enhance efforts to improve quality.[21]

Television, direct mail, billboards, print and radio media are used in promotion. Large numbers of exposures are needed to influence buyers, and the cost per exposure becomes important. Television advertising is the most expensive. In metropolitan areas, many print media are also expensive.[22] Daily newspapers and television reach a population much larger than that served by a single hospital or physician group. Only the larger systems serving several counties can efficiently advertise in these media. Radio and local print media are more geographically targeted. The cost of promotion in metropolitan areas is one advantage of integrated systems; they serve a higher fraction of the market and get more gain from expensive advertising.

Influencing health behavior

As described in Chapter 11, integrated healthcare systems are moving to promote wellness in their communities. Wellness promotion encourages healthy lifestyle and cost-effective prevention behaviors.

General promotional campaigns to all well members of the population include direct mail, media advertising, print and video material in schools and work sites. The content of these messages can include image advertising, and can be linked to promotion of certain insurance plans or primary care panels. General promotion requires very high frequency of contact. Effective strategies must overcome complex motivations to pursue the unhealthy behavior.[23] They repeat the message over and over, and use a variety of vehicles to convey and reinforce it. Wellness promotion becomes an ongoing activity, consuming a specific budget and constantly studied for opportunities to improve cost-effectiveness.

Specialized promotion is often more cost-effective for changing behavior, as Chapter 11 notes. Focused efforts on identified market segments allow more efficient communication, forming partnerships with groups interested in the target population, and tailoring of the message to the special needs of the risk group.

Managing patient expectations

Patient satisfaction is important in retaining market share and also important in malpractice claim management.[24] The most effective way to manage patient satisfaction is to identify weaknesses and meet them through continuous improvement. Special programs exist to analyze shortfalls in depth, pinpointing specific responses.[25] Programs have also been designed to recover from serious dissatisfaction.[26]

At the same time, patient expectations can be unrealistic. Media reports frequently emphasize dramatic, curative medical intervention and may overstate the power and value of high-tech care. It is important to counter these and restore realistic expectations. In reality, self-treatment and family care is effective in many conditions. In the case of self-limiting disease and terminal disease, there is often nothing healthcare professionals can add. Similarly, the use of lower skilled professionals, such as nurse practitioners in place of physicians, or primary physicians in place of specialists, offers certain advantages in both cost and effectiveness.[27] The issue in these approaches is threefold: protection against the real need for more technologically advanced care, attractive provision of the lower cost service, and persuasion and reassurance to make people comfortable with it.

Promotional techniques can help persuade and reassure. As in the case of wellness behavior and risk prevention, efforts can be either general or targeted, and targeted approaches are generally more cost-effective. For example, home and hospice care can be generally promoted with convenient services and attractive prices, but success is likely to hinge on convenience, well-trained staff who reassure family members, prompt response to calls for assistance, and incentives such as respite care. Self-care for common infectious diseases and minor injuries can be promoted and improved through telephone triage. Prompted to question for risks that the patient or a parent might overlook, triage nurses can provide reassurance and recommend simple treatments but also arrange emergency care when indicated. General promotion may overcome some of the lack of confidence in physician extenders. Specific training in reassurance and readily available backup are targeted programs to increase success. Similar promotion may be useful in reducing the customer demand for specialist care.

Targeted promotion can focus directly on the expectations of specific patient groups. For example, advance description of elective surgical procedures can identify many common complications or variations in the recovery pattern and provide instructions or reassurance about them. It can prepare the patient to accept the usual outcomes, and in some cases convince patients that the rewards of the procedure are not worth the pain, risks, and cost.[28] It is known in advertising that customers tend to perceive what they have been conditioned to expect.[29] Clinical problems associated with a high level of dissatisfaction can be identified and studied to devise more satisfactory treatment patterns. These may deliberately emphasize activities that are designed to provide symptomatic relief, such as the deliberate use of chiropractors in certain cases of low back pain.[30]

Specific high-cost problems may be addressed through complex strategies. The cost of care at the end of life, estimated to be more than 25 percent of all Medicare expenses, can be reduced without substantial change in the outcome through the use of fewer heroic measures.[31] Avoiding unnecessary heroics requires prior understanding and acceptance by patient and family, and reassurance to caregivers. A comprehensive strategy would reach patients well before their life end, allow close relatives to understand the issues and participate in the decisions, offer alternatives to heroic intervention, and build consensus and acceptance among caregivers. Every hospital admission and HMO enrollee must by law be given the opportunity to complete an advance directive informing his or her caregivers on managing the end of life.[32] The organization can stress the desirability of completing the directive, without bias toward a particular solution. If patients consider the issue, it seems likely they will improve their understanding and many will have greater comfort with lower cost measures.

The use of sites and agencies other than healthcare may allow more complete and candid discussion of the end-of-life issues, allowing patients and families to become comfortable in advance. Churches, congregate living centers, and senior recreational facilities can hold educational discussions on the question of dying. Promotion that reaches both patients and staff will improve staff understanding and acceptance as well.[33] Hospices provide not only an alternate form of treatment appropriate to specific patients; they also exemplify a philosophy of how to die. Ethics committees can be established both to supervise the strategy itself and to provide consultation to staff in complex cases. Finally, bereavement counseling can assist both families and staff with the painful emotions involved.

Marketing the Organization to Providers

Employees, physicians, donors, and volunteers enter into voluntary exchange relationships with healthcare organizations that have many similarities with customer relations. The organization wants ideally to be attractive in all these relationships; it can deal with an oversupply by being selective.

The effort to market the organization to providers begins by deliberately incorporating their viewpoint in all the various levels of decisions (Chapters 5 and 8). The opinions of current members will be an important predictor for those who may join in the future. Thus, well-managed organizations seek broad participation in decisions like the mission, vision, and strategic positioning. These statements of intent attract like-minded people and discourage those whose values are not supportive of the group's. As the goals are translated to operations, the operations themselves reveal the intent and capability of the organization. Operational realities reinforce or belie commitment to community values, and providers will seek organizations whose real values parallel their own.

The effect of specific promotional activities on providers is carefully considered in well-managed organizations. Several common public relations documents are used as much to recruit and inform members as customers. The mission and vision are usually promoted aggressively among the members. The annual report, periodic newsletters, and press releases used by local media reach providers as well as customers. Because of their interest, they are likely to be particularly sensitive to the messages. Some messages, like "Excalibur Health System is a caring organization," may be as powerful as tools to reach caregivers as they are to convince customers.

Most large healthcare organizations also promote themselves directly to provider groups. Promotional packets for potential house officers and physicians seeking primary care locations are commonplace; considerable care and expense is justified in light of the importance of the decision on both sides. Various promotional devices are used to attract clinical professionals in short supply. Many organizations advertise routinely in nursing, physical therapy, and pharmacy journals to attract new professionals.

Strategic affiliations to recruit personnel are also common. Affiliation with teaching programs increases the familiarity of graduating students. Programs to assist students with summer and part-time work affect not only the students directly involved, but their classmates who learn by word of mouth. Some institutions reach several years below graduation. Working with inner-city high schools to encourage young people to enter healing professions is popular. Like many promotional activities, it reaches two audiences: the students and the community at large.

Managing External Relationships

Scale is clearly important in marketing and management of successful healthcare organizations. Fixed cost is spread, diversification is increased, risk is shared, and customer needs are met better in large than small organizations. Offsetting these advantages are the difficulties of loss of flexibility, conflicting values among participants, and increased capital requirements. One aspect of marketing is the deliberate management of relationships with other organizations sharing some part of the goals of Figure I.1 on page 28. These relationships range from competition through several levels of contractual permanence to essentially irreversible mergers or acquisitions.

In reality, few healthcare organizations even come close to offering the full array of patient services suggested by Figure I.1 under one corporate umbrella. Health insurance and intermediary functions are often arranged by others. Prevention, nursing home care, mental health and substance abuse programs, hospices, and home care are often provided by other organizations. The physician organization may be a separate corporation or several corporations. Drugs and medical equipment are often supplied to ambulatory patients through independent organizations. The goal of well-managed organizations must be to provide the full array of services, meeting all customer needs with barrier-free relationships that make the mechanics of transfer virtually invisible to patients.

The goal requires minimizing **transaction costs**, that is, the costs of maintaining the relationship, including the costs of moving patients geographically or between corporations.[34] Ownership of the service may not be the optimal solution; the alternative is collaboration between organizations, some of which will inevitably be competitors. It now appears likely that most organizations will collaborate on several major services, of which insurance and physician organization may be the most important. The management of relationships between the components has become one of the major functions of the modern healthcare organization. Paradoxically, the issues involved in reducing transaction costs tend to be operational questions reflecting needs of participants more than the formal relationship between the units, as the following example shows.

Analyzing the healthcare marketplace

The first step to a strategy of organizational positioning is a review of all services customers need and where they get them. A simplified version of this review is given in the following example.

Modern Health Services (MHS) is an integrated health system serving a large metropolitan area (called Metropolis to protect the actual identity) and other areas. MHS has adopted a special mission to serve the poor and does more than its share of charity and under-financed care. As shown in Figure 13.8, MHS owns an unusually broad range of services in Metropolis—acute

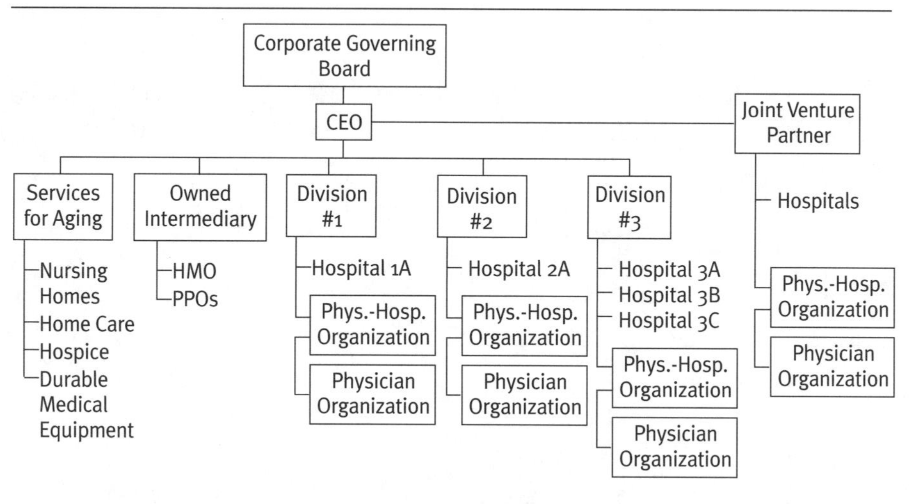

FIGURE 13.8 Organization of an Integrated Health System

Note: Each unit reporting to the CEO has its own advisory board, composed of members of its community, representatives of other units, and local community members.

inpatient facilities, mental health and substance abuse services, nursing homes, home care, hospices, and medical equipment services for the aging. It owns an HMO and PPOs, and collaborates with several local physicians' organizations. The corporation is doing well, but not dramatically so. It has a stable to slowly growing market share, positive net income, and a reasonable balance sheet. So do several other large healthcare organizations in Metropolis, representing an array from comparable integration to single purpose competitors. The fact that there are no clear competitive winners suggests that simple models like total integration or arms-length collaboration have market and organizational limitations.

Here are a few of the strategic problems facing MHS:

Geography

- The Metropolis market, shown in Figure 13.9, is about four million people, stretched over a seven-county land area that takes about 90 minutes to cross either north-south or east-west. Travel times between points are longer if freeways are not convenient.
- Central City, the geographic and historic center of Metropolis, is now only one of many residential, work, or shopping destinations. Each family has a constellation of destinations that it views as convenient, but there is a strong market preference for care near the family home.
- In contrast to their employees, many large employers operate in several geographic locations and view the market as a single entity.

Health Insurance Markets

- Blue Cross and Blue Shield (BCBS) dominates traditional insurance, which in total covers about 50 percent of the market.

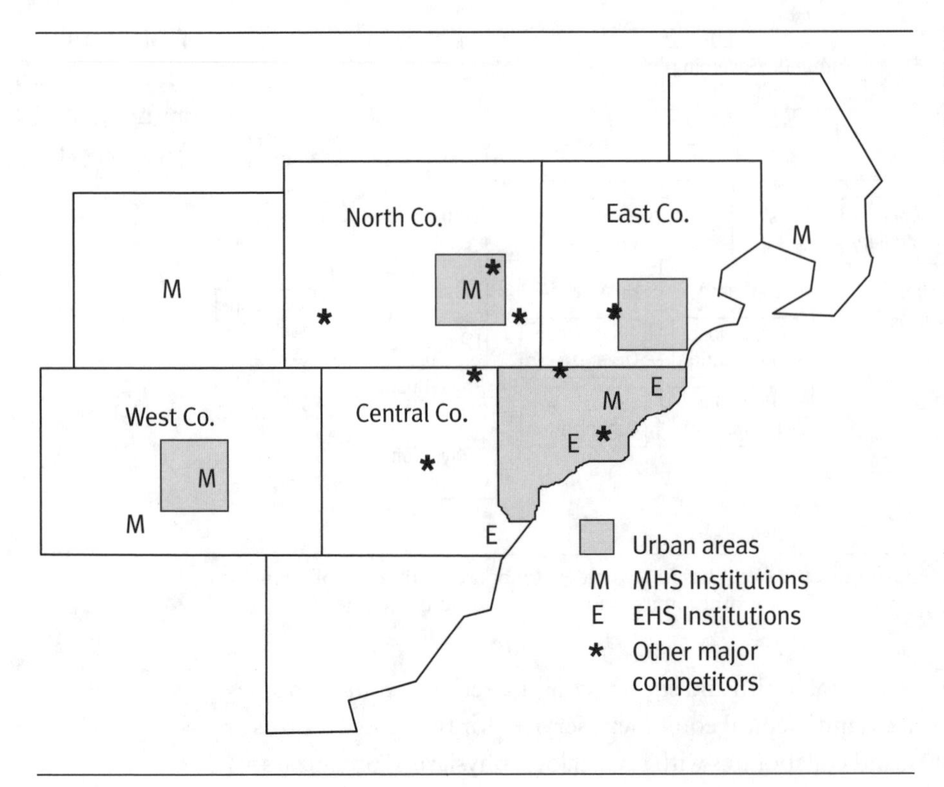

FIGURE 13.9 Metropolis Health Care Market

- Edison Health System (EHS) and BCBS dominate the HMO market, which is about 25 percent of the total population. The MHS HMO has only 15 percent of the HMO market, somewhat less than 200,000 lives.
- PPOs are relatively insignificant at around 10 percent of the total.
- Medicare subscribers are broadly distributed geographically and are almost exclusively served by traditional coverage. They constitute 10 percent of the insured, but a much larger percent of the expenditures.
- Medicaid and uninsured populations are about 10 percent of the total market but are concentrated in a few specific locations. The largest is Central City. Medicaid has moved to HMO structures; MHS is a significant participant.

Healthcare Markets

- There are six healthcare organizations, of which EHS is the largest. MHS is one of the smaller systems. The remaining competition is scattered and for the most part ineffectual.
- Smaller, focused organizations can move quickly to develop specific market strategies and high-quality operations in mental health, substance abuse, long-term care, home care, and hospices. These "independents" form the primary competition for MHS in these markets.

- Physician organizations are relatively untested. Although all the systems employ at least a few physicians, and EHS employs about half of its physicians, most care is given by small groups. MHS is a leader in developing structures among independent physicians, but its own organizations differ in commitment, maturity, and effectiveness.

Although the example is from the perspective of one healthcare organization, the analysis would be similar for its major competitors. The pressures of conflicting marketplaces that MHS faces in Metropolis are unique only in the details. Most metropolitan areas hold the same combinations of diverse geographies, overlapping markets, and varying competitors. The underlying array of complementary, competing, and collaborating organizations will be present in all and will change over time. Employers in Metropolis are convinced that costs must be controlled, and will migrate toward managed care solutions of various kinds. Other cities differ in the extent of managed care today and the commitment to the future.

MHS must "formulate programs designed to bring about exchanges of values" within Metropolis. It has discovered that unified responses to this environment simply will not work. What builds market share for a hospice in the northern suburbs has nothing to do with expanding the HMO. There are four consequence to the discovery. First, there is a strong need to decentralize and delegate so that MHS subsidiaries are effective in various geographic and service markets. The result is that each subsidiary develops its own strategies, oriented around its market and explicitly different from others. Second, tensions develop between the subsidiaries that must be solved by essentially the devices used to relate freestanding corporations. That is, a significant portion of the corporate effort must go to transaction costs, settling internal boundary disputes and in some cases making sure the subsidiaries do not become independent. The core is weakened as a result of the delegation and transaction costs. It tends to look more like an alliance and less like an integrated organization. Third, tensions also develop between MHS, its subsidiaries, and other organizations. Even an organization as large as MHS cannot ignore the possibilities of collaboration with other organizations. Effective abilities to deal with other large organizations tend to strengthen the core. But to be effective, MHS must be able to speak for all its subsidiaries. Fourth, money for capital investment is limited, and demands for capital are not. MHS must optimize the return on each investment it makes.

Developing a strategy of internal relationships

Internal opportunities

MHS has pursued a decentralized vision, with local boards for each of its major geographic areas, and separate boards for its aging services and its HMO/PPO. Each of these subsidiaries is charged with building market share, but it is also expected to work closely with other MHS corporations and to earn a small surplus. Some predictable tension lines emerge:

- The HMO, fighting aggressively for market share from regional employers, wants effective cost and quality control from the providers. The providers, operating in local markets, are more responsive to local demands for service and employment.
- Physicians, even more locally focused than MHS provider organizations, resist integration of medical and hospital care. As primary care grows in importance, tensions between primary and referral physicians mount.
- The acute care hospitals are forced to support managed care concepts even though managed care is only 25 percent of the market. Major reductions in inpatient services occur as a result.
- The hospitals are forced to mediate primary and referral physician conflicts. They start at this task with stronger ties to the specialists than to primary care.
- Perspectives of major competitors are far from uniform. For example, EHS is a friend to some MHS subsidiaries and a threat to others. Other systems are dominant in some markets but irrelevant in others. BCBS is a major source of revenue to all acute care subsidiaries and physicians, but clearly a competitor to the HMO.
- Relationships between acute care and aging services are remote. The locations and market shares of the aging services are such that it is frequently difficult to encourage transfers within MHS.

The strength of these tensions is such that members of MHS subsidiaries not infrequently wonder whether they belong to the central organization or would be better on their own. The central organization spends much, possibly most, of its time trying to align interests of various subsidiaries to meet market opportunities. The advantage of MHS over separate organizations is constantly in doubt.

To understand the marketing opportunities and devise a successful strategy for MHS, it is necessary to search aggressively for shared advantages. One way to identify these is to ask what would happen if all the subsidiaries of Figure 13.8 were granted immediate independence. The results would be something like this:

- The fundraising capability of the central organization would be lost. The subsidiaries as independents would have difficulty raising equivalent amounts of capital.
- The shared HMO would be an independent organization. It remains a distant third in a competitive marketplace, without the capital reserves or market contacts of the two leaders. It could have more difficulty implementing a successful strategy than it does now.
- Each healthcare subsidiary would face the task of negotiating new relationships with insurers and intermediaries. An advantage of collective negotiation would be lost, and most subsidiaries would move to replace it with new collective relationships.

- The physician organization problems would remain. Because no subsidiary is large enough to operate a successful HMO, they would probably move to form new allegiances protecting their physician relations. Capital shortages would make it difficult to implement long-range plans. Some might be forced to seek new affiliations to meet capital needs.
- The aging services units would see little change from independence. They would lose referral sources and would move to replace these on a geographically convenient basis.
- The opportunity to serve the poor would be substantially diminished. Much of the service to the poor is geographically specific and relies on subsidies from the earning of other areas.

The results of MHS dissolution in most cases would find the former subsidiaries making new allegiances. It is predictable that these allegiances would present problems very like those of the current MHS structure. The advantages that keep MHS in existence are:

- ability to address regional markets;
- ability to raise capital;
- ability to find and capitalize upon synergies between its operating components, such as sharing information technology and benchmarking;
- ability to sustain experimental and developmental programs that provide examples and incentives for continuous improvement; and
- ability to serve the poor.

An internal strategy

An MHS strategy must capitalize upon these advantages and avoid exacerbating the existing tensions. Such a strategy might be based on the following tenets:

- Emphasize financial stability and protection of the capital base. The central office would prescribe acceptable limits for long-range financial plans and annual budget guidelines. It would authorize and obtain capital funds.
- Encourage independent actions by subsidiaries within a framework of centralized capital generation and a market trend toward centralized healthcare finance dominated by managed care.
- Establish capital fund priorities for programs that enhance managed care capability, such as the expansion of managed care insurance, the development of information systems, or the organization of physician services.
- Support care of the disadvantaged, with explicit assignment of funds earned by the subsidiaries.
- Provide central planning and marketing databases and technical support specialists to assist subsidiaries in developing locally effective strategies.
- Use regional media to promote an MHS image with public relations, advertising, and coordinated support for local efforts.

- Assign accountability to the central office for relations with the other large organizations and regionally oriented employers and for developing regional markets.

The most critical element of the strategy is the maintenance of healthy subsidiaries. This demands certain reserved powers enforcing capital and other performance and effective measurement systems for the central unit. It also demands decentralization, allowing the subsidiaries to act as though they were independent entities in their specific markets wherever possible. Because most of the direct competitors are local, any strategy that ties the hands of local subsidiaries will fail.

Developing an external strategy

If the first part of the MHS strategy is to decentralize within explicit limits and encourage independent response to local markets, the second must be to deal centrally with the common forces of the regional market. As noted in Chapter 4, other organizations can be classified as those that compete for market share (competitors), those with whom formal agreements have been reached (allies), and those that offer noncompeting services (complementary organizations). As the complexity of MHS relationships and the Metropolis market suggest, large regional organizations tend to be all three.

Figure 13.10 shows the major current ties between Metropolis Health Care and health insurance organizations, as of 1994. Figure 13.10 is considerably simpler than reality. It illustrates the kinds of relationships that can exist and shows some important examples. Collaborative relationships between insurance intermediaries and providers and competitive relations between similar organizations are inevitable. The reality of Figure 13.10 is that most competing organizations also collaborate.

There are several levels of relationships between the organizations in Figure 13.10. Strictly speaking, all are forms of collaboration.

- *Competition* emphasizes independence, but the organizations are forced by tradition and by law to compete within a framework of rules. Products and services must be comparable, for example. Price is an important basis for comparison; quality is becoming one. Many sales are made in response to customer requests for proposals; in these, the customer outlines major parameters of the service rather than the vendor. Laws forbid collusion over price and markets and require truth in advertising.
- *Contracts* are defined agreements between parties who may be competitors in other areas to accomplish specific considerations important to each of the parties. BCBS's participating hospital agreement is an example. It sets the terms under which all the systems will provide inpatient and outpatient care to members and the price that will be paid.
- *Alliances* involve an agreement to collaborate on undefined activities such as problem solving. They permit wider ranging considerations than can be specified in contracts, but like contracts, they are still subject to laws

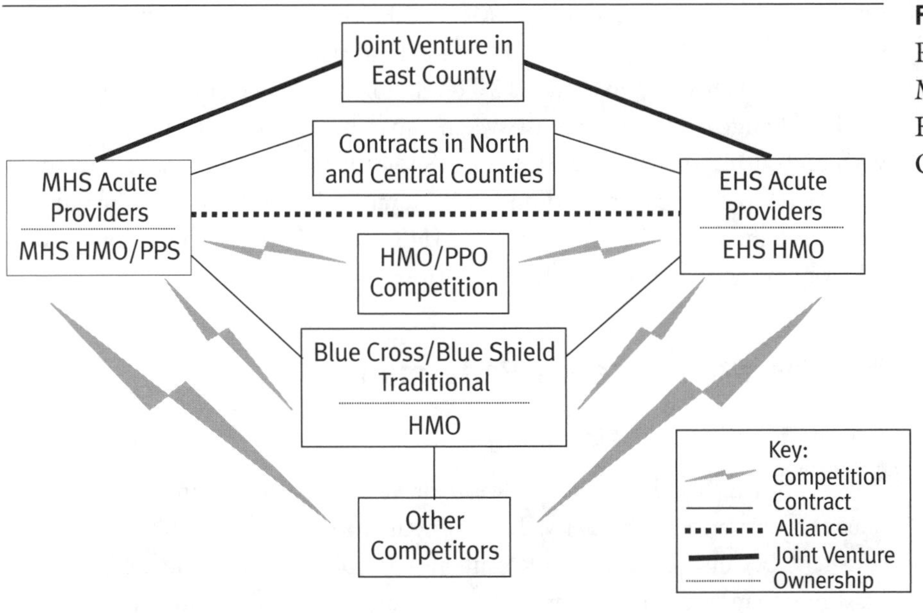

FIGURE 13.10 Relationships of Major Healthcare Organizations

governing competition and can be terminated by the parties. They are often supplemented by letters of agreement and contracts on specific activities.

- *Joint ventures* are longer-term contracts committing assets to specific goals and specific governance structures. Thus EHS and MHS have agreed to run provider facilities in the eastern suburbs through shared governance and executive activities. Termination of the agreement would be difficult, but neither party is committed to loss of autonomy outside the specific venture.
- *Joint operating agreements* are contracts of long-term affiliation just short of merger. Like mergers, they establish a new entity, but they reserve certain rights, such as the ability to dissolve the agreement or the ability to appoint certain officers, to the original participants.
- *Mergers and acquisitions* are irreversible combinations of assets and operations. Normally in a merger neither of the original parties survives; in an acquisition only one party survives.

It is easy to explain how a situation such as Figure 13.10 develops. In each collaboration, the participants seek first to meet market need, and thereby improve their own performance, and second to minimize transaction costs. Thus, relationships between competitors, such as the joint ventures that link EHS and MHS, make perfect sense. Each relationship was the lowest transaction cost opportunity the participants could find to meet specific market goals. MHS was seeking ways to reduce costs and support specialty services in the northern suburb where EHS needed facilities to match its growing HMO sales. A contract would serve the purpose; a joint venture would open opportunities to go beyond. The MHS/EHS joint venture allowed them to serve eastern markets neither had been able to penetrate on their own.

It is likely that the Figure 13.10 relationships will change steadily as the market changes. The other four systems may be forced to seek stronger ties with each other or with the MHS/EHS joint venture. All the alliances short of ownership can be dissolved; in fact, several explorations have occurred and failed. Alliances like the one between MHS and EHS may grow to ownership relations or be replaced by other affiliations.

Measures of Marketing Performance

Global Measures of Marketing

The central measures of contribution or value of a marketing program are market share and profitability. It is difficult to construct a single global assessment because both are the result not simply of marketing but the successful management of all parts of the organization. Although the measures available are incomplete, a marketing program can be assessed by most of the six dimensions used in other programs. Demand measures are difficult even to conceptualize, and output and productivity measures are incomplete. Some activities, like advertising, can be tracked with productivity measures such as cost per contact. As with planning, quality of marketing programs must be subjectively assessed in both outcomes and process contexts. Some customer satisfaction can be measured directly, but the customer for most marketing is the organization itself. Global performance like market share is important, but many elements of execution affect it as much as marketing. Costs can be captured in conventional accounting systems, with emphasis on labor, surveys and special data acquisition, and advertising costs. Costs of alliances are much more diffuse and are not likely to appear principally in marketing accounts. Although the marketing staff is small, satisfaction remains an important performance measure.

Figure 13.11 shows a set of measures for the marketing program of a large healthcare organization. Expectations are set about these measures in the annual budget exercise, and performance is assessed against expectations. Overall, considerable subjectivity is involved. Organizations can benchmark their marketing costs against similar ones, and even against other industries, but these remain imperfect guides. Many specific marketing programs, or campaigns, can be more rigorously analyzed. Their costs can be estimated, expectations established about outcomes, and actual results compared to expectations.

Campaign-Oriented Measures of Marketing

Campaigns identify specific goals such as market share or behavior change in population segments. Expectations can be set about response rates (demand),

FIGURE 13.11 Possible Measures for a Marketing Program

Dimension	Measure
Output	Advertising expenditure, reach, frequency Cost per media exposure Number of presentations, speeches Number of media references Negotiations conducted
Quality	Outcomes of negotiations Independent evaluation of content and design
Cost/Productivity	Personnel Data acquisition Advertising Outside contractors Cost per exposure, campaign, or new patient
Human Resources	Departmental employee satisfaction
Customer Satisfaction	Survey and focus group responses to media releases Satisfaction of internal customers Overall patient satisfaction Changes in demand or market share

costs, costs per response, process quality, customer satisfaction, and changes in target market share. Many of these are reasonably free of interactions with the rest of the institution, so that marketing can be directly accountable for the results. For example, an organization might identify 35 percent of a large market as generally preferring its services, and might identify several segment strategies to expand this share, such as a Medicare HMO, centers of excellence in certain referral specialties, and an expanded availability of primary care physicians. Each of these has specific measures that can be evaluated as part of a campaign. Expectations for improvement in these measures can be established and performance evaluated as shown in Figure 13.12. Much of the annual budget for marketing is directed at campaigns, and turnarounds are short enough that progress can be evaluated annually.

Advertising and public relations campaigns can be measured by **reach**, an estimate of the number of people who will see or hear a specific advertisement, and **frequency**, the average number of times each person is reached. Productivity measures are useful in these situations; it is common to calculate cost per exposure, where exposure equals reach times frequency. These are useful in guiding decisions about specific campaigns, but it is important to remember that the relationship between exposures and behavior change, such as market share, is unclear.

Surveys and direct consumer evaluations are important in assessing marketing activity, and provide both procedural and outcomes quality indicators. Major promotional campaigns should have pre- and post-campaign evaluations built in. Advertising material can be pretested on focus groups to assess its effectiveness in changing customer attitudes and expectations,

FIGURE 13.12
Measures for Specific Campaigns

Campaign	Actions	Measures
Medicare HMO	Advertising in local papers, TV, radio shows Billboards on major traffic arteries Appearances in senior centers, churches, union halls Direct mail to lists of former HMO members discontinued on retirement Direct sales to seniors indicating interest Prizes for subscribers bringing new members	Number of exposures; exposures/target audience member; cost/exposure by medium Number of public relations appearances, audience size Number of responses by phone, letter Survey of awareness and attractiveness[1] Number of subscribers, percentage of total market, cost per subscriber Surveys of subscriber satisfaction and estimate of continued subscription
Centers of excellence in orthopedics, cardiology	Preparation of data on cost per case and quality of results Publication of original research in peer-reviewed journals, distribution of reprints, feature stories in local media Direct sales to managers of local HMOs, PPOs Competitive bid for Medicare, Medicaid contracts Presentations to primary care physicians	Increase in listings or contracts for referrals from HMOs, PPOs, government programs Increased referrals of traditional insurance patients Change in total demand, cost per case Cost of campaign per new case Cost of campaign/change in profit per case
Increased primary care access	Direct mailing to physicians in primary care fellowships Coordination with presently affiliated physicians Senior executive meetings with local physicians affiliated with competitors Program of practice acquisition, expansion Introduction of nurse practitioners, with media advertising and public relations Program of office support to increase physician productivity	Number of new responses Number of new physicians recruited Number of nurse practitioners placed, demand for nurse practitioner services Patient visits/physician Delay for emergency, routine, and preventive office visits Patient satisfaction Program cost per new physician, per new visit

[1] Kotler and Clarke, *Marketing for Health Care Organizations*, 440–01.

for example. Surveys can assess name familiarity, attitudes, and several stages of acceptability up to actual changes in behavior. Focus group approaches use smaller samples but allow in-depth discussions with individuals. They will sacrifice precision in estimating specific attitudes, but expand details of the dynamics of the exchange. For example, surveys can identify how many items in wellness programs actually changed health risk behavior, while focus groups and individual interviews might reveal specific elements the customer liked or did not like. Surveys and focus groups can be conducted by an independent agency without identifying the sponsoring organization if desired.

Surveys and focus groups can be quite costly. The cost of obtaining the information must be weighed against the cost of not having it, which is also high. Misjudging patient needs or potential demand can endanger the institution; the cost of a survey to learn these needs is never that high. Maintaining objectivity is important; professional sampling techniques, questionnaire design, and administration are costly, but not as costly as an error in assessing a program. It is possible to reduce costs by combining surveys that require similar samples. Thus, a general marketing program adds expertise in assessing customer needs and exchange opportunities. It also offers opportunities to reduce costs by tying similar assessments together.[35]

Organizing the Marketing Activity

The contribution of a specialized marketing unit is technical and professional expertise; the steps involved in marketing are increasingly elaborate. Masters' degrees in business or health administration are useful beginnings, but neither program emphasizes the details of advertising or public relations. Experience with a commercial agency or a large healthcare-oriented team is highly desirable for the senior marketing people.

Consultants are available for most marketing functions. Advertising particularly is purchased from agencies with experience in design, campaign development, and media contracts. Market studies and customer surveys are often contracted to consultants. They benefit from advanced technical knowledge, and a consultant with a detailed knowledge of a geographic area can achieve better results at lower costs. The database that results from continuing study of a market is a valuable proprietary resource. Even if much of the data collection is delegated to planning or marketing consultants, the organization should make an effort to retain the data in their entirety.

Strategic marketing is rarely contracted to consultants. Negotiation is often retained as an activity of the CEO or senior staff. Consultants can be used as intermediaries or mediators, but trustees may be as effective in these roles.

Given the small size of most marketing activities, it seems likely that internal organization is a team, perhaps with designated leadership based on seniority or professional experience. Internal organization by market segment is useful, particularly when there is little overlap in specific actions. For example, the group marketing to insurance intermediaries and employers is likely to be different from that concentrating on marketing to patients. It could be established as a separate responsibility center in very large organizations.

The important organizational questions are the scope of the marketing activity and its relation to other units. There is apparently some tendency to separate public relations from the marketing activity, and a stronger one to separate marketing from planning.[36] There are inescapable ties between these activities. Marketing and planning share a database that is a major resource for the organization. The evaluation of many strategic and some programmatic opportunities requires both a marketing and a planning perspective. Marketing for a specific project and for image building should be integrated. Thus, even in larger organizations with three separate functions and accountabilities, coordination under one executive appears desirable. The three functions affect the future of the organization as a whole, and should be close to the strategic core. Reporting to the chief executive officer is most common, and most appropriate.

Figure 13.13 suggests the formal marketing accountability hierarchy for a large organization. Duties in most smaller organizations are probably a team responsibility, and most of the specific responsibility centers disappear. Members of either structure might have matrix ties to specific subsidiaries. In the very largest organizations, marketing may be decentralized to subsidiaries. Alternatively, a central marketing unit can consider itself an in-house consultant service to all parts of the organization that seek its help. It is possible to establish transfer payments for consultant services, permitting better cost allocation between subsidiaries and promoting a professional relationship between the units.

FIGURE 13.13 Formal Hierarchy for a Large Marketing Operation

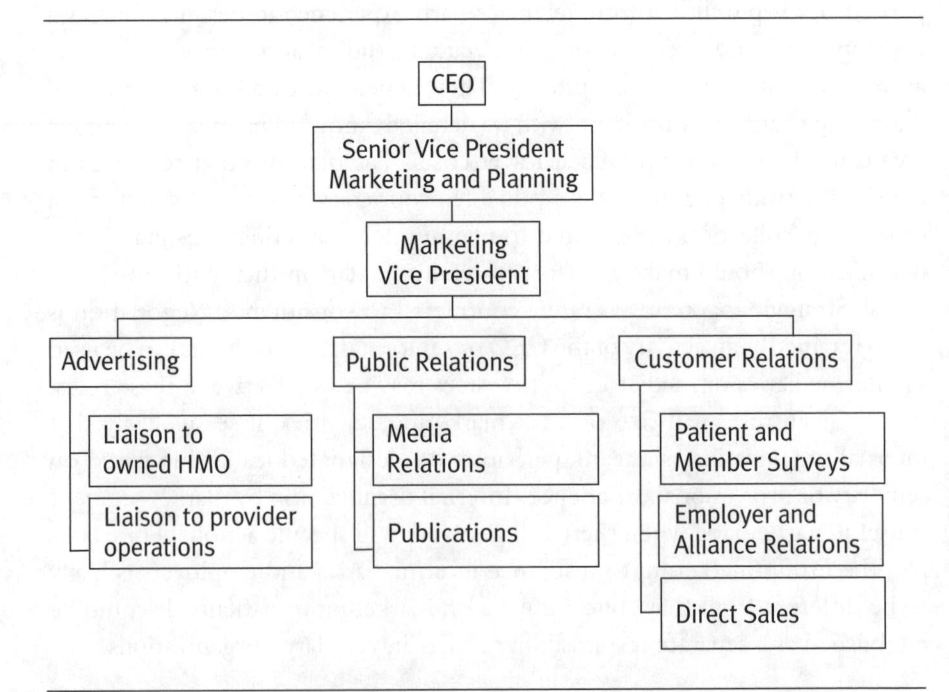

Suggested Readings

Angrisani, D. P., and R. L. Goldman. 1997. *Predicting Successful Hospital Mergers and Acquisitions: A Financial and Marketing Analytical Tool.* New York: Haworth Press.

Curtis, R., T. Kurtz, and L. S. Stepnick (eds.). 1998. *Creating Consumer Choice in Healthcare: Measuring and Communicating Health Plan Performance Information.* Chicago: Health Administration Press.

The Center for the Evaluative Clinical Sciences, Dartmouth Medical School. 1998. *Dartmouth Atlas of Health Care in the United States.* Chicago: American Hospital Publishing, Inc.

Kotler, P., and G. Armstrong. 1999. *Principles of Marketing.* Englewood Cliffs, NJ: Prentice-Hall.

Kotler, P., and R. N. Clarke. 1987. *Marketing for Health Care Organizations.* Englewood Cliffs, NJ: Prentice-Hall.

Lewton, K. L. 1995. *Public Relations in Health Care*, 2d ed. Chicago: American Hospital Association.

Simon, R. 1994. *Levers of Control: How Managers Use Innovative Control Systems to Drive Strategic Renewal.* Cambridge, MA: Harvard Business School Press.

Sturm, Jr., A. C. 1998. *The New Rules of Healthcare Marketing: 23 Strategies for Success.* Chicago: Health Administration Press.

Zajac, E. J., and T. A. D'Aunno. 1997. "Managing Strategic Alliances." In *Essentials of Health Care Management,* edited by S. M. Shortell and A. D. Kaluzny, 328–54. NY: Delmar Publishers.

Zuckerman, A. M. 1998. *Healthcare Strategic Planning: Approaches for the 21st Century.* Chicago: Health Administration Press.

Notes

1. P. Kotler and R. N. Clarke, *Marketing for Health Care Organizations.* Englewood Cliffs, NJ: Prentice-Hall, 5 (1987)
2. G. M. Naidu, A. Kleimenhagen, and G. D. Pilari, "Organization of Marketing in U.S. Hospitals: An Empirical Investigation." *Health Care Management Review* 17(4): 29–32 (1992)
3. J. A. Boscarino and S. R. Stieber, "The Future of Marketing Health Care Services." In P.D. Cooper, *Health Care Marketing: A Foundation for Managed Quality.* Gaithersburg, MD: Aspen Publishers, 71–83 (1994(
4. R. E. MacStravic, "Market Administration in Health Care Delivery." *Health Care Management Review* 14(1): 41–8 (1989)
5. Kotler and Clarke, *Marketing for Health Care Organizations,* 61–7
6. K. L. Lewton *Public Relations in Health Care.* Chicago: American Hospital Association, 133–62 (1991)
7. Kotler and Clarke, *Marketing for Health Care Organizations,* 66–7
8. R. Frasca and M. Schneider, "Press Relations: A 14-Point Plan for Enhancing the Public Image of Health Care Institutions." *Health Care Management Review* 13(4): 49–57 (1988)
9. American Medical Association, 3 Trade Reg. Rep. CCH

10. Kotler and Clarke, *Marketing for Health Care Organizations*, 25–27
11. T. Bodenheimer, and K. Sullivan, "How Large Employers Are Shaping the Health Care Marketplace." *New England Journal of Medicine* 338(14): 1003–7, (Apr 2, 1998); 338(15): 1084–7 (Apr 9, 1998)
12. C. Ngeo, "The First Gatekeeper: Healthcare Ads Target Women as Key Decision Makers." *Modern Healthcare* 28(27): 34 (Jul 6, 1998)
13. J. R. Galagher, "Listening to the Consumer: Implications of a Statewide Study of North Carolinians." *Journal of Health Care Marketing* 9(4): 56–60 (1989)
14. P. M. Lane and J. D. Lindquist, "Hospital Choice: A Summary of the Key Empirical and Hypothetical Findings of the 1980s." *Journal of Health Care Marketing* 8(4): 5–20 (1988)
15. J. A. Chilingerian, "New Directions for Hospital Strategic Management: The Market for Efficient Care." *Health Care Management Review* 17(4): 73–80 (1988)
16. R. E. MacStravic, "Market Administration in Health Care Delivery." *Health Care Management Review* 14(1): 41–8 (1989)
17. S. Dawson, "Health Care Consumption and Consumer Social Class: A Different Look at the Patient." *Journal of Health Care Marketing* 9(3): 15–25 (1989)
18. J. John and G. Miaoulis, "A Model for Understanding Benefit Segmentation in Preventive Health Care." *Health Care Management Review* 17(2): 21–32 (1992)
19. A. G. Woodside, R. L. Nielsen, F. Walters, and G. D. Muller, "Preference Segmentation of Health Care Services: The Old-Fashioneds, Value Conscious, Affluents, and Professional Want-It-Alls." *Journal of Health Care Marketing* 8(2): 14–24 (1988)
20. S. MacStravic, "Reverse and Double Reverse Marketing for Health Care Organizations." *Health Care Management Review* 18(3): 53–8 (1993)
21. S. B. Schweikhart, S. Strasser, and M. R. Kennedy, "Service Recovery in Health Services Organizations." *Hospital & Health Services Administration* 38(1): 3–22 (1993)
22. Kotler and Clarke, *Marketing for Health Care Organizations*, 428–63
23. R. P. Hill, "The Growing Threat of AIDS: How Marketers Must Respond." *Journal of Health Care Marketing* 9(2): 9–12 (1989)
24. S. MacStravic, "Use Marketing to Reduce Malpractice Costs in Health Care." *Health Care Management Review* 14(4): 51–6 (1989)
25. L. R. Burns and L. R. Beach, "The Quality Improvement Strategy." *Health Care Management Review* 19(2): 21–31 (1994)
26. S. B. Schwiekhart, "Service Recovery in Health Services Organizations: Hospitals and Health Services Administration 38(1): 3–21 (Spring, 1993)
27. S. Barger and P. Rosenfeld, "Models in Community Health Care: Findings from a National Study of Community Nursing Centers." *Nursing and Health Care* 14(8): 426–31 (October, 1993)
28. F. J. Fowler, Jr., J. E. Wennberg, R. P. Timothy, M. J. Barry, A. G. Mulley, Jr., and D. Hanley, "Symptom Status and Quality of Life Following Prostatectomy." *JAMA* 259(20): 3018–22 (May 27, 1998)
29. R. E. MacStravic, "Market Administration in Health Care Delivery." *Health Care Management Review* 14(1): 51–6 (1989)

30. P. Curtis and G. Bove, "Family Physicians, Chiropractors, and Back Pain." *Journal of Family Practice* 35(5): 551–55 (November, 1992)
31. J. D. Lubitz and G. F. Riley, "Trends in Medicare Payments in the Last Year of Life." *New England Journal of Medicine* 328(15):1092–6 (April 15, 1993)
32. "Practicing the PSDA [Patient Self-Determination Act]," Special Supplement, *Hastings Center Report*, 21(5): S1–S16 (September-October, 1991)
33. R. E. MacStravic, "Market Administration in Health Care Delivery." *Health Care Management Review* 14(1): 51–6 (1989)
34. S. S. Mick, *Innovations in Health Care Delivery: Insights of Organization Theory.* San Francisco, CA: Jossey Bass Publishers, 207–40 (1990)
35. Kotler and Clarke, *Marketing for Health Care Organizations*, 428–63
36. G. M. Naidu, A. Kleimenhagen, and G. D. Pilari, "Organization of Marketing in U.S. Hospitals: An Empirical Investigation." *Health Care Management Review* 17(4): 29–32 (1992)

CHAPTER

14

THE FINANCE SYSTEM

The finance system of the modern healthcare organization controls all the assets, collects all the revenue, arranges all the funding, settles all the financial obligations, and makes a major contribution to information collection and cost control. It includes accounting as well as finance and is headed by a professional with training and experience in both fields who is usually the second or third most powerful person in the organization. The extensive role of finance of healthcare organizations is no different in purpose or function from other industries, although some of the approaches are modified to accommodate not-for-profit structures and health insurance contracts.

This chapter describes the contribution finance makes to other systems, those tasks that it must do to make the whole succeed. Finance and accounting are subject to much study, regulation, and standardization. Comprehensive texts describe the overall operation of the system. Laws, regulations, contracts, and standard practice control what is done in countless specific situations. Much of this is effectively monitored by the processes themselves and by a unique characteristic of the financial system, the annual outside audit. The audit itself, almost always conducted by one of a few national firms, is a major force toward standardization. The chapter will assume that these standards have been met, and emphasize the activities that distinguish the most successful healthcare organizations, principally strategic financial planning, provision of capital, and cost monitoring and reporting. The chapter outline follows the usual pattern of purpose and function, performance measures, personnel, and organization.

Purpose

The purposes of the finance system are to support the enterprise by:

1. recording and reporting transactions that change the value of the firm;
2. guarding assets and resources against theft, waste, or loss;
3. assisting operations in setting and achieving cost and revenue improvements;
4. assisting governance in short-term and long-term planning; and
5. arranging capital funding to implement governance decisions.

These five purposes are accomplished through two general functions: controllership, incorporating the first three, and financial management, incorporating the last two. The activities supporting these functions are shown in Figure 14.1. Although the list is lengthy and complex, most of the activities can be easily associated with one or two of the five purposes.

Controllership Functions

Financial Accounting

Accounting fulfills a direct obligation to the owners and the public, to record and report all transactions affecting the value of the firm. It establishes the number and value of all financial exchanges. The activity itself is organized by purpose into financial accounting and managerial accounting. Most of the data recording occurs in financial accounting. Completing these two functions keeps finance personnel involved in most areas of the organization.

The purpose of financial accounting is to state as accurately as possible the position of the firm in terms of the value of its assets, the equity residual to its owners, and the change in value occurring in each accounting period. Financial accounting generates the familiar balance sheet, operating statement, and cash flow statement that are basic management information for all corporations and are required public documents for most. It records each financial transaction of the organization and its subsidiaries.

Revenue accounting

Revenue accounting records all the healthcare organization's cash acquisition. In the United States, patient care revenue is almost universally organized by individual **patient ledger**, a detailed record of the individual services or supplies rendered to each patient. Only some government healthcare organizations do not maintain patient ledgers. Individual charges are associated with each entry to calculate revenue, but the charges have become meaningless under aggregate payment contracts.

The custom of individual ledger entry began in an era when patients and insurers paid fee-for-service charges established by the provider for each item. Many insurers, led by the federal Medicare program, moved to cost-based revenue structures for hospitals in the 1960s and 1970s, but an individual ledger was still required. That system failed to control costs and was abandoned beginning in 1983 in favor of prospective payment systems that unilaterally established prices for inpatient care. Payments for hospitals were based on larger aggregates representing episodes of care—the disease-specific discharge, or DRG for inpatients, and global payments for some outpatient care. HMOs moved to per diem payments (a lump sum per day of care, including all services), DRGs, or capitation, a monthly payment for each patient at risk entirely separate from the number or identity of individual patients receiving care.[1]

The movement away from fee-for-service payment divorced actual revenue from individual items of care. The ledger remained the method of

FIGURE 14.1 Functions of the Financial System

Function	Activity	Purpose
Controllership		
Financial Accounting	Maintain basic financial data and reports	Establish value of organization
Managerial Accounting	Prepare cost data used in continuous improvement, capital proposals, and pricing	Support management decisions and continuous improvement
Budgeting	Promulgate budget guidelines and budget packages	Assist line management to meet market needs
	Forecast major demand measures	Support governing board decisions
	Compile operating, financial, and capital budgets	
Reporting and Control	Disclosure of financial information	Report to owners and external stakeholders
	Routine reports on operations	Support line management in monitoring
	Special studies for planning and evaluation	Support continuous improvement
Protection of Assets	Inurement Audits Compliance review	Guard against loss and diversion of property
		Comply with contractual requirements
Financial Management		
Financial Planning	Long-range financial plan	Support the governing board in strategic positioning
		Test mission and vision against market reality
		Establish budget guidelines
Pricing Clinical Services	Develop pricing strategy and support specific price negotiations	Support maximum revenue to the institution and its physicians
Financial Structures	Multiple corporate structures	Increase investment
		Contain risk
Securing Long-Term Funds	Management of debt	Minimize cost of capital
	Management of joint ventures, stock and equity accounts	Maximize return on assets
Managing Short-Term Assets and Liabilities	Working capital management	Minimize cost of working capital

charging patients and insurers who paid amounts related to the posted charge. In the mid-1990s, about one-quarter of all inpatient care and most outpatient care was still paid on a fee-related basis. The ledger was also built into many aggregate payment schemes to identify catastrophically expensive cases called "outliers," which qualified for special additional payments.

At the same time, the managerial importance of the ledger has increased because of its detailed tally of services used. Modern computer programs permit virtually limitless specification of detail, down to individual doses of drugs and hours or minutes of professional service. Ledgers can be aggregated to build databases of resource utilization; they also support a clinical abstract containing summaries of diagnosis and treatment. The ledger is closely related to the medical record data processing systems described in Chapter 17 and has emerged as the principal source of data for achieving clinical economy and quality control.

The following are the major components of information from patient ledgers:

- *Counts of resources used*, available at the individual patient level and in sets reflecting both intermediate and final product groupings.
- *Gross revenue*. The counts of services times the charge requested for each service. It can also be summed by functional or patient group; such sums are useful when a realistic price is substituted for the charge.
- *Revenue adjustments*. The differences between gross revenue and what is actually received are posted at the level of detail supported by the payment. Under DRG and negotiated fee payments, individual patient ledgers are adjusted, but not the detail. Write-offs for charity and bad debts are also handled at the patient level. In the case of capitation payment, the discount cannot be calculated for the individual patient, but must be applied to the group of ledgers covered by the HMO contract.
- *Net revenue*. The income actually received, as opposed to what is initially posted; it is equal to gross revenue minus adjustments. Net revenue is available at the level of adjustment.

The structure of revenue accounting and the information available at various levels of aggregation are shown in Figure 14.2.

Accounting is also made for **non-operating revenue**. Income generated from non-patient care activities, including investments in securities and earnings from unrelated businesses. It is an important contribution to overall profit for many healthcare organizations.

Expenditures accounting

Accounting for expenditures reports all disbursement of funds and simultaneously generates basic information on costs. Cost ledgers show the quantities and prices of items purchased or disbursed. Thus, the payroll system generates paychecks, records of hours worked by employee, and data on labor costs; the

Ledger Level	Activity Counts	Gross Revenue	Aggregate Payment Adjustment	Capitation Payment Adjustment	Net Revenue
Individual Item	Yes	Yes	No	No	No
Patient	Yes	Yes	Yes	No	No
Responsibility Center	Yes	Yes	No	No	No
Disease Group	Yes	Yes	Yes	No	Yes
Payor Group	Yes	Yes	Yes	Yes	Yes
Accounting Period	Yes	Yes	Yes	Yes	Yes

FIGURE 14.2 Revenue Account Organization and Availability of Information

accounts payable system issues checks for purchased goods and services and provides counts of quantities used and data on cost of supplies.

Expenditures accounting is organized according to the formal accountability hierarchy, down to the level of responsibility centers (RCs) (Chapter 5). Within each RC, expenditures are classified by the kind of resource purchased, principally labor, supplies, equipment and facilities, and other. Aggregates of cost or quantity are available for each category under automated recording schemes.

Some transactions are internal rather than external exchanges. These are called **general ledger transactions**. General ledger entries are usually expense adjustments, although revenue adjustments are possible. They adjust inventory values, assign capital costs through depreciation, and recognize other long-term transactions. They tend to reflect costs that are incurred by the organization as a whole rather than items clearly assigned to individual RCs and to deal with resources that last considerably longer than one budget or financial cycle. As a result, they must be estimated with limited accuracy at accountability hierarchy levels below that at which they occur. For example, depreciation can be accounted to individual capital items, but when the item is used for multiple activities, like a building, assignment of depreciation to each activity is based on estimates.

Figure 14.3 shows the organization and availability of expenditures accounting information. As the footnotes indicate, the precision of expenditures accounting can be expanded. Many costs are directly accounted to specific patients and care activities in areas like the operating rooms and primary care offices. They add to the accounting expense, but improve its accuracy. Unfortunately, they can never be entirely complete. Important costs, such as the environmental sanitation of the operating rooms and the liability insurance of the primary care office, are inescapably joint; that is, the costs incurred are largely unrelated to the individual services rendered or patients treated.

FIGURE 14.3
Expenditures Account Organization and Availability of Information

Ledger Level	Labor Quantities and Costs	Supplies Quantities and Costs	Equipment Quantities and Costs	General Ledger Transactions
Individual Item	Partial*	Yes†	No	No
Patient	Partial*	Yes†	No	No
Responsibility Center	Yes	Yes†	Yes	Yes
Disease Group	Partial*	Yes†	No	No
Payor Group	Partial*	Yes†	No	No
Accounting Period	Yes	Yes†	Yes	Yes

*Certain high-cost labor, such as physician and nurse practitioner time, can be accounted to the individual patient. General staff, such as clerical support, cannot practically be accounted in this way.
†Certain general supplies, such as inpatient linen, cannot practically be accounted to individual items. Most higher cost supplies, including drugs and appliances, are directly accounted.

Managerial Accounting

Managerial accounting is a deliberate effort to relate revenue and expenditures to individual services and the activities of small units or responsibility centers. Its purpose is to provide data useful in planning, setting expectations, and improving performance.[2] Opposite to financial accounting, it is oriented to produce information for internal organization uses, allowing management decisions about costs, profitability, revision, and continuation and discontinuation of services. As Figures 8.2 and 8.3 suggest, managerial accounting is complicated in healthcare organizations because revenues and costs are not aggregated, paralleling the way services are produced. There are two theoretical solutions to the problem: either accumulate the costs from individual services to revenue aggregates or disaggregate the revenue.

The question answered by managerial accounting is whether the individual service or the responsibility center operated at an acceptable level of cost. The service must simultaneously meet standards of quality and patient satisfaction, but these are not at issue in the managerial accounting data. Given a service acceptable in quality and patient satisfaction, cost must meet two tests:

1. *Profitability.* At the level of aggregation at which payment is received, cost plus an allowance for the long-run strategic goals of the organization should be less than or equal to the amount paid. (Certain services may be deliberately subsidized; this amounts to a negative allowance.)
2. *Comparability.* At the level of the production unit, or responsibility center, cost should be less than or equal to the amount management is willing

to distribute to that activity relative to others comprising the revenue aggregate. This usually must be the lowest cost available; that is,
a. The responsibility center must match competing alternatives.
b. The responsibility center should show improvement toward benchmark or best practice values.

These tests can be algebraically stated as shown in Figure 14.4.

The source of data for these tests is the financial accounting system, but because of the differences in level of aggregation, substantial manipulations and adjustments are necessary to translate the data to managerially useful forms.[3] The first step in the process for the translation involves identification of costs of each responsibility center, keeping the responsibility centers as small as possible and relating them as closely as possible to specific services used either by patients or by other RCs. Each RC must then produce its service according to the profitability and comparability criteria.

Variable, semivariable, and fixed costs

The type of cost faced by the RC is critical in understanding its management. Costs can be classified as variable, semivariable, and fixed, where the type depends on the relationship of costs to output, the number of units of service produced. Variable costs are those directly proportional to output, such as meals or supplies. Semivariable costs are related to output, but in a nonlinear way. The most common is a step function, where certain levels of output require additional costs, such as the hiring of another professional provider. Fixed costs are those independent of output; usually costs that must be incurred to produce even a single unit of output, such as facilities and equipment essential to a quality service. The algebraic and graphic relationships of cost to volume are shown in Figure 14.5.

Over long time frames and at occasional windows of opportunity, all costs become variable; the entire production process can be redesigned. Most years, the opportunity to reduce costs is restricted, and the three costs are managed in different ways. Variable costs are reduced by changing the process—using lower cost labor or supplies, or less of them, for example. Changing the demand, rather than the process, operating near but not over

FIGURE 14.4 Managerial Accounting Tests of Costs and Revenue

Test	Concept	Application Level	Algebraic Statement
1.	Profitability	Smallest unit of payment	Unit cost plus allowance for strategic goals less than or equal to unit payment
2a.	Control	RC or lowest level of accountability	Unit cost less than or equal to management allowance or budget guideline
2b.	Improvement	Lowest unit of service available	Unit cost approaching or equal to benchmark

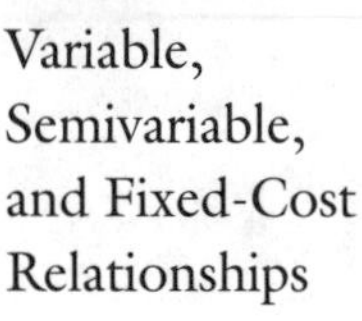

FIGURE 14.5
Variable, Semivariable, and Fixed-Cost Relationships

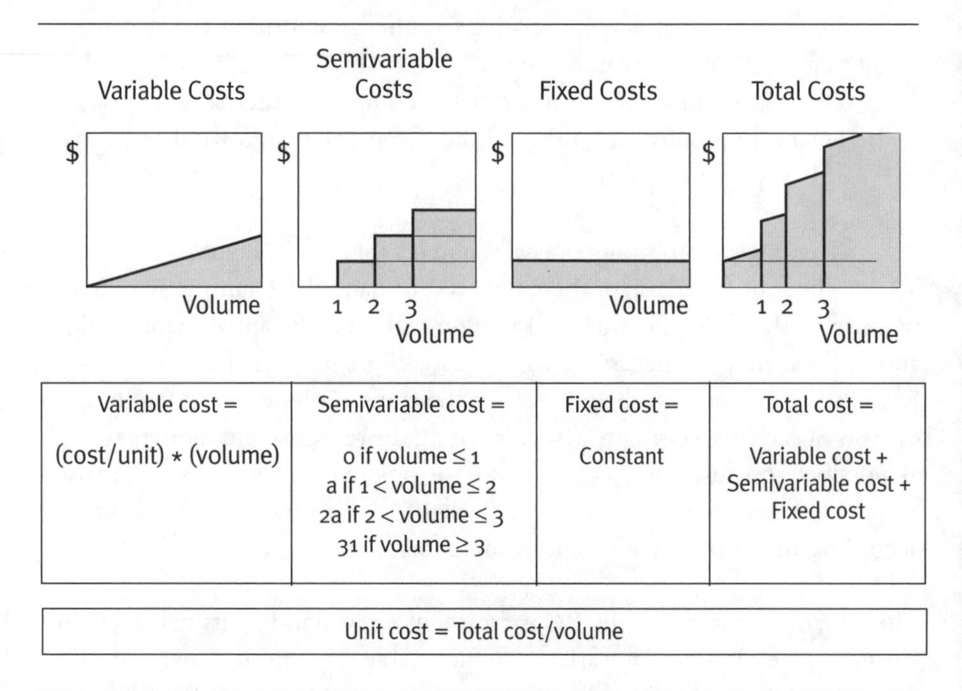

a break point reduces semivariable costs, so that the cost is distributed over as many units as possible. The nurse staffing model shown in Figure 10.5 is entirely semivariable costs; one would try to operate either just below 48 patient equivalents or just below 60 patient equivalents to minimize the cost of the BSN team leaders. Fixed costs can be reduced only by increasing volume; one would try to operate just below 60 patient equivalents to minimize the cost of the head nurse.

Marginal costs

Marginal costs are the unit costs of an additional or eliminated unit of service. They are closely related to variable costs, but when a capacity limit of a semivariable resource is reached, there can be a sudden shift in the unit cost, as the total cost graph of Figure 14.5 reflects. Whenever a fixed or semivariable resource is used at less than capacity, the marginal unit cost is exactly equal to the variable costs. Whenever the fixed or semivariable resource must be adjusted to accommodate a change in volume, the marginal cost must be specifically calculated. Marginal costs can range from near zero to very large numbers.

Marginal costs figure in planning and marketing functions of CSS (Chapter 9). The economic rules for accepting new business or discontinuing existing business relate entirely to marginal cost. New business is accepted if marginal revenue exceeds marginal costs. Existing business is discontinued when marginal revenue is less than marginal costs. A line manager seeking to optimize the overall cost performance of a responsibility center would concentrate on increasing output of services with very low marginal cost, but discouraging growth of those with high marginal costs. Demand for the services that are near a semivariable or fixed resource limit, or that have very high variable costs, would be discouraged.

Direct and indirect costs

Some costs are incurred at the point of service and are accounted directly to the responsibility center or group. The cost of supplies used directly in patient care, such as drugs or appliances, can be accounted through the RC to the patient using them. These are called **direct costs**. Other costs are incurred for large aggregates of the organization, even for the organization as a whole. Insurance, debt service, expenses of the executive office, and the operation of central services like parking and security are examples. These are called **indirect costs**, or **overhead**. Only direct costs can be controlled by a responsibility center, but every cost is direct for some RC.

Indirect costs, those services provided to another RC rather than to a patient, are an important element of healthcare. They often amount to one third of all institutional costs. A healthcare organization interested in reducing costs must follow a two-step process. First, each RC must meet the twin criteria above, producing its service at the lowest possible unit cost. Second, each RC must use as little as possible of the services from other RCs, economizing on these resources exactly as it does on purchased supplies. The managerial accounting system must assign indirect costs in a manner that promotes both goals. Historically, hospitals under cost-based reimbursement allocated indirect costs back to responsibility centers using complex formulas based on assumed relations between these costs and measures such as facility space, number of employees, total direct costs, or gross revenues.[4] The arbitrary allocation made it impossible to hold the responsibility center accountable for indirect costs. The more recent approach attempts to identify the actual transactions between RCs, cost them fairly, and make them targets for cost improvement. It is called activity-based costing.

Activity-based costing

When the basic accounting of resources is in place, it becomes possible to view some responsibility centers as independent businesses, buying and selling services to each other as well as selling them to the patient or customer. Activity-based costing does this, making it possible for the purchasing RC to make as large a fraction of its costs variable as possible.[5] The price for these internally purchased services is called a **transfer price**, which must be set by the finance activity, working with the selling RC and taking due consideration of the profitability and comparability criteria. Conceptually, the transfer price allows the buying RC to look on the purchase as a cost resource to be used as effectively as possible.[6] Software is now available to assist with this task, so that the indirect costs of any given RC can be examined and sometimes revised to transfer prices.

Transfer prices are desirable whenever they can be established, but many services can be priced only as a single annual fixed charge. Usually the problem lies with measuring the quantity of service, as in the case of governing board and executive office expenses.[7] Those services can still meet the tests of profitability and comparability. Entire systems, including information services, finance, executive management, and human resources management, are available for purchase. Mergers, acquisitions, preferred partnerships, and alliances offer ways to reduce the total operating expense of a facility, with particular attention to its overhead cost items. That is to say the twin tests of profitability and comparability must be applied at progressively higher levels of the organization as well; major units or the organization as a whole must be restructured to meet them.

Achieving accountability

The responsibility of the finance system is to produce the data for the profitability and comparability tests. The normal process in well-managed organizations is to develop forecasts of each test, refine these into expectations that are incorporated into the budget process, and monitor actual performance against expectations. The emphasis is on continuous improvement, and it requires the deliberate search for comparative data. Identifying best practices and benchmark costs is a shared activity between accounting and line management. Accounting can assist in obtaining information from other companies and in understanding the managerial accounting assumptions involved in the benchmark. Any real organization will always have an agenda of areas in which it falls short of best practice. It will set priorities for shortfalls according to their contribution to overall profit and work on as many as it can each year.

Extending ABC to final product costs

The managerial accounting system described so far is organized around the functional hierarchy—specifically, its smallest units, the RCs producing one or a few services. It produces accurate costs for the intermediate products. The accounting system must aggregate intermediate product costs to the level of final products, both to allow the profitability test for payments by disease episodes or capitation and to support the efforts of cross-functional teams working on improvement of cost and quality.[8]

A final product in healthcare almost always involves services from several different responsibility centers. Each test and treatment must be weighed in light of its contribution to the outcome; ideally only those essential to the outcome should be ordered.[9] The final product improvement team must now have data showing actual costs of treatment alternatives. The data are constructed using the patient ledgers, which identify the disease group and give the quantity of services ordered for each patient and the unit costs from each responsibility center.[10]

The final product management team is concerned with the quality, patient satisfaction, and profitability of the product. All three must be maintained to succeed.[11] (Declines in quality and satisfaction may lead to reduced volumes;

where many costs are fixed these produce drastic changes in profitability.) From the cost accounting perspective alone, the team is concerned with appropriate volumes of services and competitive costs. Figure 14.6 shows the assembly of final product costs from managerial accounting data initially organized by responsibility center. Part A of Figure 14.6 shows total direct and indirect costs, but conceptually, each final product team should have data on fixed and variable direct cost components and estimates of marginal costs arising from its actions. These are shown in Part B. The cost savings the final product team will achieve with various reductions will be closer to the variable costs. Reducing laboratory tests from 25 to 20 will save only $2.50, not worth the effort to discuss it. Sending mother and baby home a day early will save only $130, not the $1,800 per day of total direct costs. Part B also shows that if there is room to expand the number of deliveries without encountering any semivariable boundaries, the marginal cost of an additional delivery will be only $642.50. Strategically, an effort to build market share might be much more rewarding than an effort to cut costs.

In reality, there are several unsolved problems in providing Figure 14.6 data.[12] Marginal costs remain approximations in most situations. Well-managed organizations can provide estimates of current direct and indirect costs and the likely impact of changes in quantities of services upon the total cost. The estimates of direct costs are often questionable for small, high-volume services like the laboratory tests in Figure 14.6, but these are not important targets.

The final product team concentrates on the areas where important cost savings or quality improvements appear likely. It endeavors to reach consensus on a protocol that represents the most appropriate way to treat the typical patient in the group and applies the Figure 14.4 tests of profitability, control, and improvement against that protocol. The approach has proven highly productive.[13]

Budgeting

Budgeting and reporting deal with expectation setting and achievement, the basic engine for continuous improvement and competitive operation. They rest on effective managerial accounting and financial planning. Leading organizations now include expectations on several dimensions of performance, as discussed in Chapters 6 and 9, but cost budgeting remains a central part of the annual exercise. Reporting to responsibility center managers includes reliable and specific historic cost data, accurate forecasts of demand, output, and productivity, and comparative data. Budgeting of final products and accountability of final product teams, the action that creates a formal matrix organization, has become widespread as the service unit concept has spread. A section of the finance system, the budget office, generally coordinates budget development and reporting.

FIGURE 14.6 Estimating Final Product Cost from Responsibility Center Data

A. General Model

RC unit direct cost	*	Volume used in final product	=	Final product direct cost element
RC unit indirect cost	*	Volume used in final product	=	Final product indirect cost element
Central and governance indirect costs			=	Allocated indirect costs
Sum of all final product cost elements			=	Final product cost

Obstetrics Example

Delivery room cost per use*	$1250	*	1	=	$1,250.00
Postpartum care cost per day*	$ 550	*	2 days	=	$1,100.00
Nursery care cost per day*	$ 300	*	2 days	=	$ 600.00
Laboratory cost per test*	$4.50	*	25 tests	=	$ 112.50
Drug (1) cost per dose*	$5.75	*	12 doses	=	$ 69.00
Drug (2) cost per dose*	$18.50	*	4 doses	=	$ 74.00
Indirect costs	Allocated				$1,200.00
TOTAL				=	$4,405.50

B. Variable Cost Model

RC unit variable cost	*	Volume used in final product	=	Final product variable cost element
Allocated RC fixed cost for each service			=	Fixed cost elements
Central and governance indirect costs (fixed)			=	Allocated indirect costs
Sum of all final product cost elements			=	Final product cost

Obstetrics Example

Delivery room cost per use	$250		*	1	=	$250.00
Postpartum care cost per day	$100		*	2 days	=	$200.00
Nursery care cost per day	$ 30		*	2 days	=	$ 60.00
Laboratory cost per test	$.50		*	25 tests	=	$ 12.50
Drug (1) cost per dose	$5.00		*	12 doses	=	$60.00
Drug (2) cost per dose	$15.00		*	4 doses	=	$60.00
TOTAL VARIABLE COSTS		Delivery				$642.50
Fixed costs	Allocated					
Delivery		$1,000.00				
Postpartum		$ 900.00				
Nursery		$ 540.00				
Laboratory		$ 100.00				
Pharmacy		$ 23.00				$2,563.00
Indirect costs	Allocated					$1,200.00
TOTAL					=	$4,405.50

*Includes RC indirect costs

Budget components

The budget for a healthcare organization is a full, detailed description of expected financial transactions, by accounting period, for at least an entire year. Because it takes time to develop, the forecast must cover about 18 months into the future. Well-run institutions budget a second or even a third year in preliminary terms as part of their yearly budget cycle. The review of future expectations is useful to them in making smooth progress toward their financial goals.

Figure 14.7 shows the major budgets and their relationship to the finance system purposes of operational improvement, planning, and funds acquisition.

The **operating budgets** are made up of the following:

- Responsibility center **expenditure budgets**, or **cost budgets**, include anticipated costs by reporting period, responsibility center, and kind of resource. Costs are often identified as fixed, semivariable, or variable. Anticipated volumes of demand or output are now incorporated into cost budgets, and productivity measures are calculated. Indirect costs are sometimes shown, but the emphasis is on direct costs controllable by the responsibility center or unit.
- Aggregate expenditures budgets, successive "roll ups," or aggregates, summarize larger sections of the organization paralleling the functional hierarchy.
- **Revenue budgets** based on net revenue reflect expected income and profits at final product and service line levels. With the increase in

FIGURE 14.7 Major Budgets and Their Relation to Financial Goals

Budget	Contents	Use
Functional operating budget	RC expense budget	One-year or two-year plan of acceptable RC operation
	Non-financial performance expectations	
Service line operating budget	Service line expense and revenue budget	One-year or two-year plan of acceptable service line operation
	Non-financial performance expectations	
New programs and capital budget	Approved capital expenditures and funding	Manage investments in capital equipment and facilities
Financial budget	Detailed pro forma of corporate income, expense, and balance sheet	Verify budget guidelines and confirm LRFP
Cash budget	Projection of monthly cash flows	Manage working capital

aggregated revenue, revenue budgets are rarely accurate at RC levels. For that reason, leading institutions are now reporting revenues only at aggregates that can be held accountable.
- **Final product budgets** of cost and revenue for DRGs and capitated costs per member per month. These are the first step in holding cross-functional teams accountable.[14]

The **financial budgets** are composed of the following:

- **Income and expense budget**, sometimes called a "profit plan,"[15] expected net income and expenses incurred by the organization as a whole.
- Budgeted financial statements, sometimes called **"pro forma"** statements, establishing the financial position of the organization. Pro formas show not only the amounts of cash the organization will need, but also the anticipated sources of funds for several future years.
- **Cash flow budget**, estimates of cash income and outgo by period, used by finance in cash and liability management.
- **New programs and capital budget**, lists of proposed capital expenditures and new or significantly revised programs, with their implications for the operating and cash budgets by period and responsibility center. The new programs and capital budget includes all anticipated expenditures for facilities and equipment, as well as sources of funds for them. New programs and revisions of services are considered as part of the capital budget, even though they involve revenue and operating costs as well as capital. This permits initial consideration of a status quo operating budget and more rigorous evaluation of both existing and proposed components.

Primary unit operating budgets

Responsibility center and accountable cross-functional team budgets specify expectations in enough detail to serve as an unambiguous guide to the RC or team managing the activity; for each month of the coming fiscal year, by type of resource. Leading institutions now include expectations for quality, patient satisfaction, employee, and physician satisfaction developed from non-accounting data as well as demand, output, and productivity expectations developed largely from accounting data. Revenue is budgeted if it can be accurately reported and is within the control of the accountable unit. Comparative and competitive data is reported as available.

The budget can be **flexible**, that is, based on changing variable costs to meet an expectation for a steady unit cost, called a **standard cost**, or **fixed,** based on prior demand forecasts for the period and meeting an expected total cost. Flexible budgets are useful in analyzing variation; part of the variation can be attributed to changes in demand or output, and part to changes in the use of resources. Supply budgets are often flexible. Flexible budgets for labor costs require the line manager to predict demand changes and adjust staffing to them.[16] There are few RCs in which they are feasible in healthcare organizations, because of the difficulty of accurate day-to day-demand forecasting and of adjusting staffing.

The major sources of budget expectations are as follows:

- Demand is forecast for major elements such as managed care members, primary care contacts, emergency visits, hospitalizations, births, and surgeries. These events can be accurately forecast in most large operations by statistical analysis of market trends, combined with judgments of executive personnel. Forecasts for more detailed care elements are derived from those for major elements. They are developed first by the budget office and then refined for each unit by line personnel. The initial forecast is for continuation of past activities; it is then modified by actions taken on new programs and capital.
- Output forecasts are derived from the demand forecast by the RC. The usual expectation is that 100 percent of demand will be met, so that the two numbers are equal. Demand may be turned away in some situations, such as an appropriateness review or unexpected changes in the patient's condition. In other situations, output may exceed demand because of repeated work or additional services conditional on the initial results.
- Costs are forecast by type of resource from history, with independent assessment of trends in prices of purchased goods and services. The purchasing usually prepares the price forecast for supplies, human resources for personnel, and finance for indirect cost items. The initial cost forecast is based on a continuation of past activities. The RC is responsible for improvements in unit costs and volumes developed by study of operations during the year. These are part of continuous improvement activities and are frequently necessary to meet constraints on the total increase for the entire institution. The improvements may depend on new programs and capital actions.

  It is sometimes useful to reconsider the entire operation of a unit, in an effort to establish an optimally efficient operation that can be used as a benchmark or as the basis for a new program request. This process, called zero-based budgeting, does not appear fruitful as a routine approach.[17] External benchmarks and market needs are usually a more effective way to gain continuous improvement.
- Productivity is calculated mechanically as the ratios of costs to output. Both physical and dollar values are important. Productivity estimates are often compared to benchmarks and historical values and used to identify improvement opportunities.
- Revenue, when applicable, is forecast from the output forecasts and anticipated prices. (Pricing is discussed under financial management.)

Budget guidelines

All budgets must be subject to constraints based on the profitability and comparative criteria. The governing board develops guidelines from the long-range financial plan. The guidelines are expressed first for the organization as a whole, and then for progressively smaller aggregates. It is not necessary to hold each aggregate to the same profit margin; some units can be deliberately subsidized and others held to higher standards. Many religious healthcare organizations subsidize units meeting the needs of the poor, for example. Final product guidelines can be based on prevailing prices, such as the Medicare payment per DRG, with an appropriate allowance for profit. In RCs where revenue estimates are problematic, emphasis shifts to cost guidelines. Typical cost guidelines for RCs are stated in historical or benchmark terms, such as "No increase in unit cost," "Decrease by *x* percent each year to reach benchmark unit cost in three years." The unit should be involved in setting the guideline, and the sum of all the guidelines must balance against the revenue forecast. Some organizations use two guidelines, one for minimally acceptable performance, and a second stretch guideline for exceptional achievement. Incentives are established for exceptional effort.

Developing the operating budget

The budget development process is supported by the finance system, which is responsible for reaching an acceptable solution within a specified time frame. It follows an annual cycle that develops information from the environment down to the RC or cross-functional team. The cycle is shown in Figure 14.8. Completing the cycle takes about six months and demands substantial effort by every manager and executive, as well as members of the governing board. During the remainder of the year, managers can focus on the analysis of operations and development of improved methods, so that these are ready for implementation with the next cycle.

The process is managed by "packages," specific bundles of information that are transferred from one unit or level to another, and timetables, which set deadlines for package transfers.[18] The package concept allows the budget office to route information to the correct location, permitting many different teams in the healthcare organization to work at once. Figure 14.9 shows the major steps, although the process is usually more complex than the figure indicates. As a general rule, there is a specific information package for each RC or unit at each step, although later rounds of revision tend to focus on only a few unresolved areas.

The actual calculation is now computerized. Units have direct access to their own electronic files and can change physical cost and some demand elements at will up to the package deadlines. At that time, they must submit the packages to central control, where aggregates are calculated and values checked against historic records for errors or potential difficulties.

The following are guidelines for a well-run budget process:

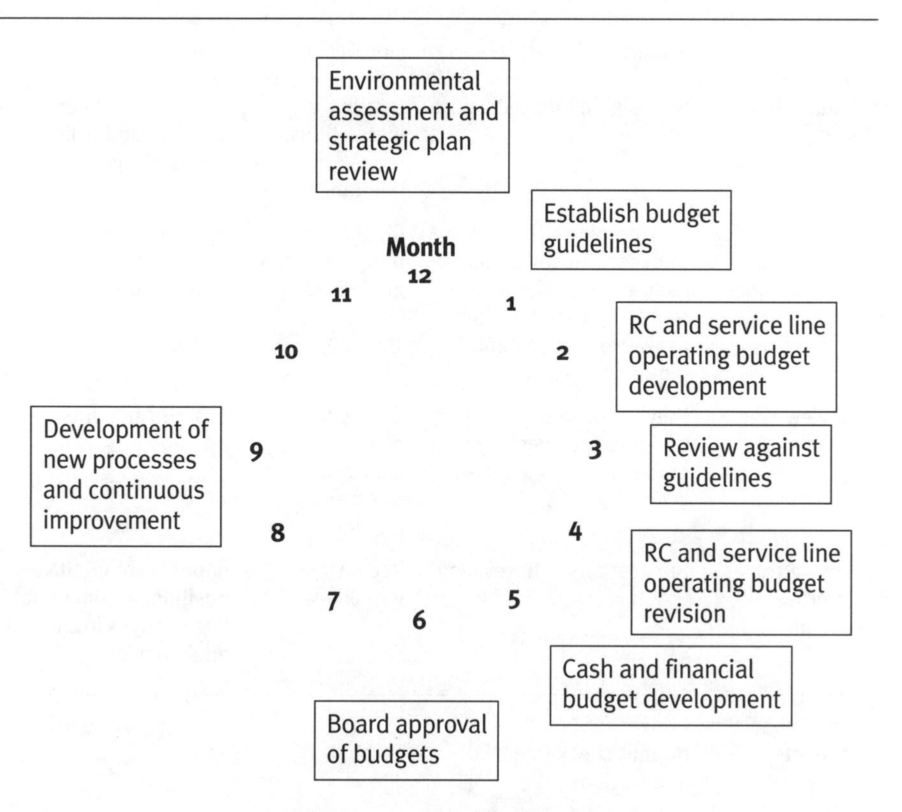

FIGURE 14.8
Annual Budget Cycle

1. The parts of the budget must constitute an integral whole. The planned activities must be consistent with each other, the strategic plan and long-range financial plan, and the annual environmental survey.
2. Budget guidelines are a major force in gaining consistency and timely progress. These include
   a. market-based forecasts of net revenue;
   b. a minimum acceptable return from operations established from the strategic plan and the long-range financial plan;
   c. a limit on increase in total cost derived from revenue minus return; and
   d. a maximum allowable capital expenditure.
3. The budget for capital expenses and new programs is separately developed and approved. It simplifies the dialogue for the expense budget and
   a. permits ad hoc debate on the relative value of programs;
   b. allows the approval of new programs and even replacement capital to be adjusted quickly as conditions change;
   c. encourages deletion proposals for obsolete or uneconomical programs; and
   d. permits the use of new programs as rewards for achieving cost and efficiency goals.

FIGURE 14.9 Major Steps in Developing Operations Budgets

Month	Finance Activity	Line Activity	Intent
1. Establish budget guidelines	Set volume forecasts, cost changes	Distribute instructions, forms, and timetables	Provide targets and information for line managers' guidance
2. RC and service line budget development	Provide more detailed forecasts, historical and comparative information to RCs and service lines; answer questions and requests for advice	Develop budgets within guidelines	Specify realistic operational expectations for coming year
3. Review against guidelines	Tally proposed operating budgets and check against guidelines	Consider possible improvements or "stretch" budgets	Ensure competitive operation
4. Revise to improve compliance	Suggest areas for revision	Reconsider guidelines	Improve competitive position; accommodate late changes in external environment
5. Develop cash and financial budgets	Develop complete budget for board review; double check financial implications		Prepare integrated package for board action
6. Board approval of budgets	Recommendation of final budget to board		Final review
7–11. Development of new processes and continuous improvement	Report on performance against budget; provide benchmark information and guidance on improvement opportunities; assist in evaluating new processes	Develop improved processes; execute plan-do-check of Shewhart cycle	Find opportunities to improve competitive position
12. Environmental assessment and strategic plan review	Present long-range forecasts, market analysis, evaluation of current mission and vision	Review and understand competitive environment	Develop consensus on organization needs, environmental conditions; reiterate relevant policy on quality, human resources, and operations

4. Line managers receive training in advance covering the budget philosophy, the importance of the outcomes expectations, the reasons for being given the opportunity to propose expectations rather than being forced to accept those of others, and the value of incorporating the viewpoints of work group members.
5. Continuous improvement is the norm. Benchmarking is routine, and

achievement of benchmark performance clearly rewarded. An RC can assume that, if nothing else changed, next year's budget would redo last year's work with slightly fewer resources because its people would have the advantage of practice and study of improvement possibilities.

6. The quality of data and the preparation of information by the budget office are important contributions to success, measured both by time to completion and usefulness of result. These should be improved from year to year, building on past work.
7. The budget process itself is subject to continuous improvement. It should be made more rigorous over time. An organization having difficulty establishing or meeting its budget is well advised to limit its attention to elementary concepts, concentrating on getting guidelines, forecasts, and improvement processes established and accepted. A well-run organization with many years' budgeting experience will do flexible budgeting, activity-based costing, and stretch scenarios. It also would have extended the detail of its reporting, both by type of resource and number of RCs. Similar growth in sophistication would occur in the capital and new programs budget.
8. RCs and cross-functional teams must participate in budget development. They should fully understand the market forces and planning processes leading to the budget guidelines. They should be able to anticipate the general direction of the guidelines for at least two years in the future. They should be trained in process analysis and continuous improvement and encouraged to work throughout the year in preparation for next year's budget needs.
9. Line managers must accept the final decisions and be convinced of their realism.[19] Executive staff and senior managers are responsible for resolving conflicts. If finance or other technical support groups impose solutions, the stage is set for failure, continued dissent, and dissatisfaction.
10. An organization-wide dialogue should go on about the market, the guidelines, and the continuous improvement program. Such a dialogue is probably essential to allow the matrix approach, and gain effective collaboration between the traditional RCs and the newer cross-functional teams. The effectiveness of the dialogue is more important than issues of data quality or process sophistication. When an effective dialogue exists, quality and sophistication often improve as a result. Without effective dialogue, there is a constant danger of having the RCs adopt an adversarial or destructive approach to the budget.[20]

Developing the new programs and capital budget

The governing board authorizes new programs and capital requests, including equipment replacement through the new programs and capital budget. Each potential investment is developed as a programmatic proposal (Chapters 9 and 12). Proposals are ranked competitively by line teams, as shown in Figure 9.8, and the final approval must accommodate the capital expenditure budget guideline. The approved proposals will constitute the budget for new programs and capital expenditures and as such will affect the revenue, cost, and cash flow budgets.

The criterion for all capital investment is optimization of long-term exchange relationships between the institution and its community. For the organization to thrive, new projects, expansions, and replacement of old investments must always be selected on the basis of this criterion, which must balance both member (internal) needs and patient (external) needs. The nature of professional behavior is such that the best managers and clinicians will always have proposals that cannot be funded, so considerable tension surrounds the selection process. The process must not only identify the best proposals, but also seem equitable to organization members.

Finance is a good choice to manage the competitive review process. Their technical skills prevent distortion of costs or benefits, and they are relatively unbiased. The following steps are helpful:

1. Proposals accumulated during the year are submitted to ad hoc committees within each of the major functional hierarchies and service lines. The task of these committees is to rank the proposals submitted.
2. Ranking should follow established guidelines for both process and criteria:
   a. A process that allows each committee member a secret vote on the rank is preferable, because it reduces recrimination, collusion, and status differentials.
   b. Membership on the committee should reflect contribution to the organization's mission, but it should also offer broad opportunity to reward successful managers. High turnover of individuals is desirable, as long as the representation of various groups is kept constant.
   c. Discussion and debate should focus on the criterion of optimizing the organization's exchange relationships, rather than the gain of a particular group or unit.
3. Second review by an executive-level committee with representation weighted to clinical systems should integrate the rankings of the initial committees.
4. The planning committee of the board may accept the initial rankings or may refer back for reconsideration. In rare cases, it may revise the original rankings, but it should do this only after discussion with the proposal supporters. It recommends funding of the higher ranked proposals on the list, selecting those that fulfill the capital budget guideline.
5. The finance committee reviews the planning committee's recommendation. Disagreement between the two committees is resolved by discussion or referred to the full board.
6. Acceptance by the board is normally at the time of adoption of the operating budget. Contingent acceptance is possible and often desirable.

Thus, a proposal may be accepted if cash flows at midyear reach a specified level, or if demand for certain services exceeds expectations.

The capital budget process requires extensive automation. There are a large number of proposals, and they are frequently combined or modified. While full descriptions are not easily computerized, a brief summary and a business plan can be entered for each. The competitive process is rigorous, and many proposals are withdrawn for further study. When the proposals are approved and implemented they often affect operating budgets. Even after approval, the details of implementation can change. Automation facilitates management of the active list of proposals, the approved budget, implementation, and modification of operating budgets.

Reporting and Control

Several kinds of cost and revenue details are reported to other systems by finance, including public disclosure, reports on budget performance, cost studies, and special or ad hoc analyses.

Disclosure of financial information

Financial accounting provides a basic set of data that generates financial reports for owners, lenders, payors, and other exchange partners. Three main reports have become standard for healthcare organizations and most other non-governmental enterprises.[21] They are the balance sheet; the income, or profit and loss, statement; and the statement of sources and uses of funds. A fourth, the statement of changes in fund balances, was added in 1990.[22] These summarize the financial activities and situation of the organization in a form now almost universal in the business world. They are usually issued monthly or quarterly to the board and monthly to the executive office.

The financial statements are a critical report to the governing board, which is obligated to monitor performance and protection of assets on behalf of the owners. Annually, the board receives the audited, final versions of these statements. They constitute the record of the board's own financial management and the discharge of its obligation to exercise fiscal prudence.

The audited annual statements are also the basis for most of the organization's financial communication with the outside world. HMOs and intermediaries often demand access to provider organization finances as a condition of payment. Audited income statements and balance sheets must be reported to the federal government as a condition of participation in Medicare. Once filed, they are accessible to the public under the Freedom of Information Act. Several states now require public release of financial reports as well. Healthcare organizations issuing bonds on public markets are also required to reveal standard financial information, plus pro formas forecasting their performance in future years. They make these public to support sale of bonds.

Well-managed healthcare organizations deliberately publish their financial reports as part of their program of community relations. Subsidiaries of integrated systems, both for-profit and not-for-profit, are not automatically required to disclose their financial information, but many multihospital organizations operating in several communities make them public as a basic community relations gesture.

Routine reports to accountable units

The controller provides monthly reports to general management, from the RC to the governing board, to assist them in achieving expectations. The purpose of the reports is to allow management to identify and correct any deviation from the budget expectations. When deviations occur, the lowest level of management affected normally corrects them. Higher levels enter only if the first efforts are ineffective. Finance personnel are involved only if there are questions of accounting or forecasts.

The design, content, and delivery of these reports are a major part of the controller's job. The reports should:

- Correspond exactly to the budgets, both in definition and time. (A common error is to report accrued rather than actual data for calendar months, creating a noticeable distortion because of varying numbers of weekend days. One solution is to avoid accruals; another is to use a 13-month year.)
- Be delivered promptly, within a few days of actual events.
- Be clearly and usefully presented. (A common problem is excess information, confusing the control purpose of the report with an archival one. Line managers who request a copy of the archive should receive it, but the control report focuses on material elements.)
- Present both physical and dollar measures on labor and other major costs.
- Be available to each person in the formal organization for his or her exact area of accountability.
- Condense information so that it is both automatically summarized from lower hierarchies and presented with equal economy at all levels. (This means that the COO's report is about the same length as a typical RC's. It usually follows very similar design.)
- Emphasize financially important variation so that major problems can be identified quickly.

Reports on product costs

The accounting for final product cost follows the process outlined in Figure 14.6. The reports should contain expectation and actual values for the following:

- counts of individual services;
- total net revenues and unit revenues by group;
- activity-based costs of the intermediate products;
- profit; and
- a method for identifying marginal costs so that the relationship between cost and changes in volume of each final product can be determined.

The reports present a serious challenge to the accounting system. First, final product costs require software capable of correctly grouping patients by final product and handling numerically burdensome calculations. (One must not overlook the scale of the activity. There are several hundred final products and several thousand intermediate products.) This problem is now largely met with expanded clinical information on the patient ledger and database management systems. Second, as indicated above, calculations of indirect and marginal costs are complex and subjective. Considerable dialogue must accompany final product reports if the limitations of the reports are to be understood by the cross-functional teams. Such an understanding is necessary to gain their acceptance and motivate them toward continuous improvement.

Thus, final product costing becomes a matter of preparing estimates or approximations using the best available data and methods, and improving upon accuracy with time. Because of the difficulties, costs are prepared routinely only for service lines and products that make large contributions to revenue. Other final product reports, such as those potentially affected by some proposed change, can be prepared on a special study basis. As time passes, the approximations will be improved and the routine coverage will be extended.

Reports on planning and special studies

Financial data are also essential to analyze operations, construct estimates for new or improved activities, and evaluate capital investment opportunities. Common uses include:

- developing new budget expectations, particularly when the operating conditions have changed;
- establishing prices of intermediate products in situations where these are sold directly, and negotiating prices of final products with third parties;
- comparing local production with outside purchase, often called make or buy decisions;
- comparing alternative methods, particularly those substituting capital for labor;
- ranking cost saving opportunities to identify promising areas in which to eliminate or reduce use; and
- estimating the impact on costs of expanding or contracting a product or service.

Information for these purposes is produced on demand, rather than by a routine schedule. The accounting function includes the maintenance of a cost data archive to explore specific questions, retrieval of relevant information, consultation on the limitations and applications of the data, and assistance in developing forecasts and expectations for new equipment and new operational processes. The level of detail required by specific proposals often calls for specific supplementary cost studies and extrapolation beyond normally recorded levels. A well-managed accounting operation produces information as required and offers consultative assistance in understanding both accounting and financial implications of specific decisions. Ideally, finance personnel work directly with RCs and teams, helping them identify fruitful avenues of investigation, develop useful proposals, and translate operational changes to accounting and financial implications.

Protection of Assets

Any corporate entity is required to maintain control of all its properties for its owners. The governing board and members of management are individually and severally responsible for prudent protection of assets, including avoidance of inurement.

Physical assets

Generally, the protection of the physical assets is considered part of the function of the plant system, assigned to security, maintenance, and materials management. Prudent purchasing practices are included in the responsibilities of materials management. The risk of misappropriation of assets is probably greater than the risks of theft or destruction by outside sources. The finance system is responsible the physical protection of cash, securities, and receivables, for ensuring that plant and equipment were used as anticipated, and for estimating the actual loss of physical property. The major risks it guards against are:

- unjustified free or unbilled service to patients;
- embezzlement of cash in the collections process;
- bribes and kickbacks in purchasing arrangements;
- supervision of financial conflicts of interest among governing board members and officers;
- diversion or theft of supplies and equipment;
- falsified employment and hours; and
- purchase of supplies or equipment without appropriate authorization.

All organizations face continuing real losses of assets, and acceptable performance requires continuing diligence. Most well-run organizations find that control of assets can safely be delegated to the finance system with only brief annual review. This is because a sound and well-understood program has been developed for the purpose; it has five parts:

1. Detailed, written procedures govern the handling of the various assets and transactions. These procedures primarily rely on the division of functions between two or more individuals and the routine reporting of checks and balances to protect assets. It is common to assign responsibility for authorizing the transaction (a payment or a charge) to line managers and responsibility for collecting or disbursing funds to accounting personnel.

2. Adequate written records and accounting systems document the actual use of assets.
3. Special attention is paid to collections and cashiering. Significant efforts must be made to ensure that third parties and individuals pay promptly and fully. Payment in cash and checks must be protected against embezzlement. Carefully designed systems to ensure prompt collection and protect both receivables and cash rely heavily on the principle of division of functions and on calculations designed to verify completion of transactions.
4. Adherence to risk control procedures and documentation requirements is monitored through internal auditors, who usually report directly to the CFO.
5. Annual outside audits verify both adherence to procedure and validity of reported outcome.

Inurement

Inurement is the diversion of funds to persons in governance or management as a result of their position of trust. Not-for-profit structure requires that no individual benefit from service to the corporation beyond any stipulated salary or compensation. For-profit structure has an analogous protection against exploitation of stockholders by directors. Under these rules, directors, officers, or trustees may not engage in business that allows them to derive financial advantage from their governing board role. The corporation is not enjoined from doing business with a board member, if such business and board membership are in the owners' interests. Thus, the key word is "advantage."

To protect against inurement, the institution must establish, and the CFO must enforce, policies that reduce financial conflict of interest. These policies have two parts. First, every governing board member and officer is required to file an annual disclosure statement identifying all their financial interests and potentially conflicting commitments, including membership on other voluntary boards. Second, members are expected to divorce themselves from any specific decision or action that involves their interests or conflicting affiliations. Well-run organizations achieve this by making the point well in advance of any specific application and by selecting members who understand both the law and the ethics.

The rule applies as well to physicians, but its application is more complex (see Chapter 8 for a complete discussion). Contracts with physicians may not offer financial incentives to refer or admit patients, except in certain types of HMO incentives. They also may not extend tax exemption to physicians in private practice. Thus, all physician contracts must be reviewed for compliance. Tax exemption rules vary by state, but Medicare fraud and abuse regulations are national.

Auditing

Programs to protect against loss, diversion, and inurement are audited routinely, first by an internal audit group and second by outside auditors.

Internal auditors use a variety of monitoring devices to detect changes in physical assets and cash, or departure from accepted practice. They pay particular attention to known areas of high risk, such as receivables and collections, payrolls, prices of purchased items, and supplies with street value. Internal auditors also review accounting practices and procedures and monitor compliance.

Outside auditors certify the financial statements to be correct, usually on a fiscal year basis. The federal government requires an audit as a condition of participation for Medicare, and many intermediaries have similar requirements. Lenders require annual audits before and during the period of any loan. The audit emphasizes areas of known high risk. It is common to use sampling techniques, with attention focused in proportion to the risk involved. Auditors are expected to maintain a deliberate distance from internal employees being audited, including the internal auditors, and to use objective methods to ascertain the accuracy of reported values for balance sheet items. They are also expected to review accounting processes and to suggest changes that will improve accounting accuracy.

Berman and Weeks note that the external auditor's "primary concern is not the needs of internal management but rather the needs of external agencies and organizations. . . ." In addition, "The value and usefulness of an independent auditor lie as much in business convention as they do in operational control."[23] Their point is well taken. External auditors make a prudent survey of the accuracy of records. Although this includes review of protection of assets, it does not in any sense include either budgeting or financial management. For protection of assets as well as for cost control, the best control systems are continuous and internal rather than episodic and external. The external controls imposed by the auditor are secondary and designed to ensure that the primary systems are working.

The governing board's role is to select the outside auditors, receive their report and review it carefully, and take action to correct any deficiencies noted. Considerable care in selecting and instructing the auditor is justified. The auditor should be accountable directly to the board's finance committee. The firm should be free of any other financial relationship to the organization. Technically, this means that any consultants should be hired from a different firm than the one handling the audit. While sound, this rule is frequently breached. It is unacceptable, however, to use a firm represented on the governing board. The accountants' code of ethics states:

> Any direct financial interest or material indirect financial interest is prohibited as is any relationship to the client, such as . . . voting trustee, director, officer, or key employee.[24]

While the governing board might override the conflict of interest for banking, groceries, or the practice of medicine, it seems both unwise and unnecessary to do so for the audit. The distance and independence of the auditor are an integral part of the audit's success.

The audit committee of the governing board, usually including only the outside directors who serve as chair, finance chair, treasurer, or secretary should formulate instructions to the auditor. The instructions for audits of protection of assets should be reviewed and revised annually. The revisions can bring different aspects of the asset protection system under scrutiny each year. The instructions should be based in part on advice from the CEO and CFO but should be confidential between the finance committee and the auditor.

The report goes directly to the audit committee. Thus the auditors are free to comment upon the CEO and CFO as well as others. The auditors' comments on both problems with the accounts and weaknesses identified in the asset protection policies are included in a document called the management letter, which accompanies the audited financial reports. The audit committee should hear an oral summary and discussion of the management letter. The expectation for the management letter is "no deficiencies," and it is usually achieved. The board should formally accept both the reports and the letter. Well-run healthcare organizations have little trouble with this system. The success of this system means that governance groups and CFOs of well-run organizations need spend little time on asset protection activity, despite its complexity and importance.

Financial Management Functions

The financial management function projects future financial needs, arranges to meet them, and manages the organization's assets and liabilities in ways that increase its profitability. Financial management in this sense is relatively recent, arising from the increased revenue base created by Medicare, Medicaid, and widespread private health insurance, and from the opportunities for obtaining credit and equity that these created. Before 1970, hospitals had two sources of funds: retained earnings and gifts. The growth of public corporations, bonded indebtedness issued and reissued to minimize interest costs, and deliberate investment in joint ventures for profit is as telling a story of the healthcare industry as the development of heart transplants. Even traditionally not-for-profit organizations now engage in a broad spectrum of financing opportunities. The five components of financial management—financial planning, pricing, management of intercorporate transfers, long-term capital acquisition, and management of short-term assets and liabilities—are now essential to survival.

Financial Planning

Financial management is a forward-looking activity with a long time horizon. It begins with the generation of a long-range financial plan (LRFP), continues with the translation of plan values to budget guidelines, and results in establishing the institution's ability to acquire capital funds through debt or equity.

Developing the LRFP

The LRFP incorporates the expected future income and expense for every element of the strategic plan, specifying the amount and the time of its occurrence. Although the accuracy of the estimates deteriorates in distant years because of the uncertainty involved, large financial requirements must be accommodated even though they are many years distant. Some activities of the LRFP, such as bond repayments and major facility replacement, require financial planning horizons up to 30 years. Most of the attention is focused on the first three to five years, where the irreversible decisions will be made.

Financial planning is now commonly done with specialized software and counsel from a respected accounting firm. A financial planning model generates pro forma statements of income, asset and liability position, and cash flow for each of the future years.[25] Assumptions about cost, price, and market share trends, and expenditures expected from the planning scenarios (Chapter 12) are input by the finance staff, possibly with members of the finance committee of the governing board. For as many scenarios as can be practically accommodated, the computer program will produce pro forma statements. These can be evaluated by means of **ratio analysis**,[26] which compares various aspects of the financial statements, such as the ratio of debt to equity, debt service to cash flow, debt service to income, and so on. The ratios can be subjectively assessed and compared to published data to judge:

- cost and reasonableness of borrowing from various sources;
- cost improvements required to meet market constraints on revenue;
- cash flow required to support debt service;
- identity and magnitude of various financial risks; and
- overall prudence of the financial management.

Good financial planning will consider as many alternate assumptions as possible in terms of their impact on the long-range plan. Various assumptions might address:

- the impact of the business cycle;
- proposed federal and state legislation;
- trends in health insurance coverage and benefits;
- donation, grant, and subsidized funding sources;
- alternative debt structures and timing; and
- opportunities for joint ventures and equity capitalization.

The LRFP should also evaluate the widest possible variety of scenarios. These might include operational changes speeding up or slowing down some programs, combining programs, and even abandoning some. They might also include financing changes revising debt structure, changing profit margin requirements, acquiring new equity investors. They may include acquisition or divestiture of some units or even the merger or closure of the institution. The objective is to identify the optimum operating condition consistent with the mission and vision, and to evaluate that condition in terms of its acceptability. Unacceptable results can force a complete reevaluation of the strategic position.

As indicated in Chapter 3, the financial plan is a critical reality check for the organization. Figure 14.10 shows the tests and the kinds of rethinking necessary to make the strategic plan fit financial realities. All of the tests in Figure 14.10 reflect market conditions involving health insurance buyers, competitors, and financial markets. The financial ratios, which reflect earnings relative to investment and various operational indicators common to all businesses, provide a way to test healthcare performance against the larger world. Bond rating agencies use the ratios and other financial statement data to issue public ratings of the risk associated with long-term debt. Lower ratings (higher risks) bring higher interest costs on debt. A similar but less formal process operates with equity capital. Thus, the institution's ability to borrow money or acquire for-profit capital is directly dependent on its ability to execute a competitive long-range financial plan.

The ideal is a strategic plan that generates operating costs substantially below available prices; when that occurs the organization has a steady stream of profits. It can invest the funds in growth, capturing an increasing market share, and it can amplify growth with borrowed or invested capital. The ideal is not often achieved. The well-managed organization uses the plan to recognize danger signals in advance and makes the necessary adjustment. Several principles guide their actions, and are weighed as the plan is considered and adopted:

- The recurring question addressed is what profit, or return from operations, the organization should seek. Well-run, not-for-profit

FIGURE 14.10 Tests and Adjustments in Financial Planning

Test	External Source	Adjustment Required
Debt ratios	Bond market	Keep debt within bond rating limits
Price	Buyers and intermediaries	Keep price competitive
Earnings	Bond and equity investment markets	Keep cash flow within bond rating limits
Demand and market share	Competitor analysis	Keep volume forecast consistent with competitor and market conditions
Cost	Benchmarks Competition	Keep cost at or below (revenue – profit)

healthcare organizations have tended to seek returns in the range of 5 percent of total costs. Large for-profit organizations seek before-tax returns two to three times that high. Healthcare organizations should seek to maintain similar levels, allowing for their tax advantage.

- The criteria for investment decisions are biased toward liquidity and away from risk, as indicated in Figure 14.10. The bias toward liquidity means that each project and scenario must justify itself in terms of community benefit. There are three basic causes of increased risk:
  1. Poor prior management has reduced the organization's financial capacity.
  2. Individual proposals are inherently risky.
  3. Too large a fraction of proposals are funded.
- Well-run organizations guard against the first by using the financial plan and budget guidelines effectively. They meet the second through the programmatic planning process and competitive review, and the third by adhering to the capital investment guideline.
- Portions of the available investment funds can be earmarked for strategic purposes, such as maintenance of current operations, development of new markets, expansion of primary care affiliations, or development of information systems. Earmarking establishes a multi-year level for the category as a whole and forces evaluation of proposals within the category.
- Investment timing is frequently important. Well-run organizations avoid borrowing at peak interest rates and refinance to take advantage of low rates.

Setting the budget guidelines

The LRFP is used to establish the budget guidelines. The senior management team develops forecasts of market share, price, and revenue and prepares a recommendation translating the cash and profit requirements of the plan to the guidelines for profit, costs, and capital expenditures. The finance committee of the governing board discusses the recommendation and alternatives and recommends the guidelines to the board as a whole. The board's action establishes the forthcoming budget and is a more critical step than the final approval, which is often reduced to a formality. Substantial departure from the plan threatens the financial security of the organization and cannot be accepted as prudent.

Pricing Clinical Services

The extent to which the vendor has the ability to set the sales price is a measure of the existence of a monopoly. Healthcare in fact held a strong monopoly for several decades, and the recent turmoil is the result of losing that monopoly. The market now determines the overall price level, but the institution must have a systematic pricing response that integrates its strategic position, financial needs, and marketing realities. The board and senior management team develop broad guidelines, and line managers working with marketing and finance spell out the details.

Major buyers, such as Medicare, Medicaid, and large commercial buyers, tend to set their prices and the structure they will use to pay. For example, traditional Medicare pays inpatient hospital care on DRGs, rehabilitation and inpatient mental health services on institutional costs, and most outpatient care on institutional charges. In each case, physicians are paid according to fee schedules. The terms are promulgated by Medicare and are not negotiable. Buyers with less power in the marketplace are willing to negotiate both the structure and the level. A small fraction of cases assume the institution and its physicians will have a structure and a price schedule, and they expect to pay it.

A pricing strategy must address the following questions:

1. What forms or pricing structures does the institution prefer?
2. What is the strategic position with regard to offering price?
3. What range of negotiated prices will the institution accept, and who is authorized to negotiate?

Pricing structures

Pricing structures range from fee-for-service (the institutional portion is called "charges"), through various levels of aggregate payments such as DRGs or global fees, to capitation and incentive systems based on collective performance. Fee-for-service imposes no integration on the providers; the institution and each caregiver can set or accept the price. As aggregate systems are introduced, the decisions become more integrated, and disease management risk is transferred to the providers. Figure 14.11 shows the major options for pricing structures as sequential levels of risk taking and requirements for integration of the institution and its medical staff. All but level 1 require some degree of increased collaboration; collaboration must increase along with risk. Most organizations will accept any level because the result of declining a contract is loss of market share. The institution and its physicians try to negotiate toward a small set of models at each level. Each unique clause adds to the contract management problems. If the buyer insists on a specific clause, the organization must understand how it will implement that clause without impairing quality of care or profitability.

Pricing strategy

Competing organizations strive for advantage on price and service, but they often have a choice on the weighting of the two. Price-oriented strategies attempt to win market share by offering below average prices and limiting service; service-oriented strategies do the opposite. Mass market strategies must balance the two. Most healthcare organizations are mass market, but niche opportunities open up for both price and service emphasis. In large markets, a niche can be substantial. "Carriage trade" healthcare organizations exist in a number of large cities, pursuing a high-price, high-service, largely fee-for-service clientele. Large organizations can adopt multiple strategies,

FIGURE 14.11 Pricing Structures for Healthcare Contracts

Level	Structure	Example	Risk	Integration
1	Fee-for-service/charges	Cash payments, traditional and catastrophic health insurance	None beyond normal business risks	Traditional physician/hospital relationship
2	Negotiated fees and charges for individual items of service	PPO contracts, some traditional Blue Cross and Blue Shield contracts	Normal business risks plus constraints imposed by contract limits	Traditional physician/hospital relationship
3	Fees and charges for episodes of care negotiated separately between institution and physicians	DRGs, traditional Medicare fee contracts, some traditional Blue Cross and Blue Shield contracts	Institution is at risk for the unit costs of services and quantities of services ordered by physicians within the episode; physician has no additional risk	Institution must gain physician cooperation to meet its risk
4	Fees and charges for episodes of care negotiated jointly between institution and physicians	Global fees: single price contracts for discrete episodes of care such as cardiovascular surgery or chemotherapy	Both physician and institution at risk for the cost of the episode	Demands physician/institution collaboration on cost per episode
5	Fees and charges negotiated jointly and subject to a group incentive	HMO contracts with penalties or bonuses for meeting utilization targets	Physician and institution at limited risk for the cost and appropriateness of care	Demands physician/institution collaboration on cost per episode, utilization, and disease incidence
6	Capitation	HMO contracts independent of disease incidence or actual costs of treatment	Physician and institution at unlimited risk for the cost of the episode and appropriateness of care	Demands physician/institution collaboration on cost per episode, utilization, and disease incidence

operating low-cost clinics in poor neighborhoods and high service offices in wealthy ones. The shared services must be mass market.

Any successful pricing strategy must include the physician perspective, and those that include advanced levels must include physicians in strategy formulation. At level 1, individual physicians operate what are essentially niche businesses. They can locate practices, select patients, set prices, and maintain a cordial, but arm's length, relationship with colleagues and the institution. Advanced levels force more integration not only between each physician and the institution, but also between physicians. A pricing strategy to assume risk must be related to an organization development strategy; otherwise the risk will not be effectively managed. The two might be accomplished in parallel, through an institution-wide managing task force and a series of service line work groups. A broad range of knowledge will be required, including

CSS managers, financial analysts, and representatives of buyers and practicing physicians. The time frame is several years, allowing for individual learning and the development of the integrated skills represented in protocols and service lines. Once the strategy is set, it tends to become permanent. Investments made in learning, promotion and sales, and contract management are not easily reversed.

Price negotiations

Through the 1990s, the market has been thrusting higher level contracts on physicians and institutions, forcing them to gain the consensus and skills to handle risks. Negotiations are partly a test of wills, where the outcome is shifted by the relative strength of the parties. Thus, the attractiveness of the healthcare organization and the solidity of its relationship with its physicians are important on the one hand, and the size of the patient group, the presence of alternative sources, and the resolve of the purchaser are important on the other. Successful negotiations also depend on:

- advance preparation, including a full understanding of the range of feasible outcomes, a fact base of the financial and other consequences of various alternatives, and a priority ranking of desired terms;
- flexibility and a willingness to explore innovative solutions that might benefit both parties; and
- operating capability that supports a broad range of feasible solutions and builds organizational attractiveness.

The bargaining team must have the support of the groups directly involved in the final contract, as well as members combining a detailed knowledge of the issues and demonstrated bargaining skill. While models where the physician organization and the institution must separately approve the results of negotiations are common, many organizations have moved to "single signature contracting" where the team is authorized in advance to accept all offers that fall within certain broad limits. Negotiations that fail to meet the single signature limits can still be referred for approval.

The single signature approach is attractive in markets with many intermediaries because it allows a prompt response and helps encourage uniformity. On the other hand, deliberate, extensive, and continuing negotiations may be more fruitful in areas where only a few intermediaries control the market. These lead to a preferred partnership relationship with the intermediary that can be used to explore points of difficulty and identify changes that would support improvement toward mutual goals (Chapter 13).

Financial Management of Multicorporate Structures

As noted in Chapter 5, many healthcare organizations are now multicorporate structures. Both for-profit and not-for-profit legal entities are permitted to form new corporations, invest in other corporations, and reverse these actions by sale or liquidation. Except for the restrictions of antitrust, there is no limit on the amount or percentage of the investment involved; it can range from negligible to wholly owned. Any combination of for-profit and not-for-profit entities is possible. The tax obligations of each corporation are considered individually as the structures develop.

The major financial benefits of multiple corporate structures are:

- *Capital opportunities.* Holding companies offer scale and diversification attractive to bond buyers. As a result, they will accept lower interest. Subsidiary corporations offer opportunities not only to dedicate capital, but also to raise new capital through borrowing or equity. Activities attractive to equity capital can be pursued only through a for-profit structure, but a not-for-profit parent corporation can form a for-profit subsidiary.
- *Reward.* Separate for-profit corporations allow various groups to invest in activities of interest to them, and to receive financial reward for the success of those activities.
- *Risk.* The liabilities and obligations of the owned or subsidiary corporation cannot generally be transferred to the parent. (There are certain exceptions, and the law in this area is changing.) Thus, the parent risks only those assets actually invested in the subsidiary.
- *Taxation.* Not-for-profit corporations can be taxed on certain activities, and for-profit corporations can respond to incentives built into the tax law with nontaxable actions. Separate corporations can frequently be designed with a view toward minimizing the overall tax obligation.

Well-managed healthcare organizations use multicorporate structures as tools to achieve specific ends. There is no theoretical or demonstrated general advantage to one structure over another. In fact, operational differences between organizations depend more on how the structure is implemented than the specific form. Thus, new corporate relationships arise because they offer improved ways to meet strategic objectives or implement specific plans. The finance system has the obligation of identifying, evaluating, and recommending these opportunities.

Within limits of accepted accounting practice, Medicare fraud and abuse provisions, and IRS regulation, funds can be transferred between corporations by transfer of earnings or by charges for services. In multicorporate situations, the parent institution may participate in equity funding and receive rewards from it. It may also sell or buy services from the subsidiary at a fair market price. A relatively common example is a healthcare organization exempt from taxes under Section 501(c)(3) of the Internal Revenue Code forming a for-profit corporation with outside investors and then contracting with that corporation to carry out certain activities. The organization reduces its capital requirement, retains control of the cost and quality of services, and expects to earn profits from its ownership position.

Charges for the contractual services between parent-subsidiary corporations are a form of transfer pricing.[27] The transfer price is clearly important to the organization, other shareholders, and the IRS. It is often possible to make substantial impact on financial reports by carefully adjusting charges. Many integrated healthcare organizations pursue these manipulations as a tax avoidance strategy. Unfortunately, the best tax strategy may not fairly reflect operational conditions and may establish negative incentives for management. Strategies based on accurate assessment of costs and profits have more long-run potential.[28] These attempt to reflect the operation of each subsidiary as if it were a freestanding organization in a competitive market with others. The accounting techniques are analogous to those used in activity-based costing. Along with their other advantages, this approach provides the basis of a defense against charges of fraud and abuse.

Securing and Managing Long-Term Funds

Finance is responsible for managing all loans, bonds, and equity capital. It evaluates alternative financing means, develops a financial strategy to implement the strategic plan, and recommends the best solution to the governing board. It arranges placement of debt and prepares supporting financial information and pro formas, and it manages repayment schedules, mandatory reserves, and other elements of debt obligation. It monitors the financial markets for opportunities to restructure financing. It manages endowments of not-for-profit healthcare organizations.

The LRFP is used to develop capital needs and sources, including prospectuses for borrowing and equity funding and plans for soliciting capital donations. Most changes in the long-term funds involve large sums of money and are done through bond issues or new corporations with equity financing. Hospitals relied largely on donated capital from both government and private sources prior to 1970. Borrowing became the overwhelming source of capitalization under cost-based reimbursement through the early 1980s. The stimulus of competition promoted a number of innovative financial solutions, including equity funding and the development of multicorporate structures.[29]

Debt and equity capitalization

Successful not-for-profit healthcare organizations have accumulated substantial equity, but they can increase equity only from donations and retained earnings. Because these are limited, borrowing, principally long-term tax-exempt bonds, will remain an important form of capital finance. The typical community hospital held long-term debt amounting to close to 50 percent of its assets.[30] Many well-managed organizations will deliberately manage their LRFP and operations to attract funds at advantageous rates. The organization that demonstrates good results in finance is preferred in the financial marketplace, and attention is paid to the elements of quality and market attractiveness supporting those results. The organization can maintain that favored position in the long run only to the extent that it invests prudently to enhance its own customer base. Either excess borrowing or insufficient investment can diminish the chance of success in the long run. Leverage, the ratio of debt to equity finance, is critical. A great many corporations of substantial size and reputation have foundered because they incurred excessive debt.

Equity finance is generally appropriate for working capital and the support of developmental expenses, whereas debt tends to be used to finance real property and long-term assets. Equity is also useful in joint ventures, allowing the partners to be rewarded for successful risk taking. In general the riskier the enterprise, the more likely and appropriate is equity finance. Investors generally expect returns commensurate with their risk. Venture capitalists, willing to support new and untested ideas, do so in the expectation of returns substantially in excess of anything available in lending markets. Tax laws are quite important in equity finance, both from the point of view of the corporation and that of the investor.

Well-managed healthcare organizations exercise extreme prudence in equity finance. Evidence suggests that there are a great many dangers. Half of all newly formed for-profit corporations are bankrupt within 12 months; it is said that half of the balance fail to survive the next economic downturn. Thus, prudence demands small, diversified investments limited to amounts that the organization could lose without seriously impairing its mission. Still, the rewards for successful use of equity financing through joint ventures are appealing, and this model will probably grow in popularity.

Figure 14.12 shows a simplified example to clarify the complex financial and operational issues involved in capital funds acquisition. A certain healthcare organization might plan to spend $50 million over the next three years to expand primary care and outpatient services. It anticipates a handsome increase in net income of $10 million per year from the new service, with relatively small risk that income will fall below that level. It has several sources for the $50 million. It could use reserves from prior earnings. It could seek tax-exempt bonds, in which case it would pay about 8 percent interest. It could create a for-profit joint venture with its physicians or with another corporation, and raise part of the money from equity investment. Finally, it could combine any or all of these approaches.

The use of debt finance can increase the project attractiveness substantially, and the use of a joint venture partner can reduce the capital requirement. The combination of the two would allow the institution to start the project with a minimum investment of its own capital, and an appealing return on the capital, if earnings match expectations. If they fall short, the bond interest is fixed and the entire drop is borne by the equity investors. In some cases the partner can reduce the risks. For example, a partnership with a physician organization to provide the service would commit the physicians to the project's success.

Scenario	HCO Equity Investment	Earnings from Project	Bond Interest Paid*	Net HCO Income $/Year†	% ROI‡
I. 100% from HCO	$50	$10	0	$10	20%
II. 50% bonds, 50% equity	$25	$10	$2	$8	32%
III. 50% bonds, 25% retained earn, 25% Joint Venture Equity	$12.5	$10	$2	$4	32%

*Bond interest 8%
†(Project earnings – Bond interest) × (HCO equity share)
‡Net earnings from project as percentage of HCO investment

FIGURE 14.12 Implications of Alternative Funding Sources for Ambulatory Care Project at HCO, Inc. (millions of dollars)

The number of questions and assumptions required even in this simple example indicates the complexity and challenge of the exercise. Obviously, accurate forecasts of volume, costs, revenues, and effects on other services are essential, even though opening is several years away. These matters must be addressed in the proposal for the venture, as discussed in Chapters 12. In addition, financial assumptions must be made about the following:

- *Price and volume interactions for the new service.* Careful understanding of the market tolerance for prices and the risks involved if demand does not meet expectations are essential to evaluate the project and the financing mechanisms.
- *Costs of alternative sources of capital.* Each of the sources has different costs and obligations built into it. The use of retained earnings may impair the organization's ability to meet other needs, such as the replacement of equipment, or increase in market share by other means, such as the acquisition of competitors. Bonds will have an interest rate dependent on the market at the time of sale, the organization's overall financial position, and federal tax policy. Organizations that have been prudently managed in the past will have advantages for all kinds of capital. They will have more retained earnings, will have lower bond interest and more debt capacity, and will be more attractive to outside investors.
- *Impact of the financing on other strategic goals.* The financing may affect competitors or partners in ways advantageous to the organization. A joint venture with primary care physicians may provide an avenue to affiliate them more closely with the organization and may improve the ability to recruit. The result may be higher market share and an increased overall profitability. A joint venture with a potential competitor may reduce risk and expand resources simultaneously.
- *Tax implications.* If ordinary income taxes apply, they will be approximately 40 percent of earnings, enough to make substantial

differences in the results. A tax adviser may be able to find precedents that establish the tax obligations of the various structures, or it may be necessary to seek a letter from the IRS.

The LRFP financial model will be employed to test outcomes not only for the expected conditions but for a range of possible futures. Each major funding avenue will be explored several times, under varying assumptions. Consultants will advise on approaches, assumptions, and implications. The financial results will be evaluated against the marketing and operational considerations. The final solution is likely to draw on all three sources of funds. Scenario IV looks attractive because it allows the institution to limit its capital investment, preserves retained earnings for other uses, and still yields a handsome return. It can be recommended to the board with widespread support from the participants.

Managing endowments

Most not-for-profit healthcare organizations have acquired endowments or permanent charitable funds. The funds can be invested for growth or income. The assistance of professional investment managers is advisable. Larger organizations use several different managers. The organization must evaluate its overall investment strategy weighing its risk versus potential earnings. In general, permanently endowed funds return about 5 percent per year, after protecting the corpus against inflation. The return is often dedicated to specific charitable purposes such as research, education, and charity care.

Managing Short-Term Assets and Liabilities

Any operation requires **working capital**, funds that are used to cover expenses made in advance of payment for services. The finance system manages these transactions to maximum advantage for the organization.

Working capital management deals in terms of days. Income can be obtained by moving assets rapidly. Cash is never left in non–interest-bearing accounts. Other liquid assets are placed where they will obtain the highest return consistent with risk and the length of time available. (Large sums of money can be invested for small interest returns on an overnight basis.) Accounts receivable and inventories are minimized because they earn no return. Accounts payable, payroll, and other short-term debts are settled exactly when due, allowing the organization to use the funds involved as long as possible.

Short-term borrowing is available to healthcare organizations. Bank loans are the most common source. Short-term borrowing is minimized because it costs money. At the same time, however, costs of borrowing need to be compared to opportunity costs of liquidating assets or failing to meet liabilities in a timely fashion. The objective is to reduce total costs of working capital, rather than to avoid borrowing per se.

Personnel and Organization

Various skilled and unskilled personnel work in the finance system of even a small healthcare organization. Many of these people perform tasks that are indistinguishable from those in any other corporation, while others perform tasks that require extensive familiarity with healthcare. Chief financial officers and their staffs develop specifications for these jobs, sometimes in consultation with the outside auditor. On-the-job training is often practical at lower levels, but supervisory people now usually have advanced degrees in accounting or finance. Recruitment of unskilled personnel is rarely difficult.

Skilled personnel, especially those with healthcare experience, are often in short supply. There is a chronic shortage of CFOs. Recruitment should always be national, health-specific knowledge should be highly prized, and the governing board should be directly involved in the CFO selection. Job specifications for CFO tend not to depend on the size of the organization. Sustaining qualified professional financial management in small organizations is a severe problem and one that may underlie more mergers and contract management than is recognized. Contract financial management is available through firms providing general management. Auditing firms do not accept responsibility for financial system operations—to do so would destroy their objectivity as auditors—but they do provide substantial ongoing consultation on financial matters to organizations of all sizes.

The Chief Financial Officer

The chief financial officer is accountable for the operation of the finance systems, including the financial management functions, and advises the CEO and the governing board on finance issues. The CFO or a deputy also assumes the duties of an employed treasurer in commercial corporations, collections, disbursement, asset control, and management of debt and equity. The healthcare organization treasurer is frequently a trustee who serves principally as chairman of the finance committee. The lack of separation between finance and treasury theoretically increases the risk of defalcation, but convincing evidence of risk is lacking and organizations protect themselves by security bonds and reliance on the external audit.

Training and skills

The skills for a CFO include a master's degree in management or business and a certificate in public accountancy (CPA). Neither are mandatory; able managers continue to arise from experience alone. However, it is increasingly likely that a person seriously interested in becoming a CFO will have found an opportunity to earn one or both. Experience is more important than formal education or certification. The CFO of a well-run healthcare organization should have substantial experience that includes exposure to the finance systems of several organizations, familiarity with all functions of the finance system, and demonstrated ability to assist line management in budgeting, cost analysis, and financial planning. Evidence of technical skill is important and can be supported both by specimens of work and by references. Evidence of interpersonal skills, particularly the ability to work with people outside the finance department, is also important and can be supported by references. The larger public accounting firms often assist in finding CFOs and, not surprisingly, are also a major source of supply. The recruitment team should include senior management, senior physician management, and governing board representation.

Organization of the Finance System

Within the finance unit

The organization of the finance system, like many of its procedures, is dictated by its functions and has been thoroughly codified. Because of the use of separation of activities to protect assets, many aspects of the organization are fixed. The two critical functions, cost control and financial management, require relatively small numbers of people, with the largest numbers of personnel being in various aspects of patient accounting and collections. Figure 14.13 shows a typical organization pattern.

Other structures are possible. Financial management in smaller organizations might be provided by the CFO with an ad hoc team. Figure 14.13 reflects the assignments of information systems, admitting and registration, and materials management to other parts of the organization (Chapters 16 and 17). In smaller organizations, one or all of these activities might be assigned to the finance system.

FIGURE 14.13 Organization of the Finance System

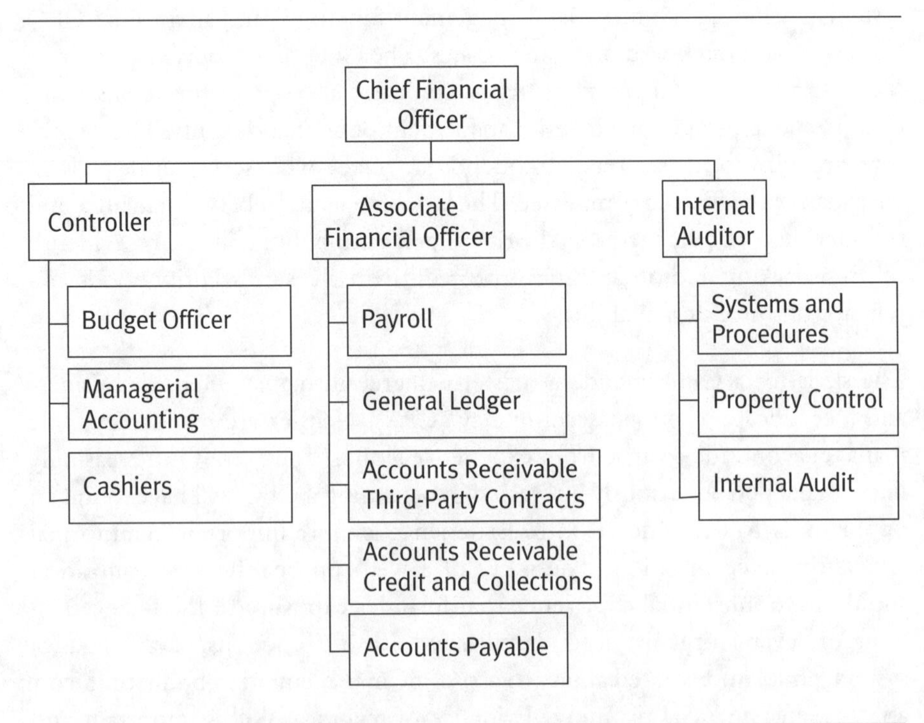

Relation of finance to line

Almost every part of the organization shown in Figure 14.13 is in direct daily contact with the rest of the healthcare organization, often over sensitive matters. The key to success is maintaining a professional, productive level of exchange. Clear, convenient systems and forms make routine information gathering as efficient as possible. Orientation and training sessions for finance personnel at all levels helps them understand clinical procedures and participate in continuous improvement projects. Finance personnel in budgeting and cost accounting relate constantly to line individuals and teams. Well-designed processes and training in consensus building make these interactions effective. It should be universally understood that line management is responsible for setting, achieving, and departing from expectations. Finance personnel provide data and interpret them; they do not enforce budget discipline.

Relation of finance to the governing board and CEO

The finance system relates directly to the governing board through the finance committee, and the CFO often represents the senior management team on the committee.

Finance committee

In this and preceding chapters, several tasks have been specifically identified for the finance committee of the board:

- assist in selecting the CFO;
- annually review the long-range financial plan and recommend the final version to the full board;
- recommend the budget guidelines to the full board;
- recommend pricing policies to the full board;
- review the proposed annual budget and recommend it to the full board;
- set the hurdle rate for capital investments;
- set the final priorities and recommend the capital and new programs budget to the board; and
- receive the monthly or quarterly report comparing operations to expectations.

The list makes it clear why membership on the finance committee is time-consuming and intellectually demanding. Members are important at meetings of the full board as well, and there are often overlapping appointments or joint meetings with the planning committee. In addition, the finance committee has routine obligations to approve the healthcare organization's banks and financial contracts, the specific bond or stock offerings, and the sale of assets and approval of contracts over predetermined levels. The list above can easily fill 10 or 11 fast-paced meetings each year. Virtually the entire staff work for the finance committee is prepared by finance personnel.

Audit committee

Key members of the finance committee are usually on the audit committee, where they select and instruct the external auditor and receive the report and management letter. The CFO and other employees should never serve on the audit committee, so that it is free to pursue any possible question raised by the auditor. Trustees with conflicts of interest over financial matters should be excluded for the same reason.

Measures of Performance

The finance activity can be measured on several of the standard dimensions, but the identification of the parameters, particularly demand and output, is confusing and arbitrary. A practical approach concentrates on four areas in which finance makes its major contributions to the healthcare organization's success:

1. costs for which finance is directly accountable;
2. collection of revenue and management of liquid assets;
3. technical quality of information, reporting, and consultative services; and
4. customer satisfaction with information, reporting, and consultative services.

Cost Measures

Labor and contract services

The finance system has a significant number of employees, consumes much of the computing resource, and often has significant outside contracts for consultation and other services. All of these are costs that should be budgeted, as with any other unit. Accountability can be carried to responsibility centers, as shown in Figure 14.13.

Working capital requirements

Working capital costs are incurred in short-term borrowing, inventories, and accounts receivable. Inventory management is often assigned to the plant system, but it is measured in "turns" per year: average inventory cost divided by supplies used per year. Short-term borrowing is measured by the net annual interest payments. The cost of receivables is measured in "days outstanding": average dollar value of accounts receivables divided by average receivables posted per day. The total working capital requirement is measured in days or simply as a percentage of annual expenditures. These numbers can now be easily benchmarked.

A medium-sized healthcare system spending $500 million annually with a 13-week average billing cycle and a four-week inventory cycle requires about $150 million in working capital, which will cost $6 million per year in interest paid or foregone from investments, the equivalent of about 100 full-time employees.

Other capital costs

Most healthcare organizations now borrow funds for various purposes and simultaneously hold long-term investments. The earnings on investments and costs of borrowing are determined in part by the quality of financial planning and financial management. The amounts, timing, and sources of funds determine the costs for a specific project. All of these activities are under the control of the CFO, who should establish and achieve expectations for investment earnings and the cost of capital as part of his or her annual budgets.

Revenue Management Measures

Operating revenue adjustments

Effective management can reduce revenue adjustments, principally contractual allowances for each third-party contract, bad debts, and charity. Price strategy reduces contractual allowances. More aggressive collection policies reduce bad debts. Accurate posting increases total revenue. Careful case review and pursuit of welfare and other third-party coverage can limit charity allowances.

An expectation should be established for each allowance, and the appropriate RC of the finance group should be held accountable. Benchmarks will be difficult to find; each institution is unique in most of these measures.

Nonoperating income

Healthcare organizations have a variety of sources of income other than those connected with patient care. Most such income is in rents, dividends, and interest earned, but income from unrelated business is also common. There should be expectations for all major types and sources of nonoperating income, and the chief financial officer should be held accountable for these. Many of these income sources are taxable. Successful management maximizes the return after taxes.

Net profit from operations

The expectation for net profit is one of the key elements of the long-range financial plan and is one of the expectations set in the annual budget guidelines. The CFO, the COO, and the CEO share accountability for meeting it. Net profit can be volatile, but large well-managed organizations appear to be able to meet expectations most of the time. The net profit figure is dependent on volume, which is well outside the control of the CFO. While some sensitivity to the difficulty of achieving the net profit expectation is in order, the importance of the measure must be recognized. No other statistic so clearly reflects the long-term health of the organization.

Technical Quality of Financial Services

The external audit and the management letter provide qualitative assessment of large groups of finance activities. Managerial accounting, budgeting, and reporting are not covered by the audit. Neither is the LRFP. These activities are no less critical to success in the long run, however, and there should be expectations for their quality.

Quality of managerial accounting

Internal assessment of the quality of all managerial accounting services requires some ingenuity, but is feasible. Senior finance personnel are equipped to judge the assumptions involved and, if necessary, to audit results. Work done for major proposals and large scale continuous improvement projects can be audited by a second member of the finance group. Outside consultants can be hired explicitly to review internal work. Professional associations and alliances with noncompeting institutions can be used to compare methods and guidelines, and possibly to audit specific projects. At least a subjective evaluation of the quality of work should be prepared annually. It can be used with the customer satisfaction evaluation to establish an improvement agenda.

Quality of the financial plan

Only subjective judgment of the quality of the long-range financial plan is practical. Worse, the people who made the plan are likely to be the ones evaluating it; nonetheless, the importance of periodic review should be obvious. By the time objective tests are available, the organization's existence may be endangered. The following are process criteria met by successful organizations:

- The plan is clear, concise, internally consistent, and consistent with the long-range plan.
- Assumptions and their implications are specified.
- Prudent and reasonable sources have been used to develop external trends, and a variety of opinion has been reviewed whenever possible.
- External events requiring modification are unforeseen by competitors as well as this organization.
- The plan is well-received by outsiders such as consultants, bond rating agencies, and investment bankers.
- The plan develops contingencies on major, unpredictable future events.

As with managerial accounting, professional associations and noncompetitive alliances can help with educational programs and methods.

Customer Satisfaction

External customers

The finance system has a number of contacts with members of the community and should carry these out in ways that reflect positively on the healthcare organization. Patient satisfaction surveys usually include questions about finance services. Many healthcare organizations now sell accounting and financial management services to physicians. Physician satisfaction is measured by market share and surveys. The finance system establishes the image of the organization in a certain sector of the community, including banks, government agencies, self-insuring employers, and insurance carriers. These relationships can be reviewed annually using a letter or phone call from a member of the executive office not directly connected with finance.

Quality of services to line managers

The finance system has a clientele for its internal budgeting and reporting activities in the general managers who must use the information. Services to line management are critical to the continuous improvement program. Their criticisms of it should be heeded, particularly when they deal with the accuracy and timeliness of the information. Concerns with conciseness, clarity, and level of specification are also important. Advice from finance personnel to general managers is also a sensitive matter, and direct assessment of the opinion of general managers about such advice is wise. Formal surveys are appropriate, as are established avenues for complaints and questions that go through a section of the executive office not involved in finance. That unit can hold discussions and review sessions as well.

Suggested Readings

Cokins, G. 1996. *Activity-Based Cost Management: Making It Work. A Manager's Guide to Implementing and Sustaining an Effective ABC System*. Chicago: Irwin Professional Publishing.

Gapenski, L. C. 1998. *Healthcare Finance: An Introduction to Accounting and Financial Management*. Chicago: Health Administration Press.

Hilton, R. W. 1998. *Managerial Accounting*, 4th ed. New York: McGraw-Hill.

Nowicki, M. 1998. *The Financial Management of Hospitals and Healthcare Organizations*. Chicago: Health Administration Press.

Swieringa, R. J., and R. H. Mancur. 1975. *Some Effects of Participative Budgeting on Managerial Behavior*. New York: National Association of Accountants.

Withrow, S. C. 1999. *Managing Healthcare Compliance*. Chicago: Health Administration Press.

Zelman, W., M. McCue, and A. Millikan. 1998. *Financial Management of Health Care Organizations*. Malden, MA: Blackwell Business.

Notes

1. P. H. Campbell, J. Hoch and D. Kouba, *Physician Compensation: A Guidebook for Community and Migrant Health Centers*. Rockville, MD: U.S. Department of Health and Human Services, Health Resources and Administration, Bureau of Healthcare Delivery Assistance (May, 1990)
2. R. W. Hilton, *Managerial Accounting*, 2nd ed. New York: McGraw-Hill (1994)
3. T. R. Prince, *Financial Reporting and Cost Control for Health Care Entities*. Chicago: Health Administration Press, pp. 219–288 (1992)
4. *Ibid*, pp. 89–378
5. G. Cokins, *Activity-Based Cost Management: Making It Work. A Manager's Guide to Implementing and Sustaining an Effective ABC System*. Chicago: Irwin Professional (1996)
6. R. A. Stiles and S. S. Mick, "What is the Cost of Controlling Quality? Activity-Based Cost Accounting Offers an Answer." *Hospital & Health Services Administration* 42(2), p. 193–204 (1997)
7. R. W. Hilton, *Managerial Accounting*, 2nd ed. New York: McGraw-Hill, pp. 618–26 (1994)
8. B. C. James, "Implementing Practice Guidelines Through Clinical Quality Improvement." *Frontiers of Health Services Management* 10(1), pp. 3–37 (Fall, 1993)
9. S. G. Gabram, et al, "Why Activity-Based Costing Works." *Physician Executive* 23(6), p. 31–7 (1997)

10. M. F. Berlin, et al, "RVU Costing Applications." *Healthcare Financial Management* 51(11), pp. 73–4 (1997); M. F. Berlin, B. P. Faber, and L. M. Berlin, "RVU Costing in a Medical Group Practice." *Healthcare Financial Management* 51(10), pp. 80–1 (1997)
11. K. Castaneda-Mendez, "Value-Based Cost Management: The Foundation of a Balanced Performance Measurement System." *Journal for Healthcare Quality* 19(4), pp. 6–9 (1997)
12. J. R. Griffith, D. G. Smith, and J. R. C. Wheeler, "Continuous Improvement of Strategic Information Systems: Concepts and Issues." *Health Care Management Review* 19(2), pp. 43–53 (1994)
13. B. C. James, "Implementing Practice Guidelines Through Clinical Quality Improvement." *Frontiers of Health Services Management* 10(1), pp. 3–37 (Fall, 1993)
14. G. B. Voss, et al, "Cost-Variance Analysis by DRGs; A Technique for Clinical Budget Analysis." *Health Policy* 39(2), pp. 153–66 (1997)
15. R. W. Hilton, *Managerial Accounting*, 2nd ed. New York: McGraw-Hill, pp. 374–375 (1994)
16. *Ibid*, pp. 502–525
17. W. O. Cleverley, *Essentials of Health Care Finance*, 3rd ed. Gaithersburg, MD: Aspen Publishers Inc., pp. 298–310 (1992)
18. H. J. Berman and L. E. Weeks, *The Financial Management of Hospitals*, 8th ed. Chicago: Health Administration Press, pp. 385–585 (1993)
19. M. A. Abernethy and J. U. Stoelwinder, "Budget Use, Task Uncertainty, System Goal Orientation and Sub-Unit Performance: A Test of the 'Fit' Hypothesis in Not-For-Profit Hospitals." *Accounting Organizations and Society* 16(2), pp. 105–20 (1991)
20. R. J. Swieringa and R. H. Moncur, *Some Effects of Participative Budgeting on Managerial Behavior*. New York: National Association of Accountants (1975)
21. T. R. Prince, *Financial Reporting and Cost Control for Health Care Entities*. Chicago: Health Administration Press, pp. 27–146 (1992)
22. *Ibid*, pp. 87–116
23. H. J. Berman and L. E. Weeks, *The Financial Management of Hospitals*, 8th ed. Chicago: Health Administration Press, p. 46 (1993)
24. American Institute of Certified Public Accountants, *Code of Professional Ethics*, Article 101 (1973)
25. L. C. Gapenski, *Understanding Health Care Financial Management*. Chicago: Health Administration Press, pp. 595–634 (1992)
26. *Ibid*, pp. 539–71
27. R. W. Hilton, *Managerial Accounting*, 2nd ed. New York: McGraw-Hill, pp. 618–26 (1994)
28. R. Cooper and R. S. Kaplan, "Measure Costs Right: Make the Right Decisions." *Harvard Business Review* 66(5), pp. 92–103 (September–October, 1988)
29. J. S. Coyne, "Hospital Performance in Multi-Institutional Organizations Using Financial Ratios." *Health Care Management Review* 10(4), pp. 35–55 (1985)
30. M. L. Lynn and P. Wertheim, "Key Financial Ratios Can Foretell Hospital Closures." *Healthcare Financial Management* 47(11), pp. 66–70 (November, 1993)

CHAPTER

15

INFORMATION SERVICES

Within a decade or so, doctors, nurses, and other clinical professions will use electronic systems that suggest a plan of care for each patient based on analysis of both the patient's history and detailed data about specific treatment options. The Internet will be instantly available as a resource for complex cases. Electronic systems will prompt completion of the plan, optimize schedules, order supplies, and demand follow-up of any unexpected occurrence. Complete text and statistical records will establish and monitor expectations at the individual patient level. Forecasts of patients' needs drawn from these plans will be available to each patient service unit. Aggregate data will be used to develop protocols and analyze clinical performance. As the data files evolve, all inpatient care will be supported by electronics and scientific analysis more rigorous than that applied to the most intensive care today. Outpatient management will use instantaneous communications, automated records and protocols to manage a broader range of diseases and conditions than is possible today. The concept, shown in Figure 15.1, would link all clinical activities electronically to the central healthcare database and beyond to health insurance. The database that served individual patient care would also support epidemiologic and quality measures.

Management applications will integrate information from clinical, accounting, and survey sources to support this clinical environment with continuous improvement of processes. Financial support, including both payment and audit of compliance to the insurance contract, will be fully automated through abstracts of the clinical record. Strategic, resource allocation, and organizational decisions will be based on analytic models using the archived data. New protocols will grow out of analysis of history, tested by computerized models and justified by sophisticated business plans. The improvements themselves will meld the clinical advances with the analytic ones. Heuristic algorithms will allow computers to suggest both clinical and managerial decisions. Human participation in the routine decisions will diminish; their role will shift to understanding the patient and the system itself.

If this vision is correct, most healthcare organizations are only now entering the early phases, and information services are in their infancy. In reality, nearly all the activities suggested by Figure 15.1 can be automated. Many have been automated for 30 years, several lifetimes in the information industry. The missing link, and the focus of the coming generation of managers, will be the integration of all this information as a central engine of management. Management will have a dual role as development proceeds. First, it must ensure

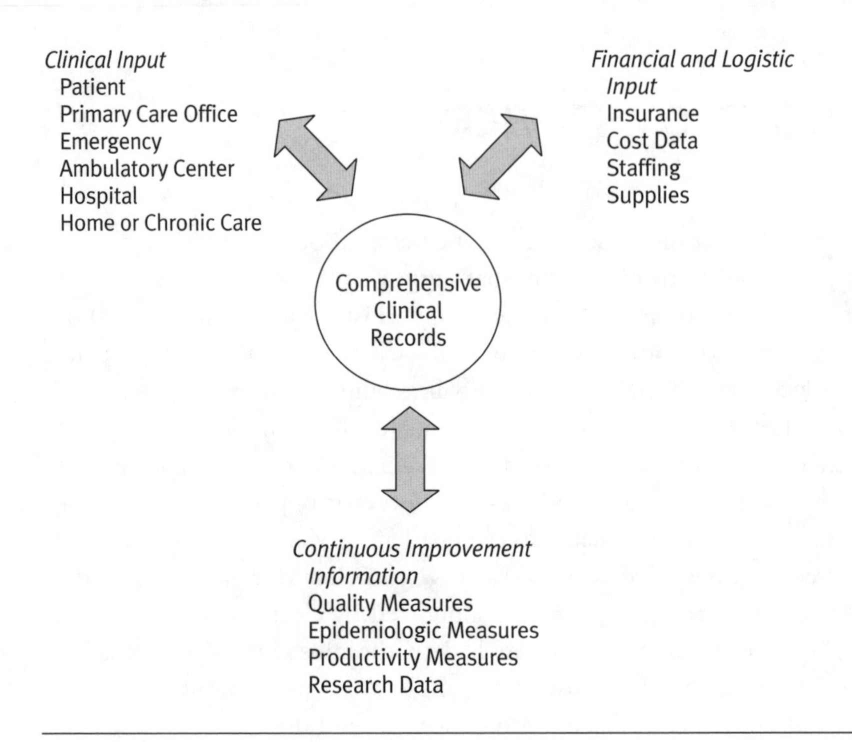

FIGURE 15.1 An Integrated Health Information System

that improvements in clinical automation meet the needs of patients, buyers, and caregivers. Second, it must encourage the managerial applications and guide organization members through the changes as efficiently and humanely as possible.

This chapter surveys the managerial challenges of the information revolution. It postulates a formally accountable information services activity with broad responsibility for all information- and communication-related support to line management, and describes definitions and purpose, functions, organization, and measures of performance.

Definitions and Purpose

Definitions

An **information system** is an automated process of capture, transmission, and recording of information that is accessible to multiple users within an organization. Under this definition, not every computer application is automatically part of an information system. A system is created when the data are routinely shared in an organizationally accessible form. As of the 1990s, most healthcare organizations have several information systems in finance, plant, and clinical services.

The various information systems must themselves be integrated if they are to provide maximum benefit to management. Much of the following discussion will deal with integrated information systems, defined as follows:

> An **integrated information system** is a set of two or more information systems organized to provide immediate electronic access to information in each.

Integration begins when the individual components of Figure 15.1 are linked together. Integration will occur over several stages of increasing sophistication in accuracy and detail, eventually permitting analysis of all the measurement dimensions discussed in Chapter 6. Recent progress has been rapid, driven both by the economic pressures exerted through managed care and by the continuing explosion in information technology. Market demands for cost control and quality assurance have led to organizational redesign, revised processes, clinical protocols, and evidence-based medicine. Many of these changes would have been impossible without the growth of computers, data exchange, and data archiving. Both of the underlying trends are expected to continue, making the growth of integrated systems inevitable. Economic pressures will not abate. Internet and intranet technologies now support telemedicine. Voice and visual transmission with speech recognition are on the current frontier.

The migration toward integrated systems has not been untroubled. Human, statistical, and technical problems must be solved as applications move from freestanding to system to integration. **Information services (IS)** is a formal organizational unit supporting the development and integration of information systems and the supply of information to points of use.

Purpose

Information services is created to be accountable for the development of integrated information systems, and for continuous improvement in information availability and use. It provides high visibility to information needs, ensures organization-wide access to reliable information, supports the infrastructure of communication, facilitates the integration of systems, and promotes effective use of information. The customers of information services are all the other units of the organization. In general, information services fulfills its purpose by stimulating the selection, design, and operation of information systems.

Functions of Information Services

The information services department or unit is accountable for five functions, as shown in Figure 15.2. These are functions that if not done impair the organization as a whole. They require a central authority and unique technical knowledge and skills. Developing and championing the information services plan is critical to justify IS strategic expenditures, and also to ensure compatibility of equipment and software. Ensuring the integrity, quality, and security of data creates a reliable information resource and protects against misuse and violation of confidentiality. Integrating information capture, communication, and routine concurrent processing is the central technical function, including the network for information transfer and the interfaces between processors necessary to smooth interaction. The archives of data quickly become a unique corporate resource that supports the "source of truth" and improves both management and clinical decisions. User training and support is an obligation of all the technical support groups, with emphasis on their area of technical expertise. For IS, the emphasis is on using computer hardware and software efficiently, improving the quality of the archived data, and recognizing new applications opportunities.

Maintain the Information Services Plan

According to Dorenfest Associates, a prominent information services consultant, healthcare organizations purchased about $13.4 billion worth of information services, software, and hardware in 1997.[1] Including labor, information systems appear to have consumed about 4 percent of operating costs of integrated healthcare systems. Additional expenditures were treated as capital expenditures. Leading organizations spend 10 to 20 percent of their net cash flow each year on IS investment, making it one of the biggest categories of capital expense. Expenditures increased at a rate of 15 percent per year from 1993 to 1997.[2]

The Dorenfest survey identifies about 35 separate kinds of software applications that are used to complete the activities shown in Figure 15.3, adapted from Figure 6.6, "Major Data Processing Systems." Although these

FIGURE 15.2
Functions of Information Services

Function	Content
Maintain the information services plan	Process that incorporates line views, establishes a prioritized agenda for progress, commits a block of capital funds for several years, and supports an annual review of specific projects
Ensure the integrity, quality, and security of data	Activity defining measures and terminology, improving data input, and guarding against inappropriate access or application
Integrate information capture and processing	Operation supporting widespread convenient access to current data, archives, and appropriate software through computers and related equipment
Archive and retrieve data	Activity capturing historic, as opposed to current, data to support management and clinical decisions in forecasting, analysis, and the design of improvements
Train and support users	Program to provide training in the use of automated systems and analytic skills; consulting service to improvement teams to assist in forecasting, analysis, modeling, trials, and improvement design

components are in place in almost all large healthcare organizations, the Dorenfest survey indicated that less than half of these institutions had integrated capability in critical areas such as patient record retrieval, financial data, clinical data, or scheduling. A third or more of these organizations reported buying plans in each of these areas.[3] The shaded areas of Figure 15.3 show these deficiencies.

The limitations are a mixture of computer and managerial issues. Patient registration, for example, is straightforward in a single site, but becomes a limitation to the development of Clinical Records and Claims, the leftmost shaded box, when it must be extended to several hundred primary care sites. Many of these sites are owned by physicians and have purchased or leased incompatible registration and claims systems. There are several conceptual solutions to this problem, but few working examples. In the middle row, automated coding is a technical reality, but accurate coding depends on accurate underlying records, a problem largely of human performance. Similarly, cost accounting is understood theoretically, but real cross-functional improvement teams cannot get the quantity and quality of information that the organizations would like them to have. The combination of failures in registration, coding, and cost accounting mean less than desirable performance in the right-hand column.

The tools for improvement are impressive, but individual rather than systematic. A directory of vendors is available from commercial sources.[4] Hardware for information systems is largely a commodity item, purchased to specification at the lowest price. Dorenfest identified 786 software vendors,

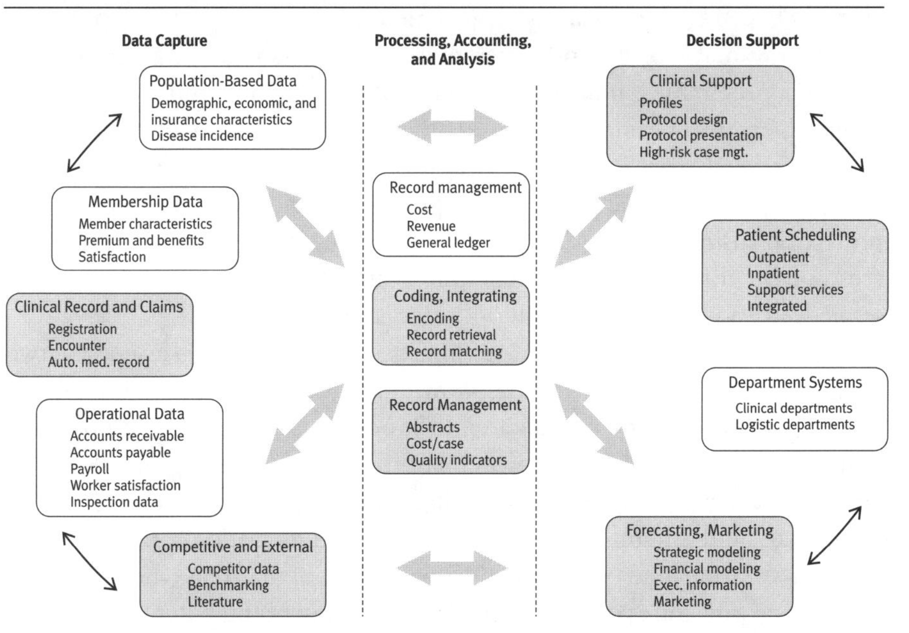

FIGURE 15.3 Important Deficiency Areas in Major Data Processing Systems

most of whom have concentrated on excellence in a single function or subfunction. Although the market is consolidating around a few suppliers, as of 1997, only 14 vendors had installations in more than 25 percent of healthcare organizations.[5] The integration of new systems is now handled largely through trade agreements and industry-wide standards. But many systems in an institution are not new. The oldest, usually inpatient billing systems, go back to the 1960s. These "legacy systems" are usually fitted to new advances by interfaces, rather than replacement of the original code. The infamous "Year 2000" or "Y2K" problem is a representative example. The original code, buried in several layers of modernization, was incapable of handling a number larger than 99. A typical healthcare organization finds itself dealing with one or more of the leaders for basic systems and integration, several of the smaller vendors for specific applications, and a large set of legacy systems. The IS plan provides continuous improvement in capability against this reality.

Strategy for the IS plan

Well-managed healthcare organizations use their IS investment as an explicit competitive strategy.[6] They believe that excellence in information handling will determine future customer decisions and market share; it is as critical to their success as quality care or convenient access.[7] They will use information to improve their healthcare product, making it more attractive than their competition. The information plan is used to establish priorities for the integrated effort, justify the overall investment, and identify the kinds of operational improvements that will result from the added information.

The strategy has two important elements: a long-term commitment and a plan to achieve operational savings and quality improvement as the investments are made. The long-term commitment is necessary because several years elapse between beginning an IS improvement to changing operating processes to take advantage of it. Both operating and IS personnel must commit to a strategy integrating information and process, and they must sustain that commitment throughout the period. Funds are earmarked in the financial plan for several years into the future, protecting a minimum investment in information from the annual ranking process described in Chapter 14. The protection ensures that funding will remain stable, that the paths to real return are thought through, and that the information investments are realistically sequenced and coordinated with operational improvements.

Translating IS investments to improved performance is essentially two different coordination activities, as shown in Figure 15.4. First, several major IS components must be coordinated to produce useful services to operating units. Different component improvements produce different profiles of these services. At the same time, the operating units support continuous improvement goals, and different goals require different information services. The IS plan is best formulated by ranking the importance of the goals (the right-hand side) to basic measures of success, market share, and profitability, and working backward to a timetable for the availability of specific services (the middle) to one for specific IS components (the left-hand side). Given the uncertainty that surrounds each decision, developing the plan is a substantial challenge and a high-risk investment. The ability to think through, gain consensus, and then implement the plan is a hidden key to leadership. Inability has contributed to many organizational failures and can be expected to contribute to many more in the coming decade.

IS Planning Process

The planning process is shown in Figure 15.5. The IS department is responsible for development and implementation of the plan, but because of the centrality of the plan to corporate success, there must be extensive operations and governance participation and approval. Environmental needs and internal operations needs are communicated from planning and operations. An advisory committee includes senior managers from those units, with strong representation from the clinical organization. The IS department must monitor technical developments in information processing, the capability of competitors, and the needs of the general environment to identify important trends.[8] The IS department selects components based on the advice of the committee and on direct surveys and discussions with specific operations units. The plan is incorporated into the organization's strategic plan and long-range financial plan.[9] These two steps require governing board action. Management of implementation other than components for particular departments is an IS responsibility. Annual progress is reviewed against the plan, which is often revised. IS and the line units share accountability for achieving the intended improvements once the new systems are installed.

IS plan content

The IS plan should be a general information strategy that specifies the performance requirements for the organization as a whole over the next three to five years and identifies the information services that will be required to achieve these levels.[10] The IS plans cover the following topics:

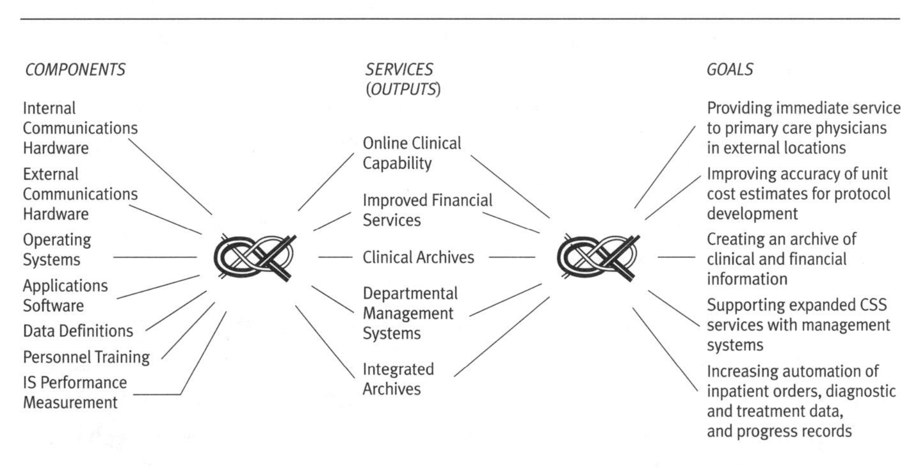

FIGURE 15.4
Elements of IS Plan

FIGURE 15.5
Information Systems Plan Development and Implementation

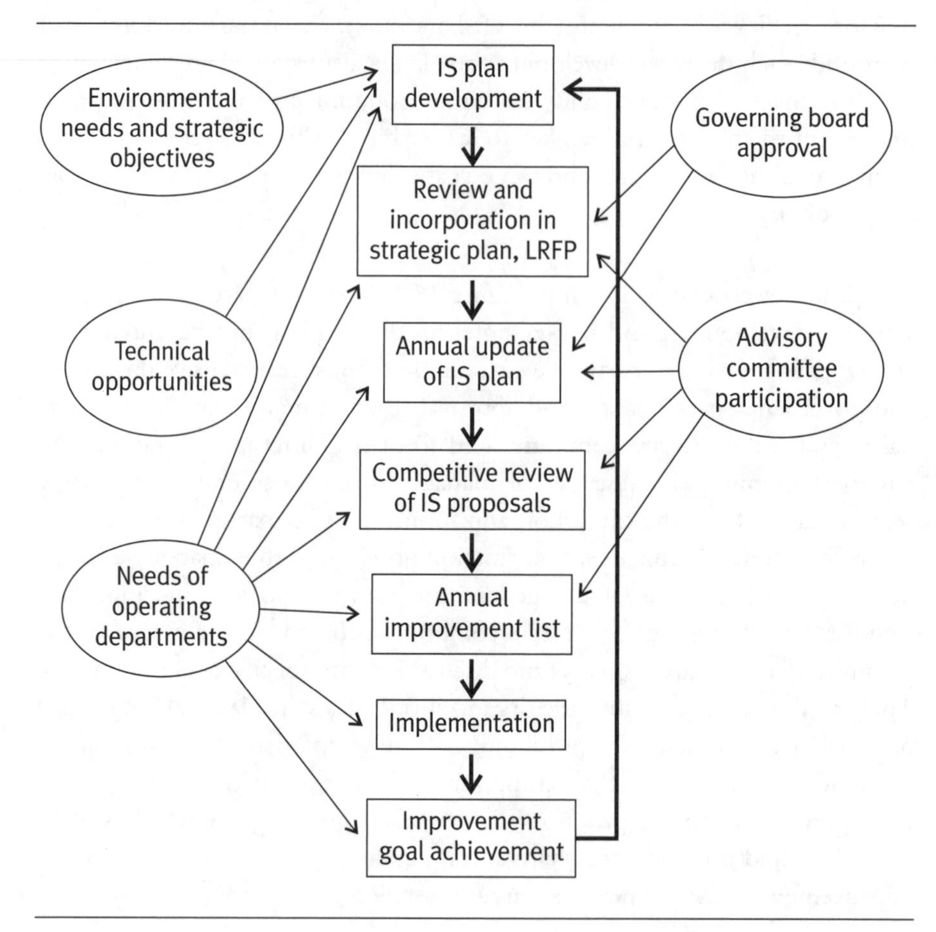

1. information goals, the market share and profitability benefits to be achieved, and the approximate timetable;
2. central hardware plans, with timetables, costs, and financing;
3. improvements in major systems capabilities, with specific timetables, costs, financing, and areas of expected benefit;
4. description of anticipated applications, sources of benefits, and coordination with improvement programs to achieve the benefits;
5. opportunity for requests from individual units, and a procedure for competitive review of unit proposals;
6. plans for system maintenance and user education; and
7. plan for annual review and updating.

Specific requests for improvements in information systems are reviewed against the IS plan, rather than through the capital and new programs budget. (In practice, many information applications that do not require major changes in IS capability can be submitted to either budget. A coordination mechanism is necessary to avoid duplication or confusion but is relatively easy to arrange.)

A sound IS planning strategy has the following characteristics:

Issues in IS planning success

1. It establishes a permanent and expansible infrastructure of communications hardware, operating systems, and uniform data definitions.
2. It identifies essential and desirable applications and rules out those opportunities that are infeasible or problematic in the specific setting. Priorities are based on the needs of the organization as a whole and weighed against the risks of technological or implementation failure.
3. It establishes benefit expectations in terms of specific IS capabilities, but also in terms of global measures of organizational performance. It identifies the operational revisions necessary to gain the benefits and the timetable for return on investment. It represents a commitment by IS and executive management to achieve the plan and its benefits.
4. It is created and implemented within a competitive time frame. The planning process is deliberately completed in time for governing board review prior to the start of the budget cycle. The implementation timetable is realistic and reliable. As with all negotiated expectations, the organization can anticipate compliance with most of the deadlines.
5. It minimizes the risk of technological failure by using tested technology. Emerging information technology moves through three phases—development, initial or "alpha site" testing, larger scale or "beta site" testing, and finally commercial availability as an established, reliable product. Significant costs can be incurred by institutions participating in alpha or beta testing through delays, breakdowns, and reconfigurations. Sharply reduced purchase prices and even royalties from future sales are not uncommon for alpha and beta sites. Even with these discounts, both the risk and the cost of failure may be higher than most institutions should accept.[11] On-site development is deliberately avoided. When essential it is usually a joint venture with a commercial vendor.
6. It recognizes the interactive nature of information systems benefits and contains opportunities for operating units to articulate their own information needs and plans. IS staff assists in development of proposals that are then judged competitively against others, in a manner similar to the new programs and capital budget review.
7. Once adopted, it is annually reviewed, updated, and extended.

Evaluating operational proposals

Information strategies are implemented through proposals for systems improvements. These arise both from IS itself, generally for the infrastructure, and from other operating units seeking process improvements. Figure 15.6 lists ten steps in the planning process for specific information services proposals. The steps in Figure 15.6 appear onerous, but it is dangerous to omit them. As is the case with other programmatic proposals (Chapter 12), well-run organizations seem to make the *preliminary* decisions in steps 1 to 3 quickly, eliminating projects with low value, or that do not support the strategy. They

FIGURE 15.6
Ten Steps in Information System Improvement

Preliminary: Easy steps that allow many possibilities to be scanned

1. Identify

Broad search for possible improvements from survey of current capabilities, market pressure, and IS strategy.

Changes should be expected to yield improved control: *Better mean or smaller variance on one or more performance dimensions, at either intermediate and final product levels.*

2. Justify

Demonstrate feasibility of the proposal:

Commercially available pharmacy management system will provide inventory control and drug use data.

Describe necessary process changes:

Dispensing and drug ordering revisions. Pharmacy Committee revises formulary and prescribing policies.

Quantify anticipated control capabilities:

Inventory costs down at least 20 percent. Better than 50/50 chance prescribing costs for high-cost drugs can be reduced by one-third.

3. Value

Estimate the worth of each control improvement:

Inventory reductions $500,000. Drug usage reductions about $300,000 per year.

Selection: Developing detailed proposals and ranking them competitively

4. Specify

List operating requirements:

Desired features and constraints

Identify and describe available products:

Descriptions for several products

Evaluate each on features, cost, compatibility, expansibility, and maintenance:

May require visits, tests, references, negotiation with vendors

5. Select Vendor

Identify the vendors offering acceptable products. This process is complicated by the fact that both valuation and product specification have several dimensions, and all must be accommodated:

A spreadsheet showing major features and relative advantages of each vendor.

Line units and IS must agree on the best vendor, integrating the various advantages and costs:

Further negotiation with vendors is possible. The vendor of choice is selected.

6. Rank Projects

An IS advisory committee of line managers with IS participation evaluates all proposals completed through step 5. It must incorporate interactions between proposals and rank orders them:

Consensus-building techniques, negotiation, and leadership are often essential.

7. Select Projects

The advisory committee compares the rank-ordered cost against the IS plan and recommends the final list to the governing board:

A rank-ordered spreadsheet presents projects, line commitments, timetables, and costs and benefits in summary form.

continued

FIGURE 15.6 continued

Installation: Installing improvements and ensuring actual performance improvement	
8. Plan Installation	The committee develops a sequential plan for installation of all approved projects, with interim achievements at specified dates: *Line and IS agreement on installation is important.* *Major projects will have a PERT chart and critical path analysis.*
9. Install	IS will monitor installation progress against the plan and will report necessary revisions to the advisory committee.
10. Confirm	IS and line managers involved will monitor performance measures against the value expectations from step 3. Opportunities to exceed expectations will be explored. Performance will be summarized for the advisory committee. IS and line managers will identify the next round of improvements.

then focus their resources on the reduced set of opportunities, make wise *selection* decisions at steps 4 to 7, and follow through *installation* in steps 8 to 10, ensuring that the operational improvements they desired really occur.

The first five steps involve a collaboration between IS and the line units directly affected by a proposal. Together they agree on the system, the benefits, and the vendor. There are often major obstacles. Communication difficulties between the line, which rarely understands information technology, and IS, which often has difficulty understanding clinical requirements and processes, must be overcome. Vendors' systems are not directly comparable. Clinical processes must often be redesigned to follow established best practices. Modification of software to accommodate local idiosyncrasies is rarely wise.

The proposals are usually quite specific as to application, effort, vendor, cost, and implementation timetable. They should be equally clear on benefits. It is impossible to allocate the benefits between the line teams that achieve them and the information system that lets them do it. The solution is to make proposals joint between IS and the line departments involved in implementation. Then both are committed, and the effort to prepare the proposal reveals and solves many of the potential problems.

Figure 15.6 uses a proposal selection process involving an IS advisory committee. The role and structure of the committee is discussed further below. Participating in IS plan development and reviewing specific proposals are the committee's two most important tasks. The committee provides a separate but similar procedure to the new programs and capital budget competition described in Chapter 14.

It is likely that success in IS planning feeds itself. Good strategies, smart selections, and effective installations give the well-run healthcare organization insights into the next round of information systems improvements. Weaker institutions make inferior strategic choices, belabor the selection process, and fail to capitalize on the installation. They find themselves with reduced choices as the delays and opportunity costs mount.

Ensure the Integrity, Quality, and Security of Data

As massive amounts of information develop, and people depend routinely on its use, the importance of uniform definitions, accurate entries, and protection against loss, theft, or corruption mount. A well-managed IS ensures these characteristics by deliberate programs controlling measures, data capture routines, and access to recorded data.

Defining terminology and measures

Any term that is used in a quantitative system must have a precise definition, and the definitions must be kept consistent across many different users. Terms like "admission," "patient day," and "unit price" appear straightforward, but in reality require specific, written definitions to avoid inconsistencies that may later prove troublesome. (For example, is a patient kept overnight in emergency an "admission"? Is a stay of less than 24 hours one day, and if so, how should it be distinguished from a stay of more than 24 hours but less than 48? Is the charge what is billed or what is collected?)

Various units of healthcare organizations are concerned with the problem of accurate definitions. Accounting has used the audit system and a national panel, the Financial Accounting Standards Board, to ensure accurate definitions of public accounts. Over many years, an elaborate system of rules has developed in general use. The American Hospital Association maintains a set of common definitions and statistics that it uses for national reporting.[12]

In clinical areas, medical records administrators and nosologists (specialists in the description and classification of disease) have labored over common medical terms, such as the identification and coding of diagnoses and procedures, for decades. The International Classification of Disease, Version 9, Clinical Modification (ICD9CM) represents the work of an international panel modified to fit national needs but allow worldwide reporting and comparison of diagnoses and procedures.[13] The DRG system is based on ICD9CM and monitored by insurance intermediaries and the federal Health Care Financing Administration. Similarly, a set of physician and outpatient procedure codes, Current Procedural Terminology (CPT), is maintained by the American Medical Association and serves as the basis for outpatient and physician billing.[14] Various professions and specialties have codes for their activities. The College of American Pathologists maintains codes for laboratory tests.[15] Therapists have formal definitions and codes for their treatments. An industry standard language, HL7, is broadly accepted for electronic clinical information.[16] The National Library of Medicine has developed a Unified Medical Language System (UMLS) to support retrieval of biomedical information from a variety of sources, linking disparate computer-based systems.[17]

In other areas definitions are embedded in business contracts and government regulation. The National Bureau of Standards maintains definitions for common measures of time, energy, temperature, distance, and weight as well as thousands of more specialized technical measures.

The first step in ensuring data quality is to compile these definitions and abide by them. But there are so many different sources that problems of conflict and omission are inevitable. A committee on measurement and definitions can ensure that all relevant national sources have been adopted, investigate potential conflicts and ambiguities, and define additional measures the institution needs.

In any case, each term that is entered into a common database or that is used by more than one unit must have a precise definition. With the growth of large-scale storage and access devices, the definitions themselves are available directly from work stations. Coding systems like ICD9CM, CPT, and DRGs are available in a variety of formats.

Data capture

The issues in the capture of information are completeness and accuracy. Missing information is as destructive as errors. The following steps insure accurate data entry:

1. Automated entry is preferable to human entry. Retrieval of information from electronic archives is superior to the human interface, which is both the most expensive and least accurate link in most data entry.
2. All important information should be edited and audited at entry to ensure accuracy. Electronic edits can be built into the capture system to eliminate omissions and keystroke errors. Edits generally are based on a single field of information; the field must contain a certain kind of data, such as certain numbers or letters, or selection from a certain list. Audits generally compare two or more fields for consistency; age, gender, and diagnosis are common examples. The extent of edits and audits depends on the centrality of the information. Key records such as initial patient registration would be subject to the most rigorous control, possibly including duplicate entry by a second worker in addition to several dozen electronic edits and audits.
3. Retrieval is preferable to re-entry. Information should be captured for electronic processing only once. Subsequent patient registrations would require re-entry of several fields of identifying information before recovering an existing entry and would update the original record with changes.

For any data capture involving information shared among organization units, IS should review the design and maintenance of capture forms or screen specifications, edits and audits, information distribution and archiving, and retrieval capability. In addition, IS has complete responsibility for the management of certain kinds of information including:

- *Patient registration and placement records.* This information includes descriptions of present, future, and immediate past patients critical to clinical communication, billing, scheduling, and communication with patients and families.
- *Files of patients' unit record numbers.* Patients are usually assigned a unique, lifetime record number that must be retrieved when the patient returns for care, even after a long absence. A special file accesses not only the patient's name and number, but several confirming attributes, such as date of birth, sex, race, and mother's name. Specialized retrieval and entry systems allow sound-oriented searches, searches by portions of the name, or by other attributes. New entries are audited against existing ones to prevent duplication.
- *Patient medical record files.* Medical records are increasingly automated. The medical records management function has become part of IS in many organizations. The files consist of five broad categories: identification and summary material, work-up and care plans, orders, order results, and notes. The order file supports the patient ledger. It and identification material are now routinely electronic. Results reporting follows after orders are automated. Clinical protocols permit automation of much of care plans and work-ups. Progress is being made on automation of case summaries and many kinds of notes.[16]
- *Patient, employee, and household surveys.* Direct querying of patient and family satisfaction has become a routine device for marketing and outcomes quality assessment. Employee and physician attitudes are important to effective recruitment and motivation, and are also surveyed frequently. Household surveys, which reach people who are not necessarily patients or who use competing sources of care, are less common, but they are important tools for understanding market preferences and market share potentials.

  To be reliable, surveys must use carefully designed protocols, rigorous sampling routines, and extensive follow-up to reduce nonresponse. Central control over the design and administration of surveys is essential to ensure accurate results and interpretation. Control can be lodged either in IS or in units most closely connected to the survey population, such as marketing for patient surveys and human resources for employee surveys.

Other units, particularly planning, finance, and human resources, have extensive responsibilities for automated databases in their areas. IS must ensure that these databases are properly accessible and usable with its own.

Maintaining confidentiality of information

IS is responsible for designing and maintaining systems to protect files against unauthorized use. Most information about specific patients and some employee records are confidential and need to be protected against unauthorized access.[17] IS must identify the confidentiality requirements and incorporate controls in operations to ensure that they are met.[18] These usually take the form of requiring user identification and restricting access to qualified users. Cards, passwords, and voice readers are used for this purpose. Confidentiality is also important in archiving and retrieval. The archive must be protected from inappropriate use and reporting must be constructed in ways that prevent inference about individuals from statistical analyses. Centralized archiving and monitoring of data uses and users protect against these dangers.[19,20] Restrictions on access to small sets of data or certain combinations of data can be built into the archive or the data retrieval system.

The issue of confidentiality is important, but relative. Many healthcare confidentiality problems are similar to other information sources that are now automated, such as driving records, credit records, and income tax files. The real question is one of the benefits of convenient access versus the risk of damage. Reasonable steps to reduce the risk seem to be all that is required to gain general acceptance. Manual systems of handling patient and personnel information were far from foolproof. There is little evidence that computers necessarily make the problem worse; properly designed, they may reduce the chance of misuse or inappropriate access. Proper design is essential, however. Unprotected electronic files can be accessed quickly, in large numbers, for a variety of improper purposes. Commercially available software incorporates substantial protections.

Protecting against loss, destruction, or sabotage

The archives and the installed software of an information system are resources of incalculable value to the organization itself. They are subject to several perils. Physical destruction or loss can result from mislabeling, theft, fire, electrical power disturbances, floods, magnetic interference, viruses, and deterioration.[21] The normal protections are duplication, separate storage, selection, and protection of sites. Thus, central processing and archiving sites are restricted to authorized personnel and are safely located. Power supplies are deliberately redundant. Routine backups are kept in separate sites.

Electronic data and software can be sabotaged by outsiders and employees, working under a variety of motivations. Protection includes personnel selection, bonding, surveillance, and auditing for employees. Outsiders are kept out by passwords and security devices and detected by activity monitors.

Commercial firms now offer both consulting services and direct assistance on data protection. A well-managed organization has a formal plan for maintaining protection and confidentiality, and a recovery plan for each of the perils. The IS department is responsible for maintaining this plan, including monitoring effectiveness, and periodic drills for specific disasters.

Integrate Information Capture and Processing

The function of data communication and processing is to ensure that all users have access to data necessary for their operations, and computing capability to use it effectively. Figure 15.7 abstracts the concept of data integration from Figure 15.2. The major sources of data, discussed in Chapter 6, each access and contribute to each other's needs and create in the process a data archive.

With the growth of decentralized computing, the emphasis of the function has shifted to design and management of integrated systems of hardware and software. The function includes support of the entire patient record system, the maintenance of central hardware and software, including communication systems, and the support of departmental hardware and software.

Supporting the patient record

The patient registration, scheduling, coding, record management, and clinical support functions of Figure 15.2 are information processes reflecting the actual care given the patient, recorded in the patient record. They register all contacts between the patient, caregivers, and the organization. A critical set of financial, legal, and demographic information is created for each episode of care. In all but the simplest encounters, this information is used concurrently by several clinical services as well as the business office. It provides the basic communication between clinical services about each patient. The activities that generate entries are decentralized to many locations in the institution, but automation permits central control of the entry screens, data edits, and data quality.

FIGURE 15.7
The Concept of Integrated Data

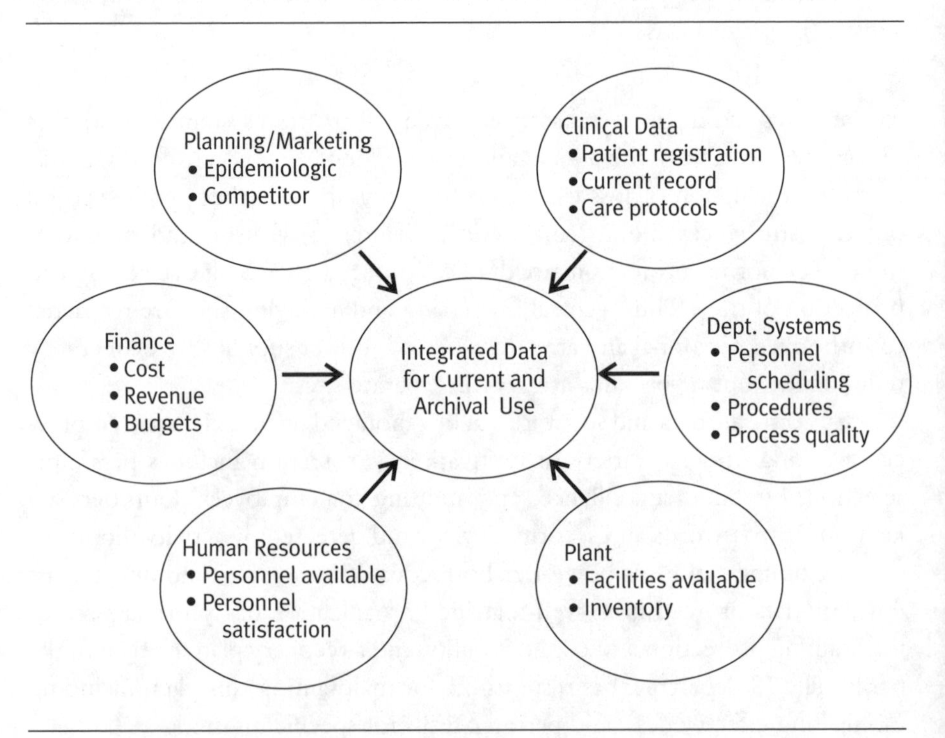

The goal of medical records management has become the automation of all the major parts of the medical record. Automation improves accuracy, permits instantaneous communication, and vastly speeds statistical summary and retrieval. Patient registration, record indexing, order entry, and results reporting systems are now at least partly automated. The frontiers of automation are in recording progress notes and other subjectively determined, patient specific information in major episodes (hospitalization and extensive outpatient care) and in data capture in the primary caregiver's office. The primary care office is often geographically remote, and the process of primary care, where 12 to 15 patients are seen per hour by each caregiver, does not accommodate extensive record keeping.

At completion of a treatment episode, the record is audited for completeness, and diagnostic and treatment codes are assigned. Major episodes, such as inpatient admissions or ambulatory surgery, are summarized. The recorded diagnoses, treatment, codes, and summary must be formally approved by the attending physician or caregiver. The data must be audited and stored, including handwritten elements as well as automated ones. Storage is organized by patient, so that a historic record is available for use at the patient's next need. The individual episode record is also the basis for almost all clinical statistics, and figures constantly in quality and process improvement activities.

The medical records function includes management of record completion and the assignment of codes. Coding and completion must precede billing; substantial revenue is involved in delays or lost records. Rigorous accuracy is essential, both to correctly identify each episode for clinical analysis and to pass audits by insurers. Incorrect codes often lead to lower priced DRG assignments, but deliberate "upcoding" is subject to severe penalties as fraud. Coding requires substantial technical knowledge, but various automated tools are now available to support the coding process.

Communications and centralized services

The personal computer (PC) makes it possible to meet most people's computational needs with a processor and storage facility on their desks. PCs available today for less than $1,000 can carry out more instructions per second than the largest known machines of a decade ago and store four billion bytes of data. (That is 750 times the size of this book.) Their widespread use means that the critical task for IS is no longer to process data or store it; it is to facilitate access and communication.

IS provides for communication by maintaining high-speed links, usually optical fibers, and by operating dedicated hardware and software. These are **local area networks** (LANs) serving individual units within about 1,000 yards of one another, and **wide area networks** (WANs) reaching across cities or around the world. **Client-server** machinery facilitates translation between alternative data formats used by the competing hardware and operating systems. Most large healthcare institutions have installed LANs serving individual hospitals and clinics. They purchase WANs connecting them together from firms specializing in WAN construction. They are beginning to use Internet and intranet to integrate various processors and databases, including telephone, facsimile, and electronic mail communication along with video and other data.

Decentralized hardware and software

Most of the hardware now used by healthcare organizations is decentralized and is part of the resources and accountability of operational units. IS supports the users by the following activities:

1. setting standards for hardware and data management and offering consultative services that help users meet their computational needs at minimum cost;
2. operating networking systems;
3. selecting widely used hardware and software, and negotiating favorable prices by bulk purchase;
4. providing maintenance service and backup equipment to standardized hardware and software; and
5. assisting with financing for proposals accepted under the IS plan.

Most software and virtually all hardware is now purchased from commercial vendors. Even large special purpose routines like inventory management, payroll and personnel systems, and general ledger systems are available from national vendors, sometimes modified for specific healthcare use. Much departmental software is available from smaller vendors. Software used in an information system must meet the IS plan; be compatible with existing hardware, software, and data standards; and be supported by the vendor to adapt to changes in hardware and operating requirements over time. (Units can purchase unsupported software for local uses short of formal information systems. Financial assistance through the IS plan and the value of purchasing contracts and local maintenance are powerful resources to convince operating units on the virtues of uniformity.)

Departmental decision support systems

It is often possible to identify recurring management decisions that can be computerized on departmental information systems. The systems handle the department record keeping, generate automatic communications such as orders and charges for other systems, maintain current or short-term archives, and undertake elementary modeling for scheduling, staffing, and inventory management.

These systems automate management decisions that formerly required substantial time and expert judgment and that were made less consistently by human beings. They become important tools for planning and budgeting as well as aids to day-to-day decision making. An example is the nursing staffing system described in Chapter 10. The system uses counts and severity measures of patient demand with data on the number and skills of nurses to establish staffing. It shows current shortages and overstaffing by unit and shift, and the optimum deployment of available nurses in terms of patient need. A second module suggests staffing levels required for given demand forecasts, estimates employment requirements, and prepares a personnel budget. A third module translates the available personnel levels into a work schedule that optimizes access to nursing care based on forecasts of volume and severity, and a fourth draws samples, prints questionnaires, and tallies results of process quality inspections. Well-managed hospitals now have departmental information systems in many areas, including clinical support services, nursing, human resources, and plant systems. They perform various tasks, but the following elements are frequently present:

- *Personnel scheduling*—work schedules for individual employees that accommodate patient care needs but are also sensitive to employee desires
- *Patient or activity scheduling*—schedules for the performance of specified work (such as housekeeping or routine maintenance) or for the optimal use of physical facilities (such as beds, operating rooms, and x-ray machinery)
- *Recording and process control*—automated tracking of orders and specimens, preparation of reports and records, and word processing
- *Inventory management*—automated re-order, distribution, and accounting for routine supplies
- *Electronic mail*—software to permit multiple users of departmental systems to communicate with each other and, through networking, with other systems
- *Educational and training programs*—automated prompts on the recommended method or procedure for new personnel or infrequent situations
- *Quality assessment*—measures of process and outcomes quality obtained by automated sample selection, questionnaire design, and statistical analysis
- *Job assignment and human resources accounting*—provisions for skill profiles of employees and for day-to-day adjustment of actual work to reflect unpredictable variation in demand for personnel

Several examples of these systems are available for a variety of clinical, human resources, and plant services. The central information service has four functions with regard to departmental decision support systems:

1. assist in the planning, design, installation, and interfacing of the departmental system;
2. provide the necessary historic and current data from other sources;
3. maintain data quality of newly input information; and
4. archive the data of general or permanent value.

Archive and Retrieve Data

Archiving is an automated by-product of integrated information capture. Each of the major systems shown in Figure 15.6 generates archives. Some of the more important are:

- *Archives of clinical activity, compiled from patient records.* These permit historical analysis of output, efficiency, and quality, and variation in performance among sites and providers.
- *Archives of population, marketing activity, patient satisfaction, and competitor behavior.* These support analyses of market needs, promotional activities, and demand.
- *Archives of personnel history, skills, and satisfaction.* These are essential to determine recruitment needs and to assist in attracting highly qualified workers and physicians.
- *Archives of cost and resource use.* These support identification of fixed, variable, and marginal costs and profitability.

These archives are essential for forecasting performance measures, for revealing potential improvements, and for modeling and evaluating them. Many proposals require data from several basic archives.

Other archives can be obtained through the internet. Medsearch, the automated indexing and abstracting service of the National Library of Medicine, is an important example. The archive contains more than 8.7 million references on clinical and healthcare journal publications, accessible by topic, author, publisher, national origin, language of publication, title, and date. An abstract of up to 250 words is available if provided by the publisher, and full text capability is being added. The archive is current generally to the actual date of publication. A team studying a specific surgical procedure could maintain an up-to-the-minute survey of published literature about it. So could a team studying healthcare-related issues, such as the organization of clinical services. Special sections cover healthcare management, nursing and clinical support services, and specific disease groups. The Centers for Disease Control, the Health Care Financing Administration, and many other federal agencies have extensive resources on line.

Archive management

Archiving depends on effective completion of the data integrity function. Given that sound data have been acquired, the archival function emphasizes easy identification and retrieval of the relevant information. Relational retrieval systems have made the recovery of information from internal archives quick and easy. However, most relational systems require specific content and format for data entry. Often only more recent archives are translated to the relational base, and older data require more elaborate retrieval methods.

Executive support systems

The monitoring function of central management is now supported by special purpose software that allows rapid access to large archives of integrated data. Executive support systems take data from several archives, organize them to parallel accountability and cross-functional team structures, and make them available for either routine or special purpose reports. The software accesses the archive, selects the measures of interest, and aggregates them to the level needed. Board and executive level reports can be prepared routinely every month, assuring consistent definitions and data sources. Graphic presentations are automated, as is table construction and labeling. Either screen, slide, or paper formats are possible. Subroutines make it possible to evaluate deviations from expectations in terms of severity, statistical significance, or duration. In screen versions, the user may "drill down" to identify the source and extent of variation.[22] In addition to performance data, archives like personnel names and addresses and employment status are routinely accessible.

Archive user support

The more complicated improvement studies require more than simply the retrieval of specific data. It is necessary to consider whether all possible archives have been included, how to relate data from different archives, and how to deal with omissions and limitations in the data. A decision support specialist familiar with archive content, user needs, and retrieval processes greatly amplifies the value of the archives. Special software may be required to link data from two or more major files. Even in the best data archives there are changes in key definitions and gaps in the data. These weaknesses must be evaluated in relation to the specific questions being asked. For example, a study of a major clinical service such as orthopedics or cardiac surgery might require data from several sources:

- final product performance integrating cost, revenue, and quality data on the major diagnosis or procedure groups in the service;
- patient satisfaction and market share data by major market segment and diagnosis;
- individual performance and satisfaction variation by provider;
- Medsearch bibliographies on important diagnosis or procedure groups;
- scheduling capabilities of clinical support services involved;
- pricing and vendor data for several expensive supply items;
- epidemiologic trends for national and local data; and
- benchmark performance of other provider units.

Most of the information will be retrieved from the archives of the sources generating it. Only the first three topics are likely to be integrated, or to need automated integration, but substantial technical and statistical issues will arise within the first three. The available time period may be different in the clinical and cost data. Is it appropriate to compare or combine the two? Critical definitions may have changed over time. Two new DRGs introduced a year ago divide what once was a single group. Is it better to use the new, or recombine them and gain more history? If there is a loss of some data, can that loss be treated as random, or was it the result of a process that acted systematically on different segments of interest? A sudden loss of demand may reflect the departure of specific surgeons. Were their caseloads similar to everyone else's, or unique? If they were unique, what change does their loss make on the performance statistics? An important part of the archival function is understanding data and computing constraints, devising ways to present the data effectively to users, and making sure the users understand the limitations.

Train and Support Users

The training and user support function includes general training programs and consultation and support for specific applications. While the training function is shared between planning, marketing, finance, and IS, the archives and existing software make IS a major contributor.

General use software

As shown in Figure 15.8, healthcare organizations use a variety of commercial software packages throughout the institution. Standardization of these packages is useful because it facilitates communication, supports cross-functional teams, and permits transfer of operators from one application to another. Selection criteria include user acceptability, compatibility, cost, and service. Microsoft has captured a large share of general applications. Much of this software is deliberately designed to be user friendly. It contains help facilities, comes with manuals, and incorporates much technical material into background that need not be mastered by the casual user. The goal is to make the technically correct analysis easy to do and easy to understand. Software convenience and clarity encourage the decision makers to make maximal use of the data.

Statistical programs make the analysis more rigorous and more reliable, avoiding false conclusions about reality. Graphic packages permit the prompt generation of colorful displays, which help many people understand the meaning of statistics. Spreadsheet software allows the construction of alternative scenarios and the search for the best solution based on the improved understanding that comes from statistical analysis and graphic display. A central activity of continuous improvement is the search for the optimal set among these numerous alternatives. Spreadsheets allow the decision makers to ask "what if" questions and trace the implications in terms of key performance variables like cost, profit, and quality.

More elaborate software for modeling several financial activities is well developed and is now available commercially. Software for examining alternative pricing decisions and designing future capital debt structures is in widespread use among well-managed institutions. Also emerging is software that addresses marketing-related issues of expansions, acquisitions, and changes in final product profiles. Although the use of financial and statistical modeling requires much expense and effort, it is rapidly becoming standard practice for all decisions at the strategic level.

An example is the development of strategies for medical staff recruitment. Word processors, calendars, and message systems are now expected as devices to communicate; they would be used to justify further study and build

FIGURE 15.8 General Use Software

Software	Use	Common Trade Names
Word processing	Text entry, formatting, archiving. Allows multiple authors for major reports, subject searches of minutes, etc.	Word WordPerfect
Spreadsheet	Repetitive calculations, graphics, some statistical analysis. Allows multiple versions of business plans, budgets, etc.	Lotus Excel
Database	Uniform entries to data sets, rapid retrieval, sorting. Allows easy segmentation of customer lists, inventories, etc.	Paradox Access FoxPro
Message	Easy posting and retrieval of messages. Allows rapid, recorded communication between many users.	Mail CC:Mail
Calendars	Agendas, schedules, contacts, and future obligations. Allows easy tracking of multiple activities, facilitates planning.	Sidekick Advantage On-Schedule
Statistical	Advanced analysis of quantitative data. Allows specialized regression and significance testing.	SAS, Systat
Graphics	Advanced presentation formatting and graphics. Allows convincing graphics, tables, and charts.	Harvard Graphics PowerPoint

an improvement team. Statistical and graphic analysis would be used to forecast population trends and patient demand statistics. The potential demand would be organized by primary and specialty care. Spreadsheet software would develop a model showing the impact of alternative locations and specialty mixes on visits, market share, admissions, requirements on clinical services, and revenues. Once the optimum location and specialty mix was determined, the results would be fed to the long-range financial plan to incorporate the impact of these decisions on overall operations.

The IS role includes:

- *Identifying the preferred vendor or vendors.* Large institutions may wish to support more than one vendor. Often institutions that have acquired or merged activities will be forced to support two or more vendors.
- *Encouraging adoption of the software.* Learning to use new software requires an investment of time and money before the advantages occur. One IS role is to encourage units to make this investment.
- *Negotiating price and supplier maintenance.* IS can arrange an organization-wide license and usually can negotiate price advantages and, in some cases, extended service.

- *Providing maintenance and updates.* While general use software requires very little maintenance, periodic updates are issued. These must be evaluated, purchased if desirable, and installed, together with whatever training is indicated.
- *Supporting the selected software with training and consultation.* IS can provide introductory training for new installations and new employees and advanced training for people making extensive applications. Similarly, it can provide assistance when problems arise. These activities are part of the larger training and consultation services discussed below.

Training programs

Users need training at two levels. New employees or new users need introductory training. Experienced users and people facing unique needs frequently require advanced training. The training should go beyond use of the software to include information about available data and approaches to analysis. The objective is not just familiarity with a tool, it is application of the tool for improved performance. Training should show how the software can be used with common CQI tools, for example. The selection and design of graphs and tables is a useful topic. Advanced training should show appropriate applications of elementary statistics, or address specific issues of recurring concern, such as advanced analysis of control chart statistics.

Training should emphasize the most efficient medium. Formal classroom instruction is one approach, most efficient when the content is relatively clear, human interaction is usually necessary, but the level of interaction is such that one instructor can assist several students. Written and electronic media are far less expensive and allow students to proceed at their own pace, but they lack human interaction. Backing them up with messages and consultation helps ensure that the students will remain motivated and make steady progress. Electronic conferences and user groups are popular. They tend to emphasize unique applications requiring considerable human interaction on a one-to-one level.

Consultation

Most large ISs offer a help desk that supplements other training activities. Experts in general software who can help users attempting specific tasks staff the desk. It is usually accessible electronically and by telephone.

More extensive consultation should also be available, although it can be provided in planning, marketing, or financial management. Although mastery of the general software is included, the subject of the consultation is more problem oriented—ways to accomplish certain analyses, interpret ambiguous results, improve graphic displays, overcome limitations in the data.

Management engineering consultation is used by many well-managed organizations. The engineers are trained in analysis of work processes, statistical and financial analysis, development of stochastic and deterministic models, field testing, and design of improved systems. Their skills include most of the areas important to an RC or cross-functional team working on an improvement. They tend to be heavy users of the archived data, and, therefore, are familiar with it and its limitations. Similarly, their training allows them to answer many of the technical questions in statistics and cost accounting.

Organization of Information Services

Well-managed healthcare organizations have sought centralization, direct accountability to top line officers, and enhanced visibility as a way to promote information services. They use a structure like that shown in Figure 15.9, with central accountability placed high in the organization as a whole. The five functions can be divided several ways but the three-part design shown has the advantage of linking similar activities into identifiable roles of roughly equal size and separate skills.

The discussion of the organization includes the roles of the chief information officer and the IS advisory committee, the major functions outlined in Figure 15.9, and the use of outside consultants and information service vendors.

Chief Information Officer

The role of an information executive or chief information officer has emerged with the growth of IS and has tended to move to a higher level within the organization. CIOs report either to the CEO, COO, or CFO and are part of the senior management team. Reporting to the CEO or COO ensures recognition of the nonfinancial aspects of information management and gives

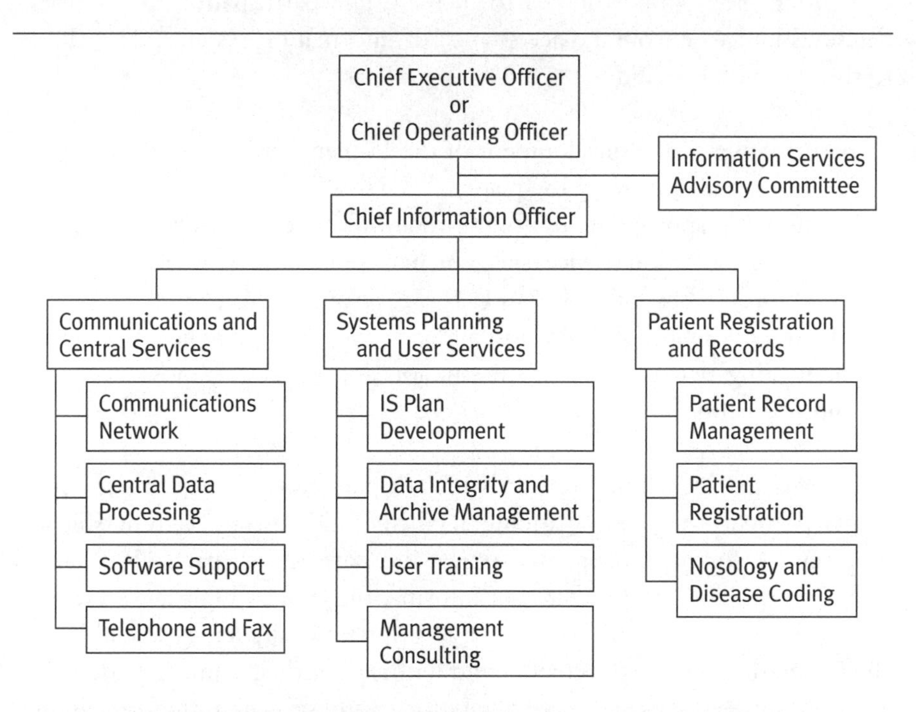

FIGURE 15.9 Organization of Information Services

the CIO equal stature with other essential operational and technical support executives. Early CIOs were masters of computer technology. The future CIO is likely to need a broad understanding of both the technology and of healthcare applications. Leadership and negotiating skills will distinguish excellence. Much of the burden of representing information needs in strategic decisions falls on CIOs. Their role in many situations will be to convince others of the power of information and encourage them to use it effectively.[23] Success will be accompanied by increased demand, and continued success will require effective service. In larger institutions, the IS itself will include several dozen employees, enough to present a management challenge.

Training for the CIO can come from several routes. Training in computer operations, management engineering, or medical records administration provides a useful beginning, but an advanced degree in management engineering, business, or health administration is valuable. Many CIOs in larger facilities have doctoral level preparation. Experience in healthcare information systems is clearly essential. Consulting experience is common in CIO backgrounds. A professional organization, CHIME, provides continuing education and similar services.[24]

Information Services Advisory Committee

A committee of key users of information services is an important adjunct to a well-run department. The committee's purposes include broad representation in the development of systems investment priorities and communication to ensure effective systems design and integration. On a different level, the committee offers opportunities to increase line participation in important decisions and to encourage acceptance of information systems. The charge to the committee includes:

1. participating in the development of the IS plan, resolving the strategic priorities, and approving the plan;
2. encouraging appropriate use of information services;
3. ranking information services investment opportunities and recommending a rank-ordered list of proposals to the governing board;
4. advising on definitions of terms; and
5. monitoring performance of the division and suggesting possible improvements.

Membership should routinely include persons from major user departments, particularly finance, planning, medicine, and nursing. Membership can be a reward for supervisory personnel who have shown particular skills in using information. The director of information services is always a member and may chair the committee. Other appropriate chairpersons would be the chief operating officer, the chief financial officer, or their immediate deputies. The committee will use a variety of task forces and subcommittees, expanding participation in smaller projects, but using its authority to coordinate these activities.[25]

Patient Registration and Records

The volume and importance of clinical data supports a separate activity with an executive who can deal directly with clinical professions. As the traditional medical records activity changes it becomes an inescapable part of an integrated information services. As retrieval technology becomes more widespread, and heuristic use of patient data files more common, the need for combined technical skills in coding, retrieval, statistics, and interpretation will make this a major center of information services. Specialists in clinical information management have a professional association, the American Health Information Management Association.[26] The association offers several levels of certification, culminating in the Registered Record Administrator, which requires specific baccalaureate education. It also offers certification programs for medical coding skills.

Communications and Central Services

The operations group is responsible for the following activities:

- operation of centralized processing and shared peripherals;
- maintenance of the communications network;
- management of the physical archive and retrieval software;
- maintenance of personal computer and work station hardware;
- maintenance of all software in common use, including mainframe and supported personal computer programs; and
- consultation on planning issues.

As the automated activities have increased in scope, the networked computer system has become more complex and the operational requirements have become more demanding. In particular, order communication requires continuous service of many more remote terminals, with a much lower tolerance of service delays. Shared data such as patient registration information is now required almost instantly through the hospital, and the goal is to make it available to ambulatory sites. Operations tolerances are very narrow. People now rely on trouble-free computing, and failures can cause massive disruptions.

The operations group is also responsible for implementing improvements. These are usually managed with project teams, and project management can be a substantial part of operations.[27] The teams can incorporate IS users and coordinate all parts of major revisions.

Systems Planning and User Services

A well-managed information services unit will have people who devote significant parts of their time to "closing the loop" of information use. Their activities will include management of the IS planning process (Figure 15.5) and assisting line teams to develop information-oriented improvements using the ten-step approach described in Figure 15.6. The user services unit can manage the archive and be accountable for decisions about data integrity and security. It can coordinate definitions, with input from patient records, accounting, and others. As the "source of truth" function has grown, it has gained increased visibility in the organization. At least one leading organization makes the archive and information manager an independent member of the senior management team, as vice president for quality improvement.[28]

Training and consultation in using information systems is a natural extension of planning and installation, and it is frequently essential to realization of benefits. Training is important both for new installations and for continued operations. Personnel turnover and systems development make ongoing training essential.

Decision support is an internal consulting activity oriented around performance improvement. Management engineers and statisticians in this unit support all forms of improvement studies. They are trained to help managers analyze operating problems and develop work methods. They are equipped to work closely with people from finance, planning, and marketing on large-scale problems.

Familiarity with the archives, the information systems, and the analytic software are important advantages for this group. Their experience with data definitions and processing routines is an added advantage. They should be able to model improvements and design field trials. Many of the existing departmental decision support systems arose from engineering studies and operations research. Conversely, their knowledge of the operating problems makes them valuable contributors to information systems planning. Management analysis requires close collaboration between the technical support activities. It can be located in a separate technical support group, or in planning/ marketing units. Placing the major analytic capability in IS ties it to a resource valued by the line managers. It gives analysts the opportunity to use computerization as a reward, overcoming perceptions of implied criticism or a threat that often accompany internal consultants.

Use of Outside Contractors

The question of outside contracting for information services is often controversial. On the one hand, there is a well-founded tradition of not allowing a critical service outside the organization itself. On the other, information services is a highly technical area where the expertise of a vendor may be of great value. It pays to understand the opportunities and hazards of outside contracting to evaluate the opportunities specifically, rather than by rule-of-thumb.

Several kinds of assistance from outside contractors are available for information services:

1. *Integrated software support.* Commercial companies develop standardized comprehensive integrated software that is usable in a great many smaller healthcare organizations. The companies providing the software also maintain it, incorporating changes imposed by outside agencies and technological advances. They sometimes offer customization services as well.
2. *Finance.* Leases and mortgages on hardware are generally available from a variety of outside sources. Software is usually available for purchase or lease from the software vendor. However, there are transaction costs in dealing with several different companies and in using general institutional debt for information systems. An outside contractor can consolidate the financing and offer a comprehensive system on a single lease.
3. *Consultation and planning.* Assistance in selecting hardware and software, analyzing current capabilities, benchmarking, and developing a plan for improvements is available from accounting firms and other consultants. Larger organizations and those where standardized solutions will not be appropriate frequently rely on independent consultants to assist them in identifying all information opportunities and selecting a coordinated package.
4. *Facilities management.* A few companies specializing in healthcare organization needs operate on-site data-processing services under contract. These companies also arrange for financing for the facilities and can be hired for consultation and planning.
5. *Joint developmental ventures.* For those healthcare organizations in a position to develop new or improved applications, collaboration with an established vendor is highly desirable. The vendor brings experience, extra personnel, capital, and a marketing capability if the development succeeds.

In a complex, rapidly moving technical field, the use of a consultant is often prudent. Consultants can assist materially with the IS plan. Few healthcare organizations have the expertise to forecast developments in hardware, software, and applications. Both management consulting firms and public accounting firms offer consulting services, as do the firms providing direct information services. There are advantages to each type of company, but the key criterion should be a record of successfully identifying rewarding applications, whether they are in the finance, clinical, or some other system of the hospital.

Integrated software services tend to be selected by smaller institutions. Relatively complete applications are available at an attractively low price. Flexibility is quite limited, and there is little customizing. Improvements must be selected from among the offerings of the company. The availability of special finance options and alternatives for computer hardware adds to the organization's supply of capital and can help lower the cost of financing generally.

Facilities management of information services has appealed to both large and small organizations. The contracting firm is expected to name a senior IS manager with technical skills and knowledge comparable to those of a manager the organization would employ. The on-site manager is supported by the broader experience and specialized knowledge of the contractor's other employees. The skills of the outside group are often useful in information services planning and systems installation. Lower level employees may work either for the contractor or the healthcare organization.

A role remains for hospital leadership. The advisory committee would remain in place. The information services plan must become a collaboration between the contractor and the institution. The contractor has no incentive to limit the hospital's choices and usually will profit from an excessive program for improvement. Thus, even with a facilities management contract, hospital governance has the responsibility and the opportunity to select improvements and pace the evolution of the information system. Some well-run organizations hire both service and consulting firms. Although the cost is high, the test of the result is in improved operations. If the information services committee can incorporate the full set of information, balance the competing viewpoints, and devise a more effective program, the cost is justified.

Measures of Performance

Performance measures for IS should cover the full set of six dimensions shown in Figure 6.2. The customers for IS include all the other systems of the organization and some outside clients, but the critical test is the ability to serve clinical departments. Performance expectations are set as they are elsewhere, using a negotiation process centered around the annual budget. Benchmarks, customer needs, and the experience of consultants will be used frequently to set expectations, but as usual, expectations must be set so that they are achieved or exceeded in the vast majority of cases. Monitoring will be important to identify future improvements, to reward the information services committee and information services personnel, and to suggest corrections in the rare cases in which expectations are not achieved.

Figure 15.10 shows an array of measures designed to assess the overall contribution, and organized by the major service units of a large IS. Most of these are derived from standard cost accounts, the operating logs detailing automated activities, and activities of the director, subordinate units, and the information services committee. Many can be automated and obtained at low cost. Some require special surveys of line managers. Several require a departmental audit. A large number of specific activity measures can be devised to supplement the list in Figure 15.10.

The measures in Figure 15.10 emphasize quality and service more than resources consumed. While resource consumption is important, the central management question for IS is not "How much are we spending?"

FIGURE 15.10 Global Measures for IS Performance

Dimension	IS Unit	Measures
Demand	Communication and central services	Peak load systems users
	System plan and user services	Requests for consultation Requests for training
	Patient registration and records	Requests for records Requests for registration
Costs	Communication and central services	Labor and supplies costs by activity Equipment costs by activity Cost of improvements
	System plan and user services	Labor costs by activity
	Patient registration and records	Labor costs
Human Resources	All	Employee recruitment and satisfaction
	Patient registration and records	Training and certification of coding personnel and record administrators
Output and Productivity	Communication and central services	Cost per user hour or contact
	System plan and user services	Cost per consultation Cost per trainee hour
	Patient registration and records	Cost per patient
Quality	Communication and central services	Machine failures Timely implementation of improvements
	System plan and user services	Comparative scope of service Audit of archive operation
	Patient registration and records	Record completeness Delay to deliver record JCAHO audit
Customer Service	Communication and central services	Peak access delay User satisfaction
	System plan and user services	Trainee satisfaction Line manager satisfaction
	Patient registration and records	Clinical service satisfaction Technical support satisfaction

but "What are we getting for the money?" The outside audit is important. While the JCAHO devotes increasing attention to IS, an annual or biennial audit by a consultant expert could address the full scope of issues and provide a comparison to similar institutions. The audit team would examine centralized operations for the adequacy of service and the appropriateness of software, hardware, and costs. It would review patient records for completeness, timeliness, and accuracy. It would evaluate the IS plan in light of achievements of others and the current state of services and archives. It would evaluate both the kinds of training and consultation available and the quality of actual work.

Suggested Readings

Antosz, L. (ed.). *Health Care Software Sourcebook.* Gaithersburg, MD: Aspen Publishers, published annually.

Austin, C. J., and S. B. Boxerman. 1997. *Information Systems for Health Services Administration*, 5th ed. Chicago: Health Administration Press.

Chapman, A. R. (ed.). 1997. *Health Care and Information Ethics: Protecting Fundamental Human Rights.* Kansas City, MO: Sheed & Ward.

Committee on Maintaining Privacy and Security in Health Care Applications of the National Information Infrastructure, Computer Science and Telecommunications Board, Commission on Physical Sciences, Mathematics, and Applications, National Research Council. 1997. *For the Record: Protecting Electronic Health Information.* Washington, DC: National Academy Press.

Duncan, K. A. 1998. *Community Health Information Systems: Lessons for the Future.* Chicago: Health Administration Press.

Kissinger, K., and S. Borchardt (eds.). 1996. *Information Technology for Integrated Health Systems: Positioning for the Future.* New York: J. Wiley.

Mattingly, R. 1997. *Management of Health Information Functions & Applications.* Albany, NY: Delmar Publishers.

McWay, D. C. 1997. *Legal Aspects of Health Information Management.* Albany, NY: Delmar Publishing.

Nicholson, L. 1999. *The Internet and Healthcare*, 2nd ed. Chicago: Health Administration Press.

Prokosch, H. U., and J. Dudeck (eds.). 1995. *Hospital Information Systems: Design and Development Characteristics, Impact and Future Architecture.* Amsterdam/New York: Elsevier.

Shapiro, J. (ed.). 1999. *Guide to Effective Healthcare Information and Management Systems and the Role of the Chief Information Officer.* Chicago: Healthcare Information and Management Systems Society.

Ziegler, R. (ed.). 1997. *Change Drivers: Information Systems for Managed Care.* Chicago: American Hospital Publishing.

Notes

1. S. Dorenfest & Associates, Ltd., *Selected Industry Findings from the Dorenfest Databases.* Chicago: Dorenfest Associates p. 81 (1998)
2. *Ibid*, pp. 81–2
3. *Ibid*, pp. 66–7
4. Aspen Reference Group and L. Antosz, ed., *Health Care Software Sourcebook.* Gaithersburg, MD: Aspen Publishers (1997)
5. Dorenfest Associates, pp. 57–8
6. J. B. Martin, A. S. Wilkins, S. K. Stawski, "The Component Alignment Model: A New Approach to Health Care Information Technology Strategic Planning." *Topics in Health Information Management* 10(1): 1–10 (Aug. 1998)
7. M. G. Kahn, "Three Perspectives on Integrated Clinical Databases." *Academic Medicine.* 72(4): 281–6, (Apr, 1997)

8. D. D. Moriarty, "Strategic Information Systems Planning for Health Service Providers." *Health Care Management Review* 17(1): 58–90 (1992)
9. J. R. Griffith, V. K. Sahney, and R. A. Mohr, *Reengineering Healthcare: Building on Continuous Quality Improvement.* Chicago: Health Administration Press (1995)
10. A. L. Lederer and V. Gardiner, "Strategic Information Systems Planning: The Method/1 Approach." *Information Systems Management* 13: 20 (Summer, 1992)
11. J. R. Griffith, *Designing 21st Century Healthcare: Leadership in Hospitals and Healthcare Systems.* Chicago: Health Administration Press, pp. 105–108 (1998)
12. American Hospital Association. *Hospital Statistics, 1993–94 edition.* Chicago: American Hospital Association, xiii–xxx (1993)
13. *International Classification of Diseases, 9th Revision, Clinical Modification*, 2nd ed. Washington, DC: U.S. Department of Health and Human Services, Health Care Financing Administration (1980)
14. *CPT 94 Physicians' Current Procedural Terminology.* Chicago: American Medical Association (1994)
15. College of American Pathologists, Committee on Professional Relations *Guidelines for Pathologists: Professional Practices* 1st ed. Skokie, IL: The College of American Pathologists (1977)
16. C. J. McDonald, "The Barriers to Electronic Medical Record Systems and How to Overcome Them." *Journal of the American Medical Informatics Association*
17. http://nlm.nih.gov. U.S. National Library of Medicine. Last updated 23 Feb. 1998.
18. Committee on Maintaining Privacy and Security in Health Care Applications of the National Information Infrastructure, Computer Science and Telecommunications Board, Commission on Physical Sciences, Mathematics, and Applications, National Research Council, *For the Record: Protecting Electronic Health Information.* Washington, DC: National Academy Press (1997)
19. A. R. Chapman, ed., *Health Care and Information Ethics: Protecting Fundamental Human Rights.* Kansas City, MO: Sheed & Ward (1997)
20. B. Wright, "Health Care and Privacy Law in Electronic Commerce." *Healthcare Financial Management* 48(1): 66, 68–70 (January, 1994)
21. Council on Scientific Affairs, American Medical Association, "Feasibility of Ensuring Confidentiality and Security of Computer-Based Patient Records." *Archives of Family Medicine* 2(5): 556–60 (May, 1993)
22. R. J. Cox, *Managing Institutional Archive: Foundational Principles and Practices.* New York: Greenwood Press (1992)
23. T. Franks, "The Strategic Advantage: Decision Support Through Executive Information Systems." *Computers in Healthcare* 12(1): 36,39 (January, 1991)
24. J. Griffin, "The Modern CIO: Forging a New Role in the Managed Care Era." *Journal of Healthcare Resource Management* 15(4):16–7, 20–1 (May, 1997)
25. College of Healthcare Information Management Executives website: www.chime-net.org/index.asp (viewed 10/2/98)
26. C. Sjoberg and T. Timpka, "Participatory Design of Information Systems in Health Care." *Journal of the American Medical Informatics Association* 5(2): 177–83, (Mar-Apr, 1998)

27. American Health Information Management Association. Chicago: website www.ahima.org/index.html. (updated: September 21, 1998)
28. K. Mahlen, "Project Administration Departments Improve Information Systems Initiatives." *Healthcare Financial Management* 51(12): 38, 40, 42, (Dec. 1997)
29. J. R. Griffith, *Designing 21st Century Healthcare.* Chicago: Health Administration Press, pp. 101–103 (1998)

CHAPTER

16

HUMAN RESOURCES SYSTEM

In 1996, healthcare organizations had nearly ten million employees, reflecting a steady increase throughout the preceding two decades.[1] The number of professions and job categories had also increased. A typical medium-sized healthcare organization employs persons in more than three dozen licensed or certified job classifications, including building trades and stationary engineers as well as clinical professions. Many of the positions are held by part-time personnel. The number of individuals employed is about 30 percent larger than the full-time equivalents (FTE) count.

In addition to **employees**, the human resources of a healthcare organization include doctors and others whose services are contracted through arrangements other than employment, and volunteers. The employed healthcare work force supports a physician group of nearly 500,000 in more than two dozen specialties.[2] Finally, healthcare organizations also use contract labor services, via long-term management contracts for whole departments and shorter contracts for specific temporary assistance. Long-term contracts are common for housekeeping, food service, and data processing. Among the shorter are consultation contracts with accounting firms and planning firms, as well as shift-by-shift requests for nurses, clerks, and other hourly workers. In total, a medium-sized healthcare organization requires more than 1,500 persons working at about 1,000 full-time jobs in about 100 different skills.

This group, referred to in earlier chapters as the "members" of the organization, constitutes the most important asset, its human resource. Regardless of the specific relationship, each member joins the organization in a voluntary exchange transaction. The member is seeking some combination of income, rewarding activity, society, and recognition. The organization is seeking services that support other exchanges. Some aspects of the exchange relationship with members deserve emphasis.

1. The members are absolutely essential to continued operation. Members' motivation and satisfaction directly affect both quality and efficiency. Unusually high motivation can provide a margin of excellence, while a few highly dissatisfied members can temporarily or occasionally disrupt operations.[3]
2. Membership, like the seeking of care, is a free choice for most people. Even those whose skills can be employed only in specific settings, like operating rooms, usually have some choice of which institution they will work at and how much work they will seek. Success in attracting and keeping

members tends to be self-sustaining; the organization with a satisfied, well-qualified member group attracts more capable and enthusiastic people. The well-run organization markets itself to its members almost as much as it markets itself to its customers.

3. The members represent only about 3 percent of the community served, but because of their close affiliation and their frequent contact with patients, they are unusually influential.
   - As a promotional force, members—both those who come into direct contact with patients and those whose unseen services determine patients' safety and satisfaction—are powerful. What they say and do for patients and visitors will have more influence on competitive standing than any media campaign the organization might contemplate.
   - As an economic force, members are also significant. Healthcare organizations are always important employers in a community. Healthcare organizations are often the largest employers in a community, even without including their affiliated physicians and their employees. Furthermore, about half the payroll represents income from outside the community, largely Social Security payments for Medicare. Finally, most of the employment opportunities are in unskilled and semi-skilled jobs. The economic impact is weighted to lower-middle-class females, a group presenting serious employment problems for many communities.
   - As a political force, members can command increased respect for the healthcare institution among elected officials of government and labor unions by demonstrating their support of it. While members are only about one-tenth as numerous as patients, their strength can be multiplied when the issue is important enough to motivate their families, as is often the case when substantial numbers of jobs are at stake.

This chapter reviews the purpose of human resources management, the functions that must be performed to sustain an effective workforce, the organization to accomplish the functions, usually called the human resources department, and the measures of success in performing the functions.

Purpose of the Human Resources System

The purpose of the **human resources system** is to plan, acquire, and maintain the skills, quality, and motivation of members consistent with fulfillment of the organization's mission. Because a properly worded mission defines community, service, and cost, this purpose accommodates both the profile of skill levels and the needs for economy defined by the governing board (Chapter 3). Motivation and quality reflect the exchange nature of membership contracts; the human resources system manages all of the monetary transactions and many of the nonmonetary rewards.

The human resources department is a major logistic support unit that provides most human resource functions for nonprofessional employees and a large share of those for professional employees. The department is a central element of a human resources system, but not all of it. The department emphasizes recruitment, training, and compensation services; other parts of the organization affect the system with workplace environments and job definitions. Doctors and volunteers are least likely to be directly affected by the human resources department, but well-run organizations are increasingly placing key functions of these groups under the department. In the well-run organization, the human resources department advises on all human resource issues, contributing technical expertise and reinforcing the workplace culture.

Functions of Human Resource Management

Levine and Tyson, reviewing the empirical literature on employee participation, noted that participation produces at least short-run gains in productivity and sometimes produces substantial long-term improvements.[4] The four characteristics that emerge from the literature as promoting productivity are:

1. some form of profit sharing or gain sharing;
2. job security and long-term employment;
3. measures to build group cohesiveness; and
4. guaranteed individual rights.[5]

These characteristics are similar to the empowerment and measurement goals of continuous quality improvement; they depend on the overall performance and culture of the organization. But given sound performance by other parts of the organization, the human resource system must accomplish six functions to support a productive workforce. As shown in Figure 16.1, these functions recruit, train, compensate, and support the member group and support continuous improvement in human resource management generally.

Work Force Planning

Work force planning allows the organization adequate time to respond to changes in the exchange environment with replacement, increases, or decreases in the numbers of members. The work force plan is a subsection of the long-range plan. It develops forecasts of the number of persons required in each skill level by year for the length of time covered by the long-range plan. It also projects available human resources including additions and attrition, even to specifying the planned retirement of key individuals.

Development of plan

The initial proposal for the work force plan should be developed using forecasts of activity from the services plan. The services plan is developed from the epidemiologic needs of the community and the long-range financial plans

FIGURE 16.1 Functions of Human Resources

Function	Description	Example
Work force planning	Development of employment needs by job category	RNs required and available by year
	Comparison with existing work force and identification of changes	Strategy for recruitment, retention, and complement reduction
Work force maintenance	Advertising, school visits, and other promotion	RN recruitment program
	Selection, orientation, and training	Credentials review
	Record of skill levels and performance	Orientation and continuous improvement courses
	Survey of satisfaction and analysis of dissatisfaction	Personnel record of RNs including special competencies
	Grievance management	Satisfaction survey and analysis
		Employee counseling and grievance mediation
Management education	Programs of supervisory training, human relations skills, continuous improvement skills	Head nurse programs in personnel policies, supervision, participation on cross-functional teams
Compensation management	Market surveys of base pay, benefits allowance, and incentives	RN pay scales, payment method, RN benefit selection, benefit cost, compensation, incentives, absenteeism records
	Record of hours worked and earnings	
	Maintenance of benefits eligibility, use, and cost	
Collective bargaining	Response to organizing drives, contract negotiation, and administration	Management of RN labor contract if any
Continuous improvement and budgeting	Analysis of employment markets, benefit trends, and work conditions	Identification of potential shortage situations, of competitive recruitment difficulties
	Development of improvement proposals for general working conditions	Proposals for improvement of benefits or work conditions
	Development of department budget and budget for fringe benefit costs	Human resources department budget and detail for benefits, costs, budgets

(Chapters 12 and 14). The work force plan technically includes, and is always coordinated with, the medical staff plan (Chapter 8). As shown in Figure 16.2, the plan should include:

- the anticipated size of the member and employee groups, by skill category, major site, and department;
- the schedule of adjustments through recruitment, retraining, attrition, and termination;
- wage and benefit cost forecasts from national projections tailored to local conditions;
- planned changes in employment or compensation policy, such as the development of incentive payments or the increased use of temporary or part-time employees; and
- preliminary estimates of the cost of operating the human resources department and fulfilling the plan.

The plan is often prepared by a task force including representatives from human resources, planning, finance, nursing, and one or two other CSSs likely to undergo extensive change. The draft is reviewed by the major medical staff specialties and employer departments, and their concerns are resolved. The revised plan is coordinated with the facilities plan because the number and

FIGURE 16.2 Illustration of Work Force Plan Content

Category	Current Supply (1999)	Need (FTE) 2000	Need (FTE) 2001	Need (FTE) 2002	Attrition per Year	Recruitment (Reduction) 2000	Recruitment (Reduction) 2001	Recruitment (Reduction) 2002
RN, Inpatient	250 FTE, 300 persons	230	210	200	50	30	30	40
RN, Outpatient	45 FTE, 60 persons	55	60	60	15	25	20	15

RN Strategy: Recruit from three local associate degree schools. Advertise in national and state journals. Offer training to facilitate transfer from inpatient to outpatient. Starting salary 10 percent below nearby metropolitan area. Emphasize health and child care, maintain education and retirement benefits. Encourage LPNs to seek further training.

Costs (2000):

Activity	**Cost per Unit**	**Cost per Employed FTE**
Recruitment/orientation	$1,250/recruit	$ 241/FTE
Personnel records, benefits management and counseling	$450/employee	$ 550/FTE
Health benefits	$2,400/employee over 20 hours/week	$ 1,627/FTE
Child care benefits	$100,000 per year*	$ 3,351/FTE
Social Security and Medicare	$ 1,950/FTE	$ 1,950/FTE
Retirement benefits	$ 1,500/FTE	$ 1,500/FTE
Vacation and absenteeism replacements	$900/employee	$ 1,102/FTE
Training programs	$700/FTE	$ 700/FTE
Total cost per FTE		**$11,021**

*Subsidy to Child Care Center. The Center is used by 30 percent of the nurses.

location of employees determine the requirements for many plant services. The final package must be consistent with the long-range financial plan. It is recommended to the governing board through the planning committee.

Using the work force plan

The work force plan must be reviewed annually as part of the environmental assessment, along with other parts of the long-range plan. The amended plan and the annual budget guidelines direct the development of even more detailed plans for the coming year. The human resources department works closely with the employing departments to specify individual compensation changes and work force adjustment. The financial implications of these actions are incorporated into the departmental budgets, which set precise expectations for the number of employees, the number of hours worked, the wage and salary costs, and the benefit costs.

Well-run organizations also use the work force plan to guide human resources policies. Among these are the timing of recruitment campaigns; guidelines for the use of temporary labor such as overtime, part-time, and contract labor; and incentive, compensation, and employee benefit design. The plan may be useful in making decisions about new programs and capital, as when the existence of a surplus work force becomes a resource for expanded services. Even such strategic decisions as mergers or vertical integration can be affected by human resource shortages and surpluses. All of these applications of the plan call for close collaboration with other executives and clinical departments. Collaboration is also desirable on short-term work force management issues, particularly training, motivation, lost time, and turnover. Improvements in these areas reduce the cost of the human resources department and can be translated into direct gains in productivity and quality by line managers.

The penalty for inadequate work force planning is loss of the time and flexibility needed to adjust to environmental changes. Many management difficulties are simpler if adequate time is available to deal with them. Inadequate warning causes hasty and disruptive action. Layoffs may be required. Recruitment is hurried and poor selections may be made. Retraining may be incomplete. Each of these actions takes its toll on workers' morale and often directly affects quality and efficiency. Although the effect of each individual case may be modest, it is long lasting and cumulative. The organization that makes repeated hasty and expedient decisions erodes its ability to compete.

Maintenance of the Work Force

Building and maintaining the best possible work force requires continuing attention to exchange relationships between the organization and its members. The organization cannot remain passive. The best people must be recruited, and they are more likely to remain with an organization that actively meets their personal needs. Investments in recruitment, retention, employee services, and programs for training supervisors in human relations become a part of the intangible benefits as perceived by the employee or member. The additional cost of well-designed programs in these areas is relatively small, but the return is very high.

Recruitment and selection

Retention of proven members is generally preferable to recruitment because the risk of dissatisfaction is lower on both sides. However, expansions, changes in services, and employee life cycles result in continuing recruitment needs at all skill levels. Equal opportunity and affirmative action laws, sound medical staff bylaws, and union contracts all require consistency in recruitment practices. A uniform protocol for recruitment establishes policies for the following activities:

1. *Position control.* Documentation of the number of FTEs approved, the identity and hours of persons hired for them, and the number of vacancies controls paychecks authorized and approval of recruitment requests, and keeps the work force at expectations established in the annual budget.
2. *Job description.* Each position must be described in enough detail to identify training, licensure, and experience requirements and to determine compensation. Descriptions are developed by the line, approved and recorded by human resources.
3. *Classification and compensation.* Wage, salary, incentive, and benefit levels must be assigned to each recruited position. These must be kept consistent with other internal positions, collective bargaining contracts, and the external market. Human resources maintains the classification and associates classes with pay scales and incentives.
4. *Job requirements.* The job description is translated to specific skills and knowledge sought with enough precision to permit equitable evaluation of applicants. Human resources assists line managers in making the translation and assessing skills.
5. *Applicant pool priorities and advertising.* Policies covering affirmative action and priority consideration of current and former employees and employees' relatives for job openings. Policies also cover the design, placement, and frequency of media advertising, including use of the organization's own newsletters and publications. Human resources generally develops and administers the policies.
6. *Initial screening.* Screening normally includes review and verification of data on the application. It may or may not include interviews. It includes a brief physical examination and may include drug testing.[6] Particularly for high-volume recruitment, screening takes place in the human resources department so that it will be uniform and inexpensive.
7. *Final selection.* Applicants who pass the initial screening are subjected to more intensive review, usually involving the immediate supervisor of the position and other line personnel. The final selection must be consistent with state and federal equal opportunity and affirmative action

requirements and with the job description and requirements. Human resources monitors compliance with these criteria.

8. *Orientation.* New employees need a variety of assistance, ranging from maps showing their work place to counseling on selecting benefit options. They should be given a mentor who can help them fit into their work group. They should learn appropriate information about the organization's mission, services, and policies to encourage their contribution and to make them spokesmen for the institution in their social group. The mentor is assigned by line personnel, but human resources usually provides the training and counseling.
9. *Probationary review.* Employees begin work with a probationary period, which concludes with a review of performance and usually an offer to join the organization on a long-term basis. Often, increased benefits and other incentives are included in the long-term offer. Line supervisors conduct the probationary review, with advice from human resources.

Modifications of the basic protocol are usually made for professional personnel and for temporary employees. Modifications for temporary employees and volunteers greatly simplify the process to reduce cost and delay, while those for professional personnel recognize that recruitment is usually from national or regional labor markets and that future colleagues should undertake most of the recruitment.

For the medical staff leaders and higher supervisory levels, search committees are frequently formed to establish the job description and requirements, encourage qualified applicants, carry out screening and selection, and assist in convincing desirable candidates to accept employment. The human resources department acts as staff for the search committee while ensuring that the intent of organization policies has been met. Well-run organizations now use human resources personnel to conduct initial reference checks and to verify licensure status and educational achievement for doctors and other professional personnel. This provides both consistency and a clearer legal record.

Healthcare organizations are subject to various regulatory and civil restrictions affecting recruitment. Federal regulations regarding equal opportunity require that there be no discrimination on the basis of sex, age, race, creed, national origin, or handicaps that do not incapacitate the individual for the specific job. Those covering affirmative action require special recruitment efforts and priority for equally qualified women, African Americans, and Hispanics. (Religious organizations may give priority to members of their faith under certain circumstances.) In addition to these constraints, organizations must follow due process, that is, fair, reasonable, and uniform rules, in judging the qualifications of attending physicians. Medical staff appointments are also subject to tests under antitrust laws (Chapter 8). Healthcare organizations are required to be able to document compliance with these rules and may be subject to civil suits by dissatisfied applicants. Monitoring and documenting compliance with these obligations is a function of the human resources department.

Workplace diversity

Most healthcare organizations strive to promote diversity in their work force.[7] They pursue affirmative action vigorously and make a deliberate effort to represent the ethnic and gender makeup of their community in their medical staff, management group, and work force.[8] They make a deliberate effort to promote women in management.[9] While this may be driven in part by law or a belief in the need for justice, it is also supported by sound marketing theories. Many people seek healthcare from caregivers who resemble them. African American doctors, nurses, and managers are important to African American patients. Increasing attention to the needs of female workers have clearly influenced the structure of employment benefits and the rules of the workplace.

Work force satisfaction and retention

Healthcare organizations now routinely survey personnel at all levels to assess general satisfaction with the work environment. The surveys must be carefully worded and administered in ways that protect the worker's anonymity. "360-degree" reviews have become popular; these surveys combine elements of satisfaction and evaluation. They allow evaluation by supervisors, subordinates, and both internal and external customers. Special problems identified from the surveys and other monitoring mechanisms are often pursued in focus groups or cross-functional groups. Well-run organizations make an effort to interview persons who are leaving. Their candid comments can be useful to eliminate or correct negative factors in the work environment. They often serve to improve the departing worker's view of the organization as well.

Human resources conducts surveys, interviews, and focus groups, and staffs cross-functional teams working on workplace problems. It analyzes and reports data and seeks benchmarks to guide line managers. It frequently counsels line managers on individual improvement opportunities.

Policies for promotion, retirement, and voluntary and involuntary termination must be similar in fairness and consistency to those for recruitment. For motivational purposes, they should be designed to make work life as attractive as possible, and they should permit selective retention of the best workers. This means that all collective actions should be planned as far in the future as possible and be announced well ahead of time. Criteria for promotion or dismissal should be clear and equitable, and loyal and able employees should be rewarded by priority in promotion and protection against termination. It also means that all policies are administered uniformly and that there is always a clear route of appeal against actions the employee views as arbitrary. Human resources participates directly in major reductions, designing actions and communications that minimize the impact. It provides counseling and appeals services in individual cases.

Employee services

Most healthcare organizations provide personal services to their employees through their human resources department on the theory that such services improve loyalty and morale and, therefore, efficiency and quality. Evidence to support the theory is limited, but the services are often required if competing employers provide them. Specific offerings are often tailored to the employees' responses. Popular programs are allowed to grow, while others are curtailed. Charges are sometimes imposed to defray the costs, but some subsidization is usual. Those commonly found include:

- Health education, health promotion, and access to personal counseling for substance abuse problems. Employee assistance programs, formally structured counseling to assist with stress management and alcohol and drug abuse, have been popular in recent years.[10] Many large companies have nurses or physicians on site to handle workplace injuries and illness;
- Infant and child care;
- Social events, often recognizing major holidays or corporate events, but also used to recognize employee contributions;
- Recreational sports; and
- Credit unions and payroll deduction for various purposes.

One theme of these activities is to build an attitude of caring and mutual support among healthcare workers, on the theory that a generally caring environment will encourage a caring response to patient and visitor needs.

Occupational safety and health

The hospital and some outpatient care sites are moderately dangerous environments for workers. The hospital contains unique or rare hazards, such as repeated exposure to low levels of radioactivity or small quantities of anesthesia gases and increased risk of infection. In practice, however, accident rates are low. Illness and injury arising from hospital work are kept to low levels by constant attention to safety.[11] The organization's dedication to personal and public health encourages this vigilance. For those who might be complacent or forgetful, two laws reinforce its importance. Workers' compensation is governed by state law. Premiums are based on settlements but also on process evidence of attention to safety. The federal **Occupational Safety and Health Act (OSHA)** establishes standards for safety in the workplace and supports inspections. Fines are levied for noncompliance.

Much of the direct control of hazards is the responsibility of the clinical and plant departments. Infection control, for example, is an important collaborative effort of housekeeping, facility maintenance, nursing, and medicine to protect the patient. Employee protection in well-run organizations stems from procedures developed for patient safety. The human resources department is usually assigned the following functions:

- monitoring federal and state regulations and professional literature on occupational safety for areas in which the organization may have hazards;

- identifying the department or group accountable for safety and compliance on each specific risk;
- keeping records and performing risk analysis, and leading improvement efforts for general or widespread exposures;
- maintaining records demonstrating compliance and responding to visits and inquiries from official agencies;
- providing or assisting training in and promotion of safe procedures; and
- negotiating contracts for workers' compensation insurance, reviewing appropriate language where the insurance is negotiated as part of broader coverage, or managing settlements where the organization self-insures.

Educational services

Human resources departments provide significant educational opportunities for employees and supervisors. In-service education is offered on topics where uniformity of understanding is desired.[12] On issues to be handled uniformly among relatively large groups, human resources personnel provide the entire program. Routine offerings are usually less than two hours long, with multiple sessions when more time is needed. Classes are limited in size, and offerings are repeated to provide greater access. Topics include:

- *Orientation.* Review of the organization's mission, history, major assets, and marketing claims, as well as policies and benefits of employment.
- *Continuous improvement and performance measurement.* Basic education in continuous improvement offered to all employees, including the reason for, meaning of, and application of concepts, including several basic tools (Chapter 6) and description of improvement team procedures.
- *Work policy changes.* Reviews covering the objectives and implications in major changes in compensation, benefits, or work rules.
- *Major new programs.* Permanent or temporary actions that affect habits and lifestyles of current workers. (New buildings, relocations, and construction dislocation are often topics.)
- *Retirement planning.* Offered to older workers to understand their retirement benefits and also to adjust to retirement lifestyles.
- *Outplacement.* To assist persons being involuntarily terminated through reductions in work force.
- *Benefits management.* Selection of options and procedures for using benefits, including efforts to minimize misuse.[13]

Clinical departments often use their own supervisors or consultants for professional topics, but human resources in larger organizations provides facilities, promotion, and logistic assistance. Human resources can collaborate with planning and finance units on organization-wide concerns such as the annual budget and continuous improvement.

Guest relations has become a prominent educational offering for human resources departments. These programs use roleplaying, games, and group discussion techniques to reinforce attitudes of caring and responsiveness to patients and visitors. Well-run organizations use the guest relations educational programs as part of a comprehensive effort; workers will respond more effectively to customer needs when their own needs are met by responsive supervision, adequate facilities and equipment, and organization policies that encourage flexibility toward customer needs.

Work force reduction

Rapid change in the healthcare industry has forced many organizations to make substantial involuntary reductions in their work forces. Because job security is an important recruitment and retention incentive, it is imperative that such reductions be handled well. Good practice pursues the following rules:

- Work force planning is used to foresee reductions as far in advance as possible, allowing natural turnover and retraining to provide much of the reduction.
- Temporary and part-time workers are reduced first.
- Personnel in supernumerary jobs are offered priority for retraining programs and positions arising in needed areas.
- Early retirement programs are used to encourage older (and often more highly compensated) employees to leave voluntarily.
- Terminations are based on seniority or well-understood rules, judiciously applied.

Using this approach has allowed many healthcare organizations to limit involuntary terminations to a level that does not seriously impair the attractiveness of the organization to others.

Grievance administration

Well-run healthcare organizations provide an authority independent of the normal accountability for employees who feel, for whatever reason, that their complaint or question has not been fully answered. Larger human resources departments often offer ombudsman-type programs providing an unbiased counselor for concerns of any kind. Personnel in these units are equipped to handle a variety of problems, from health-related issues they refer to employee assistance programs or occupational health services, to complaints about supervision or work conditions, to sexual harassment and discrimination. Most of the approaches are concerns rather than grievances when they are first presented. The function of the office is to settle them fairly and quickly, and if possible identify corrections that will prevent reoccurrence. The office's success depends on its ability to meet worker needs. It must remain flexible and independent in its orientation, yet management must heed its advice.

A few of the matters presented to ombudsman offices and line officers become formal grievances or complaints. Under collective bargaining, the union contract includes a formal grievance process that is often adversarial in nature, assuming a dispute to be resolved between worker and management. Under non-union arrangements, a grievance procedure is still necessary.

Good grievance administration begins with sound employment policies, effective education for workers and supervisors, and systems that emphasize rewards over sanctions.[14] Effective supervisory training emphasizes the importance of responding promptly to workers' questions and problems. Good supervisors have substantially fewer grievances than poor ones.

When disagreements arise, good grievance administration stimulates the following informal reactions:

- documentation of issue, location, and positions of the two parties to provide guides to preventive or corrective action;
- credible, unbiased, informal review to identify constructive solutions;
- informal negotiations that encourage flexibility and innovation in seeking a mutually satisfactory solution;
- counseling for the supervisor involved aimed at improvement of future human relations;
- settlement without formal review, either by mutual agreement or by concession on the part of the organization; and
- implementation of changes designed to prevent recurrences.

These processes are appropriate in both union and non-union environments. They should make the formal review process typically found in union contracts, leading to resolution by an outside arbitrator, unnecessary in the vast majority of cases. Grievances that go to formal review encourage an adversarial environment. Even if the concession appears relatively expensive, the organization is better off avoiding review and making an appropriate investment in the prevention of future difficulties.

Management Education

Human resources is responsible for training most line managers in three areas: facts about relevant policies and procedures, skills in human relations and supervision, and tools for budgeting and continuous improvement. Under continuous improvement approaches, more than simply mastery of tools is required. Non-health companies report substantial investments in managerial training, up to 80 hours per manager per year.[15] At least one large integrated system also makes a large investment.[16] Employees at all levels must think of themselves and the organization as continuously learning.[17] Many of these skills are delivered by other technical support units, on a "just-in-time" basis. Planning, marketing, finance, and information services personnel provide direct assistance to improvement teams when they need it. Human resources efforts may focus on the most commonly used tools and serve to emphasize the importance of the concept.

Facts about policies and procedures

Effective line supervisors are expected to answer a wide variety of questions from their workers. Many of these will be factual issues about the employment contract and the work environment. Examples are questions about compensation and benefits, incentive programs, and policies on leaves. An educational program to support the supervisors might include:

- Modern theories of human relations and supervision. Learning the supervisor's role and the importance of sound human relations. Policies and goals for the workforce, including the promotion of diversity and the elimination of sexual harassment;[18]
- In-service courses in major policies, important changes, and how to use the procedure manuals. (Leading organizations now have procedures in electronic files that can be quickly searched for the topic. The relevant policy can be quickly printed for the employee, and explained to ensure full comprehension); and
- Telephone and electronic mail access for specific questions, and personal consultation to the employee or supervisor where indicated.

Skills in human relations and supervision

Supervisory training and counseling is a particularly important human resources function. Promising workers are identified well before they are promoted and are trained in methods of supervision and effective motivation. Much of the folklore of American industry runs counter to the realities of sound first-line supervision.[19] Thus, even promising personnel need repeated reinforcement of the proper role and style. Multiple presentations using a variety of approaches and media are used to establish and reinforce basic notions: the use of rewards rather than sanctions, the importance of fairness and candor, the role of the supervisor in responding to workers' questions, and the importance of clear instructions and appropriate work environments.[20] Typical topics cover skills in orienting new people, training new skills, motivating workers, answering worker questions, disciplining, and identifying problem workers. Cases, roleplaying, recordings, films, and individual counseling are helpful in maintaining supervisor's performance.

Tools for budgeting and continuous improvement

Supervisors in continuous improvement programs need a variety of skills to identify opportunities, evaluate them, motivate their personnel, and implement the PDCA cycle. These tools are usually taught in several courses of a day or two each.[21] Budgets and capital budgets have now become complex enough that sessions on how the guidelines are generated, what sorts of improvements and proposals are appropriate, and how to handle the mechanics of preparation and submission are useful.

Human resources often organizes these programs using faculty from planning, marketing, finance, and information services. It is important to tie the mechanical skills of budgeting and continuous improvement projects to the human relations skills necessary to sustain motivation.

Compensation

Employee compensation includes direct wages and salaries, cash differentials and premiums, bonuses, retirement pensions, and a substantial number of specific benefits supported by payroll deduction or supplement. Federal law defines employment status and requires withholding of social security and income taxes from the employee and contributions by the employer.[22] Other employment benefits are automatically purchased on behalf of the employee via the payroll mechanism. Compensation constitutes more than half the expenditures of most healthcare organizations. From the organization's perspective, such a large sum of money must be protected against both fraud and waste. From the employee's perspective, accuracy regarding amount, timing, and benefit coverage should be perfect.

The growing complexity of compensation has been supported by highly sophisticated computer software, with each advance in computer capability soon translated into expanded flexibility of the compensation package. The latest developments in payroll have been increased use of bonuses and incentive compensation, as well as "cafeteria" benefits, which allow more employee choice. Well-run organizations now use payroll programs that process both pay and benefit data for three purposes: payment, monitoring and reporting, and budgeting. This software permits active management of compensation issues in the human resources department through position control, wage and salary administration, benefit administration, and pension administration.

Job analysis

Compensation programs require a description and classification of each job in the organization. The job description used to establish recruiting criteria also serves as a basis for classifying the position in a pay category. Human resources classifies the job in relation to others and establishes a pay scale for it.

Position control

The organization must protect itself against accidental or fraudulent violation of employment procedures and standards and must ensure that only duly employed persons or retirees receive compensation. This is done through a central review of the number of positions created and the persons hired to fill them, called **position control**. Creation of a position generally requires multiple approvals, ending near the level of the chief operating officer. Positions created are monitored by the human resources department to ensure compliance with recruitment, promotion, and compensation procedures and to ensure that each individual employed is assigned to a unique position.

It is important to understand the limitation of this activity; it controls the number of people employed rather than the total hours worked. The number of hours worked outside position control accountability is significant. Position control protects only against paying the wrong person, hiring in violation of established policies, and issuing double checks. It does not protect against overspending the labor budget or against errors in hours, rates, or benefit coverage.

Wage and salary administration

Most healthcare organizations operate at least two payrolls and a pension disbursement system. One payroll covers personnel hired on an hourly basis, requiring reporting of actual compensable hours for each pay period, usually two weeks. The other covers salaried, usually supervisory, personnel paid a fixed amount per period, often monthly. Contract workers, such as clinical support service physicians, are often compensated through non-payroll systems. (Benefits, withholding, and payroll deduction are usually omitted from contract compensation, although certain reporting requirements still apply.)

Wage and salary administration covers all of these disbursements for personnel costs, and includes the following activities:

- *Verification of compensable hours and compensation due.* This is applicable only to hourly personnel. The accountable department is responsible for the accuracy of hours reported, and for keeping hours within budget agreements. The task of the human resources department is to verify line authorization, the base rate, and the application of policies establishing differentials. Modern systems also identify other elements, such as location or activity, to support cost-finding activities. The data become an important resource for further analysis.
- *Compensation scales.* The well-run organization strives to be competitive in each position where comparison can be made to other employers and to treat other positions equitably. To achieve this goal, each job classification is assigned a compensation grade. The human resources department conducts or purchases periodic salary and wage surveys to establish competitive prices for representative grades. At supervisory and professional levels, these surveys cover national and regional markets. For most hourly grades the local market is surveyed.
- *Seniority, merit, and cost-of-living adjustments.* Beginning around World War II wages and salaries were adjusted annually to reflect changes in cost of living and the experience and loyalty reflected by job seniority. Calculating the amount or value of these factors and translating that into compensation at the appropriate time is the task of the human resources department. Well-run healthcare organizations are rapidly diminishing the importance of these compensation factors. Seniority and cost-of-living raises are not directly related either to the market for employment or the success of the organization. Merit raises, increases in the base pay reflecting the individual employee's skill improvements, are difficult to administer objectively[23] and tend to become automatic. Leading organizations are moving to replace all three adjustments with improved compensation scaling and performance-oriented incentive payments.

Incentive compensation

The market demand for competitive performance has made tangible reward for individual achievement desirable, and improving information systems have made it possible.[24] An organization built on rewards and the search for continued improvement is strengthened by a system of compensation that supplements personal satisfaction and professional recognition.[25] Healthcare organizations have advanced significantly toward this goal,[26,27,28] although few reports appear in published literature.

One approach is to recognize that wages and salaries should be based on market conditions, but that adjustments in compensation are most appropriately based on the employee's contribution to organizational goals. Certain constraints must be recognized in designing a system of this type:

- The resources available will depend more on the organization's overall performance than on any individual's contribution. They may be severely limited through factors outside the organization's control. The incentives must recognize this reality, emphasizing overall performance over unit or individual performance.
- Equity and objectivity will be expected in the distribution of the rewards.
- The individual's contribution will be difficult to measure.
- Group rewards attenuate the incentives to individuals. The larger the group, the greater the attenuation.
- The incentive program must avoid becoming a routine or expected part of compensation.

Well-run healthcare organizations are beginning to experiment with incentive compensation. It is likely that successful designs will have the following characteristics:

- The use of incentive compensation will begin at top executive levels and be extended to lower ranks with experience.
- Annual longevity increases will disappear as incentive pay increases.
- Incentives will be limited by difficulties in measurement and administration, but will provide a substantial portion of compensation, particularly for senior management.
- Incentives will be related to overall performance, but will be awarded to individuals based on their perceived contribution.
- Assessment of contribution will be retrospective, but will be based on achievement of improvements in expectations set in the preceding budget negotiation.

A bolder scenario is possible under continuous improvement. Where comprehensive measures covering all six dimensions of performance are available, and workers are comfortable with continuous improvement, work groups can set specific expectations and anticipate incentive payment for meeting them. "Gain sharing" approaches suggest that primary worker groups can effectively set expectations consistent with the needs of the larger organization and that the effort to do so will lead to measurable improvement in achievement. Those gains can then be used in part to reward the workers. At least one healthcare organization has followed that general model for a few years with some success.[29]

Benefits administration

Many of the social programs of Western nations are related directly or indirectly to work, through programs of payroll taxes, deductions, and entitlements. These programs are fixed in place by a combination of market forces, direct legal obligation, and tax-related incentives. Non-wage benefits are generally exempt from income and Social Security taxes, providing an automatic gain of at least 18 percent in the benefits that can be purchased for a given amount of after-tax money. Further gains stem from insurance characteristics. Life, health, accident, and disability insurance are substantially less costly when purchased on a group basis.

As a result, healthcare organizations and other employers in the United States support extensive programs of benefits, which add as much as 40 percent beyond salaries and wages to the costs of employment. (The term "fringe benefits" was common until the total cost of these programs made it obsolete.) The exact participation of each employee differs, with major differences depending on full-time or part-time status, grade, and seniority. In general, there are five major classes of employee benefits and employer obligations beyond wage compensation:

1. *Payroll taxes and deductions.* The employer is legally obligated to contribute premium taxes to Social Security for pension and Medicare benefits, as well as to collect a portion of the employee's pay for Social Security and withholding on various income taxes. Most employers also collect payroll deductions for union dues, various privileges like parking, and contributions to charities such as the United Way. Certain funds, such as uninsured healthcare expenses and child care expenses, can be exempt from income taxes by the use of pre-tax accounts. While the deductions represent only a small handling cost to the employer, they are an important convenience to the employee.
2. *Vacations, holidays, and sick leave.* Employers pay full-time and permanent employees for legal holidays, additional holidays, vacations, sick leave, and certain other time such as educational leaves, jury duty, and military reserves duty. They grant unpaid leaves for family needs, in accordance with the Family and Medical Leave Act of 1993,[30] and for other purposes as they see fit. As a result, only about 85 percent of the 2,080 hours per year nominally constituting full-time employment is actually worked by hourly workers. The non-worked time becomes a direct cost to the organization when the employee must be replaced by part-time workers or by premium pay. It also is an important factor in the cost of full-time versus part-time employees. Part-time positions often share in employment

benefits only on a drastically reduced basis. On a per-hour-worked basis, they can be significantly less costly.

3. *Voluntary insurance programs.* Health insurance is a widespread and popular entitlement of full-time employment. Retirement programs must be funded according to rules similar to those for insurance. Life insurance and travel and accident insurance are also common. Various tax advantages are available for these protections, and they are paid for by combinations of employee and employer contributions. The employer obtains a group rate that is much lower than that offered to individuals. Some employer options for these programs are not technically insurance. They are generally subject to state laws or the federal Employee Retirement Insurance Security Act (ERISA). Direct employer contributions add about 10 percent to the cost of full-time employees. They are rarely offered to employees working fewer than 20 hours per week and may be graduated to those working between half and full time.
4. *Mandatory insurance.* Employers are obligated to provide workers' compensation for injuries received at work, including both full healthcare and compensation for lost wages. They are also obligated to provide unemployment insurance, covering a portion of wages for several months following involuntary termination.
5. *Other perquisites.* A wide variety of other benefits of employment can be offered, particularly for higher professional and supervisory grades. These generally are shaped by a combination of tax and job performance considerations. Educational programs, professional society dues, and journal subscriptions are commonly included. Cars, homes, club memberships, and expense accounts are used to assist executives to participate fully in the social life of their community. The theory is that such participation increases the executives' ability to understand community desires and identify influential citizens. Added retirement benefits, actually income deferred for tax purposes, and termination settlements are used to defray the risks of leadership positions.

In managing employment benefits, the human resources department strives to maximize the ratio of gains to expenditure. Four courses of action to achieve this are characteristic of well-run departments; three of them relate to program design and one to program administration.

1. *Program design for competitive impact.* The value of a given benefit is in the eye of the employee, and demographics affect perceived value. A married mother might prefer child care to health insurance because her husband's employer already provides health insurance. A single person whose children are grown might prefer retirement benefits to life insurance. Young employees often (perhaps unwisely) prefer cash to deferred or insured benefits. Employee surveys help predict the most attractive design

of the benefit package. Flexibility is becoming more desirable as workers' needs become more diverse. Recent trends have emphasized cafeteria benefits, where each employee can select preset combinations.

2. *Program design for cost-effectiveness.* Several benefits have an insurance characteristic such that actual cost is determined by exposure to claims. Health insurance, accident insurance, and sick benefits are particularly susceptible to cost reduction by benefit design. Health insurance, by far the largest of these costs, is minimized by the use of managed care approaches, including copayments, premium sharing, and selected provider arrangements. Accident insurance premiums are reduced by limiting benefits to larger, more catastrophic events. Duplicate coverage, where the employee and the spouse who is employed elsewhere are both covered by insurance, can be eliminated to reduce cost. Costs of sick benefits can be reduced by eliminating coverage for short illnesses and by requiring certification from a physician early in the episode of coverage.
3. *Program design for tax implications.* Income tax advantages are a major factor in program design. Many advantages, such as the exemption of health insurance premiums, are deliberate legislative policy, while others appear almost accidental. Details are subject to constant adjustment through both legislation and administrative interpretations. As a result, it is necessary to review the benefit program periodically for changing tax implications, both in terms of current offerings and in terms of the desirability of additions or substitutions.
4. *Program administration.* Almost all of the benefits can be administered in ways that minimize their costs. It is necessary to provide actual benefits equitably to all employees; careless review of use may lead to widespread expansion of interpretation and benefit cost. Strict interpretation can be received well by employees if it is prompt, courteous, and accompanied by documentation in the benefit literature initially given employees. Health insurance is probably the most susceptible to poor administration. Careful claims review, enforcement of copay provisions, and coordination of spouse's coverage are known to be cost-effective. Prevention of insured perils is also fruitful. Absenteeism and on-the-job injuries are reduced by effective supervision. Accidents and health insurance usage are reduced by effective health promotion, particularly in cases of substance abuse.[31] Counseling is also believed to reduce health insurance use. Workers' compensation is reduced by improved safety on the job site and case management of expensive disabilities. Unemployment liability is reduced by better planning and use of attrition for work force reduction. Human resources management affects all these activities through employee services, supervisory training, work force planning, and occupational safety programs.

Pensions and retirement administration

Pensions and retirement benefits pose different management problems from other benefits because they are used only after the employee retires. Non-pension benefits are principally health insurance supplementing Medicare. Recent developments have led healthcare organizations to offer bonuses for early retirement as a way of adjusting the work force.

Pension design and retirement program management involve questions of benefit design and administration that are directly analogous to those of other insured benefits. Because the benefit is often not used for many years and represents a multi-decade commitment when use begins, pensions are funded by cash reserves and retiree's health insurance premiums are shown as a liability on the organization's balance sheet. As a result, pension issues also include the definition of suitable funding investments, that is, to what extent they should be divided between fixed-dollar returns and those responsive to inflation, and the management of the funds, including investment of them in the organization's own bonds or stock. Finally, pension-related issues include the motivational impact of the design on the tendency of employees to retire.

The pension itself, but not necessarily other retirement benefits, is regulated under ERISA. Regulations for ERISA specify the employer's obligation to offer pensions, to contribute to them if offered, to vest those contributions, and to fund pension liabilities through trust arrangements. These regulations leave several elements of a sound pension and retirement policy to the organization:

- the amount of pension supplementing Social Security;
- the amount, kind, and design of Medicare supplementation (capitation and other programs encouraging economical use of benefits have become more common);
- opportunities for additional contribution by employees;
- accounting for unvested liabilities (benefits not paid if the employee leaves the organization before the time required for vesting);
- funding of unvested pension liabilities;
- use of unvested funds to finance the organization's needs;
- division of investments between equity and fixed-dollar obligations and selection of those investments; and
- incentives to encourage or discourage retirement (Age 65 is an arbitrary and increasingly irrelevant standard. Federal law allows most older workers, including healthcare workers, the right to continue work without a mandatory retirement age.).

Many of these issues can be and frequently are delegated to pension management firms or fund trustees. Others are important parts of a well-planned work force management program that must be handled by the human resources system. In addition to these financial, technical, and motivational concerns, most organizations accept an obligation to provide retirement counseling, including education to help the employee manage pensions and health insurance benefits.

Retired workers represent large future liabilities. At the time of a female employee's retirement, the organization typically commits itself to pension payments and support of Medicare supplementary health insurance for a period averaging nearly 15 years. ERISA requires a trust fund to support pension payments, and the health insurance supplement payment is represented as a liability on the balance sheet. In past times of high inflation, many hospitals felt obligated to adjust pensions for very old workers because inflation has eroded their buying power below subsistence levels. Such adjustments are, by definition, not funded.

Although healthcare organizations are currently using retirement bonuses as a method of work force reduction, at other times it may pay to retain older workers. In general, they are more amenable to reduced hours, have reliable work habits, and are less likely to have unpredictable absences.

Economic, legal, and social considerations in compensation

Employment compensation, including benefits, is an exchange transaction governed primarily by an economic marketplace. It follows then, that the market is the best and usual source of information on compensation. Healthcare organizations depart from the market price for labor at their peril: a lower price may not attract enough qualified personnel, and a higher one may waste the owners' funds. Wage and salary surveys to determine market prices are available for purchase, particularly for national markets; however, continuing contact with appropriate markets is one of the important functions of the human resources system.

Legal restrictions are also important. Healthcare organizations are subject to federal and state laws governing wages, hours, and working conditions. As noted, they are also obligated to follow equal opportunity and affirmative action regulations. The human resources department is usually accountable for compliance with most of these regulations and for all records and documentation in support of compliance.

Social considerations are more complex. Many people who are concerned with healthcare are also concerned with related issues of a good society, such as the availability of meaningful work, the adequacy of low wages and pensions, the equity of payment for equivalent work, and the avoidance of exploitation of minorities or subgroups of the society. These questions are rarely straightforwardly addressed. In particular, efforts to improve compensation are often associated with reductions in the number of jobs available, possibly by reducing the competitiveness of the organization. Well-run organizations tend to do the following:

- comply with market trends;
- comply with applicable laws and regulations;

- take advantage of indirect ways to increase employment or compensation to disadvantaged groups; and
- advocate as an organization more significant redress of these important social problems.

This posture allows large healthcare organizations to play a limited role in resolving social problems. They can increase work available in inner-city areas by locating facilities there. They can provide scholarships for disadvantaged persons seeking education in health professions. They can promote the use of local contractors who employ from disadvantaged groups.

Collective Bargaining Agreements

Extent and trends in collective bargaining

Healthcare organizations are subject to both state and federal legislation governing the right of workers to organize a union for their collective representation on economic and other work-related matters. Federal legislation generally supports the existence of unions; state laws vary. As a result of the extension of federal law to hospitals and of the increased availability of funds, hospital organizing drives became more common and more successful around 1970. By 1980, 20 percent of all hospital employees were unionized. The likelihood of unionization differed significantly by state, with the northeastern states and California most likely, and was far more common in urban areas. The overall percentage unionized held stable throughout the decade, although unionization in general declined.[32] The number of certification elections (the initial step of union recognition) in healthcare organizations declined steadily throughout the 1980s, although the percentage of successful elections increased slightly, to just over 50 percent in 1991. The decline was particularly noticeable in hospitals. There were 90 successful elections per year in 1980–1982, and 40 per year in 1989–1991. A small number of decertification elections offset these.[33]

By 1990, union members were only 15 percent of the U.S. work force, down from 25 percent shortly after World War II. In hospitals, unskilled workers and building trades were the most likely to be organized. Nurses were next most likely; other clinical professionals were rarely organized. Hospitals that were organized were more likely to remain organized for several years.[34] Small and declining numbers of house officers were union members.[35] Periodic efforts to organize attending physicians gained little headway.[36]

A 1989 Supreme Court decision upheld rules by the National Labor Relations Board establishing eight job classes for unionization in all hospitals. The classes are physicians, registered nurses, all professional personnel other than doctors and nurses, technical personnel (including practical nurses and internally trained aides, assistants and technicians), skilled maintenance employees, business office clerical employees, guards, and all other employees. Any organizing vote must gain support of a majority of all the members of a given class.[37] The ruling stimulated interest in unions among most of the groups identified by the ruling, including physicians, and renewed organization efforts by unions.[38,39,40] The efforts led to more successful organizing activity in healthcare than in other industries,[41] but it did not cause major changes in the overall importance of unions.[42]

Most healthcare organizations are likely to seek a position that discourages unionization or diminishes the influence of existing unions. Such a strategy is actualized through the organization's response to work-related concerns of employees.

Work-related employee concerns

Union organization drives and collective bargaining tend to be strong where employees perceive a substantial advantage to collective representation. This perception is stimulated by evidence of careless, inconsiderate, or inequitable behavior on the part of management in any of the key concerns of the workplace: response to workers' questions, output expectations, working conditions, and pay.

It is possible to diminish both the perceived advantage and the real advantage of unionization by consistently good management. Many companies have existed for decades in highly unionized environments without ever having a significant union organization. The first step is to make certain there is little room for complaint about the key concerns of the workplace and no obvious opportunity for improvement. The union then has nothing to offer in return for its dues, and its strength is diminished. The first task of the human resources department in this regard is to achieve high-quality performance on its functions. The second is to assist other systems of the organization to do the same, and the third is to present the organization so that its performance is recognized by workers.

Organization drives and responses

Organization drives are regulated by law and have become highly formal activities. The union, the employees, and management all have rights that must be scrupulously observed. The regulatory environment presumes an adversarial proceeding. Under this presumption, management is obligated to present arguments against joining the union and to take legal actions that limit the organizers to the framework of the law. If management fails in this duty, the rights of owners and employees who do not wish union representation are not properly protected. Well-run organizations respond to organizing drives by hiring competent counsel specifically to fulfill their adversarial rights and obligations. They act on advice of counsel to the extent that it is consistent with their general strategy of fair and reasonable employee relations.

Negotiations and contract administration

Collective bargaining is usually an adversarial procedure, although collaboration with unions can and should occur. The management position should avoid confrontation as much as possible, and seek collaboration. Well-run organizations use experienced bargainers and have counsel available for the more complex formalities. Once again, management is obligated to represent owners and employees who are not represented at the bargaining table. Healthcare organizations with existing unions pursue a strategy of contract negotiation that attempts to minimize or eliminate dissent. They will accept a strike on issues that depart significantly from the current exchange environment for workers or patients, but as a strategy they avoid strikes whenever possible.

Under certain circumstances, management must pursue contracts that reduce income or employment for union members. Two rules govern such a case: it must apply equally to nonunion workers, and it must be well justified by external forces in the exchange environment.

Contract administration is approached in a similar vein, but the adversarial characteristic of organizing and bargaining should not carry over into the workplace. The objective is to comply fully with the contract but to minimize an adversarial environment that uses the contract as a source of controversy. Considerable supervisory education is necessary to implement this policy. Supervisors should know the contract and abide by it, but whenever possible their actions should be governed by fundamental concerns of human relations and personnel management. Any distinction between unionized and nonunionized groups should be minimized.

Continuous Improvement and Budgeting

The human resources department is obligated to support continuous improvement in its own unit and throughout the organization, and to prepare a budget for its own activities consistent with collective needs. Its customers are both employees and employing units. Leading thought in human resources management places great emphasis on this function; it is regarded as the central contribution of the unit.[43]

Continuous improvement

The competitive environment will demand extraordinary efforts to improve human relations.[44] Most healthcare organizations must make major improvements in labor efficiency and cost. The best will understand that the loyalty, skill, and motivation of the work force are also critical and that any effort to address the problems of costs must involve increasing the contribution and the compensation of many workers. Pursuing these concepts will improve efficiency while simultaneously making workers more valuable to themselves and to the organization. At the other extreme, badly managed organizations will take hasty, ill-considered actions devastating those persons who are terminated and demoralizing those who remain. The demoralization will generate problems of cost, quality, and attractiveness to patients and qualified professionals.

Continuous improvement of human relations begins with competency in each of the functions of the human resources system. It includes information systems for retrieval and analysis of human resources data and measures of performance for the human resources department itself, emphasizing service to other systems and outcomes quality. As shown in Figure 16.3, there are usually several opportunities to expand human resources services. When the indicator directly measures the workforce, as in the employee satisfaction and labor cost illustration in Figure 16.3, the human resources opportunity is clear. Even if the opportunity is in operational performance improvement, training and motivational issues may be the underlying cause.

Human resources has extensive obligations to support continuous improvement in other units. These include advising on personnel requirements and recruiting, resetting wage and salary levels, and assisting with training programs. Most important, they include continuous reinforcement of the motivating factors for improvement, particularly empowerment. Empowerment

FIGURE 16.3 Typical External Improvements for Human Resources Services

Indicator	Opportunity	Example
Employee satisfaction variance	Identify special causes and address each individually	Improve employee amenities Special training for supervisors with low employee satisfaction
Inadequate operational performance improvement	Support line review of causes	Focus groups on motivation Seek evidence of worker dissatisfaction Review incentive programs
High health insurance costs	Promote more cost-effective program	Revise health insurance benefits Install managed care Promote healthy lifestyles
Labor costs over benchmark	Support orderly employment reduction	Curtail hiring in surplus categories Design and offer early retirement program Start cross-training and retraining programs

FIGURE 16.4 Typical Internal Improvements for Human Resources Services

Indicator	Opportunity	Example
Potential RN shortage	Expand RN recruitment program	Install expanded part-time RN program, emphasizing retraining, child care, flexible hours
High benefits cost	Redesign benefit package	Cafeteria benefits with elimination of extremely high cost elements
Low incentive payments	Redesign incentive pay program	Expand eligibility for incentives, improve measurement of contribution

is easily destroyed by authoritarian supervisory practices.[45] Motivation drops quickly when these develop. Human resources must monitor, counsel, and train constantly to support an effective program.

The internal continuous improvement of human resources is designed to anticipate line needs and be ready for them as they arise. Improving internal information systems, particularly those associated with work force planning and management, are examples. Recruitment, benefits, regular and incentive compensation, and outcomes measures of work force maintenance can be benchmarked against competitors and non-healthcare service organizations. Programs for special work groups can be redesigned or invented. Because these programs should be anticipatory, there may be no direct measure of need for them. Figure 16.4 gives some common examples.

Budget development

Human resources is responsible for its own budget covering all six dimensions of performance. Figure 16.5 indicates the measures and some likely management questions to be reviewed in the budget for each dimension.

It is important to establish realistic constraints on cost. The department almost never generates revenue. Its costs and services can sometimes be benchmarked against similar institutions, but one benchmark is the price of outside contracts. It is possible to purchase human resources individual services from commercial vendors. Some companies provide complete work force management. Thus, many of the discussions of appropriate levels of quality and unit cost revolve around competitive sources for equivalent services. It is possible to sell human resources services to line departments on a scheme of transfer pricing (Chapter 14). While this approach may result in economies, it may also unduly dampen demand for services. The costs of inadequate training and counseling to line departments may be unreasonably high. Even

FIGURE 16.5 Issues in Human Resources Budget Development

Dimension	Possible Issues
Demand	Hours of training provided per employee Adequacy of coverage of training programs, counseling, recruitment assistance
Cost	Comparison of costs with history and similar organizations
Human Resources	Satisfaction and performance of department's own employees
Output/ Efficiency	Comparison of output to demand Comparison of cost per hire, cost/employee to competitors and similar organizations
Quality	Comparison to competition, other service organizations
Customer Satisfaction	Employee satisfaction with benefits, training programs, etc. Supervisor satisfaction with department

so, demands, outputs, and unit costs of specific human resources services are important and should be studied as part of the budget.

Organization and Personnel

Human Resources Management as a Profession

Human resources management emerged as a profession after World War II, in response to the complexities created by union contracts, wage and hour laws, and benefits management. Healthcare organizations were sheltered from these developments for several years, but as the need arose healthcare organizations moved to establish an identifiable human resources system and to hire specially trained leadership for it. Although there is no public certification for the profession, there is an identifiable curriculum of formal education and a recognizable pattern of professional experience. Healthcare practitioners have an association, the American Society for Healthcare Human Resources, a unit of the American Hospital Association. Well-run organizations now recruit their human resources director or vice president from persons with experience in the profession generally and preferably with experience in healthcare. Larger organizations often have several professionals. Professional training and experience contribute to mastery of the several areas in which laws, precedents, specialized skills, or unique knowledge define appropriate actions.

Organization of the Human Resources Department

Internal organization

The human resources department is organized by function, in order to take advantage of the specialized skills applicable to its more time-consuming activities. Figure 16.6 shows a typical accountability hierarchy for a larger organization with labor union contracts. Smaller organizations must accomplish the same functions with fewer people. They do so by combining the responsibility centers shown on the lower row. (Collective bargaining is less common in smaller institutions.)

In very large organizations, human resources tends to be decentralized by work site. While some activities, such as information processing, can be centrally managed, others require frequent contact with employees and supervisors. A central office can monitor planning, support more elaborate educational programs, and maintain uniformity of compensation, benefits, and collective bargaining. Decentralized representatives available in each site concentrate on implementation of these programs and issues of work force maintenance and continuous improvement. Work force planning is generally handled by an ad hoc team led by the vice president for human resources. While various sites must participate as well as various work groups, a centralized approach maximizes the opportunities for promotion and relocation without layoff.

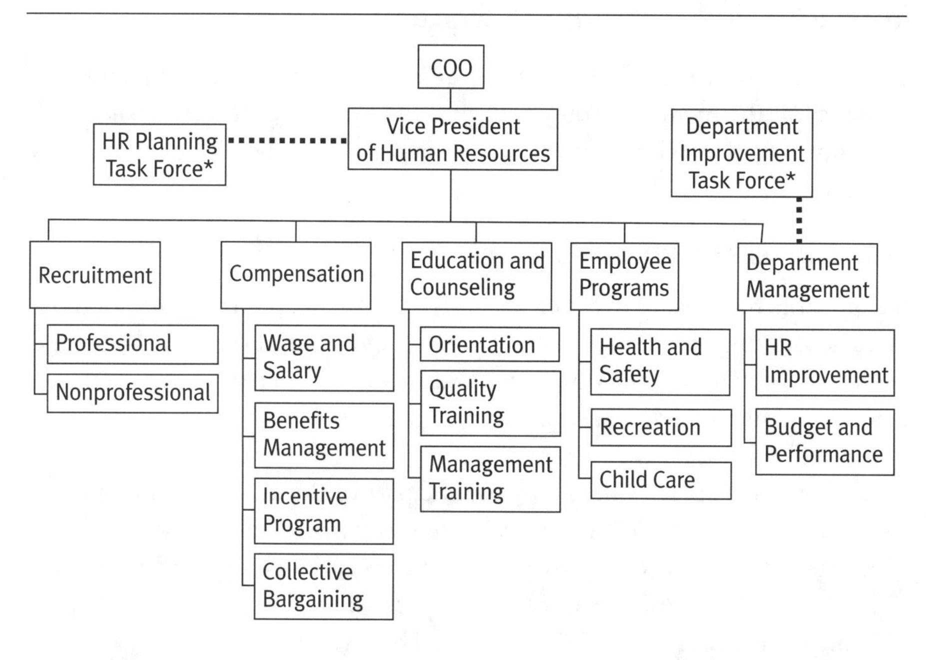

FIGURE 16.6 Organization of a Large Human Resources Department

*Task forces draw on department members and outsiders as indicated.
Dotted lines show chairs.

Division of responsibility with other systems

The more controversial organizational problems relate to the division of human resources functions between the department and the unit accountable for the member's costs and output. Whether the human resources department is involved or not, the functions of the human resources system must be performed for all organization members. By the same token, all members require supervision by and assistance from their accountable unit. Thus, the question of the exact domain of the human resources department is inevitably a matter of judgment.

Well-run organizations have identified the question as one of appropriate joint contribution to the needs of the member. They seek the solution not in the assignment of functions to either the line or the human resources department, but rather in the identification of the amount and kind of contribution each unit can make in completing each function. This approach recognizes that the goal is to perform each function well for each member of the work force and that the human resources system must be a collaboration between the department and the line unit involved. In judging the assignment of specific functions, one bears in mind the human resources department's contributions: uniformity, economy, and specialized human resources skills. The operating unit's contributions are professional and technical knowledge of the specific tasks.

Measures and Information Systems

Quantitative assessment of human resources must address the state and performance of the member group as well as the human resources department. The human resources department is the "source of truth" on human resources measures.[46]

Measurement of Human Resource

It is possible to measure many characteristics of the workforce using sophisticated accounting, personnel record keeping, and satisfaction surveys. Precise definitions of the concepts being measured are easily obtained from accounting practice and standard definitions. Figure 16.7 lists many of the commonly used measures for assessing the membership.

Membership assessment is a routine part of the annual environmental assessment. The values for measures in the four dimensions can be compared with benchmarks and comparable organizations and with their own history.

Measurement of the human resources department obviously begins with the measures shown in Figure 16.7. The level of achievement on these measures is an outcomes quality measure for the department; the state of the workforce is its principal product. An additional set of measures is important in assessing the department itself, as shown in Figure 16.8.

Cost measurement of the human resources activity and its components is relatively straightforward. Concerns are sometimes raised about the cost of time spent in human resources activity by personnel not in the human resources department, an amount that would not normally be captured by the accounting system. Examples are time spent in training or participating in task forces with a direct human resources goal. These concerns assume that time spent on these activities results in lost production elsewhere. In fact,

FIGURE 16.7 Measures of the Human Resources Department

Dimension	Measure
Demand	New hires per year Unfilled positions
Costs and Efficiency	Number of workers Full- and part-time hours paid Overtime, differential, and incentive payments Benefits costs by benefit Human resources department costs
Quality	Skill levels and cross-training Recruitment of chosen candidates Examination scores Analysis of voluntary terminations
Satisfaction	Employee satisfaction Turnover and absenteeism Grievances

FIGURE 16.8
Measures of Human Resources' Functional Effectiveness

Dimension	Concept	Representative Measures
Demand	Request for human resources department service	Requests for training and counseling services Requests for recruitment Delay in filling positions Number of employees
Cost	Resources consumed in department operation	Department costs by functional account Physical resources used by department
Human resources	The work force in the department	Satisfaction, turnover, absenteeism within the department
Output/ efficiency	Cost/unit of service	Cost per hire, employee, training hour, paychecks issued, etc.
Quality	Quality of department services	Time to fill open positions Results of training Audit of services Service error rates
Customer satisfaction	Services as viewed by employees and supervisors	Surveys of member satisfaction with human resources

the premise may be false; the morale or skills improvement resulting from participation may cause production increases rather than decreases.

Customer satisfaction measures are easily obtained in conjunction with other member surveys. Focus groups or task forces may provide supplementary information. Quality measures can be developed for specific activities, such as benefit administration and paycheck errors. Recruitment is often measured by the time to fill positions, and the percentage of top-ranked candidates actually recruited. Process measures, such as the percentage of eligible members participating in various programs, or the content and presentation of educational materials can be developed.

Most of the measures of departmental performance can be benchmarked. It is useful to compare performance with other service industries, rather than strictly within healthcare.

Information Systems

Structure

The information systems of human resources management are built around seven core files of information, as shown in Figure 16.9. These files record the status of the human resource—personnel counts, qualifications, compensation, and vacancies—and the activity—unit costs, satisfaction, turnover, absenteeism,

FIGURE 16.9 Core Files of the Human Resources Information System

File	Uses
Position Control (list of approved full-time and part-time positions by location, classification)	Provides a basic check on number and kinds of people employed
Personnel Record (personal data, training, employment record, hearings record, benefits use)	Provides tax and employment data aggregated for descriptions
Work Force Plan (record of future positions and expected personnel)	Shows changes needed in work force
Payroll (current work hours or status, wage or salary level)	Generates paychecks Provides labor cost accounting
Employee Satisfaction (results of surveys by location, class)	Assesses employee satisfaction
Training Schedules and Participation (record of training programs and attendance)	Generates training output statistics and individual records
Benefits Selection and Utilization (record of employee selection and use of services)	Benefits management and cost control

grievances, and training. Many of the files are automated. Actions such as employment, training, anniversary reviews, promotion, or termination are electronically captured, along with data generated by payroll systems.

Ethical issues

Important ethical questions are raised in connection with the information in these files. The records involved are usually viewed as confidential. At the simplest ethical level, human resources files, like patient records, must be guarded against unauthorized access and misuse.

More serious questions arise when basic concerns have been met. Reduction of dissatisfaction, turnover, absenteeism, grievances, accidents, and illness is a socially useful goal of human resources management. It is clearly proper, even desirable, to study variations as measures of supervisory effectiveness that can be improved by systems redesign, counseling, and education. Yet, actions based on worker characteristics such as age, sex, or race or records such as illness and grievances can be illegal and are often ethically questionable. Some facts, such as drug test data, are potentially destructive, and the database cannot be made error free. Some companies have attempted to deny employment opportunities in situations in which there was high risk of occupational injury. For example, such an approach would deny employment in operating rooms to female nurses in their childbearing years because there are known pregnancy risks related to exposure to anesthesia.

One must note that in almost all cases harm results from the misuse of information rather than the acquisition of it. In fact, knowledge of age-, sex-, and race-related hazards can only be deduced from studies of their specific impact. Thus, denial of the value of all or part of the information potential is also unethical—it permits the organization to do less than it should on behalf of all workers. A sound policy must balance the advantages of investigation against its dangers. These rules help:

- Information access is limited to a necessary minimum group. Those with access are taught the importance of confidentiality and the organization's expectation that individuals' rights will be protected.
- Formal approval must be sought for studies of individual characteristics affecting personnel performance. Often a specific committee including members of the organization's ethics committee reviews each study. Criteria for approval include protection of individual rights, scientific reliability, and evidence of potential benefit.
- Actions taken to improve performance are reward oriented rather than sanction oriented. Considerable effort is made to find nonrestrictive solutions. (In the operating room example, avoidance of the more dangerous gases would be one such solution, improved air handling another, and concentrating use in one location a third. While none of these may be practical, all should be considered before a restrictive employment policy is established.)
- When used, sanctions or restrictions offer the individual the greatest possible freedom of choice. The right of the individual to take an informed risk should be respected, although it may not reduce the organization's ultimate liability. (In the operating room example, a nurse may accept employment with a full explanation of the risks as they are currently known. The complex probabilities of pregnancy, stillbirth, and infant deformity clearly depend on her personal lifestyle and intentions. Weighing them would be the nurse's moral obligation. Legally, the organization's liability for later injury might be reduced by evidence that full information was supplied about the hazards involved, although such an outcome is uncertain.)

Suggested Readings

Carter, C. C. 1994. *Human Resources Management and the Total Quality Imperative.* New York: American Management Association.

Dreachslin, J. 1996. *Diversity Leadership.* Chicago: Health Administration Press.

Fottler, M. D., S. R. Hernandez, and C. L. Joiner (eds.). 1994. *Strategic Management of Human Resources in Health Services Organizations,* 2nd ed. Albany, NY: Delmar Publishers.

Jackson, S. E., and Associates (eds.). 1992. *Diversity in the Workplace: Human Resources Initiatives.* New York: Guilford Press.

Pfeffer, J. 1994. *Competitive Advantage Through People: Unleashing the Power of the Work Force.* Boston: Harvard Business School Press.

Sibson, R. E. 1998. *Compensation*, 5th ed. NY: AMACOM Books.

U.S. Department of Labor. 1993. *Framework for a Comprehensive Health and Safety Program in the Hospital Environment.* Washington, DC: U.S. Department of Labor, Occupational Safety and Health Administration, Directorate of Technical Support, Office of Occupational Health Nursing.

Notes

1. U.S. Bureau of the Census, *Statistical Abstracts of the U.S., 1997,* 117th ed. Washington, DC: U.S. Bureau of the Census, Table 662 (1997)
2. J. P. Weiner, "Forecasting the Effects of Health Reform on U.S. Physician Workforce Requirement: Evidence from HMO Staffing Patterns." *Journal of the American Medical Association* 272(3), pp. 222–30 (July 20, 1994)
3. J. Pfeffer, *Competitive Advantage Through People: Unleashing the Power of the Work Force.* Boston: Harvard Business School Press, Ch. 2 pp. 27–65 (1994)
4. D. I. Levine and L. D. Tyson, "Participation, Productivity, and the Firm's Environment." In A. S. Blinder, ed., *Paying for Productivity.* Washington, DC: The Brookings Institution pp. 183–243 (1990)
5. *Ibid*, p. 205
6. J. W. Fenton, Jr., and J. L. Kinard, "A Study of Substance Abuse Testing in Patient Care Facilities." *Health Care Management Review* 18(4), pp. 87–95 (Fall, 1993)
7. S. Cejka, "The Changing Healthcare Workforce: A Call for Managing Diversity." *Healthcare Executive* 8(2), pp. 20–3 (March–April, 1993)
8. S. E. Jackson and Associates, eds., *Diversity in the Workplace: Human Resources Initiatives.* New York: Guilford Press (1992)
9. A. M. Rizzo and C. Mendez, *The Integration of Women in Management: A Guide for Human Resources and Management Development Specialists.* New York: Quorum Books (1990)
10. J. C. Howard and D. Szczerbacki, "Employee Assistance Programs in the Hospital Industry." *Health Care Management Review* 13, pp. 73–9 (Spring, 1988)
11. U.S. Department of Labor, "Framework for a Comprehensive Health and Safety Program in the Hospital Environment." Washington, DC: U.S. Dept. of Labor, Occupational Safety and Health Administration, Directorate of Technical Support, Office of Occupational Health Nursing (1993)
12. K. N. Wexley and J. Hinrich, eds., *Developing Human Resources.* Washington, DC: Bureau of National Affairs (1991)
13. M. L. Finkel, "Evaluate and Communicate Health Care Benefits." *Employee Benefits Journal* 22(4), pp. 29–34 (December, 1997)
14. C. R. McConnell, "Behavior Improvement: A Two-Track Program for the Correction of Employee Problems." *Health Care Supervisor* 11(3), pp. 70–80 (March, 1993)
15. E. A. McColgan, "How Fidelity Invests in Service Professionals." *Harvard Business Review* 75(1), pp. 137–43 (January–February, 1997)

16. J. R. Griffith, *Designing 21st Century Healthcare: Leadership in Hospitals and Healthcare Systems.* Chicago: Health Administration Press, pp.183–4 (1998)
17. D. A. Garvin, "Building a Learning Organization." *Harvard Business Review* 71(4), pp. 78–91 (July–August, 1993)
18. R. K. Robinson, G. M. Franklin, and R. L. Fink, "Sexual Harassment at Work: Issues and Answers for Health Care Administrators." *Hospital & Health Services Administration* 38(2), pp. 167–80 (Summer, 1993)
19. E. Jansen, D. Eccles, and G. N. Chandler, "Innovation and Restrictive Conformity Among Hospital Employees: Individual Outcomes and Organizational Considerations." *Hospital & Health Services Administration* 39(1), pp. 63–80 (Spring, 1994)
20. J. F. Manzoni and J. L. Barsoux, "The Set-up-to-Fail Syndrome." *Harvard Business Review* 76(2), pp. 101–13 (March–April, 1998)
21. C. C. Carter, *Human Resources Management and the Total Quality Imperative.* New York: American Management Association (1994)
22. W. B. Moore and C. D. Groth, "Independent Contractors or Employees? Reducing Reclassification Risks." *Healthcare Financial Management* 47(5), pp. 118, 120–4 (May, 1993)
23. M. T. Kane, "The Assessment of Professional Competence." *Evaluation and the Health Professions* 15(2), pp. 63–82 (June, 1992)
24. R. E. Sibson, *Compensation*, 5th ed. New York: AMACOM Books (1998)
25. D.I. Levine and L.D. Tyson, "Participation, Productivity, and the Firm's Environment." In A. S. Blinder, ed., *Paying for Productivity.* Washington, DC: The Brookings Institution, pp. 183–243 (1990)
26. A. Barbusca and M. Cleek, "Measuring Gain-Sharing Dividends in Acute Care Hospitals." *Health Care Management Review* 19(1), pp. 28–33 (Winter, 1994)
27. S. Laverty, B. J. Hogan, and L. A. Lawrence, "Designing an Incentive Compensation Program That Works." *Healthcare Financial Management* 52(1), pp. 56–9 (January, 1998)
28. J. R. Griffith, *Designing 21st Century Healthcare: Leadership in Hospitals and Healthcare Systems.* Chicago: Health Administration Press, pp.111, 184 (1998)
29. J. R. Griffith, *Designing 21st Century Healthcare: Leadership in Hospitals and Healthcare Systems.* Chicago: Health Administration Press, pp.111 (1998)
30. R. W. Luecke, R. J. Wise, and M. S. List, "Ramifications of the Family and Medical Leave Act of 1993." *Healthcare Financial Management* 47(8), pp. 32, 36, 38 (August, 1993)
31. J. W. Fenton, Jr., and J. L. Kinard, "A Study of Substance Abuse Testing in Patient Care Facilities." *Health Care Management Review* 18(4), pp. 87–95 (Fall, 1993)
32. R. Tomsho, "Mounting Sense of Job Malaise Prompts More Healthcare Workers to Join Unions." *Wall Street Journal*, B1 (June 9, 1994)
33. C. Scott and C. M. Lowery, "Union Election Activity in the Health Care Industry." *Health Care Management Review* 19(1), pp. 18–27 (Winter, 1994)
34. C. J. Scott and J. Simpson, "Union Election Activity in the Hospital Industry." *Health Care Management Review* 14(4), pp. 21–8 (Fall, 1989)
35. G. J. Bazzoli, "Changes in Resident Physicians' Collective Bargaining Outcomes as Union Strength Declines." *Medical Care* 26(3), pp. 263–77 (March, 1988)

36. *McGraw-Hill's Washington Report on Medicine & Health* 40 (February 24, 1986)
37. C. R. Gullett and M. J. Kroll, "Rule Making and the National Labor Relations Board: Implications for the Health Care Industry." *Health Care Management Review* 15(2), pp. 61–5 (Spring, 1990)
38. D. Burda, "Service Employees International Union Accelerates Organizing Drives in Wake of Ruling on Bargaining Units." *Modern Healthcare* 21(19), p. 7 (May 13, 1991); L. Perry, "$500,000 Added to Nurses Unionizing Efforts." *Modern Healthcare* 21(14), p. 14 (April, 1991)
39. M. L. Ile, "From the Office of the General Counsel, Collective Negotiation and Physician Unions." *Journal of the American Medical Association* 3: 262(17), p. 2444 (November 3, 1989)
40. L. V. Sobol and J. O. Hepner, "Physician Unions: Any Doctor Can Join, But Who Can Bargain Collectively?" *Hospital & Health Services Administration* 35(3), pp. 327–40 (Fall, 1990)
41. C. Scott and C. M. Lowery, "Union Election Activity in the Health Care Industry." *Health Care Management Review* 19, pp. 18–27 (Winter, 1994)
42. M. H. Cimini and C. J. Muhl, "Labor-Management Bargaining in 1994." *Monthly Labor Review* 118, pp. 23–39 (January, 1995)
43. D. Ulrich, "A New Mandate for Human Resources." *Harvard Business Review* 76(1), pp. 124–34 (January–February, 1998)
44. J. Barnsley, L. Lemieux-Charles, and M. M. McKinney, "Integrating Learning into Integrated Delivery Systems." *Health Care Management Review* 23(1), pp. 18–28 (Winter, 1998)
45. C. Argyris, "Empowerment: The Emperor's New Clothes." *Harvard Business Review* 76(3), pp. 98–105 (May–June, 1998)
46. R. Galford, "Why Doesn't This HR Department Get Any Respect?" *Harvard Business Review* 76(2), pp. 24–6 (March–April, 1998)

CHAPTER

17

PLANT SYSTEM

Large healthcare organizations have several different plants and plant-related services. Figure 17.1 shows the major facilities of an integrated healthcare system. At the simplest level, a number of primary care sites that are deliberately distributed throughout the community provide the usual medical office amenities. These facilities have few needs beyond those of other small service facilities. At the other extreme, the acute hospital provides complete environmental support not only for patients, but for staff and visitors as well. It provides all the services of a large hotel or office building, but with unusual hazards and narrower tolerances. It must have extra supplies of power and water to allow it to operate through disruptions of those services. It requires narrower tolerances on temperature, humidity, air quality, cleanliness, and wastes. It has relatively higher volumes of human traffic, particularly during the night hours. Because of its traffic, it has high risks of personal and property safety. It deals with highly specialized equipment, expensive and dangerous supplies, and biological, chemical, and radiologic contaminants.

The plant system must meet all of these needs. It is the second largest system in terms of personnel. Housekeeping and food service often rank just behind the largest clinical departments in employees and costs. Consistent with the plan of the book, this chapter attempts to describe the **plant system** as it contributes to the other four systems of governance, finance, clinical, and human resources. It emphasizes what the chief operating officer and the heads of the clinical departments expect from plant services. The focus is on:

- purpose of the plant system;
- functions that must be performed, with attention to the total requirement rather than the part traditionally assigned to plant departments;
- skills and organization required in plant systems; and
- measures that show how well the job has been done and areas needing improvement.

There is a substantial library on the components of plant systems that this chapter does not replace. Some of the more general works are cited at the end of the chapter.

Purpose of the Plant System

The plant and the plant services determine in large part what impressions people form about the healthcare organization. They are thus an important

FIGURE 17.1
Facility and Supply Characteristics of Integrated Health Systems

Activity	Facility	Non-Health Counterpart	Special Needs
Primary care	Small office	Small retail store	X-ray machine Drugs and clinical supplies Clinical waste removal
Outpatient specialty care	Medical office building	Shopping mall	Special electrical and radiologic requirements Drugs and clinical supplies Clinical waste removal
Long-term care	Nursing home	Motel	Extra fire safety and disability assistance Drugs and clinical supplies Clinical waste removal Pathogenic organisms Special air handling
Acute and intensive care	Hospital	Hotel	Extra fire safety and disability assistance Drugs and clinical supplies 24-hour security High traffic volumes Dangerous chemicals High-voltage radiology Radioactive products Clinical waste removal Pathogenic organisms Special air handling Emergency power

element in promotional activity, not only in regard to patients but also in the recruitment of hospital team members. Beyond the minimum required for safety, the well-managed organization strives to operate a plant system that is reliable, convenient, attractive, and yet economical because these are the expectations of members and customers.

Smooth, continuous operation of plant services is occasionally a matter of life and death. Several hazards, including fire, chemicals, radiation, infection, and criminal violence, can be life threatening to employees, visitors, and patients. The well-run organization uses carefully designed, conscientiously maintained programs to reduce these risks to near vanishing.

> The purpose of the plant system is to provide the complete physical environment required for the mission, including all buildings, equipment, and supplies; to protect organization members and visitors against all hazards arising within the healthcare environment; and to maintain reliable plant services at satisfactory levels of economy, attractiveness, and convenience.

Functions

The numerous activities that constitute the plant system can be grouped into seven major categories, as shown in Figure 17.2. It is noteworthy that the plant system goes well beyond the physical plant itself. It includes the management of all supplies, and it relates to all services providing the environmental requirements for medical care. These range from lawn mowing and snow removal through security guards and signage to the life-support environments of surgery and intensive care. The range and variety of activities constitutes the challenge of managing the system. Everything must be done well, from the smallest primary care office to the inpatient intensive care unit.

Facilities Planning and Space Allocation

Facilities planning

Plant operation begins with adequate planning for space and fixed equipment. Healthcare plants are built for their users; thus, plans begin with identifying specific needs and architectural specifications. They continue through the management of construction contracts and the life cycle of maintenance, renovation, and eventual replacement.

FIGURE 17.2 Functions of the Plant System

Function	Activities	Examples
Facilities planning	Planning, building, acquiring, and divesting facilities	Facilities plan Construction and renovation management Facilities leasing and purchase Space allocation
Facilities operation	Operation of buildings, utilities, and equipment	Repairs and routine upkeep Heat, air, and power services
Clinical engineering	Purchase, installation, and maintenance of clinical equipment	Magnetic resonance Laser surgery Respirator
Maintenance services	Housekeeping, groundskeeping, and environmental safety	Cleaning Decorating Snow removal Safety inspections Waste management
Guest services	Support for workers, patients, and visitors	Parking Food service Security services
Supplies services	Materials management	Clinical supplies Drugs X-ray film Anesthesia gases
Continuous improvement and budgeting	Coordination with other systems, service improvement, annual budget	Patient transport Cleaning schedules Energy conservation

As shown in Figure 17.3, the facilities plan begins with an estimate of the space needs of each service or activity proposed in the services plan. Space needs must be described by location, special requirements, and size. Need is compared to available space, and deficits are met at the lowest cost. Conversion, renovation, acquisition by sale or lease, and new construction are the four major ways of meeting needs. Conversion, the simple reassignment of space from one activity to another, is the least expensive, but so many healthcare needs require specific locations and requirements that renovation, acquisition, or construction are frequently necessary. The final facilities plan shows the future location of all services and documents the renovation, acquisition, or construction necessary in terms of specific actions, timetables, and costs.

Forecasting space requirements

Given a forecast of demand for a service, space requirements are forecast from one of two simple models. Where demand can be scheduled or delayed until service is available:

$$(1)\ \text{Facility Required} = (\text{Units of Demand/Time Period}) \times (\text{Space Required per Unit of Demand}) \times (1/\text{Load Factor})$$

FIGURE 17.3
Facilities Planning Process

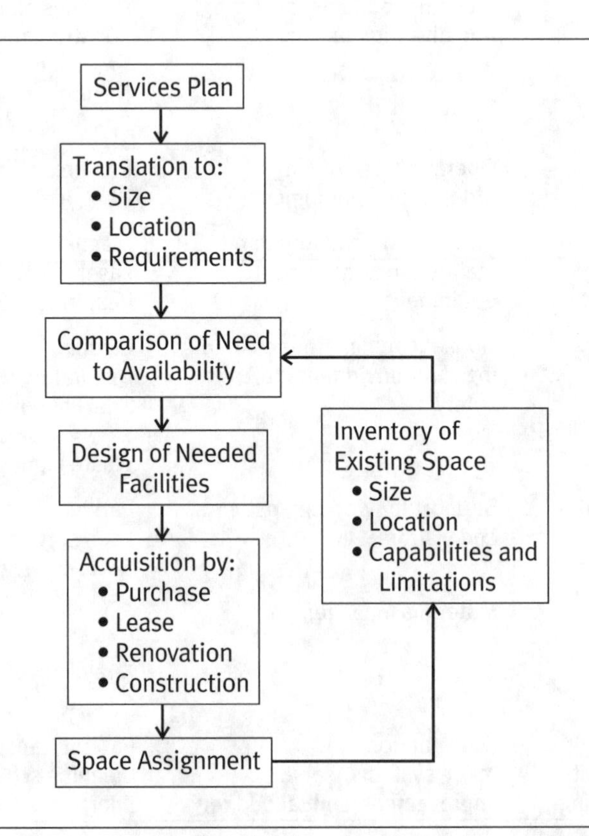

or, where demand must be met without delay (see the discussion of stochastic models in Chapter 6):

(2) Facility Required = Maximum Units of Demand in Single Time Period × (Space Required per Unit of Demand)

The units of demand are the number of patients or services expected in a real time period, the space/unit is the amount of facility required by each patient or service, and the load factor is an allowance for facility idle time. Space required per unit of demand is often measured in specific time and facility dimensions, as machine hours/treatment or bed days/patient.

For example, for schedulable treatments and admissions, the number of treatment rooms required is:

Treatment Rooms = Treatments/Week
× Hours/Treatment
× (1/(Hours Available/Room-Week))

and the number of inpatient beds required is:

Beds Required = Admissions/Year
× Bed-Days/Admission
× (1/(Bed-Days Available/Bed))

But because Bed Days/Admission is the same as Length of Stay, and Bed-Days Available/Bed is the same as Occupancy:

Beds Required = Admissions/Year
× Length of Stay
× 1/Occupancy)

For stochastic services requiring immediate service:

Number of Delivery Rooms = Maximum Number of Mothers in One Hour
× One Room/Mother

The load factor accommodates the time a facility is idle, and is always less than 1.0. Idle time has three sources: time not acceptable to customers, such as holidays and nights; time required for maintenance; and time required as standby for emergency. It is usually possible to schedule maintenance in times of low demand, effectively combining the first two elements. Most physical facilities must have some allowance for peak loads. The load factor becomes a tradeoff between occupancy and market considerations. For example, most inpatient beds can be operated in the low 90 percent occupancies, although many organizations are more comfortable with a lower percentage. Facilities where emergency demand is often encountered, such as obstetrics and coronary care, must be sized to accommodate patient need and will operate at much lower occupancy.

Methods for the actual calculation will get quite complex. Often several methods of forecasting are used to improve confidence in the forecast. For example, surgeries will be categorized by type of room and square feet required. Each type of room will have several sources of demand that are forecast separately. Duration of operations will be studied through industrial engineering techniques. Tradeoffs will be required between specific room designs and room locations and between current efficiency and future flexibility. A room designed for a certain specialty might be highly inefficient for other demand. Tradeoffs must also be evaluated between the efficiency of high load factors and the increased customer and member satisfaction and safety of lower levels. A simulation model might be constructed to evaluate tradeoffs between alternative designs and load factors.

Renovation, construction, and acquisition

Implementing the facilities plan requires a comprehensive program of real estate and building management. The plan indicates the requirements and the way they will be met. These statements must be expanded into specifications and drawings for both space and fixed equipment, and translated to reality by completion of work. Real estate must sometimes be acquired, contracts let, progress maintained, and results inspected and approved before the facility can be occupied. In large projects, several years elapse between approval of the facilities plan and opening day.

Real estate is acquired through purchase or lease. It is possible to lease all or part of a facility, including a single lease for a building and equipment designed and constructed specifically for the healthcare organization. The selection of purchase or lease is a matter of financial management (Chapter 14).

Major construction and renovation usually call for extensive outside contracting. The traditional approach is to retain an architect, a construction management firm, and a general contractor. Construction financed directly by public funds, such as that of public hospitals, usually must be contracted via formal competitive bids. Private organizations frequently prefer more flexible arrangements, negotiating contracts with selected vendors. Recent innovations have simplified the contracts by combining various elements; turnkey construction involves a single contract to deliver the finished facility. Advantages of speed and flexibility are cited, and it is likely that costs can be reduced if the healthcare organization is well prepared and supervises the process carefully.

Smaller renovation projects are often handled by internal staff. As an interim step, the organization can provide design and construction management, preparing the plans and contracting with specific subcontractors.

All parts of healthcare facilities are subject to safety and convenience regulations, with patient care areas having the highest standards. Most of the regulations are contained in the ***Life Safety Code*** and other codes developed by the National Fire Protection Association.[1,2] **Licensure**, JCAHO, and Medicare certification requirements enforce compliance.[3] Facilities must also comply with federal standards for handicapped access.[4]

These regulations require routine inspection and maintenance. They often dictate important specifications of new construction. They require revision of previously approved construction when a renovation is made to the general area containing conditions no longer in compliance with the current code. They occasionally require renovation specifically to meet changes in the code. The length of time before compliance with current codes becomes mandatory is variable, depending on the severity of the hazard. The degree of departure from current code is an important factor in renovation and remodeling plans.

Regardless of the size or complexity of the project, any project to change the use of space should be carefully planned in advance and closely managed as it evolves. A sound program includes:

1. review of the space and equipment needs forecast;
2. identification of special needs;
3. trial of alternative layouts, designs, and equipment configurations;
4. development of a written plan and specifications;
5. review of code requirements and plans for compliance;
6. approval of plan and specifications by the operating unit;
7. development of a timetable and PERT chart identifying critical elements of the construction;
8. contracting or formal designation of work crew and accountability;
9. ongoing review of work against specifications and timetable; and
10. final review, acceptance, and approval of occupancy.

Space allocation

The criterion for allocating existing space is conceptually simple. Each space should be used or disposed of in the way that optimizes achievement of the organization's mission. In reality, this criterion is quite difficult to apply. Activities tend to expand to fill the available space. As a result, there are always complaints of shortages of space and an agenda of possible reallocations or expansions. When activities shrink, the space is often difficult to recover and reuse. Space is highly valuable and unique; the third floor is not identical to the first. Space also confers prestige and symbolic rewards; space next to the doctors' lounge is more prestigious than space adjacent to the employment office. As a result, space allocation decisions tend to be strenuously contested.

Well-run organizations address this problem by incorporating space use and facility needs into their long-range planning, developing a facilities plan that translates the service decisions to specific available or needed space. The plan describes necessary additions or reductions in the space inventory. Each unit seeking substantial additional space or renovation must prepare a formal request and gain approval from the space office before submitting a new program or capital proposal following the procedures outlined in Chapter 12. The following guidelines assist in space management:

- Space management is assigned to a single office that permits occupancy and controls access to space.
- A key function of the space management office is the preparation of the long-range facilities plan. Planning and marketing staff assist in the preparation. The draft plan is derived from the services plan, and the final version becomes part of the planning package. The facilities plan includes:
  - forecasts of specific commitments for existing and approved space;
  - plans for acquisition of land, buildings, and equipment as indicated;
  - renovation and refurbishing requirements for existing space;
  - plant revisions indicated by approved new services and technology, the physician recruitment plan, and the human resources plan; and
  - plans for new construction.
- The cost of the facilities plan is incorporated into the long-range financial plan and annual review and approval processes. This step ensures a realistic financial plan.
- Specific space allocation decisions are made as part of the planning process to ensure widespread understanding of the decisions.
- The plant department implements acquisition, construction, and renovation. Details of interior design are reviewed and approved by units that will be using the space.

Facility Operations

The important components of facilities operations are shown in Figure 17.4. A substantial amount of plant system activity is devoted to maintaining and repairing the physical plant and its major equipment. Utilities services for healthcare institutions are often more demanding than for non-healthcare facilities. The cost of energy failures is so high that electrical and steam systems are usually built with substantial redundancy.

Maintenance and repair services

The objective of maintenance and repair services is to keep the facility and its equipment like new, so that patients, visitors, and staff perceive the environment positively or neutrally. The goal is achieved by emphasizing preventive maintenance. When the cost of downtime is included, it is usually preferable to fix or replace equipment before it is broken. Well-managed plant systems schedule preventive maintenance for all the mechanical services. A significant fraction of mechanics' time is devoted to preventive maintenance, and adherence to the schedule is one of the measures of the quality of the department's work. Similarly, they inspect plant conditions such as floor and wall coverings, plumbing, roofs, and structural members regularly and schedule repair or replacement as they show deterioration.

The technical requirements dictate that contracts with outside vendors be used to maintain many of the more specialized items. Contracts should weigh responsiveness and downtime appropriately and should be for relatively short periods, to permit prompt change of vendor if necessary. One issue

FIGURE 17.4
Facilty Operations—Buildings, Utilities, and Equipment

Maintenance and Repair Services	Utilities Services
Plant maintenance and refurbishing Preventive maintenance Repair of conventional equipment Maintenance of nonclinical, technical equipment • Vehicles • Laundry machinery • Elevators • Heating, steam, and air conditioning equipment • Other	Electrical service • Backup service • Emergency generation • Cogeneration Heating and air conditioning • Routine needs • High pressure steam • Special air control problems Communications support • Telephone, television, and computer wiring • Radio communication • Pneumatic tube systems • Robot delivery systems Patient-related utilities • Oxygen • Suction

is the question of who should initiate and supervise maintenance contracts. Well-run organizations tend to place the responsibility on the line unit using the equipment, if only one unit uses the equipment. The plant department is accountable for equipment in general use, such as elevators, heating, and air conditioning. Actual contracting for all equipment maintenance is centralized through materials management, which must consult with the accountable units.

The accountable unit is also responsible for initiating requests for replacement. These occur when the equipment is more expensive to maintain than replace, or when new technology offers substantial improvements in operating costs. In the case of critical equipment such as elevators and power supplies, it occurs when the risk of significant downtime reaches critical levels. The risk of significant downtime is highly subjective. Outside consultants are often used to evaluate costly equipment.

Provision of utilities

Utilities for most outpatient offices are no different from other commercial buildings, but inpatient hospitals operate sophisticated utility systems that provide air, steam, and water at several temperatures and pressures and filter some air to reduce bacterial contamination.[5] They also provide multiple safeguards against failure because of the extreme consequences. For example, hospitals supply high-pressure steam for sterilizing and laundry equipment. The use of higher pressures requires continuous surveillance by a licensed boiler operator. Operating rooms use specially filtered air, and several sites have unique air temperature control problems. As a result utilities are more elaborate than those usually found in public buildings.

Electrical systems are particularly complex. Feeds from two or three substations are desirable, approaching the hospital from opposite directions.[6]

In addition, the hospital must have on-site generating capability to sustain emergency surgery, respirators, safety lights, and communications. Several areas must switch to the emergency supply automatically, requiring them to be separable from other, less critical uses.[7]

Some healthcare organizations use their heating boilers to generate electrical power, a practice called cogeneration. The local system is integrated with the public utility supplying electricity, and the utility buys any surplus power. Alternatively, the organization may buy steam from the utility for facilities located close to a generating plant, avoiding the cost of maintaining its own boiler.

Several other problems complicate the hospital's utility supply. Most hospitals pipe oxygen and suction to all patient care areas. Many also pipe nitrous oxide to surgical areas. Many hospitals use pneumatic tubes to transport small items such as paper records, drugs, and specimens. A few use automated robot cart systems to transport larger supplies.

Clinical Engineering

Integrated healthcare organizations require a wide variety of specialized clinical equipment that must be maintained near optimum operating characteristics and repaired or replaced as indicated. Apparatus like ventilators, magnetic resonance imagers, ultrasounds, multichannel chemical analyzers, electronic monitoring equipment, heart and lung pumps, and surgical lasers has become commonplace. The acquisition, maintenance, and replacement of this equipment is often assigned to professionally trained clinical engineers.[8] Their understanding of purposes, mechanics, hazards, and requirements allows them to increase the reliability of the machinery and reduce operating costs.[9,10,11]

The role of clinical engineering includes the following activities:

- assisting the user department or group to develop specifications, review competing sources, and select clinical equipment;[11]
- verifying that power, weight, size, and safety requirements are met;
- contracting for maintenance, or arranging training for internal maintenance personnel;
- periodic inspection of equipment for safety and effectiveness; and
- developing plans for replacement when necessary.

Maintenance Services

The array of activities involved in housekeeping, groundskeeping, and environmental control is shown in Figure 17.5. These activities must be performed in compliance with a variety of federal regulations established by OSHA and the Environmental Protection Agency.[12]

Housekeeping	Groundskeeping
Interior decorating	Landscaping
Routine cleaning	Grounds maintenance
• General patient areas	
• High-risk patient areas	**Environmental Safety**
• Non-patient areas	Physical control of chemical, biological, and radiological hazards
Special problem areas	• Contaminant storage
• Odor control	• Contaminant waste removal
• Sound control	• Special cleaning and emergency procedures
Waste Management	Facility safety
Solid waste removal	• Inspection and hazard identification
Clinical waste removal	• Hazard correction
Recycling	

FIGURE 17.5 Maintenance Services—Housekeeping, Groundskeeping, and Environmental Safety

Housekeeping and groundskeeping

Housekeeping and groundskeeping must maintain campuses in the millions of square feet efficiently at standards ensuring bacterial and other hazard control. Some services, such as snow removal and exterior lighting, must be round the clock. In well-run organizations these activities are conducted to explicit standards of quality and are monitored by inspectors using formal survey methods. These activities also interact with important programs for environmental safety. Continuous improvement, training, and carefully specified equipment and supplies are used to attain high levels of cleanliness and safety.

Cleaning and landscape services are frequently subcontracted. The most common contracts are for management-level services. The outside firm supplies procedures, training, and supervision; the workers are hourly employees. Large organizations, and those with access to central services for training and development of methods, may be able to justify their own management.

Decorating and landscaping are done with an understanding both of public taste and of the cost of specific materials. Colors, fabrics, and designs are selected both for comfort and durability.[13] The best decorating creates an attractive ambiance, but is made of materials that do not show wear and are durable and easy to clean. Careful initial design leads to higher capital costs, but lower operating costs and greater user satisfaction. It is believed to contribute to patient recovery.[14]

Waste management

Environmental needs and hazards in clinical wastes have complicated the problem of waste management. Waste disposal must meet increasingly stringent governmental standards protecting the safety of landfills, water supplies, and air. Many cities require segregation of nonclinical wastes to permit recycling. Federal and state laws govern burning and shipment of wastes. A federal law governs handling of clinical wastes.[15] Although evidence that clinical wastes are particularly hazardous outside the institution is lacking, they must receive special handling from source to ultimate disposition.[16]

Within the healthcare organization, wastes must be handled correctly and efficiently.[17,18] Clinical wastes are a known hazard for hepatitis and AIDS contamination. Specially designed systems for waste management must be taught to general housekeeping personnel.[19,20] Interim storage is usually required before shipment to the final site. Healthcare organizations usually contract for waste removal, but the handler must be certified for clinical wastes.

Environmental safety

There are four basic approaches to control of hazardous materials. These approaches must be coordinated between different units in most healthcare organizations.

1. *Restricting exposure at the source.* Good design and good procedures for use reduce chemical contamination. The cheapest way to deal with a specific chemical contaminant is frequently to replace it. Many of the chemicals used in healthcare organizations are selected as part of the clinical diagnosis and treatment, however, so review of the necessity for using dangerous chemicals is often a medical question.

   Restricting exposure to bacteriological contaminants is more difficult, and building design and operation are frequently important. Air and water handling systems can be made almost completely safe. Special handling is necessary for contaminated wastes. Human vectors in the spread of infection are harder to control, and they include both caregivers and plant personnel. Special gowns and techniques are used to protect workers and to prevent the spread of infection to other patients. Development of comprehensive control systems and monitoring of actual infection rates is a clinical function usually assigned to an infection control committee. It is wise to have at least one plant person on the infection committee. Larger organizations may have persons from plant operations, housekeeping, and central supply services available to consult with the infection committee.
2. *Cleaning and removal.* Cleaning methods must reflect the need for bacterial and chemical decontamination. The housekeeping department is usually responsible for cleaning and removing hazardous substances. All horizontal surfaces are major sources of bacterial cross-contamination; in some areas, such as the operating rooms, more extensive attention is needed. There are occasionally special problems of chemical contamination as well, such as from the use of radioactive isotopes.
3. *Attention to exposed patients, visitors, and staff.* Trauma or infection results from exposure to contaminants, which can occur either during patient treatment or afterward, handling or disposing of equipment. Although much public attention has been given to AIDS, hepatitis is actually a more serious threat to hospital workers and also occurs much more frequently among patients. Healthcare organizations must provide workers' compensation for any employee injury resulting from exposure. Although workers are entitled to their choice of physician, many organizations use a clinical member of the infection committee to examine

any person believed to be injured and to provide care to those who will accept it. Concentrating cases in a single doctor provides continuity and promotes thorough understanding of hospital hazards.

4. *Epidemiological analysis of failures.* Epidemiological studies are an important part of an infection control program. Studies of the incidence of specific illnesses can detect incipient epidemics and may be the only way to reveal certain problems of chemical contamination. The information necessary for epidemiological studies frequently requires the assistance of a physician. The work requires special training in epidemiology. It is often assigned to a member of the infection committee.

Guest Services

Large numbers of patients, visitors, and staff become the guests of healthcare organizations and require a variety of physical services. People expect to come to a facility; park; find what they want; get certain amenities such as waiting areas, lounges, and possibly food; and leave without even recognizing that they have received service. Those telephoning expect a similarly complete, prompt, and unobtrusive response. The organization's attractiveness is diminished if the services listed in Figure 17.6 are either inadequate or intrusive. The personnel delivering the services are in constant contact with the organization's important constituencies. Their effect on customer and member satisfaction is almost as great as nursing's.

Guest services frequently involve multiple locations and small work groups, but they require coordinated management and a significant investment in centrally operated support systems. For example, receptionists and security personnel need current knowledge of the location of each inpatient and each special event or activity. Coordinated management of guest services stresses the importance of a satisfactory overall impression. It may also contribute to efficiency by allowing overlapping functions to be eliminated. Relations with housekeeping, security, and plant operations also require coordination.

Reception and messenger services

In a large healthcare organization, several dozen people have reception jobs that involve primarily meeting and guiding the organization's guests. Signs and display of telephone numbers (as in the yellow pages) aid efficient routing.

Patients and large physical items must be moved around the organization, and training in guest relations, emergency medical needs, and hospital geography are necessary to do the job well. Larger organizations have circulating vans connecting various sites. These move workers, patients, and some supplies promptly and inexpensively. Because requests for transportation are often random and because it is difficult to supervise messengers, there are important efficiencies in pooling messenger needs. Very large organizations may have more than one pool, but smaller ones usually combine all messenger and reception activities under one supervisor.

FIGURE 17.6 Guest Services—Work Force, Patient, and Visitor Support

Security Services	Communication and Transportation Services
Guards	Telephone and television service
Employee identification	Messenger service
Facility inspection and and monitoring	Tube transport systems
	Reception and guidance
Food Service	Signage
Cafeteria and vending service	Parking
Patient food service	Telephone reception and paging
Routine patient service	
Therapeutic diets	

Security services

Security services are necessary in most settings to protect employees, visitors, patients, and property. There is a recognized hazard of theft, property destruction, and personal injury to workers and visitors. The hazard is particularly high in urban areas. High-quality security services are preventive. Security involves controlling access to the hospital, monitoring traffic flow, employee identification, and lighting to create an environment both reassuring to guests and discouraging to persons with destructive intentions.[21] Television and emergency call systems amplify the scope of surveillance.[22,23] Employee education is helpful in promoting safe behavior and prompt reporting of questionable events. Special attention must be given to high-risk areas such as the emergency room[24] and parking.[25]

Uniformed guards are the final element of a high-quality program, not the initial one. They serve to provide a visible symbol of authority, to respond to questions and concerns, and to provide emergency assistance in those infrequent events that exceed the capability of reception personnel.

Security is frequently a contract service, although it obviously must be coordinated with local police and fire service. Municipal units sometimes provide the contract service, particularly in government hospitals. Not-for-profit healthcare organizations usually do not pay local taxes in support of local fire and police service; as a result, there is often a question about the extent to which taxpayer services should be provided. Some states have imposed fees on not-for-profit organizations to reflect public services provided.

Emergency assistance should normally follow a previously developed security plan. The recurring major hazards of public areas should be addressed in the plan. These include armed and unarmed criminals, political protesters, and mentally impaired persons; bomb threats, fires, and serious accidents involving damage or release of toxic materials. The security plan for major community disasters is particularly taxing and is part of the hospital disaster plan (Chapter 4).

Food service

The preparation of food for patients, staff, and guests has become a service similar to the food services of hotels, airlines, and resorts, rather than a clinical service. It must be conducted to high standards of quality, beginning with control of bacterial hazards and safety in preparation and distribution. Several foods are ideal media for bacterial growth. Employee hand washing and medical examinations are important to avoid systematic bacterial contamination. Further, careful food handling is necessary to prevent acute food poisoning. Kitchens include an unusual number of burn, fall, and injury hazards. Food service must also provide inexpensive, nutritious, appealing, and tasty meals that encourage good eating habits. It must supply them to remote locations and, either directly or by arrangement with nursing, deliver them to many people who are partially incapacitated.

Hospitals typically offer a choice of entrees, appetizers, and desserts to each patient on census. Patient meals must also be provided to a variety of clinical specifications. Soft, low-sodium, and sodium-free diets account for up to half of all patient meals; however, bulk foods meeting these specifications can be prepared by personnel without clinical training. In addition to patient meals, about an equal number are provided to staff and guests, usually in cafeterias. Visitors and employees expect greater variety, a range of prices, and service at odd hours. It is common to operate a snack bar or coffee shop and a variety of vending machines offering snack food and soft drinks.

These concerns are relatively easy to meet through sound general procedures. Food service is frequently contracted. Contract food suppliers meet the quality and cost constraints through centralized menu planning, well-developed training programs for workers and managers, and careful attention to work methods. Nutritional education and consultation and the preparation of special diets to meet medical needs is available through the clinical dietetics service. These professional nutritionists have an important advisory role in menu planning, but they have limited contact with the mass feeding operation.

Materials Management Services

Healthcare organizations typically spend nearly 10 percent of their budget for supplies. Like other industries, they use office supplies, foodstuffs, linens and uniforms, fuels, paints, hardware, and cleaning supplies. They also use implants, whole blood, specialized dressings, single-purpose medical tools, and a large variety of drugs. Most supply costs are represented in the following inventory groups, which are either large volumes of inexpensive items, like foodstuffs, or relatively small volumes of very expensive items, like implants:

- surgical supplies and implants;
- pharmaceuticals, intravenous solutions, and anesthesia gases;
- foodstuffs;
- linen; and
- dressings, kits, and supplies for patient care.

Improving the materials management function

Materials management concentrates almost all supplies purchases under a single unit of the organization that is responsible for meeting standards of quality and service at a minimum total cost. The materials management function includes the activities shown in Figure 17.7. Many of these items conflict with one another. For example, larger order quantities save delivery costs but increase warehouse costs, and cheaper distribution systems may increase user dissatisfaction or waste. Thus, the problem of materials management is to design systems of acquisition that achieve the lowest overall costs, rather than simply purchasing at the cheapest price.

Specification of supplies is a critical component of materials management. Working with line personnel, materials management personnel strive to standardize similar items, establish criteria for appropriate quality, and eliminate unnecessary purchases.[26] Reducing the number of items purchased reduces the number of orders that must be placed and the inventories that are required. It may eliminate unnecessarily expensive items. Examination of the application and alternative approaches may lead to improved methods and new supply specifications. For example, disposables may be compared to equipment that is processed for reuse. Materials management personnel estimate the cost of disposable and reusable alternatives and assist in selecting the more cost-effective.

Most important, the larger volumes of standardized materials can be controlled more carefully for quality and used to negotiate lower prices. The purchasing process itself uses longer-term contracting and competitive bidding to reduce prices. Most well-managed organizations now use **group purchasing**, cooperatives that use the collective buying power of several organizations to leverage prices downward. In addition, vendors contribute to the cost of the materials handling system. Automation of inventories, ordering, and billing reduces handling costs. "Just in time" deliveries are calculated

FIGURE 17.7 Materials Management Activities

Material Selection and Control
Specifications for cost-effective supplies
Standardization of items
Reduction in the number of items

Purchasing
Standardized purchasing procedures
Competitive bid
Annual or periodic contracts
Group purchasing contracts

Receipt, Storage, and Protection
Reduction of inventory size
Control of shipment size and frequency
Reduction of handling
Reduction of damage or theft
Economical warehouse operation

Processing
Elimination of processing by purchase or contract
Improved processing methods
Reduced reprocessing or turnaround time

Distribution
Elimination or automation of ordering
Improved delivery methods
Reduced end-user inventories
Reduced waste and unauthorized usage

Revenue Enhancement and Cost Accounting
Uniform records of supplies usage

to keep inventories at near-zero levels. Most major vendors supply just-in-time service, effectively bearing the cost of inventory management as part of their activities rather than the healthcare organization's.[27] Some large vendors offer comprehensive materials management, providing a complete service at competitive costs.[28] Recent innovations have included risk-sharing incentives in these contracts.[29]

Significant savings are possible in materials handling systems.[30] These systems receive, inspect, and store supplies, receive and fill orders, and record usage. Routine sampling of received goods assures quality. Centralized storage protects against theft and damage. Division of duties guards against embezzlement and accounting fraud. Usage records and automated delivery systems reduce or eliminate inventories at the point of use and are designed to achieve low-cost handling. Materials management includes the design of distribution systems and the maintenance of usage records. Automatic resupply reduces time spent by end users ordering and checking supplies. Some bulk supplies are now delivered by robots to reduce costs.[31] Finally, automated records of supplies used provide data for cost analysis, and in cases where individual payments are made for the supplies, posting of account receivables.

Continuous Improvement and Budgeting

Like all other systems of the healthcare organization, the plant system must explicitly devote time to improving quality and efficiency of service. Plant systems have undergone substantial revision in recent years. Materials management programs, energy conservation programs, environmental hazard controls, and security services are vastly different from a decade ago. That trend will continue in the decade to come. The cycle of identifying, studying, and improving processes, and incorporating the improvement into the next annual budget, will be a fixture of plant systems management. Much of the improvement activity will involve coordination of services with other units. Much of it will also involve longer-term activities, such as revisions centered around capital replacement.

The improvement cycle

The cycle of improvement and budget development and achievement is shown in Figure 17.8. A key function of leadership is to stimulate the cycle. The goal is to have several improvement concepts in process, completing a few each year to meet externally imposed budget standards, so that each year's budget is both acceptable and achievable.

Well-run organizations now hold plant services responsible for meeting market demands. The other systems and their employees join patients and families as explicit customers. Satisfaction of customer requirements, including both price and quality, is the consuming goal. The plant system operates as a service organization for the rest of the world, as a resort hotel might. Like the hotel, it views itself as one of many alternatives where customers could spend their money. Measurement of achievement, revision of methods and

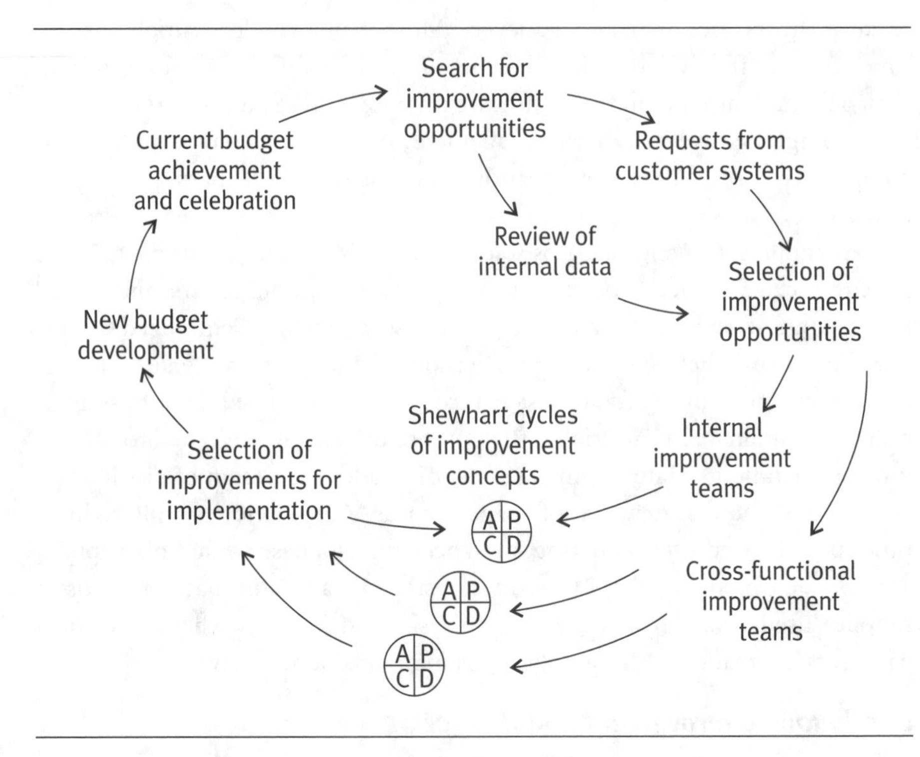

FIGURE 17.8 Cycle of Continuous Improvement and Budgeting for the Plant System

equipment, annual expectation setting, training, and reward are the tools for improving service.

Attractive, convenient, comfortable plant services are a competitive asset. Without them, market share may fall. As it does, volume declines, forcing fixed costs per discharge up. Thus, final product efficiency may depend as much on the quality of plant service as on its cost. Ingenuity and effort are necessary to avoid reducing quality of plant service under severe cost constraints. Organizations may at times wish to increase plant system costs to gain an advantage in the market.

The well-run organization is moving rapidly toward comprehensive performance measurement, which allows direct comparison with alternative sources or desired performance levels. A housekeeping service, for example, can compare its cost to outside contractors' and its customer satisfaction ratings to external benchmarks or internal goals. It conducts process quality review and can identify variation in its own performance as well as compare itself to industry standards. It surveys its staff and collects data on absenteeism and turnover that can also be compared to industry standards. (See "Measures of Performance," below.)

At the same time, the department is evaluated by the other systems of the organization and is receptive to the needs of those systems. Requests for cross-training, revised scheduling, special cleaning needs are welcomed, and handled as marketing opportunities. Out of the internal review and the requests of the customer systems comes the agenda for improvement. The department pursues that agenda constantly, through internal studies and participation in cross-functional task forces.

Many issues in final product efficiency relate to the coordination of services between clinical services and plant services. New food service systems must coordinate with nursing; patient transportation must adapt to new diagnostic services; new supplies and methods of assembling supplies must be revised for new nursing intermediate product protocols. These improvements are designed by cross-functional teams or by internal teams of clinical services that will require close cooperation by plant systems units. The opportunity to participate on these teams is valuable in two senses. First, the cognitive exchange of information leads to a better result. Second, the participants on the team gain insight into the underlying customer needs. They come away from the process understanding why the improvement was necessary, and more committed to making it work.

Cross-functional team membership is now assigned to the lowest level of personnel capable of addressing the issue. This is often the workers themselves. Food service workers participate on the cross-functional team designing a new food service. (The team will also have membership from nursing, materials management, and clinical nutrition.) The assignment brings a practical perspective not previously available, but more important it demonstrates empowerment to the work group and provides an opportunity to reward work group leadership.

Most improvements are related to changes in work methods rather than better motivation of workers. New methods resulting from cross-functional teams must be explained and sold to plant workers. Internal improvements usually involve changes in equipment and methods. The way in which new methods and equipment are introduced is often critical to their success. The improvement process should follow the Shewhart cycle of Plan, Do, Check, Act (Chapter 2). Improvements from cross-functional teams should be explained, justified, and demonstrated to plant workers as part of their implementation. Understanding and acceptance of the plant workers is essential to success.

Internal improvement teams should be composed mainly of workers. The function of the supervisor is ideally to coach, motivate, and make the opportunity clear. Retraining of workers is often critical to success of the new method. Part of the Check activity involves identifying new methods and learning how to teach them.

The annual budget establishes goals for each dimension of performance for each responsibility center. The next year's goals must meet price and quality standards imposed by the larger organization by implementing improvements developed during the year. An aggressive continuous improvement program should allow most plant units to meet the budget requirements. The challenge should be in finding the improvements for the subsequent year, not in making the proposed budget. Most units should be able to celebrate achieving the current budget as a motivation to work on the next. Failure to improve, or to remain competitive with alternate suppliers, suggests the need to restructure the service or to change suppliers.

Evaluating long-term opportunities

Opportunities to restructure plant services arise when the organization faces major change, such as new partnerships or facility replacement. Windows of opportunity arise that close as commitments are made. For example, consider an organization that has operated its own laundry for many years. Its existing equipment is still useful, but aging and already less efficient than current models. As long as the equipment is still serviceable, contract laundry services may not be price competitive, but when the organization faces a major investment to replace that equipment contract services are suddenly more attractive. Similarly, an opportunity to use the existing laundry space for more productive activities may make contract service more attractive. The alternative use is also a window; the need will be met in other ways if the laundry site is not promptly evaluated.

Major windows of opportunity are usually two or three years long, covering several budget cycles. They must be identified as part of the facilities plan, evaluated, and accommodated by plant system management. The annual environmental assessment should include review of the facilities and equipment plan and explicit evaluation of opportunities to purchase plant services from outside vendors. The review will require collaboration among facilities planning and space allocation people and the planning unit. The plant system managers must be cognizant of the review and of the basic principle, that any plant service is retained only when it is more effective than an outside contractor. When the decision is made to revise a plant service, effective programs to make the necessary conversions require careful planning in themselves.

Personnel Requirements and Organization

Personnel Requirements

Managers and professional personnel

There are few widely recognized educational programs in plant management. The professional societies have not offered registration as a qualification for employment, but they do suggest that active membership should be a criterion.[32] As a result, job descriptions depend heavily on prior experience. Contract management firms have extensive on-the-job training and may be the best source of managers.

A bachelor's degree in engineering is generally considered necessary for facility operation managers, particularly if construction responsibilities are included. Some large organizations also employ architects, a profession with both formal education and licensure. Although there are licensure requirements for professional engineers and architects in consultative practice, the requirements do not apply to employment situations. Clinical equipment engineers generally have bachelor's engineering degrees, and specialized programs are available.[33,34]

Materials managers should acquire general business knowledge. Course work in law and business is certainly an asset, but much of the needed knowledge can also be acquired by well-supervised experience. Security managers frequently have active police experience and at least bachelor's degrees in their field. Food service managers have bachelor's degrees and extensive experience in bulk food preparation.

Several professions are involved in environmental safety. Infection control is often the concern of a medical or nonmedical epidemiologist. Both have formal educational requirements. The physician is frequently privileged in communicable disease and in any case should be subject to routine credentials review. Organizations with high-voltage radiation therapy services usually employ a radiation physicist who can also assist with radiation safety. Large organizations employ toxicologists to assist with control of chemical contamination. There is an engineering specialty known as safety engineering. Consultative services are available in many of these areas. The local public health department may also have useful resources.

Employees

The traditional building trades and stationary engineers provide apprenticeships. They are usually licensed by local or state authorities, but licensure is not mandatory for employees under appropriate supervision. Security personnel are frequently former police and may have attended college programs in police work. Job descriptions in these fields normally require the appropriate license or certificate and consider relevant prior experience favorably. All other employees are recruited as unskilled labor or, in the case of materials management, clerical labor.

Training and Incentives

Cost-effective plant services require both preparation of employees to do the work and incentives for doing it well. The plant system has a variety of training needs for both employees and supervisors. It also requires a system of nonmonetary and monetary incentives to motivate its personnel.

Training needs

Most plant employees need explicit training in how to do their jobs. As methods and equipment become more sophisticated, a worker who does not fully understand both what must be done and how to do it cannot produce at a competitive level. As a result, sound plant systems programs teach new workers and retrain old ones on an ongoing basis. In addition to job content, purpose, and method, employee training for several plant areas must include guest relations. As participation on improvement teams increases, workers must be trained in continuous improvement fundamentals.

Supervisors need all these skills, including mastery of the work methods. At least one of the contract housekeeping services, ServiceMaster, insists that all its supervisors including the company president spend a week doing the most menial housekeeping jobs. In addition, supervisors need explicit training in supervision. Conventional wisdom about the supervisory process is quite different from empirically tested models of what supervision should be. The folklore of the boss who gives orders and has special privileges must be replaced with an understanding of a supportive leader who is obligated to find answers to employee questions. Formal education, including case studies and role playing, establishes the desired model. Constant reinforcement is necessary to keep it in place. Supervisors also need advanced training in continuous improvement and training in budgeting.

These training programs must all be carried out at a high school level, and in many communities they must accommodate several languages. The emphasis is on action, practice, graphics, and only lastly words. The training programs all present important opportunities to build the employee's pride in craftsmanship and loyalty to the organization.

Increasing incentives and rewards

If attention is paid to measures, goals, and methods, the gains from reward systems are greatly increased, both for the worker and for the hospital. Three desirable guidelines are that most expectations should be met, rewards for good performance should be frequent and generous, and sanctions should be rare. (Not surprisingly, this is as true for the plant system as for the medical staff.)

The most important incentives are nonmonetary. Pride of achievement is probably the most important. It is supported by prompt reporting of formal measures, well-designed methods, appropriate training, and responsive supervision. Recognition of achievement includes both verbal and nonverbal responses of the supervisor. The amount of recognition should be tailored to the level of achievement: any positive response should be recognized by the supervisor, above average results by coworkers, and extraordinary achievement by the organization at large. The supervisor is critical in pride of achievement and recognition.

Explicit monetary incentives, beyond the basic contract for compensation and employment, appear to play a relatively minor role in motivating workers. For example, they cannot overcome disincentives from poor supplies or inadequate training. Nor do they effectively replace pride of achievement. They are most powerful as supplements to nonmonetary incentives, where even a small payment serves to show the seriousness of management intent. Monetary incentives can be dysfunctional when they encourage unneeded output or disregard of customer wants. They can be defeated by the workers, who can exaggerate supply and equipment problems and create grievances.

Use of Contract Services

Healthcare organizations contract extensively for plant services. Smaller organizations have relied on building management firms for facility services and a variety of specialized vendors for equipment maintenance. Larger organizations contracted for specialized equipment like elevators and services like groundskeeping. Major construction is almost always contracted. It is not surprising, therefore, that when specific technologies began to emerge for laundry, housekeeping, specialized equipment maintenance, food service, and security, healthcare organizations turned quickly to contracts that provided inexpensive access to them.

The trend in plant services has been away from ownership and toward contract service for some years, and it is likely to continue. The movement in healthcare organizations parallels one in industry in general.[35] The following sections review the advantages and disadvantages of contracting, varieties of contract arrangements, and guidelines for successful contracting.

Advantages and disadvantages to contracting

The advantage of contracting is access to the contractor's repository of specialized knowledge. A contractor like ServiceMaster, which provides housekeeping and food services to about 1,800 healthcare organizations,[36] quickly acquires an experience base in its areas that exceeds even the largest healthcare organization's. By specializing in a function and building up experience and activity in that area, the contractor can:

- develop a cadre of experienced people equipped to solve whatever problems may arise;
- develop more efficient methods:
  - specify better tasks, tools, and supplies
  - train personnel more effectively
  - develop more precise measures of quality and efficiency;
- develop and implement software:
  - improve scheduling
  - develop quality control
  - capture and analyze cost and use data;
- learn more effective ways of motivating personnel; and
- take advantage of larger volumes:
  - gain lower prices on supplies and equipment
  - support more cost-effective substitution of capital for labor.

The list is the same set of factors that supports any industrial specialization. Different services have different profiles of specific advantages. In each case, success is proved by growth in the marketplace. Several forms of contracting have met this test.

The disadvantage of contracting is potential loss of control of performance. Incomplete or incorrect specification of the desired service may lead to excessive cost or dissatisfaction. Ineffective supervision of the contract by the healthcare organization may lead to suboptimal achievement of its terms. The savings may not be passed back to the healthcare organization. Monopoly or ineffective negotiation may leave most of the savings with the supplier. Successful contract suppliers grow and may not be as efficient as they once were. Growth can create personnel shortages, unexpected problems, overcommitment, inflexibility, and loss of motivation.

Thus, there is always a point of equilibrium at which contracting and not contracting are equally appealing. The equilibrium is subject to adjustment with changing conditions. It is quite possible that two almost identical organizations will reach opposite conclusions about contracting.

Extent of contracting

Service contracts vary in scope and duration. The simplest are short-term, task-oriented contracts, such as consulting arrangements or equipment repair contracts. The most complex are long-term commitments for multiple tasks or even for a general purpose. A large-scale construction contract or a contract to operate an entire hospital is an example. Awarding and administering service contracts depends on their duration, complexity, and uniqueness. Operating units can negotiate simple contracts directly with materials management personnel. A contract for hospital operation or a major construction project would require governing board action. In between, contracts for managing the major functions, shown in Figure 17.2, can be managed by the executive group.

The list of actual contracts between healthcare organizations and service firms is quite long, and growing. The service corporation is usually a for-profit company, and is often a national corporation. Examples include:

- contracts for specified discrete tasks, such as job classification and salary surveys, preventive maintenance, or construction;
- sporadic or infrequent services, such as snow removal, equipment evaluation, or consultation on specific problems;
- contracts for general equipment maintenance or updates;
- contracts for clinical equipment maintenance or updates;[37]
- contracts for continuing services, such as housekeeping, food service, laundry, data processing, and security; and
- contracts for complete functions, such as comprehensive materials management services, turnkey construction, or complete facility management.

All forms of contracting seem to have been increasing, but the last four have risen from near zero to a substantial fraction of hospital expenditures. Although exact figures are difficult to obtain, the total is probably 3 to 5 percent of hospital expenditures, approaching $20 billion a year.

Criteria for successful contracting

Well-run organizations negotiate contracts in a way that will exploit the advantages and disadvantages to their overall benefit. This is not necessarily to the supplier's disadvantage; the best contracts are frequently those in which both parties win. The following conditions make a successful result more likely:[38]

1. The organization has a full, clear, and realistic understanding of the service desired:
   a. Descriptions of the scope of work are unambiguous.
   b. Systems are in place to measure supplier's performance with regard to demand, output, quality, and cost.
   c. Quantitative expectations on these parameters have been developed from history or benchmarking.
2. There is a competitive market. Several suppliers have records of effective performance in similar situations and demonstrate both interest and capability in the service to be performed.
3. Resources that the healthcare organization must supply are available:
   a. Facilities and equipment are scheduled for the contractor's use.
   b. Systems for supplying orders and other necessary communications are in place.
   c. Terms, methods, and personnel for contract supervision can be specified.
   d. Programs for the transfer of activity have been developed.
4. The contractor will identify a manager who has both skills and rank appropriate to the scope of the contracted work.
5. An initial request for proposals is used to evaluate suppliers and to improve the quality of the specifications:
   a. Invitations include all potentially qualified bidders.
   b. Initial specifications avoid accidental or arbitrary restriction of bidders or of potential gains. The scope of work is pragmatically defined to cover items that are essential to the organization and also achievable by a satisfactory number of bidders.
   c. Suppliers are encouraged to respond with modifications or extensions of the initial specifications; these can be evaluated on their merits.
   d. Further discussion with suppliers can help develop the best possible final specifications.
6. Qualified suppliers are selected from the initial round and asked to submit more detailed proposals, including competitive prices.
   a. Sufficient bidders are invited to the second round to encourage competitive pricing.
   b. Format for the final proposal is specified closely enough to permit direct comparison of bids.
   c. Opportunity to price alternatives and options separately remains.

d. Contract length is kept to a relatively short period, or termination on short warning is permitted, to provide continuing incentive for achieving the hospital's expectations.

Steps 5 and 6 normally apply only to complex, long-term contracts.

The difficulty with these criteria is that they fail to cover realistic situations in which the organization is justified in seeking a service contract. They say, in effect, that when there are several well-managed suppliers, an organization with a service that is already well managed can negotiate a good contract. While this is true enough, it overlooks situations in which the organization must correct serious weaknesses in plant systems services and situations in which one dominant service contractor has developed an exceptional record. Some issues to consider in those situations are as follows:

- Initial competition can be against the organization's own performance. Renewals present a problem. Either benchmarks must be found, independent consultants used, or the renewal must be subjectively evaluated. The possibility of restoring internal service at a future date should be explicitly evaluated.
- The expertise of the supplier can often be used to strengthen the expectations and establish measures of performance. This can be done either through negotiations, short-term consulting contracts prior to a longer-term commitment, or contracts that specify the development or improvement of performance measures. Contracts for improvement of performance generally contain incentive payments or penalties.
- A poorly run organization or service may have to sacrifice price for quality improvement.
- An organization that assists a new company or pioneers in new areas of contract services should anticipate extra benefits in the form of price reduction or profit sharing on future sales.

Organization of Plant Services

Comprehensive accountability

Traditionally, larger healthcare organizations have had chief engineers, purchasing agents, housekeepers, security officers, food service heads, and central supply supervisors with departmental status reporting independently to deputy or chief operating officers. Communications services and other support activities tended to be assigned expediently. Comprehensive plant accountability, that is, concentrating plant services under one manager reporting to the COO, seems to have been rare, but it is likely to become more common.

Plant systems organization should be flexible for organization size and extent of outside contracting. Figure 17.9 shows a general model for plant systems organization in a large healthcare organization. Any element on

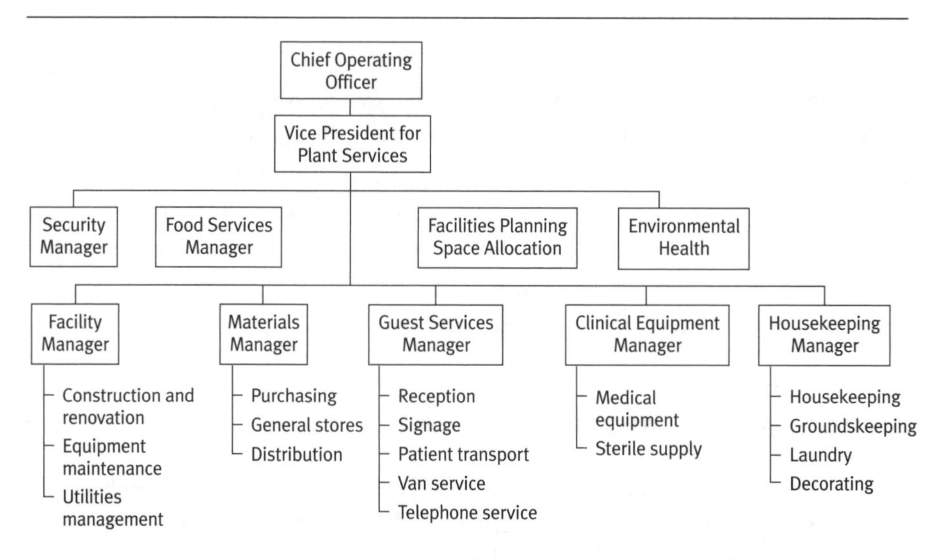

FIGURE 17.9 Plant Systems Organization for Larger Organizations

Figure 17.9 can be contracted to an outside firm, including the vice president for Plant Services.

The assignment of several small activities of Figure 17.9 is debatable.[39] Some or all of guest services and housekeeping can be assigned to facilities operation, for example. Alternatively, guest services and security can be merged. Laundry can be elevated to a manager level, and probably will be if the institution operates its own laundry.

Smaller organizations will be more likely to use contract services. They must still provide the full array of services, and finding specialists in all the areas is expensive and often difficult. In general, the simpler activities such as food service, housekeeping, or security are easier to contract, while the most complicated ones, such as facility operations and materials management, are more difficult. The risk of an unsatisfactory contract rises with the complexity of the assignment. Facility planning and space allocation is the most problematic and most likely to be retained internally.

The most debatable question appears to be the organizational locus of materials management. Surprisingly, leading materials managers themselves feel that the "importance placed on materials management . . . was related more to who reports to the materials manager than to whom the material manager reports. . . ."[40] One option would be to treat the unit as part of finance, but this places product delivery in what is otherwise an information-processing activity, creating few promotional opportunities for the successful manager. The concept of separation of duties to discourage fraud and abuse also militates against the close association of materials control and accounting. A second option would be for the materials manager to report directly to the COO. A third is the hierarchy suggested here, reporting to the manager of plant services, who reports to the COO.

Within the materials management organization itself there seems to be virtue in centralization of authority. The managers surveyed by Holmgren and Wentz saw all plant services except housekeeping, security, and plant operations as their "ideal" domain.[41] They also believed they should control all inventories, including drugs and foodstuffs, although they conceded the need for clinical functions in the dietary and pharmacy departments. Although materials management can easily include supervision of annual contracting for housekeeping and similar services, it seems unlikely that other guest services would be grouped with materials services.

Measures of Performance

Plant services must first be reliable and safe, then satisfactory to hospital members and visitors, and finally efficient. Measures for the six dimensions are well developed and can usually be transferred easily from industrial sites or between hospitals. Human resources and customer satisfaction measures are similar to operating units, recognizing that all the other units of the organization are customers of plant services, along with patients, families, and other guests.

Measures of Output and Demand

Output and demand for plant system services are usually measured identically; output is simply that portion of demand that is filled. Demand is measured differently for each of the functions of the plant system, using various combinations of patient or service requests, specific facility required, and duration, as reflected in the examples shown in Figure 17.10.

To establish resource expectations, it is necessary to forecast demand. This is usually possible by analysis of historic data on the incidence and duration of demand for each identified physical resource. Peak loads are frequently

FIGURE 17.10 Examples of Demand Measures for Plant System Functions

Service Request	Incidence Measure	Duration Measure
Surgery cleanup	Number of cases	Minutes/case
Heating/air conditioning	Degree–days	N/A
General housekeeping	Square footage	Minutes/square foot
Specialized housekeeping	Square footage by type	Minutes/square foot by type
Safety inspection	Specific type	Hours/inspection
Meal service	Meals/day by type	N/A
Security and reception	Personnel by location	Hours/day
Supplies	Units by type	N/A

important. Analysis of cyclic fluctuation and frequency distributions or ranges are frequently required to set sound resource expectations.

Many activities of the plant system require short-term forecasts, with horizons ranging from hours to months. Efficiency in supply and service processes such as housekeeping, heating, and food service depends on careful adjustment to variation in demand. Well-run organizations are supplying current estimates of demand for services like these from order entry and nursing scheduling systems. (Several kinds of service are related to patient acuity.) It is likely that, in the future, patient scheduling systems will be used to forecast demand for these services.

Inventory management calls for slightly longer-term forecasts. The key to efficiency and quality of service is accurate forecasts of demand at the most detailed level possible. These forecasts can be used to operate exchange cart deliveries, minimizing out-of-stock items and emergency trips, and to maintain optimum inventory levels and ordering cycles. The preparation of these forecasts is normally the obligation of the materials management unit, with guidance from finance and planning. Experienced materials managers can often make useful, subjective refinements to statistically prepared forecasts.

Measures of Resource Consumption and Efficiency

Personnel, supplies, and capital resources are all important in plant services. The costs and physical units of all the resources involved should first be accounted to a plant system responsibility center. Each plant responsibility center can be held accountable for the total cost of operating its unit, including labor, materials, and capital costs consumed by the unit, as well as purchase price, inventory level, and wastage of inventoried supplies.

Standard cost accounting practices have some important limitations. Capital costs are accounted at straight-line depreciation of original purchase price, without interest, often resulting in substantial understatement. Inventory costs are rarely adjusted for the value of money invested in inventory. Only the most elaborate cost accounting systems incorporate all the other costs of maintaining the plant service. A rental concept of capital (that is, the current market cost to rent the facility or equipment involved) may be more useful, particularly in deciding whether to continue operating plant system units or to contract services. Similarly, inventory-handling costs include the interest earned on capital invested in inventory.

Fixed and variable costs

Flexible budgeting and variable cost identification are particularly appropriate for plant units with high variability in demand, such as food service, laundry service, and heating. Fixed cost elements, that is, those not sensitive to changes in demand are budgeted annually and minimized principally through changes in work processes. In the case of variable cost items, including some labor costs and most supplies consumed, the plant responsibility center manager can be held accountable for units used and price, while operating managers are responsible for volume. By identifying the elements of cost variation, one can deal with each as a separate management problem.

When the goods or services are used by another responsibility center, a separate accounting transfers the cost incurred to the user. Transfer pricing (Chapter 14) can be used to distribute the cost to the users. Final product costs representing services actually sold to patients or their insurers are aggregated from user costs, as shown in Figure 17.11. This system permits triple accountability for the costs. The using responsibility center is accountable chiefly for the quantities used. A cross-functional team can evaluate the final product cost in light of competitive prices.

Some problems become easier with a final product approach. While the intermediate efficiency of certain responsibility centers remains problematic, many final product cost efficiencies, such as security costs per discharge or space management cost per discharge, are easily measured. Most important, it is final product efficiency that meets exchange demands and, therefore, must be used to guide the expectations for each plant service unit. That is, the true performance requirements for a plant system are set by exchange demands, the price the public is willing to pay for the service. Efforts to understand efficiency requirements in terms of history or technology rather than willingness to pay can be seriously misleading.

Measures of Human Resources

Well-managed plant systems can retain stable productive work forces despite relatively low wages for most jobs. The secret lies in the quality of training and supervision, and the appropriate use of nonmonetary and monetary incentives. The quality, loyalty, and attitude of the work force can all be measured. Personnel records show training program completion, absenteeism, and disciplinary incidents. Turnover and recruitment statistics show loyalty. (The workers themselves recruit to fill many jobs.) Attitudes are assessed by periodic survey, as they are for other systems.

FIGURE 17.11 Sequence of Cost Accounting and Resource Management

	Plant Responsibility Center	**User Responsibility Center**	**Final Product Responsibility**
Cost Accounting	Labor + Supplies consumed + Capital consumed + Supplies purchased for others Total cost Output units Transfer Price	Transfer price × Number units consumed User cost of service Final product units Final product cost/unit	Sum of Final product costs/unit by final product Cost/final product
Accountability	↑ ↓	↑ ↓	↑ ↓
Benchmark or Reference	Cost of equivalent purchased service	Operation of comparable centers	Price offered by buyer or intermediary

Measures of Quality

Plant systems generally are not lacking for quality measures. The major sources are users, outside inspectors, inside inspectors, and work records; the number and variety of examples has grown steadily in recent years. The JCAHO includes a thorough review of structural measures of plant safety and has moved to emphasize performance statistics for plant services.[42,43] Internal audits of plant systems are recommended.[44] Line managers, particularly in nursing, should be encouraged to report any maintenance failure that is likely to reduce patient satisfaction or safety promptly. Repeated reports on the same problem indicate a major deficiency in quality. Figure 17.12 shows important measures of quality that are available to almost any healthcare organization.

Process measures are useful in monitoring day-to-day activity. Inspections are critical to laundry, food service, supplies, maintenance, and housekeeping. Subjective judgment is usually required, but it is improved by clear statements of process standards for cleanliness, temperature, taste, appearance, and so on. The frequency of inspection is adjusted to the level of performance, and performance is improved by training and methods rather than negative feedback. Work reports, like incident reports, reveal correctable problem areas in plant maintenance and materials management.

Back orders, incomplete work, and delays in filling orders can be reported as incidents or as ratios of days' work outstanding. These are essentially failure statistics, and they need to be classified by severity or importance. Being out of stock, particularly of critical items, can be treated similarly. Many utilities

FIGURE 17.12 Measures of Quality for Plant Systems

Type	Approaches	Examples
Outcomes	Surveys	Visitor and staff satisfaction
	Incident counts	Falls, complaints
	User complaints	Cleanliness/repair problems reported by user departments
Process	Raw materials inspection	Compliance to purchase specification
	Service/product inspections	Food preparation, patient food tray, telephone response delay
	Contract compliance	On-time supplies delivery
	Supply failures	Back-ordered items
	Inventory waste	Losses of supplies
	Schedule failures	Delays in patient transport Construction deadlines
	Automated monitoring	Temperature and humidity control
Structure	Plant inspections	Licensure survey
	Equipment inspections	Elevator maintenance
	Worker qualifications	Stationary engineer coverage

services are now automated, so permanent records exist of environmental conditions. Under automated order systems and electronic accounting of supplies use from exchange carts, out-of-stock items and backorders can be reported automatically as well.

Establishing Constraints and Expectations

The plant system, like any other part of the healthcare organization, must operate in recognition of buyer and patient imposed limits on costs and quality. Expectations should be set for all performance measures after careful consideration of benchmarks, competition, user satisfaction data, and current capability. It is a relatively simple matter to generate comparative data for many plant service responsibility centers. Benchmarks and scientific standards for these values are widely available. numerous consultants offer information on labor standards for laundries, kitchens, and the like, and cost standards for energy use, construction, renovation, and security. Constraints on costs are derived from two sources: the competitive prices of outside vendors and the internal needs developed from the budget guidelines. The former are preferable wherever they can be obtained.

The existence of comprehensive measures for plant services makes comparison with outside vendors important. While exceptions may be made in the short run, or when the stability of outside suppliers is questionable, as a general rule, no plant service should be operated internally that can be supplied as well in the long run from outside sources. Thus, expectations for cost, quality, and satisfaction measures of internally operated plant services should meet or exceed those of outside suppliers.

Suggested Readings

Joint Commission on Accreditation of Healthcare Organizations. 1990. *Emergency Preparedness: When the Disaster Strikes,* Plant Technology & Safety Management Series. No. 2. Oakbrook Terrace, IL: JCAHO.

Framework for a Comprehensive Health and Safety Program in the Hospital Environment. 1993. Washington, DC: U.S. Department of Labor, Occupational Safety and Health Administration, Directorate of Technical Support, Office of Occupational Health Nursing.

American Institute of Architects Academy of Architecture for Health, with assistance from the U.S. Dept. of Health and Human Services [ed]. 1996. *Guidelines for Design and Construction of Hospital and Health Care Facilities,* 1996–97. Washington, DC: American Institute of Architects Press.

Bennett, J. V., and P. S. Brachman (eds.). 1998. *Hospital Infections,* 4th ed. Philadelphia: Lippincott-Raven.

Malkin, J. 1992. *Hospital Interior Architecture: Creating Healing Environment for Special Patient Populations.* New York: Van Nostrand Reinhold.

O'Reilly, J. T., P. Hagan, P. de la Cruz, et al. 1996. *Environmental and Workplace Safety: A Guide for University, Hospital, and School Managers.* New York: Van Nostrand Reinhold.

Tomasik, K. M. 1989. *Plant, Technology & Safety Management Handbook: Safety Management, Life Safety Management, Equipment Management, Utilities Management,* 2nd ed. Chicago: Joint Commission on Accreditation of Healthcare Organizations.

Notes

1. National Fire Protection Association, *Code for Safety to Life from Fire in Buildings and Structures* Boston: The Association, (published annually). See also other NFPA publications, such as *Health Care Facilities Handbook,* 3rd ed. (1990)
2. L. L. Neibauer, Codes Put Greater Emphasis on Life Safety, *Consulting-Specifying Engineer* 7(5 Suppl 2), 18–20, 23 (April 1990)
3. D. Erickson, B. Berek, and G. Mills, "Complying with Current Joint Commission Statement of Conditions (Soc) Requirements." *Healthcare Facilities Management Series* p 1–10 (January 1997)
4. "Americans with Disabilities Act (ADA) Accessibility Guidelines for Buildings and Facilities, Architectural and Transportation Barriers Compliance Board, Final Guidelines." *Federal Register* 56(144): 35408–542 (Jul 26, 1991)
5. "Controlling Ambient Biohazards; What You Can't See Can Hurt." *Healthcare Hazardous Materials Management* 7(6): 6–8 (March, 1994)
6. J. A. Sather, "Health Care Facilities Demand Reliable Electrical Distribution Systems" *Consulting-Specifying Engineer* 7(2): 34–9 (February, 1990)
7. I. Lazar, "Standby Power for Critical Areas: Hospitals." *Consulting-Specifying Engineer* 7(2): 50–5 (Feb, 1990); D.L. Stymiest, "Managing Hospital Emergency Power Testing Programs." *Healthcare Facilities Management Series* p 1–16, (April, 1997)
8. D. K. Wilder, "Clinical Engineering Support for the Critical Care Unit." *Critical Care Clinics* 9(3): 501–9 (July, 1993)
9. M. L. Dickerson and M. E. Jackson, "Technology Management: A Perspective on System Support, Procurement, and Replacement Planning." *Journal of Clinical Engineering* 17(2): 129–36 (March–April, 1992)
10. J. T. Anderson, "A Risk-Related Preventive Maintenance System." *Journal of Clinical Engineering* 17(1): 65–8 (Jan–Feb, 1992)
11. N. Cram, J. Groves, and L. Foster, "Technology Assessment—A Survey of the Clinical Engineer's Role Within the Hospital." *Journal of Clinical Engineering* 22(6): 373–82, (Nov–Dec, 1997)
12. A. R. Turk, "Health Care Safety Management: A Regulatory Update for 1997." *Healthcare Facilities Management Series* p 1–27 (March, 1997)
13. J. Malkin, "Beyond Interior Design." *Health Facilities Management* 6(11): 18–22, 24–5 (November, 1993)
14. R. S. Ulrich, "Effects of Interior Design on Wellness: Theory and Recent Scientific Research," *Journal of Health Care Interior Design* 3: 97–109 (1991)
15. "Hazardous Waste Management System: Identification and Listing of Hazardous Waste—EPA. Final Rule and Response to Comments." *Federal Register* 57(1): 12–4(January 2, 1992)
16. J. H. Keene, "Medical Waste: A Minimal Hazard." *Infection Control and Hospital Epidemiology* 12(11): 682–5 (Nov, 1991)

17. A. N. Hayne and L. T. Peoples, "Analysis of an Organization's Waste Stream," *Hospital Materiel Management Quarterly* 14(3): 46–55 (February, 1993)
18. J. Studnicki, "The Medical Waste Audit: A Framework for Hospitals to Appraise Options and Financial Implications." *Health Progress* 73(2): 68–74, 77 (March, 1992)
19. P. Hebert, A. Stechman, B. Snyder, and R. Gralla, "Design and Implementation Issues in Training Staff to Do Primary Prevention of HIV in Acute Care Settings." *International Conference on AIDS* 6(3): 312 (June, 1990)
20. J. M. Golden, Jr., "Safety and Health Compliance for Hazmat. The "HAZWOPER" (Worker Protection Standards for Hazardous Waste Operations and Emergency Response) Standard." *Journal of Emergency Medical Services* 16(10): 28–31, 33 (October, 1991)
21. "Special Report, Violence in Hospitals: What Are the Causes? Why Is It Increasing? How Is It Being Confronted?" *Hospital Security and Safety Management* 13(9): 5–10 (January, 1993)
22. "Special Report, Update on EAS (electronic article surveillance) Systems: Protecting Against Patient Wandering, Infant Abduction, Property Theft." *Hospital Security and Safety Management* 14(6): 5–9 (October, 1993)
23. "Special Report, Upgrading Security: Hospitals Opt for New Equipment; New Approaches; Heavy Investments in Additional Patient, Employee Protection." *Hospital Security and Safety Management* 15(3): 5–9 (July 1994)
24. G. L. Ellis, D. A. Dehart, C. Black, and M. J. Gula, "Owens A Ed Security: A National Telephone Survey." *American Journal of Emergency Medicine* 12(2): 155–9 (March, 1994)
25. "Special Report, Hospitals and Parking Security: Shoring up a Major Crime Locale." *Hospital Security and Safety Management* 14(7): 5–9 (November, 1993)
26. M. S. Weiss, "How to Ensure Supplier Quality from Your Supplier Management Program." *Hospital Materiel Management Quarterly* 19(3):1–10, (1998)
27. G. C. Kim and M. J. Schniederjans, "Empirical Comparison of Just-in-Time and Stockless Materiel Management Systems in the Health Care Industry," *Hospital Materiel Management Quarterly* 14(4): 65–74 (May, 1993)
28. J. C. Kowalski, "CEOs and CFOs Express Concern about Materials Management." *Healthcare Financial Management* 52(5): 56–60, (May, 1998)
29. *Ibid*, "Controlling Supply Expenses Through Capitated Supply Contracting." *Healthcare Financial Management* 51(7): 74–6, 79, (July, 1997)
30. R. C. Schuweiler. "The Cost Management Organization: The Next Step for Materiel Management." *Journal of Healthcare Resource Management* 15(5): 11–8, (June, 1997)
31. P. Cappa, "Outfitting Your Hospital for the New Wave of Robots." *Journal of Healthcare Materiel Management* 12(6): 33–4, 37–8 (June, 1994)
32. American Hospital Association, *Hospital Engineering Handbook*. Chicago: AHA pp. 20–21 (1974); J. H. Holmgren and W. J. Wentz, *Material Management and Purchasing for the Health Care Facility*. Chicago: Health Administration Press, 243–49 (1982)
33. S. M. Majercik, "The BMET (biomedical equipment technician) Career:

Academic Curricula, Hospital Needs, & Employee Perceptions." *Journal of Clinical Engineering* 16(5): 393–402 (September-October, 1991)
34. W. A. Morse, "Career Opportunities in Clinical Engineering." *Journal of Clinical Engineering* 17(4): 303–11 (July–August 1992)
35. J. B. Quinn, T. L. Doorley, and P. C. Paquette, "Beyond Products: Services-Based Strategy." *Harvard Business Review* 68(2): 58–60, 64–6, 68 (March–April 1990)
36. ServiceMaster website: www.servicemaster.com (Oct. 8, 1998)
37. C. L. Tudor and C. R. Gemmill, "Third-Party Capital Equipment Management Cuts Costs." *Healthcare Financial Management* 43(4): 32–6, 38 (April 1994)
38. L. T. McAuley, "Administrative and Operational Responsibilities in Contract Management." *Topics in Health Care Financing* 20(2): 76–81 (Winter, 1993)
39. M. Frize and M. Shaffer, "Clinical Engineering in Today's Hospital: Perspectives of the Administrator and the Clinical Engineer," *Hospital & Health Services Administration* 36(2): 285–305 (Summer, 1991)
40. Hol Hogren and Wentz, *Material Management and Purchasing for the Health Care Facility*. Chicago: Health Administration Press, 6 (1982)
41. *Ibid*, 6.
42. O. R. Keil, "The Joint Commission's Agenda for Change: What Does It Mean for Equipment Managers?" *Biomedical Instrumentation and Technology* 28(1): 14–7 (January–February 1994)
43. E. Weisman, "The Agenda for Change: Performance Focus Alters JCAHO's Survey Process." *Health Facilities Management* 7(1): 16 18–9 (January, 1994); 7(2): 26 28–31 (February, 1994)
44. L. Duplechan, "The Internal Environmental Audit: A Practical Plan for Hospitals." *Healthcare Facilities Management Series* 1–24 (July, 1993)

GLOSSARY

360-degree reviews. Formal evaluations of performance by subordinates, superiors, and customers of the individual or unit.

Accountability. The notion that the organization can rely on the individual to fulfill a specific, prearranged expectation.

Activity-based costing. A process whereby costs for final products and service lines are established by reaggregating unit costs from contributing services.

Acuity. A measure of how sick patients are, used to establish nurse staffing needs.

Ad hoc committee. A committee formed to address a specific purpose, for a specified time period.

Alliances. Relations between organizations that are entered into primarily for strategic purposes.

American College of Healthcare Executives (ACHE). The leading professional association for healthcare managers.

American Osteopathic Association (AOA). A voluntary national organization of osteopathic physicians. AOA offers inspection and accreditation services similar to those of the Joint Commission on Accreditation of Healthcare Organizations.

Ancillary services. See *Clinical support services.*

Appropriate care. Care for which expected health benefits exceed negative consequences.

Attending physicians. Those doctors having the privilege of using the hospital for patient care.

Attributes measures.

Bar chart. A display of differing values by some useful dimension, such as day of week, operator, site, or patient group.

Benchmark The best known value for a specific measure, from any source.

Best practice. A process used to generate a benchmark.

Blue Cross and Blue Shield Plans. A locally managed health insurer participating in the national Blue Cross-Blue Shield Association.

Boundary spanning. Activities through which the organization selects its exchanges looking outward to define what the organization must do to thrive.

Budget guidelines. Desirable levels of key financial indicators established at the start of the budget process by the governing board.

Bureaucratic organization. A form of human endeavor in which groups of individuals bring different skills to bear on a single objective in accordance with a formal structure of authority and responsibility.

Business units. Activities for which healthcare organizations create separate hierarchies. They may include non-healthcare activities, such as health insurance. See *Service lines.*

Capitation. A method of compensating caregivers that pays a fixed dollar amount for each month the patient remains under contract with a particular provider, regardless of the amount of care the patient uses.

Care plans. Expectations for the care of individual patients, normally aggregates of several intermediate product protocols.

Case manager. An individual who coordinates and oversees other healthcare professionals in finding the most effective method of caring for specific patients.

Cash flow budget. Estimates of cash income and outgo by period.

Cause and effect diagrams. These show relationships between complex flows and allow teams to identify components, test them as specific causes, and focus their investigation.

Census. Number of patients in a hospital or unit.

Centralized structures. Organizations that retain much control in the parent unit.

Certificates of need (CON). Franchises for new services and construction or renovation of hospitals or related facilities, issued by many states.

Charitable organizations. Organizations with tax-exempt status distributing funds and other resources for charitable purposes.

Chief executive officer (CEO). The agent of the governing board holding the formal accountability for the entire organization.

Client-servers. Computing machinery that makes it possible for multiple users to be in communication at the same time, and facilitates translation between alternative data formats used by the competing hardware and operating systems.

Clinic rounds. Educational review of cases in an outpatient setting or clinic.

Clinical expectation. A consensus reached on the correct professional response to a specific, recurring situation in patient care.

Clinical nurse practitioner. Nurse with extra training who accepts additional clinical responsibility for medical diagnosis or treatment.

Clinical support service. (1) A unit organized around one or more medical specialties or clinical professions providing individual patient care on order of an attending physician, such as laboratory or physical therapy; (2) a general community service, such as health education, immunization, and screening, under the general guidance of the medical staff.

Clinical system. The part of a healthcare organization that provides hands-on patient care and monitors it to ensure both quality and effectiveness.

Closed [medical] staff. A medical staff organization that is not open to licensed physicians generally (e.g., medical staffs organized around employed groups or university faculties).

Collateral organization. The broad group of organizational activities, such as committees, conferences, task forces, and retreats, that are established for the purpose of attacking problems crossing several organizational units.

Common provider entity. A single entity of physicians and hospitals willing to accept full payment from an insurance carrier or intermediary for a "bundle" of provider services and distribute it as indicated. See also *Medical service organization.*

Community. A group of geographically related individuals and organizations sharing some resources. Healthcare organizations are usually among the shared resources of a community.

Community hospitals. A short-stay general or specialty (e.g., women's children's, eye, orthopedic) hospital, excluding those owned by the federal government.

Community-focused strategic management. The notion that the organization repeatedly asks itself the questions—What is our community's goal, why, and how does the organization best serve it?—and uses the answers to select among business opportunities.

Conjoint medical staff. A flexible and pluralistic relationship between doctors and the hospital that assumes increasingly close affiliation. Combines the requirements of a "privileged medical staff," with formal planning for physician recruitment and ongoing participation in operating and strategic decisions.

Constraints. Limits on the range of acceptable operating conditions.

Continuous improvement. A concept of the organization setting expectations that it can and will achieve, but that will be set at a better level each year.

Control chart. A run chart with the addition of statistical quality control limits.

Controlled substances. Drugs regulated by the federal government, such as narcotics.

Conviction. Characteristic indicating that a decision or proposal is persuasive; that is, most members of the organization will be convinced that it is realistic, and they as individuals will have a successful future.

Copayment. Insurance clause that requires a fraction of the benefit costs to be paid by the patient.

Corporate model. A theory of organization emphasizing a powerful chief executive, resembling the prevailing styles of large industrial and commercial corporations.

Cost budgets. Anticipated volumes of demand or output with emphasis on direct costs controllable by the responsibility center or unit.

Credentialing. The process of privilege review.

Current procedural terminology (CPT).

Customers. Exchange partners who use the services of the organization and generally compensate the organization for those services (e.g., patients). Also, by extension, other units within the hospital that rely on a particular unit for service.

Cybernetic. A characteristic of organizations reflecting purposive search: the establishment of goals, measurement of progress, and correction of activity to improve progress. (From cybernos, helmsman).

Decentralized structures. Those that allow much power in subsidiary, as opposed to central units.

Decision support systems (DSS). Information recovery systems that provide rapid retrieval of selected data from multiple files or archives.

Deductible. Insurance clause that defers benefit until a specific amount has been spent by the patient. It is a standard feature of catastrophic or major medical insurance contracts, where it serves to rule out routine medical expenses.

Demand. Requests for service.

Department. A unit of the accountability hierarchy, such as "housekeeping department." Also an organization of doctors in a major specialty, as in "obstetrics department."

Deterministic models. Those that deal with future events as fixed numbers, rather than as random events subject to a predictable variance.

Diagnosis-related groups (DRGs). Groups of inpatient discharges with final diagnoses that are similar clinically and in resource consumption. Used as a basis of payment by the Medicare program and, as a result, widely accepted by others.

Direct costs. The costs of resources used directly in an activity that can be controlled through the unit accountable for the activity.

Discharge planning. A part of the patient management guidelines and the nursing care plan that identifies the expected discharge data and coordinates the various services necessary to achieve the target.

Efficiency. (1) The return or output achieved for a given level of input or resources; (2) the ratio of output to input, or input to output. See also *Productivity.*

Elective. Demand that can be met at an indefinite time.

Employees. Exchange partners compensated by salary and wages.

Empowerment. Achievement of the ability to influence working conditions and service policies. Usually applied to lower level managers and nonmanagerial personnel.

Endogenous events. Those largely within the control of an operator.

Environmental assessment. A corporate activity identifying changes in the environment, and perspectives of others in the community on these changes, with particular attention to those changes affecting customers, competitors, and members of the hospital.

Equal employment opportunity agencies. Government agencies that monitor the rights of member groups are among those entitled to access to the healthcare organization and its records.

Evidence-based medicine. The concept that ideal medical treatment is supported by careful and systematic evaluation emphasizing rigorous controlled trials.

Exchange partners. Individuals or groups participating in exchanges with the hospital.

Exchange. A mutual or reciprocal transfer that occurs when both parties believe themselves to benefit from it. It results in a relationship between an organization and its environment, such as employment, sales, donations, purchases, etc.

Executive. Informally, a manager who participates in the strategic functions of the organization or who supervises several levels of managers.

Exogenous events. Those that are largely outside the control of a line operator.

Expectations. (1) Work goals for organization units and their members; (2) specific statements summarizing agreed upon dimensions of performance.

Expenditure budgets. Costs anticipated by reporting period, responsibility center, and natural account.

External auditor. An external reviewer who attests that the accounting practices followed by the organization are sound, and that the financial reports fairly represent the state of the business.

Final product budgets. The cost and revenue for DRGs and capitated costs per member per month.

Final products. Sets of clinical services reaching generally recognized end points in the process of care, such as hospital discharge, or care for an individual for a discrete illness or an extended period of time.

Financial budgets. Expectations of future financial performance composed of income and expense budget, budgeted financial statements, cash flow budget, new programs and capital budget.

First-line supervisor. See *Responsibility center manager.*

Fishbone diagrams. See *Cause and effect diagrams.*

Fixed budget. A cost budget that establishes expectations each period that are independent of variation in demand. The expectation is expressed in terms of total cost rather than unit cost.

Flexible budget. A cost budget that establishes expectations for each period that depend on variation in demand. The expectation is expressed in terms of unit cost rather than total cost.

Flow process charts.

Forecasts. Predictions of future operating environments.

Formal organization. Organizations that grant authority over certain activities, are held accountable for certain results, and compensate participants for their effort.

For-profit hospitals. Those owned by private corporations that declare dividends or otherwise distribute profits to individuals. Also called investor owned. They are usually community hospitals.

Frequency. In advertising, the average number of times each person is reached by a specific advertisement.

General ledger transactions. Financial transactions that are internal rather than external exchanges. They often deal with resources that last considerably longer than one budget or financial period.

Global fee. A compensation plan whereby the institution receives a single payment that it must then distribute to itself and its physician partners.

Governance system. The part of a healthcare organization that monitors the outside environment, selects appropriate alternatives, and negotiates the implementation of these alternatives with others inside and outside the hospital.

Government hospitals. Hospitals owned by federal, state, or local governments.

Government regulatory agencies. Agencies with established authority over healthcare activities—licensing agencies and rate-regulating commissions are examples.

Gross revenue. The sum of all posted charges in a specified time period.

Group purchasing. Alliances that use the collective buying power of several organizations to leverage prices downward.

Groups without walls or **"virtually integrated groups."** Physician organizations that allow their members to continue traditional practice, and they do not immediately change geographic coverage.

Guideline. See *Patient management protocol.*

Hawthorne effect. A series of experiments that showed that the fact of experimentation and the attention it drew could improve performance, independent of the experiment itself.

Health maintenance organization (HMO). A form of health insurance emphasizing comprehensive care under a single insurance premium, designed to eliminate unnecessary costs and to improve quality and acceptability of service through sharing of risk for the cost of care.

Health promotion. Activities to change patient or customer behavior regarding health.

Healthcare organization.

Hierarchical organization.

Histogram. A graphic display grouping individual values that shows the relative frequency of each group.

Home care agencies. Organizations providing care in the home.

Homeostasis. In biology a "state of physiological equilibrium produced by a balance of functions and of chemical composition within a organism" and more generally a "tendency toward relatively stable equilibrium between interdependent elements."

Horizontal integration. Integration of organizations providing the same kind of service, such as two hospitals or two clinics.

Hospital-based specialists. Those physicians providing consultative care to attending physicians, such as pathologists, radiologists, and anesthesiologists.

House officers. Licensed doctors pursuing postgraduate education.

Human resources system. The part of a healthcare organization that recruits and supports the hospital's employees and other workers, such as doctors and volunteers.

Human subjects committee. A committee reviewing research activities for potential dangers to patients.

Hurdle rate. A requirement for a minimum positive return, expressed as a percentage of net revenue.

Image. Reputation of the organization.

Implicit profit. The difference between revenues at the transfer price and costs.

Incident report. Written report of an untoward event that raises the possibility of liability of the organization.

Income and expense budget. Expected net income and expenses incurred by the organization as a whole.

Indemnity insurance. Insurance benefit design that pays cash benefits for specific services received, as opposed to ensuring the service itself. HMOs provide service benefits; catastrophic and preferred provider plans often provide indemnity coverage.

Independent physicians association (IPA). Health maintenance organization paying its affiliated doctors on a basis other than salary.

Independent practice association (IPA). Health maintenance organization paying its affiliated doctors on a basis other than salary.

Indirect costs. Costs incurred for large aggregates of the organization, even for the organization as a whole. Insurance, debt services, expenses of the executive office, and the operation of central services like parking and security are examples.

Influence. The ability to affect an organization's or an activity's success. Influence is usually gained by controlling a resource.

Influentials. Exchange partners having above-average influence on the affairs of the organization.

Informal organizations. Human behavior where groups of people share information and gratification, make partnerships and friendships, and divide and specialize the work.

Information services (IS). A formal organizational unit supporting the development and integration of information systems and the supply of information to points of use.

Information system. An automated process of capture, transmission, and recording of information that is permanently accessible to the organization as a whole.

Insurance carrier. An intermediary bearing insurance risk.

Integrated health system. An organization that strives deliberately to meet the full spectrum of the health needs of its community.

Integrated information system. A set of two or more information systems organized to provide immediate electronic access to information in each.

Intermediary. A payment or management agent for healthcare insurance (e.g., Medicare intermediaries) who pay providers as agents for the U.S. Health Care Financing Administration.

Intermediate product protocol. Consensus expectation that establishes the normal set of activities and performance for an intermediate product.

Intermediate product. A procedure that is a part of care, such as a surgical operation.

Inurement rules. Rules that protect against the distribution of assets of a community corporation to individuals or small groups within the community.

Inurement. Dispersal of corporate funds to an individual. Particularly, illegal dispersal of funds of a not-for-profit corporation, or dispersal of funds to persons in governance or management.

Joint Commission on Accreditation of Healthcare Organizations (JCAHO). A national organization of representatives of healthcare providers: American College of Physicians, American College of Surgeons, American Hospital Association, American Medical Association, and consumer representatives. The JCAHO offers inspection and accreditation on quality of operations to hospitals, home care agencies, long-term care facilities, and integrated health systems.

Licensure. Government approval to perform specified activities.

Life Safety Code. Safety and convenience regulations developed by the National Fire Protection Association.

Line units. Units of the accountability hierarchy directly concerned with the principal product or outcome of the organization. In healthcare organizations, these are the clinical units: the medicine, nursing, and the clinical support services.

Local area networks (LANs). Computer links serve individual units within about 1,000 yards of one another.

Long-range planning. The series of resource allocation decisions implementing vision and strategies over several future years.

Long-range financial plan (LRFP). A projection of revenues, cost, cash flow, assets, debt, and equity agreed on as a multiyear goal.

Long-range plans. Documents that record decisions made, usually in the form of actions or events that are expected to occur at specific future times.

Long-term care facilities. Healthcare facilities for the chronic sick, such as nursing homes.

Make or buy decisions. Services planning decisions that evaluate owning and operating a service (make) versus contracting with an outside vendor (buy).

Managed care. Collective label for a broad range of changes in the financing mechanisms for healthcare that transfer the costs back to providers, such as doctors and hospitals, and to users, patients and their families.

Management letter. Comments of external auditors to the governing board that accompany their audited financial report.

Managerial accounting. A deliberate effort to relate revenue and expenditures to individual services and the activities of responsibility centers.

Marginal costs. Costs that vary with a change in condition such as a new process or a shift in demand.

Market-oriented. A style of management identifying the interests of the community and searching for ways the hospital can meet them.

Market share. The percentage of total demand in a market served by an organization.

Marketing. (1) In common usage, generally implies sales, promotional, or advertising activity, but in professional texts and journals, also incorporates the entire set of activities and processes normally ascribed to planning, plus those relating to sales and promotion. (2) The deliberate effort to establish fruitful relationships with exchange partners, not just to customers, but to all exchanges, including employees and other community agencies.

Matrix organizations. Organizations where RCs or middle managers have explicit, permanent, dual accountability. Reporting can be developed around any pair of the potential conflict points: geography, time, skill or profession, task or patient.

Media. Press, radio, television, and purchased advertising provide communications with exchange partners.

Medicaid agency. The state agency handling claims and payments for Medicaid.

Medicaid. Governmental assistance for care of the poor and, occasionally, the near-poor established through the state/federal program included in Public Law 89-97, Title 19.

Medical service organization (MSO). A formal group of providers including at least a hospital and doctors, able to contract for care to be rendered to specified groups of patients.

Medical staff bylaws. A formal statement of the governance procedures of the medical staff.

Medical staff members. Physicians, dentists, psychologists, podiatrists, etc., admitted to practice in the healthcare organization.

Medical staff organization. The structure that both represents and governs medical staff members.

Medical staff recruitment plan. An element of the long-range plan establishing both the size of the medical staff and the services the hospital will provide.

Medicare intermediary. The private agency handling claims and payments for the federal Medicare programs. Often the local Blue Cross and Blue Shield Plan.

Medicare. Social Security health insurance for the aged established by Public Law 89-97, Title 18.

Members. Those people who participate in the hospital's closed system activities. Members are employees, doctors, trustees, other volunteers, and other nonemployed providers of care, chiefly dentists, psychologists, and podiatrists.

Mental hospitals. Inpatient providers emphasizing mental illness and substance abuse care.

Middle managers. Persons with supervisory authority over several responsibility centers, supervised in turn by executives.

Mission statement. A statement of the good or benefit the healthcare organization intends to contribute, couched in terms of an identified community, a set of services, and a specific level of cost or finance.

Modal specialists. Those who treat the largest percentage of patients with the disease or condition.

Model. A simplified representation of reality that can be manipulated to test various hypotheses about the future.

Monte Carlo simulation. A computerized test of a stochastic model by repeated trial.

Multi-unit organization.

Natural accounts. The kinds of resources purchased, principally labor, supplies, equipment and facilities, and other.

Net revenue. Income actually received as opposed to what is initially posted; equal to gross revenue minus adjustments for bad debts, charity, and discounts to third parties.

Networks. Associations or affiliations among exchange partners with similar interests.

New programs and capital budget. Lists of proposed capital expenditures and new or significantly revised programs, with their implications for the operating and cash budgets by period and responsibility center.

Nominating committee. A standing committee of the governing board that proposes candidates for membership and key offices.

Non-operating revenue. Income generated from nonpatient care activities, including investments in securities and earnings from unrelated businesses.

Not-for-profit hospitals. Hospitals operated with federal tax exemption for community rather than stakeholder benefit.

Nurse anesthetist. Nurse with special training who administers anesthesia.

Nurse clinician. Nurse with advanced training and certification in diagnosis and treatment. Nurse clinicians can substitute for physicians under appropriate guidance.

Nurse midwife. Nurse with special training who practices uncomplicated obstetrics.

Nurse practitioner. Specialist in the nursing problems of patients with certain diseases, or in specific departments such as pediatrics or medicine.

Nursing. The provision of physical, emotional, and educational services to support or improve patients' equilibrium with their environment and to help the patients regain independence as rapidly as possible.

Objective function. A quantitative statement of the relationship between events and desired results.

Occupational Safety and Heath Administration (OSHA). Government agency that monitors the health and safety of employees.

Open [medical] staff. Medical staffs that extended privileges to any licensed physician. Now obsolete. Also applied informally to any medical staff that is not "closed."

Open system. Pattern of relationships and dependencies that connect the organization to its environment.

Operating budgets. These are made up of responsibility center cost budgets, aggregate expenditures budgets, revenue budgets, final product budgets, and cash budgets.

Operating core. The accountability hierarchies that serve the central purpose of the organization (traditionally line units).

Operating system. A process or specified plan for achieving an organizational goal.

Opportunity cost. The cost of committing a resource and thereby eliminating it from other potential uses or opportunities. Opportunity costs do not appear in accounting records.

Optimization. Allocation of scarce resources to maximize achievement of some good or benefit.

Organization culture. Behavioral styles and values broadly accepted within an organization. Often unwritten and traditional.

Outcomes measure. Performance measure that assesses the quality of the final product or outcome of care. Most measures are in the form of counts or rates (counts divided by the total population at risk) and are treated as attributes measures.

Outreach program. Program or strategy to reach a new population or market, particularly a program for prevention that reaches individuals who are not necessarily patients.

Outsourcing. Practice of purchasing or contracting for clinical or support services as an alternative to producing them within the organization.

Overhead. See *Indirect costs.*

Pareto analysis. A bar chart format, with the items rank ordered on a dependent variable such as cost, profit, or satisfaction, that examines the components of a problem in terms of their contribution to it.

Patient ledger. Account of the charges rendered to an individual patient.

Patient management protocol. A formally established expectation that defines the normal steps or processes in the care of a clinically-related group of patients. Protocols specify the intermediate products and outcomes quality goals for care, and by implication, the cost.

Peer review. Any review of professional performance by members of the same profession.

Peer review organization (PRO). External agency that audits the quality of care and use of insurance benefits by individual physicians and patients for Medicare and other insurers.

Physician organization. A formal relationship between physicians that includes arrangements for contracting with health insurers and may extend to shared services. Often serves to represent physicians in a physician hospital organization.

Physician-hospital organization (PHO). A formal organization melding the interests of the community hospital and its physicians. It has equal or near equal representation of hospital and physician directors and allows the partners to collaborate for fee-for-service and managed care financing.

Plan Do Check Act (PDCA). An approach to problem solving characterized by careful study of the problem (Plan), a proposal for revision (Do), a trial (Check), and implementation (Act).

Planning. The process of making resource allocation decisions about the future, particularly the process of involving organization members and selecting among alternative courses of action.

Plant [operations] system. The part of a healthcare organization that operates and maintains the physical facilities and equipment.

Point of service (POS). A healthcare financing plan that offers unlimited choice of provider with substantial financial incentives to use a preferred panel of providers.

Position control. A system controlling the number of positions created and identifying specific persons hired to fill them.

Power. Influence that is relative among partners and variable across time and place.

Preferred provider organization (PPO). A healthcare financing plan that encourages subscribers to seek care from selected hospitals, doctors, and other providers with whom it has established a contract. PPOs are often intermediary arrangements with insurance risk remaining with the employer. They may or may not include care management.

Prevention. Direct interventions during the care process or separate from it, to avoid or reduce disease or disability.

Primary care practitioners. Doctors in family practice, general internal medicine, pediatrics, nurse practitioners, and midwives. May also include psychiatrists and emergency care physicians.

Primary care. The first point of contact between the patient and the healthcare system. Primary caregivers identify diagnoses, provide treatment directly for most problems, and select appropriate specialists for the balance.

Primary prevention. Activities that takes place before the disease occurs to eliminate or reduce its occurrence.

Privileges. Rights granted annually to physicians and affiliate staff members to perform specified kinds of care in the hospital.

Pro forma. A forecast of financial statements, establishing the future financial position of the organization for a given set of operating conditions or decisions.

Process. The series of actions or steps that transform inputs to outputs.

Productivity. The ratio of inputs (resources) to outputs, or vice versa (e.g., "Cost per discharge," "Tests per worker-hour"). See also *Efficiency*.

Professional review organizations (PROs). Organizations led by doctors that do not insure or provide care but that audit the quality of care and the use of insurance benefits for Medicare and other insurers.

Programmatic proposals. Proposals for resource allocation usually arising from the units or departments, tending to affect only the nominating department, which are intended for inclusion in the new programs and capital budget.

Prospective payment system (PPS). Nationally promulgated price structure for Medicare patients.

Protocol. See *Patient management protocol.*

Providers. Institutional and personal caregivers such as doctors, hospitals, nurses, etc.

Quality of care. The degree to which health services for individuals and populations increase the likelihood of desired health outcomes and are consistent with current professional knowledge.

Quality. The value or contribution of the output as defined by, or on behalf of, the customer.

Radar chart. A report designed to give a quick visual summary of multiple dimensions or measurements. Measures are expressed relative to established expectations allowing a uniform reporting for very diverse measures. Also called a "spider diagram."

Ratio analysis. A method of evaluating the financial condition of the firm by examining the relative size of various aspects of financial statements.

Reach. In advertising, an estimate of the number of people who will see or hear a specific advertisement.

Realism. Characteristic indicating that a decision or proposal will meet the test of competition or will lead to a successful future for the enterprise.

Referral specialties. Physicians that receive many or all of their patients on referral from other physicians.

Relative value scales. Scales expressing the relative value of individual services such as laboratory tests or physician's care activities.

Reserved powers. Powers held permanently by the central corporate board.

Resource allocation decisions. The commitment to expend resources in certain directions.

Resource dependency. The concept that suggests that organizations depend on their ability to attract resources such as financial support of customers and the efforts of employees.

Responsibility center (RC). The smallest formal unit of organizational activity, usually the first level at which a supervisor is formally designated.

Responsibility center manager (RCM). The supervisor of a responsibility center. Also called a "primary monitor" or "first-line supervisor."

Revenue budgets. Expectations of future income.

Run chart. A display of performance data over time to show trends and variation.

Scale. The size and scope of an organization.

Scatter diagram. A graphic device for showing association between two measures.

Scenarios. Various ways to improve the strengths, weaknesses, opportunities, and threats (SWOT) proposed and evaluated against the environmental assessment. Alternative perceptions of future actions and performance.

Secondary prevention. Activities that reduce the consequences of existing disease, often by early detection and treatment.

Section. In medical organizations, an organization of members of a given subspecialty.

Segmentation. The deliberate effort to separate markets by the message to which they will respond.

Self-perpetuating boards. Governing boards that themselves select new members and successors.

Senior management team. The CEO and the managers reporting directly to the CEO.

Sensitivity analysis. Analysis of the impact of changed exogenous events, usually developing (in modeling) most favorable, expected, and least favorable scenarios to show the robustness of a proposal and indicate the degree of risk involved.

Service lines. Units of the operating core that are designed around patient-focused care for related disease groups, or that include non-healthcare activities, such as health insurance.

Severity scales. Generalized scales that can adjust for variation in patient condition.

Shewhart cycle. See *Plan Do Check Act (PCDA).*

Staff units. Units of the accountability hierarchy that serve technical or support activites for the line.

Stakeholders. Individuals or groups who can affect the success of the organization. Also called "influentials."

Standard cost. An established expectation for unit cost, usually based on process analysis or best practice.

Standing committee. A permanent committee, established in the bylaws of the corporation or similar basic documents.

Stochastic models. Those incorporating chance variation in the analysis and evaluation of the solutions.

Strategic apex. The uppermost levels of a bureaucratic organization concerned principally with functions of governance, planning, and finance.

Strategic opportunities. Opportunities that involve quantum shifts in service capabilities or market share, usually by interaction with competitors, large-scale capital investments, and revisions to several line activities.

Strategic planning. A process reviewing the mission, environmental surveillance, and previous planning decisions used to establish major goals and nonrecurring resource allocation decisions.

Strategic position. Mission, ownership, scope of activity, location, and partners of the organization.

Strategy. The systematic response to the changing conditions surrounding an enterprise. The concept of strategic management implies deliberate guidance toward an explicit purpose.

Structural measures. Measures of compliance with static expectations, such as those relating to physical facilities or the formal training of individuals.

Supercontrollers. Managers who supervise responsibility center managers.

Suppliers. Exchange partners for goods and services such as supplies and utilities.

Surveillance. See *Environmental assessment.*

Technical and **Logistic Support.** Units of the formal organization that support the operating core. Historically called "staff units."

Tertiary prevention. Activities that reduce or avoid complications or sequelae in existing disease or disability.

Third-party administrators (TPAs). Organizations that process claims and sometimes also control use of benefits for employers who are carrying their own insurance. See also *Intermediaries.*

Transaction costs. The costs of maintaining a relationship, including the costs of communication, negotiation, etc.

Transfer price. Imputed revenue for a good or service transferred between two units of the same organization, such as housekeeping services provided to nursing units. Where the service is not sold directly to the public, the price is established by complex cost accounting and comparison against available market information.

Trustees. Members of the governing board of not-for-profit healthcare organizations who volunteer their time to the healthcare organization, their only compensation being the satisfaction they achieve from their work. The title reflects their acceptance of the assets in trust for the community.

Urgent. Demand that may be met within a few days but that cannot be deferred indefinitely.

Variables measures. Performance measures that can take a continuous range of values, as contrasted to attributes measures that can take only two values (e.g., pass/fail).

Vertical integration. The affiliation of organizations providing different kinds of service, such as hospital care, ambulatory care, long-term care, and social services.

Vision statement. An expansion of the mission that expresses values, intentions, philosophy, and organizational self-image.

Volunteers. People who volunteer their time to the healthcare organization, their only compensation being the satisfaction they achieve from their work.

Wide area networks (WANs). Computer communication that reaches across cities or around the world.

Work group leader. An individual formally responsible for helping the group achieve its goals. A first-line supervisor.

Work groups. See *Responsibility center*.

Working capital. The amount of cash required to support operations for the period of delay in collecting revenue.

Index

ABOUT THE AUTHOR

John R. Griffith, M.B.A., FACHE, is the Andrew Pattullo Collegiate Professor, Department of Health Management and Policy, School of Public Health, The University of Michigan. A graduate of Johns Hopkins University and the University of Chicago, he was director of the program and Bureau of Hospital Administration at The University of Michigan from 1970 to 1982, and chair of his department from 1987 to 1991.

Professor Griffith has been at Michigan since 1960. He is an educator of graduate students and practicing healthcare executives. He has served as chair of the Association of University Programs in Health Administration and as a commissioner for the Accrediting Commission on Education in Health Services Administration. He is active as a consultant to numerous private and public organizations. He was an Examiner, Malcolm Baldridge National Quality Award, 1997–1999.

He is the author of numerous publications, including *Designing 21st Century Healthcare: Leadership in Hospitals and Healthcare Systems.* The first edition of *The Well-Managed Healthcare Organization* won the ACHE Hamilton Prize for book of the year in 1987.

Professor Griffith was awarded the Gold Medal of the American College of Healthcare Executives in 1992. He has also been recognized with the John Mannix Award of the Cleveland Hospital Council, the Edgar Hayhow and Dean Conley Prizes of ACHE, and citations from the Michigan Hospital Association and the Governor of Michigan.

Professor Griffith is a director of The Allegiance Corporation, a physician-hospital organization serving Ann Arbor. He is a member of the National Advisory Board of Family Road, a company devoted to improved maternal and child care. He speaks and consults widely on the development of voluntary healthcare systems.